Hormones in Normal and Abnormal Human Tissues

Hormones in Normal and Abnormal Human Tissues

Volume 2

Editors
K. Fotherby S. B. Pal

Walter de Gruyter · Berlin · New York 1981

Editors:
K. Fotherby, Ph. D., F.R.I.C.,
Department of Steroid Biochemistry
Royal Postgraduate Medical School
University of London
Ducane Road
London W 120 HS, U. K.

S. B. Pal, D. Phil., Dr. rer. biol. hum., M. I. Biol.
Universität Ulm
Department für Innere Medizin
Steinhövelstrasse 9
D 7900 Ulm/Donau
F. R. Germany

CIP-Kurztitelaufnahme der Deutschen Bibliothek

Hormones in normal and abnormal human tissues
ed. by K. Fotherby; S. B. Pal. – Berlin; New York: de Gruyter.
NE: Fotherby, Kenneth [Hrsg.]
Vol. 2 (1981).
ISBN 3-11-008541-0

Library of Congress Cataloging in Publication Data

Hormones in normal and abnormal human tissues.

Bibliography: v. 1, p.
Includes index.
1. Hormones. 2. Hormones, Ectopic.
I. Fotherby, K., 1927- II. Pal, S. B., 1928-
[DNLM: 1. Hormones. 2. Disease. WK 102 H8127]
QP571.H663 616.4 80-27070
ISBN 3-11-008541-0 (v. 2)

 Printing: Karl Gerike, Berlin. – Binding: Lüderitz & Bauer, Buchgewerbe GmbH, Berlin.– Printed in Germany

PREFACE

With the development during the past decade of immunoassay techniques particularly radioimmunoassay, it has been possible to measure with accuracy the circulating levels of most non-polypeptide hormones although some problems still exist in regard to the measurement of polypeptide and protein hormones. Some of these problems are outlined in these monographs. The techniques used so far have enabled the accumulation of a large amount of information on the levels of these hormones in normal subjects, on changes in various pathological and therapeutic conditions and on the factors controlling the secretion of these hormones. For the non-polypeptide hormones the pathways for their biosynthesis have been elucidated by a number of different techniques. Biosynthetic schemes can be drawn up for a number of species, although there are still many gaps and points needing further substantiation, even for the biosynthesis in human tissues. For most of the polypeptide hormones the biosynthetic pathways and the factors controlling these are still incomplete. Most of these different aspects are touched upon in the various chapters in these volumes. However, we have tried to place the emphasis on the concentration of the various hormones in tissues; those where they are produced and those where they might localise and produce an effect and how these levels are modified under varying circumstances. Little information is available on these points and we hope that these volumes will provide a summary of existing knowledge which will be useful to research workers in various branches of endocrinology.

In particular, we have asked contributors to deal in their articles mainly with available information about the human and only to include results from other species where they are relevant to the human situation. We think that these volumes are the only monographs devoted mainly to this topic. As for Volume 1, we are grateful to the distinguished contributors for agreeing to undertake the task that was set and we are also grateful to Walter de Gruyter for their willingness to take on the responsibility of publishing these volumes and to Dr. R. Weber, who will ensure their speedy publication.

K. Fotherby S. B. Pal

November 1980.

CONTRIBUTORS

Numbers in parentheses indicate the page on which the authors' articles begin

E.-E. Baulieu, Unité de Recherches sur le Métabolisme Moléculaire et la Physio-Pathologie des Stéroides de l'Institut National de la Recherche Médicale, Hôpital de Bicêtre, 78, rue du Général Leclerc, 94270 - Bicêtre, France (25).

K. D. Buchanan, Department of Medicine, Queen's University, Belfast BT9 7BL, Northern Ireland, U.K. (187).

I. D. Caterson, The London Hospital Medical College, University of London, Department of Biochemistry, Turner Street, London E1 2AD, England, U.K. (101).

G. Concolino, Istituto di Clinica Medica Generale e Terapia Medica V, Università degli Studi, Rome, Italy (397).

C. Conti, Istituto di Clinica Medica Generale e Terapia Medica V, Università degli Studi, Rome, Italy (397).

R. P. Davis, Department of Laboratory Medicine, The Miriam Hospital, and Division of Biological and Medical Sciences, Brown University, Providence, Rhode Island, U.S.A. (71).

Danièle Duval, Biochimie PCEM, Université de Nice, Petit Valrose, Avenue J. Vallot, 06034 - Nice Cedex, France (25).

R. Emiliozzi, Biochimie PCEM, Université de Nice, Petit Valrose, Avenue J. Vallot, 06034 - Nice Cedex, France (25).

R. W. J. Flanagan, Department of Medicine, Queen's University, Belfast BT9 7BL, Northern Ireland, U.K. (187).

Mary L. Forsling, Department of Physiology, Windeyer Building, Middlesex Hospital Medical School, London, U.K. (1).

L. A. Frohman, Division of Endocrinology and Metabolism, Department of Medicine, Michael Reese Hospital and Medical Center and the University of Chicago, Chicago, Illinois 60616, U.S.A. (415).

J. E. Gerich, Endocrine Research Unit, Departments of Medicine and Physiology, Mayo Medical School and Mayo Clinic, Rochester, Minnesota 55901, U.S.A. (475).

Jody Ginsberg, Department of Medicine, Welsh National School of Medicine, Cardiff, CF4 4XN, U.K. (519).

R. Hall, Department of Medicine, Welsh National School of Medicine, Cardiff, CF4 4XN, U.K. (519).

J. Harmon, Biochemistry of Gene Expression Section, Laboratory of Biochemistry, National Cancer Institute, NIH, Bethesda, Maryland 20205, U.S.A. (437).

G. Hennen, Endocrinologie Clinique et Expérimentale, Institut de Médecine, Université de Liège, Liège, Belgium (123).

R. W. Henry, Department of Medicine, Queen's University, Belfast BT9 7BL, Northern Ireland (369).

M. F. Holick, Endocrine Unit, Massachusetts General Hospital, Boston, MA 02114, U.S.A. (223).

C. P. Lantos, Departamento de Química Biológica, Laboratorio de Esteroides and Programa de Regulacion Hormonal y Metabólica, Buenos Aires, Argentina (131).

G. Maghuin-Rogister, Endocrinologie Clinique et Expérimentale, Institut de Médecine, Université de Liège, Liège, Belgium (123).

J. C. Mason, Department of Biochemistry, Queen's University, Belfast BT9 7BL, Northern Ireland (369).

T. J. McKenna, Department of Endocrinology, St. Vincent's Hospital, Elm Park, Dublin 4, Ireland (339).

Sandra M. McLachlan, Department of Medicine, University of Newcastle upon Tyne, Newcastle upon Tyne, NE1 4LP, U.K. (519).

Christine Mercier-Bodard, Unité de Recherches sur le Métabolisme Moléculaire et la Physio-Pathologie des Stéroides de l'Institut National de la Recherche Médicale, Hôpital de Bicêtre, 78, rue du Général Leclerc, 94270 - Bicêtre, France (25).

D. J. Morris, Department of Laboratory Medicine, The Miriam Hospital, and Division of Biological and Medical Sciences, Brown University, Providence, Rhode Island, U.S.A. (71).

J. J. Morton, Medical Research Council, Blood Pressure Unit, Western Infirmary, Glasgow, Scotland, U.K. (1).

R. F. Murphy, Department of Biochemistry, Queen's University, Belfast BT9 7BL, Northern Ireland, U.K. (187, 369).

M. Norman, Department of Chemical Pathology, King's College Hospital Medical School, Denmark Hill, London, SE5 8RX, U.K. (437).

J. R. Pasqualini, CNRS Steroid Hormone Research Unit, Foundation for Hormone Research, 26 Boulevard Brune, 75014 Paris, France (251).

I. B. Perlstein, Veterans Administration Hospital, St. Louis, Missouri 63125, U.S.A. (281).

B. N. Premachandra, Veterans Administration Hospital, St. Louis, Missouri 63125, U.S.A. (281).

B. Rees Smith, Department of Medicine, Welsh National School of Medicine, Cardiff, CF4 4XN, U.K. (519).

J. M. Renoir, Unité de Recherches sur le Métabolisme Moléculaire et la Physio-Pathologie des Stéroides de l'Institut National de la Recherche Médicale, Hôpital de Bicêtre, 78, rue du Général Leclerc, 94270 - Bicêtre, France (25).

Carole Rickards, Department of Medicine, Welsh National School of Medicine, Cardiff, CF4 4XN, U.K. (519).

G. L. Robertson, Veterans Administration Medical Center and Indiana University School of Medicine, Indianapolis, Indiana, U.S.A. (165).

F. Sciarra, Istituto di Clinica Medica Generale e Terapia Medica V, Università degli Studi, Rome, Italy (397).

V. R. Soman, Department of Medicine, Yale University School of Medicine, New Haven, Connecticut 06510, U.S.A. (49).

C. Sumida, CNRS Steroid Hormone Research Unit, Foundation for Hormone Research, 26 Boulevard Brune, 75014 Paris, France (251).

Marta Szabo, Division of Endocrinology and Metabolism, Department of Medicine, Michael Reese Hospital and Medical Center and the University of Chicago, Chicago, Illinois 60616, U.S.A. (415).

K. W. Taylor, The London Hospital Medical College, University of London, Department of Biochemistry, Turner Street, London E1 2AD, England, U.K. (101).

E. B. Thompson, Biochemistry of Gene Expression Section, Laboratory of Biochemistry, National Cancer Institute, NIH, Bethesda, Maryland 20205, U.S.A. (437).

Kelley Williams, Veterans Administration Hospital, St. Louis, Missouri 63125, U.S.A. (281).

R. L. Zerbe, Veterans Administration Medical Center and Indiana University School of Medicine, Indianapolis, Indiana, U.S.A. (165).

CONTENTS

NEUROHYPOPHYSIAL PEPTIDES

Mary L. Forsling
Department of Physiology, Windeyer Building, Middlesex Hospital Medical School, London, U.K.

J. J. Morton
Medical Research Council, Blood Pressure Unit, Western Infirmary, Glasgow, Scotland, U.K.

Introduction

Neurohypophysial hormones, antidiuretic hormone (ADH) and oxytocin, have a unique position in endocrinology being the first to have their amino acid sequence determined and to be synthesised (1, 2). Extracts of posterior lobe were prepared as long ago as the beginning of this century and the activities, pressor and antidiuretic for ADH (3, 4) and oxytocic and milk ejecting for oxytocin (5, 6) were identified. It has also been suspected that oxytocin may play a role in sodium excretion (7). In addition, recent studies have indicated two other major areas in which ADH may be important, namely, in memory and learning (8) and in glycogenolysis in the liver (9). Both hormones are nonapeptides (see Figure 1) and are very similar in structure differing merely at residues three and eight. Their molecular weight is thus a little over 1,000. Initial estimates of the so-called Van Dyke protein gave a weight of 20-30,000, but it now appears that this protein represented a preparation of the hormone in association with the "carrier protein" neurophysin. The neurophysins comprise a group of proteins of molecular weight 10-12,000. Three neurophysins have been described in most species studied, two major components, one associated with oxytocin, one with ADH and a third

Hormones in Normal and Abnormal Human Tissues, Vol. II

Cys - Tyr - Phe - Gln - Asn - Cys - Pro - Arg - Gly NH_2

S ———————— S

Vasopressin

Cys - Tyr - Ile - Gln - Asn - Cys - Pro - Leu - Gly NH_2

S ———————— S

Oxytocin

Fig. 1 Amino acid sequence of ADH (Vasopressin) and Oxytocin

minor component, which appears to be derived from one of the other neurophysins. Unfortunately, there is no uniform nomenclature. In general, the two major components have been termed neurophysins I and II but Robinson (10) has suggested that terminology be based on the release of the peptide, as for example "nicotine-stimulated neurophysin", while some (11) believe it should be based on the chemical structure for example, MESL neurophysin (Ala-Met-Ser-Asp-Leu-Glu-Leu-Arg-neurophysin).

No clear physiological function has been established for the neurophysins. They may act as carriers within the neurohypophysial system, but it appears that the hormones exist in the unbound form in the circulation.

Assay Techniques

In common with all hormones, advances in knowledge of physiology and pathology have come with the development of a sensitive reliable assay technique. For most hormones this has been provided by radioimmunoassay. However, for the neurohypophysial hormones it is only relatively recently that reliable immunoassays have been established and many studies have utilised bioassays (12). Bioassays for ADH have in large depended on either the pressor or antidiuretic activity in the mammals. The pressor assay, generally performed in the pithed or ganglion blocked rat, is relatively insensitive and it is the antidiuretic assay, combined with a prior extraction, which allows determination of the hormone in plasma. Similarly for oxytocin there is available a relatively insensitive assay employing the ability of the hormone to cause contractions of isolated uterine muscle preparations. More sensitive assays use the action on the mammary gland, either monitoring the contraction of strips of mammary tissue _in vitro_ or the milk ejecting activity _in vivo_, but again a prior extraction step is required for plasma assays. These bioassays are relatively specific but a number of tests to exclude non-specificity should be performed. It should be possible to destroy or inhibit biological activity by incubating the extract containing neurohypophysial hormones with either thioglycollate, trypsin or a specific antiserum. Special care is needed with tissue extracts, in particular, extracts of tumour tissue when additional tests may be performed. Thus as well as monitoring antidiuretic activity, it is desirable to record parameters such as blood pressure which may influence urine flow and to establish if the extract will inhibit a mannitol diuresis (13). Using such assays, plasma ADH concentrations in normally hydrated subjects of the order of 1-4 μU/ml (2.4-10.6 pmol l^{-1}) have been reported, while extracts of normal tissue contain less than 0.1 pmol g^{-1} tissue. Circulating concentrations of oxytocin are generally undetectable and there is little or no data available on the amounts sequestered in normal tissue. Neurophysin circulates in concentrations of 0.1-1.0 ng ml^{-1} and material cross-reacting with anti-neurophysin antiserum has been found in renal and uterine extracts prepared from the pig (14) and rat (15).

On the whole, the results of immunoassay have been found to correlate well with those of bioassay (56, also see Figure 2) although on occasions immunoassay may give considerably higher values. This is especially true of extracts of urine (16) and of tumour tissue (Forsling, unpublished observations). The results of any given immunoassay are of course dependent on the antiserum used as exemplified by the studies of Thomas and Lee (17). The most successful immunization regimes have employed as the immunogen, ADH (or oxytocin) coupled to a protein such as rabbit or bovine albumin (97) or thyroglobulin, though more exotic proteins have been used (18). The radioligand ^{125}I ADH is commonly prepared using the chloramine T method of Hunter and Greenwood (19) and less commonly using a solid phase lacto-peroxidase method (95). In common with most immunoassays, coated charcoal or second antibody is for the most part used to separate bound from free hormone.

Specific assays are also available for the various neurophysins. Initially assays were established using preparations containing neurophysins I and II and generally from bovine material. Techniques have now been developed for specific neurophysins from a number of species including man. Such assays indicate that stimuli such as haemorrhage and syncope which are associated with ADH release are also accompanied by neurophysin I (or nicotine-stimulated neurophysin) (20). The relationship between neurophysin II and oxytocin is not, however, so clear cut. While this last mentioned neurophysin is released during parturition when oxytocin release is at its peak, concentrations are also elevated during pregnancy and oestrogen administration when high concentrations of oxytocin have not generally been found.

Synthesis of Hormones

A model has been developed for the synthesis of ADH within the neurohypophysis and it may be assumed that a similar model

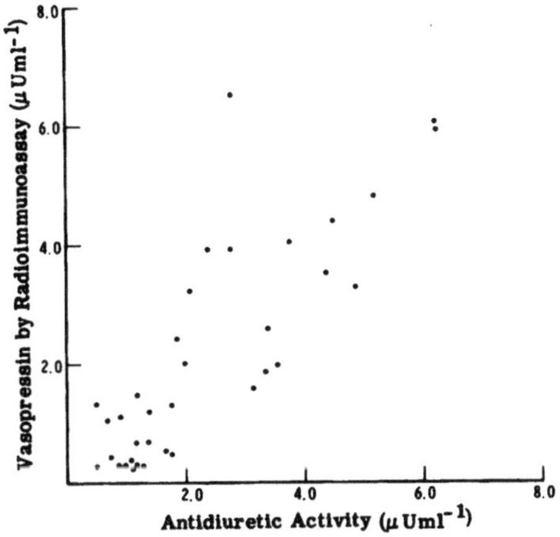

Fig. 2 Concentration of ADH (Vasopressin) in human plasma determined by bioassay and radioimmunoassay after infusion of the hormone (unpublished data)

applies also to the synthesis of oxytocin. Much of our knowledge of the synthetic mechanisms involved has come from the elegant and extensive work of Sachs and his collaborators. Again, ADH was the first hormone for which synthesis via an initial precursor protein was clearly demonstrated. Sachs (21, 22), using an infusion of $[^{35}S]$ cysteine into the third ventricle of anaesthetised dogs showed that the label was incorporated into posterior pituitary peptides. There was, however, a lag period of 1-1 $^1/_2$ h before the label appeared in the hormones and if puromycin were given towards the end of this lag period it had no effect, whereas if given before the label, it completely blocked production of the labelled hormone. This led Takabatake and Sachs to the conclusion that the neurohypophysial hormones were formed as part of a larger molecule and were then separated after its release from the ribosome. More recently, confirmation of synthesis of vasopressin within the hypothalamic nuclei has come from studies employing organ cultures. The ability to maintain functionally active endocrine cells _in vitro_ for considerable periods of time provides a unique opportunity for studying hormone production. This is of particular value when a comparison of tumour-derived products with their normal counterparts is required. Vasopressin was the first neurosecretory hormone for which synthesis in culture was demonstrated when, in 1971, Sachs, Goodman, Osinchack and McKelvy (23) reported that it was possible to maintain an explant of guinea pig anterior hypothalamus containing the supraoptic nucleus for two weeks. Using vigorous purifying techniques they were able to demonstrate that the explant could incorporate tritiated proline, phenylalanine and tyrosine into ADH. Subsequently, it was possible to maintain supraoptic nucleus neurones in culture (24) and to establish a clone of mouse hypothalamic cells which synthesized ADH (25). More recently, the intact hypothalamo-hypophysial complex was cultured (26) which allowed the transport of the hormone to the posterior lobe to be followed.

In the later studies synthesis of neurophysin was also followed and was found to parallel that of vasopressin. Sachs demonstrated that neurophysin, like ADH synthesised in the form of a precursor. When hypothalamic slices from a dog which had previously received an intraventricular infusion of $[^{35}S]$ cysteine were incubated in situ radioactively labelled neurophysin and hormone appeared in parallel in the tissue. The radioactively labelled hormone and neurophysins also appeared in parallel in the neural lobe $1-1^1/_2$ h after injection of radioactive tracer into the cerebrospinal fluid (27, 28, 96). All these results raise the possibility that the neurohypophysial hormones are synthesised together with their respective neurophysins in the form of a common precursor molecule. For the newly synthesized material to reach the neural lobe within $1-1^1/_2$ h, means that once packaged within neurosecretory granules it is transported down the axon at a rate of 3-4 mm h^{-1}, which is some ten times faster than normal axoplasmic flow. Evidence suggests that neurotubules may be involved in the process (29). The fact that the labelled hormone appears in the posterior lobe in so short a time also confirms the suggestion of Sachs that vasopressin is formed from the precursor during transport from the perikaryon in the hypothalamus to the neurosecretory terminals. Additional evidence for this hypothesis has come from Gainer and his coworkers (30, 31, 32) who monitored the protein fractions into which [^{35}S] cysteine was incorporated after injection close to the supraoptic nucleus. Initially, radioactivity was confined to a component of molecular weight 20,000 and was found in the median eminence, a region in which ADH containing fibres were found, 1 h after injection and in the posterior pituitary 30 min. later. Progressively the radioactivity in the 20,000 weight component fell while that of a 12,000 weight peak increased. An intermediate of molecular weight 17,000 was also formed. Furthermore, these proteins could be precipitated by antineurophysin antibodies. Pickering (33) has speculated on the nature of the precursor pointing out that the simplest form would be a polypeptide in which the two components were linked by a single covalent bond either through the NH_2-terminal or -COOH terminal of the hormone.

It has been suggested that the neurosecretory granules follow a predetermined route going first to the release site and those which are not released pass to the storage site (34). Release of hormone is through exocytosis (35) and is a calcium-dependent process (36). There has been some debate as to whether hormone release is by exocytosis or diffusion but most of the evidence, including the parallel release of ADH (37), favours exocytosis. This possibility has been strengthened recently by elegant freeze fracture studies (38). Freeze fracture was used (39) to study the membrane events occurring during hormone release in preparations of the neurohypophysis taken from dehydrated rats. Circular depressions, often containing granule core material that represented sites of exocytosis could be demonstrated in the cytoplasmic face. Sites of endocytosis or membrane internalization were less clearly defined. It has been suggested that endocytosis results in the formation of the clustered microvesicles that are seen in the neurohypophysial axons, but recent evidence (40, 41) indicates that membrane recapture takes place by a process that involves the formation of large vacuolar structures.

Release of ADH is in response to an action potential. In common with the release of secretory products in general calcium plays an essential role in excitation-secretion coupling in the neurohypophysis. The data of Nordman and Dyball (42) suggests that the arrival of action potentials at the nerve terminals produces a sodium-dependent depolarization followed by the opening of a calcium channel similar to the "late" calcium channel described in the squid axon (43). The resultant increase in the intracellular calcium concentrations facilitates hormone release. Hall and Simon (44)have developed a simple model to describe calcium-induced exocytosis based on the action of calcium on the membrane charge. Calcium was described as aiding membrane fusion in two ways. First, it promotes the approach of the granule to the presynaptic membrane and second, it lowers the energy of the flat state relative to the curved state so that the two membranes fuse. Thorn et al (36), however, believe it likely that calcium interacts with specific proteins at the plasma membrane. They also point out that some mechanism must exist to normalize the intracellular calcium concentration. Cyclic nucleotides have also been implicated in vasopressin release (45).

Once released into the circulation, studies on neurophysin binding constants (46), plasma binding and volumes of distribution (47) suggest that ADH and oxytocin circulate in the blood in the unbound form. The hormones are cleared rapidly from the circulation, the half-time of disappearance being less than 10 min in man (47, 48). The main sites of clearance are the liver and kidney (16). Clearance of ADH is close to GFR, but recent work (49) indicates that clearance is not solely dependent on glomerular filtration but that a postglomerular mechanism is also involved.

Once the neurohypophysial hormones reach their target tissue they bind to specific receptors on the cell membrane. Receptors for neurohypophysial hormones have been described in a number of tissues for example kidney for ADH (50) and uterus (51) and fat cells (52). At a cellular level, the best understood response to neurohypophysial hormones in mammals is the antidiuretic response to ADH. As with most peptide hormones cyclic AMP plays a role and there is good evidence that microtubules and microfilaments are involved (53).

The Syndrome of Inappropriate Secretion of ADH

Clinical conditions associated with under and over production of any given hormone have yielded much information as to its physiological function. However, this has not been true for the neurohypophysial hormones. No conditions have been described in which oxytocin secretion is impaired or altered and until recently diabetes insipidus was the only disease associated with changes in ADH secretion. However, a syndrome associated with increased ADH secretion has now been identified, the syndrome of inappropriate production of ADH (SIADH or the Schwartz-Bartter syndrome) (54). The nature of the changes seen in this syndrome were predicted (55) when Pitressin was administered chronically to a group of control subjects. The syndrome is characterised by a low plasma sodium, concentrations to 110 mmol l^{-1} and below being reported, but a relatively concentrated urine. With this degree of hyponatraemia the clinical signs of water intoxication are observed. Other features are an increase in extracellular fluid volume, an inability to excrete a water load normally, but otherwise normal renal and adrenal function. Both elevated plasma concentrations (56, 72) and increased vasopressin excretion (57) have been reported in these patients and also failure to suppress plasma vasopressin on water loading (58). These last authors found that the patients, all of whom had cancer, responded normally to a water load following successful treatment with chemotherapy, but not if there was no tumour regression. The condition has been described in association with a number of conditions (59) including central nervous system disease, respiratory disease, myxoedema, porphyria and in association with the administration of certain drugs including the anti-neoplastic drug vincristine and fluphenazine. In addition, there are an increasing number of reports of inappropriate ADH secretion in patients with various types of cancer and in particular with oat cell carcinoma of the bronchus. Of over fifty individual cases of SIADH associated with bronchogenic carcinoma, in which plasma ADH has been measured, all but three had elevated plasma concentrations. The exceptions are in a report (62) in which only one out of four cases had an elevated plasma concentration. The overwhelming evidence to date supports the original suggestion (60) that the hyponatraemia associated with bronchial carcinoma results from a raised plasma concentration of ADH or a substance biologically similar to it. Initially, the inappropriate ADH secretion was related to the effect of brain metastases and/or the pressure of mediastinum tumour mass on the thoracic vagus nerves, bringing about posterior pituitary release of ADH (60). The first important piece of evidence that the excess ADH was coming from the tumour mass and not the neurohypophysis was provided by Amatruda, Mulrow, Gallagher and Sawyer (61) who demonstrated antidiuretic activity in extracts of an oat cell bronchial tumour from a patient with SIADH. Since that time many reports have appeared describing the measurement of ADH by bioassay or radioimmunoassay in tumour tissue from patients with SIADH and lung cancer (see Table 1). The majority of these confirm the original observation and support the notion that the excess circulating ADH originates from the tumour.

Not only is it likely that the tumour secretes ADH, but it is probable that it also synthesises it prior to secretion, rather than acquiring it by a non-specific effect from the circulation (65). The strongest evidence in favour of tumour synthesis comes from a study (66) which demonstrated the incorporation of tritiated phenylalanine into vasopressin following *in vitro* incubation with tumour slices obtained from a patient with SIADH. Other evidence in favour of synthesis comes from

Table 1. LITERATURE SURVEY of ADH ACTIVITY in TUMOUR TISSUE from PATIENTS with SIADH ASSOCIATED with BRONCHOGENIC CARCINOMA

Tumour	Assay	Antidiuretic Activity μU/mg dry wt.	Comments	Ref.
Lung, (oat cell, 1 case)	B10	70 - 350	Nothing in other tissue	61
Lung (undifferentiated, 1 case)*	B10	6 - 8	Normal tissue 0 - 0.1μU/mg	86
Lung (oat cell, 1 case)	B10	10	-	87
Lung (oat cell, 1 case)	B10	7,000	-	88
Lung (oat cell, 1 case)	RIA	142μU/mg wet wt.	Normal pituitary 0.8 - 11μU/mg wet wt.	76
Lung (oat cell, 6 cases)	B10	4 - 75	Normal lung < 1μU/mg. Nothing in tumour of one patient	89
Lung (oat cell, 1 case)	B10	18	Normal pituitary 33μU/mg dry wt.	90
Lung (oat cell, 5 cases)	B10	20 - 150	-	74
Lung (oat cell, 8 cases; giant cell, 1 case)	B10 +	130 - 763	Activity detected in only four of nine cases - normal pituitary 85mU/mg.	91
Pancreas (adenocarcinoma, 1 case) *	RIA	47	Nothing detected in primary tumour	91
Lung (oat cell, 1 case)	B10	9.0	-	92
Lung (oat cell, 1 case)	B10	200	-	75
Pancreas (adenocarcinoma, 1case)	B10 RIA	290,000 380,000	Oxytocin positive, 50,000μU/mg dry wt.	77
Lung (oat cell, 1 case)	B10	525	-	93
Lung (oat cell, 1 case)	B10	40	Oxytocin positive	81
Lung (oat cell, 6 cases)	B10	50,000 - 80,000	Neurophysin positive	69, 70 94
Lung (undifferentiated, 1 case)	RIA	23.5	-	66
Lung (oat cell, 1 case)	RIA	29 in primary 1.2 in metastasis	Bioassay gave lower values, oxytocin and neurophysin positive	71
Lung (oat cell, 1 case)	B10	21 in primary 27 in metastasis	-	67
Lung (oat cell, 10 cases)	RIA	4 - 432μU/mg wet wt. in primary 2 - 25μU/mg wet wt. in metastasis	Normal tissue < 0.2μU/mg Pituitary 2560 - 5280μU/mg wet wt.	63
Lung (oat cell, 3 cases)	RIA	11 - 66μU/mg wet wt. in primary 61 - 63μU/mg wet wt. in metastasis	ADH undetectable in non-SIADH tumours, < 0.2μU/mg	64

* metastasis

the observation (67) that the zone of active tumour growth contained most of the antidiuretic activity, while the central necrotic and peripheral areas were relatively depleted of activity. The fact that not all tumours contain ADH activity (63, 64) argues against a non-specific accumulation of ADH and is compatible with the notion that certain tumour types possess a mechanism for its synthesis. The possibility that the manner of tumour ADH synthesis and storage may be similar to that existing in the neurohypophysis is based on a number of observed similarities; the detection of a large molecular weight ADH binding protein in the culture medium of cells from an anaplastic tumour (68), the detection of neurophysin in tumour tissue from patients with SIADH (69, 70, 71) and the presence of secretory granules in tumour tissue similar to those found in the neurohypophysis (66, 71).

Fluid deprivation in nine patients with SIADH and lung cancer increased circulating vasopressin (72). While factors such as changes in plasma volume, glomerular filtration and tumour progression were considered more likely to account for this observation, the possibility that there may be a degree of physiological control of ADH secretion from tumour tissue was raised. This possibility has previously been discussed (62) and the detection of a neurophysin-like polypeptide in tumours from patients with SIADH (69, 70, 71) was considered to lend support to this idea. However, physiological control seems unlikely in view of the need for the tumour to be appropriately innervated with cells capable of acting as osmoreceptors or baroreceptors. Tumour secretion of ADH is generally considered to be autonomous and probably occurs following cell death (73). Nonetheless, the tumour concentration of ADH may govern the plasma level (67, 73). This is supported by the observation (63) of a statistical relationship between tumour and plasma concentrations of ADH. However, the biological significance of this relationship should be interpreted with caution in view of the fact that tumour extracts also contained a variable percentage of immunological activity which did not behave chromatographically like synthetic ADH. While it would seem unlikely that the relatively low levels of tumour ADH could determine the very high plasma concentrations seen in some patients, the much greater mass of tumour tissue could result in absolute amounts many times greater than in the neurohypophysis. Consequently tumour mass, as well as tumour concentration, would influence the rate of release of ADH and consequently the plasma concentration.

The chemical characterisation of the ADH-like material produced by ectopic secretion remains undetermined because the relatively low tissue concentrations necessitates the use of large amounts of material, often difficult to obtain, to provide adequate quantities of purified hormone for analysis. The probability that the material present in tumour tissue is the same as the naturally occurring antidiuretic hormone (arginine vasopressin, AVP) is based on a number of pharmacological similarities (74). These include the presence of vasopressor and milk ejecting properties as well as antidiuretic activity and its inactivation by pregnancy plasma, trypsin, chymotrypsin and thioglycollate. It is also immunologically similar as evidenced by its detection using radioimmunoassay methods (Table 1). Chromatographic studies on Sephadex G-25 (74, 75) demonstrated that the majority of antidiuretic activity eluted with a mobility similar to that of pure AVP. Utiger (76) eluted a single lung tumour extract from a column of Sephadex G-50 and found that 83% of the immunological activity eluted in the AVP position. In another study (63), a mean of 65% of the immunological activity from seven primary tumours ran with a mobility similar to that for synthetic AVP following G-25 chromatography. There are therefore biological, enzymic, immunological and physical similarities to posterior pituitary AVP. It should be pointed out, however, that there may be quantitative differences between the biological and immunological measurements as shown by the much smaller amounts of antidiuretic activitiy compared to immunological activity in the tumour of a patient with multiple hormone secretion (71). Also after Sephadex chromatography of tumour extracts, Morton et al (63) found that as well as a main peak which eluted in the same position as synthetic AVP and which contained similar amounts of ADH whether measured by pressor, antidiuretic or immunoassay, there were two smaller peaks which eluted in higher molecular weight positions and which contained much smaller amounts of pressor and antidiuretic activity as compared to immunological activity. In addition, much lower plasma ADH concentrations, as measured by antidiuretic assay were found in a group of cancer patients with inappropriate ADH secretion, than have generally been reported using immunoassay techniques (58).

As evidenced from most studies (Table 1) ectopic ADH secretion is invariably confined to bronchogenic tumours of the small undifferentiated oat cell type. Exceptions have been reported, but these are very few. Two incidences of ADH activity from adenocarcinomas of the pancreas have been reported (77, 91) but in one of these (77) the histology was complicated by the accompanying presence of an oat cell tumour. The release of ADH from cultured cells obtained from an anaplastic carcinoma of the uterus was also reported (68), and an elevated plasma ADH in a patient with a squamous cell tumour (72). However, this latter patient had a normal serum sodium concentration and ectopic secretion was not confirmed as the ADH content of the tumour was not measured.

Azzopardi, Freeman and Poole (78) reported that the incidence of ectopic ADH secretion as indicated by the clinical syndrome of inappropriate ADH secretion in all forms of bronchogenic carcinoma was low (1-2%) and it has been suggested (79) that when small oat cell tumours alone are considered the incidence rises to only 7%. However, with the advent of both bioassay and immunoassay techniques for measuring plasma and tissue ADH, the notion has been forwarded that ectopic ADH secretion may be much more prevalent than previously thought, even in patients without overt hyponatraemia. This possibility arose from the observation (63) of tumour ADH activity in two patients with small cell tumours who did not have overt hyponatraemia.

A similar finding in three patients was reported (67); and a statistically higher mean plasma ADH concentration in patients with bronchial carcinoma, without hyponatraemia, than in normal subjects was also shown (72). Forsling et al (58) reported inappropriate plasma ADH concentrations in 35% of patients with untreated oat cell carcinoma of the lung. Kelly and Morton (64), however, were able to detect tumour ADH in only three of thirty-two patients with bronchogenic carcinoma, implying that ectopic secretion is not a common feature of the disease. This study would suggest that ectopic ADH secretion occurs in less than 10% of all patients with bronchogenic carcinoma, and that when it does occur it is restricted to patients with undifferentiated small cell tumours. The likelihood of an even lower incidence cannot be dismissed and certainly it seems to be less obvious than other tumour hormones, particularly ACTH (80). Few reports of tumour oxytocin activity have been published (71, 77, 81). One reason for this may be that oxytocin is only active during pregnancy and consequently would not be clinically evident. However, Vorherr (73) was unable to detect any oxytocic activity in malignant tumours from over twenty patients, and the question remains as to why some tumours appear to secrete ADH without oxytocin, a peptide differing in only two amino acids and which shares a similar synthetic pathway in the neurohypophysis.

To date there are two main theories which attempt to explain the basic mechanism of ectopic hormone production. The first of these is the 'random derepression' hypothesis (82) which suggests that with the onset of neoplasia a random derepression of the genome takes place resulting in the synthesis, among other things, of biologically active peptide hormones. This theory would require, firstly, that the more undifferentiated or anaplastic a tumour, the more likely it is to produce ectopic hormones; secondly, that the hormones produced would be structurally similar to those naturally occurring; and thirdly, that all or a large proportion of undifferentiated tumours would produce ectopic hormones. As far as ADH is concerned, investigations have shown the first and possibly the second requirements to be correct. However, the theory cannot account for the fact that only a small proportion of undifferentiated tumours appear capable of producing ADH (64). The 'endocrine cell' hypothesis suggests that ectopic hormones are derived from residual endocrine cells which, following the onset of malignancy, switch their genetic and cellular function to the production of ectopic hormones. The main cellular contenders for this role are the APUD cells (83) and the paracrine system of Feyrter (84). As applied to ADH it has been suggested that residual endocrine cells of this type may be present in lung tissue, their function being to produce a vasoactive lung peptide (VLP) (79). Neither hypothesis is mutually exclusive and the concept of derepression in tumours derived from para-endocrine cells would appear, at least, to be in agreement with many, if not all, the observations relating to ADH secretion.

SIADH associated with carcinoma of the bronchus is generally well understood and its clinical management, once diagnosed, presents no great problem. The endocrine syndrome itself plays no part in the prognosis of the patient, which is determined by the underlying neoplasm. Any application of ectopic hormone measurements must therefore be either as an aid to diagnosis or as an indicator of the effectiveness of tumour therapy. Before the first possibility can proceed, it will be essential to determine accurately the prevalence and histological specificity of ectopic secretion for individual hormones. From present information, the incidence of ADH secretion would appear to be low, and as such, its usefulness as an indicator of bronchial carcinoma would seem limited. Its contribution may lie in being one of a number of tumour hormone markers which, taken together, would cover a much higher proportion of cancer patients. Studies using plasma ADH measurements as a marker for bronchial carcinoma have been reported (85), but it should be emphasised that it remains to be proved whether the measurement of ADH or any other ectopic hormone is capable of detecting tumours earlier than techniques already in use. A more immediate application may be as a means of assessing the effectiveness of treatment in reducing the tumour mass. As discussed, it is likely that tumour mass, as well as tumour hormone concentration, is a determinant of the circulating hormone level, and as such any reduction in mass after therapy would be reflected in a fall in the plasma hormone concentration.

From the biochemical standpoint, future investigations will be directed towards the determination of the exact chemical structure of the ADH-like substance produced by the tumour. This, in turn, depending on whether it is the same as the naturally occurring peptide, should shed light on the mechanisms of the cellular and genetic changes which result in its synthesis.

References

1. Du Vigneaud, V., Ressler, Ch.J.M., Swan, C.W., Roberts, P.G., Katsoyannis, P.G., Gordon, S.: The synthesis of an octapeptide amide with the hormonal activity of oxytocin. J. Am. chem. Soc. 75, 4879-4880 (1953).

2. Du Vigneaud, V., Gish, D.T., Katsoyannis, P.G.: A synthetic preparation possessing biological properties associated with arginine vasopressin. J. Am. chem. Soc. 76, 4751-4752 (1954).

3. Howell, W.H.: The physiological effects of extracts of the hypophysis, cerebri and infundibular body. J. exp. Med. 3, 245-258 (1898).

4. Magnus, R., Schafer, E.A.: The action of pituitary extracts upon the kidney. J. Physiol., Lond. 27, IX-X (1901).

5. Dale, H.H.: On some physiological actions of ergot. J. Physiol., Lond. 34, 163-206 (1906).

6. Ott, I., Scott, C.: The action of infundibulin upon the mammary secretion. Proceedings of the Society for Experimental Biology (New York) 8, 48-49 (1910).

7. Jacobson, H.M., Kellog, R.H.: Isotonic NaCl diuresis in rats: antidiuresis and chloruresis produced by posterior pituitary extracts. Am. J. Physiol. 184, 376-389 (1956).

8. De Vied, D., Bohus, B., Van Ree, J.M., Urban, I., Van Wimersa-Griedanns, T.B.: The neurohypophysial hormones and behaviour. In: "Neurohypophysis", Eds. Moses, A.M., Share, L., Karger, Basel, pp. 201-210 (1977).

9. Hems, D.A., Whitton, P.D.: Stimulation by vasopressin of glycogen breakdown and gluconeogenesis in the perfused rat liver. Biochem. J. 136, 705-709 (1973).

10. Robinson, A.G.: Radioimmunoassay of neurophysin proteins, utilization of specific neurophysin assays to demonstrate independent secretion of different neurophysins in vivo. Ann. N.Y. Acad. Sci. 248, 246-256 (1975).

11. Chauvet, M.T., Chauvet, J., Acher, R.: Phylogeny of sheep neurophysins: partial amino acid sequence of a sheep neurophysin. FEBS Letts. 52, 212-215 (1975).

12. Chard, T., Forsling, M.L.: Bioassay and radioimmunoassay of oxytocin and vasopressin. In: "Hormones in Human Blood" Ed. Antoniades, H.N., Harvard University Press, Cambridge, Mass. pp. 485-516 (1976).

13. Fabian, M.I., Forsling, M.L., Jones, J.J., Lee, J.: The antidiuretic material detected in human body fluids and tumour tissue. J. Physiol. (Lond.), 195, 6P-7P (1968).

14. Ginsburg, M., Jayasena, K.: The occurrence of antigen reacting to antibody to porcine neurophysin. J. Physiol. (Lond.), 197, 53-63 (1968).

15. Ciarochi, F.F., Haluszczak, C., Robinson, A.G.: Neurophysin activity and dynamics in the rat. Proceedings of the 58th Meeting of the Endocrine Society, p. 234 (1976).

16. Forsling, M.L.: In: "Antidiuretic Hormone", Ed. Horrobin, D.F., Eden Press, Montreal, pp. 18-24 (1976).

17. Thomas, T.H., Lee, M.R.: The specificity of antisera for the radioimmunoassay of arginine vasopressin in human plasma and urine during water loading and dehydration. Clin. Sci. 51, 525-536 (1976).

18. Moore, G., Lutterodt, A., Burford, G., Lederis, K.: Highly specific antiserum for arginine vasopressin. Endocrinology 101, 1421-1435 (1977).

19. Hunter, W.M., Greenwood, F.C.: Preparation of iodine-131 labelled human growth hormone of high specific activity. Nature (Lond.), 194, 495-496 (1962).

20. Robinson, A.G.: The neurophysins in health and disease. In: "Clinics in Endocrinology and Metabolism", Ed. Besser, G.M., pp. 261-275 (1977).

21. Sachs, H.: Vasopressin biosynthesis. II. Incorporation of ^{35}S cysteine into vasopressin and protein associated with cell fractions. J. Neurochem. 10, 299-311 (1963).

22. Takabatake, Y., Sachs, H.: Vasopressin biosynthesis III. In vitro studies. Endocrinology 75, 934-942 (1964).

23. Sachs, H., Goodman, R., Osinchack, J., McKelvy, J.: Supraoptic neurosecretory neurones of the guinea pig in organ culture. Biosynthesis of vasopressin and neurophysin. Proc. natn. Acad. Sci. U.S.A. 68, 2782-2786 (1971).

24. Marks, B.H., Sakai, K.K., George, J.M., Koestner, A.: Effects of catecholamines on supraoptic neurones in culture. In: "Frontiers in Catecholamine Research", Eds. Usdin, Earl., Snyder, S.H., Pergamon Press, London, pp. 811-813 (1973).

25. De Vitry, F., Camier, M., Czernichow, P., Benda, P., Cohen, P., Tixier-Vidal, I.V.: Establishment of a close of mouse hypothalamic neurosecretory cells synthesising vasopressin and neurophysin. Proc. natn. Acad. Sci. U.S.A. 71, 3575-3579 (1974).

26. Pearson, D., Shainberg, A., Osinchack, J., Sachs, H.: The hypothalamo-neurohypophysial complex in organ culture: morphologic and biochemical characteristics. Endocrinology 96, 982-993 (1975).

27. Norstrom, A., Sjostrand, J.: Transport and turnover of neurohypophysial proteins of the rat. J. Neurochem. 18, 2007-2016 (1971).

28. Jones, C.W., Pickering, B.T.: Intra-axonal transport and turnover of the neurohypophysial hormones in the rat. J. Physiol. (Lond.) 227, 553-564 (1972).

29. Flament-Durand, J., Couck, A-M., Dustin, P.: Studies on the transport of secretory granules in the magnocellular hypothalamic neurones of the rat II. Action of vincristine on axonal flow and neurotubules in the paraventricular and supraoptic nuclei. Cell Tissue Research 164, 1-9 (1975).

30. Gainer, H., Sarne, Y., Brownstein, M.J.: Neurophysin biosynthesis: conversion of a putative precursor during axonal transport. Science 195, 1354-1356 (1977).

31. Brownstein, M.J., Robinson, A.G., Gainer, H.: Immunological identification of rat neurophysin precursors. Nature (Lond.) 269, 259-261 (1977).

32. Brownstein, M.J., Gainer, H.: Neurophysin biosynthesis in normal rats and in rats with hereditary diabetes insipidus. Proc. natn. Acad. Sci. U.S.A. 74, 4046-4049 (1977).

33. Pickering, B.T.: The neurosecretory neurone: a model system for the study of secretion. Essays in Biochemistry 14, 45-81 (1978).

34. Heap, P.F., Jones, C.W., Morris, J.F., Pickering, B.T.: Movement of neurosecretory product through the anatomical compartments of the neural lobe of the pituitary gland. Cell Tissue Research 156, 483-497 (1975).

35. Douglas, W.W.: Mechanisms of release of neurohypophysial hormones: stimulus-secretion coupling. In: "Handbook of Physiology", section 7, vol. IV, The Pituitary Gland and its Neuroendocrine Control, Part I. Eds. Knobil, E., Sawyer, W.H., American Physiological Society, Washington, pp. 191-224 (1974).

36. Thorn, N.A., Russell, J.T., Torp-Pederson, C., Treiman, M.: Calcium and neurosecretion. Ann. N.Y. Acad. Sci. 307, 618-639 (1978).

37. Forsling, M.L., Martin, M.J., Sturdy, J.C., Burton, A.M.: Observations on the release and clearance of neurohypophysial hormones in the rat. J. Endocr. 57, 307-315 (1973).

38. Theodosis, D.T., Dreifuss, J.J.: Ultrastructural evidence for exo-endocytosis in the neurohypophysis. In: "Neurohypophysis", Eds. Moses, M., Share, L., Karger, Basel, pp. 88-94 (1977).

39. Theodosis, D.T., Dreifuss, J.J., Orci, L.: A freeze-fracture study of membrane events during neurohypophysial secretion. J. Cell Biol. 78, 542-553 (1978).

40. Nordmann, J.J., Morris, J.F.: Membrane retrieval at neurosecretory axon endings. Nature (Lond.) 261, 723-725 (1976).

41. Theodosis, D.T., Dreifuss, J.J., Orci, L.: Two classes of microvesicles in the neurohypophysis. Brain Res. 123, 159-163 (1977).

42. Nordmann, J.J., Dyball, R.E.J.: Effects of veratridine on Ca fluxes and the release of oxytocin and vasopressin from the isolated rat neurohypophysis. J. gen. Physiol. 72, 297-304 (1978).

43. Baker, P.F., Meves, H., Ridgeway, E.B.: Effects of manganese and other agents on the calcium uptake that follows depolarization of squid axons. J. Physiol. (Lond.) 231, 511-526 (1973).

44. Hall, J.E., Simon, S.A.: A simple model for calcium-induced exocytosis. Biochim. biophys. Acta 436, 613-616 (1976).

45. Mathison, R., Lederis, K.: Cyclic nucleotides in the hypothalamo-neurohypophysial system and the release of vasopressin. In: "Neurohypophysis", Eds. Moses, M., Share, L., Karger, Basel, pp. 110-117 (1977).

46. Breslow, E., Walter, R.: Binding properties of bovine neurophysins I and II: an equilibrium dialysis study. Molecular Pharmacology 8, 75-81 (1972).

47. Fabian, M.I., Forsling, M.L., Jones, J.J., Pryor, J.S.: The clearance and antidiuretic potency of neurohypophysial hormones in man and their plasma binding and stability. J. Physiol. (Lond.) 204, 653-668 (1969).

48. Lauson, H.D.: Metabolism of neurohypophysial hormones. In: "Handbook of Physiology", section 7, vol. IV, The Pituitary Gland, Part I, Eds. Sawyer, W.H., Knobil, E., American Physiological Society, Washington, pp. 287-393 (1974).

49. Shade, R.E., Share, L.: Renal vasopressin clearance with reductions in renal blood flow in the dog. Am. J. Physiol. 232, F341-F347 (1977).

50. Jard, S., Bockaert, J.: Stimulus-response coupling in neurohypophysial peptide target cells. Physiol. Rev. 55, 489-536 (1975).

51. Soloff, M.S., Swartz, T.L., Steinberg, A.H.: Oxytocin receptors in human uterus. J. clin. Endocrinol. Metab. 38, 1052-1056 (1974).

52. Bonne, D., Cohen, P.: Characterisation of oxytocin receptors on isolated rat fat cells. Europ. J. Biochem. 56, 295-303 (1975).

53. Forsling, M.L.: In: "Antidiuretic Hormone", Vol. III, Ed. Horrobin, D.F., Eden Press, Montreal, pp. 87-99 (1979).

54. Bartter, F.C.: The syndrome of inappropriate secretion of antidiuretic hormone (SIADH). Disease-a-Month (Chicago), Nov., 1-47 (1973).

55. Leaf, A., Bartter, F.C., Santos, R.F., Wrong, O.: Evidence in man that urinary electrolyte loss induced by pitressin is a function of water retention. J. clin. Invest. 32, 868-878 (1953).

56. Morton, J.J., Padfield, P.L., Forsling, M.L.: A radioimmunoassay for plasma arginine vasopressin in man and dog: application to physiological and pathological states. J. Endocr. 65,411-424 (1975).

57. Edwards, C.R.: Vasopressin and oxytocin in health and disease. In: "Clinics in Endocrinology and Metabolism", Ed. Besser, G.M., 6, pp. 223-259 (1977).

58. Forsling, M.L., Gilby, E.D., Bondy, P.K.: Plasma vasopressin concentrations in oat cell lung cancer. J. Endocr. 71, 76P (1976).

59. Uhlich, E.: Das syndrom der inadequäten ADH-sekretion (SIADH) "Schwartz-Bartter Syndrom". Klin. Wochenschr. 55, 307-315 (1977).

60. Schwartz, W.B., Bennett, W., Curelop, S., Bartter, F.C.: A syndrome of renal sodium loss and hyponatraemia probably resulting from inappropriate secretion of antidiuretic hormone. Am. J. Med. 23, 529-542 (1957).

61. Amatruda, T.T., Mulrow, P.J., Gallagher, J.C., Sawyer, W.H.: Carcinoma of the lung with inappropriate antidiuresis. Demonstration of antidiuretic-hormone-like activity in tumour extracts. New Engl. J. Med. 269, 544-549 (1963).

62. Baumann, G., Lopez-Amor, E., Dingman, J.F.: Plasma arginine vasopressin in the syndrome of inappropriate antidiuretic hormone secretion. Am. J. Med. 52, 19-24 (1972).

63. Morton, J.J., Kelly, P., Padfield, P.L.: Antidiuretic hormone in bronchogenic carcinoma. Clin. Endocr. 9, 357-370 (1978).

64. Kelly, P., Morton, J.J.: Antidiuretic hormone immunoactivity in tumour tissue from patients with bronchogenic carcinoma (with and without hyponatraemia). Clin. Endocr. (in press).

65. Unger, R.H., Lochner, J.D., Eisentraut, A.M.: Identification of insulin and glucagon in a bronchogenic metastasis. J. clin. Endocr. 24, 823-831 (1964).

66. George, J.M., Capen, C.C., Phillips, A.S.: Biosynthesis of vasopressin in vitro and ultrastructure of a bronchogenic carcinoma. J. clin. Invest. 51, 141-148 (1972).

67. Vorherr, H., Vorherr, U.F., McConnell, T.S., Goldberg, N.M., Kornfeld, M., Jordan, S.W.: Localisation and origin of antidiuretic principle in para-endocrine-active malignant tumors. Oncology 29, 201-218 (1974).

68. Martin, T.J., Greenberg, P.B., Beck, C., Johnston, C.I.: Peptide hormone synthesis by human tissue in cell culture. In: Proceedings of the 4th International Congress of Endocrinology, Excerpta Medica, Amsterdam, pp. 1198-1204 (1972).

69. Hamilton, B.P.M., Upton, G.V., Amatruda, T.T.: Evidence for the presence of neurophysin in tumors producing the syndrome of inappropriate antidiuresis. J. clin. Endocrinol. Metab. 35, 764-767 (1972).

70. Hamilton, B.P.M.: Presence of neurophysin proteins in tumors associated with the syndrome of inappropriate ADH secretion. Ann. N.Y. Acad. Sci. 248, 153-156 (1975).

71. Rees, L.H., Bloomfield, G.A., Rees, G.M., Corrin, B., Franks, L.M., Ratcliffe, J.G.: Multiple hormones in a bronchial tumor. J. clin. Endocrinol. Metab. 38, 1090-1097 (1974).

72. Padfield, P.L., Morton, J.J., Brown, J.J., Lever, A.F., Robertson, J.I.S., Wood, M., Fox, R.: Plasma arginine vasopressin in the syndrome of antidiuretic hormone excess associated with bronchogenic carcinoma. Am. J. Med. 61, 825-831 (1976).

73. Vorherr, H.: Para-endocrine tumor activity with emphasis on ectopic ADH secretion. Oncology 29, 382-416 (1974).

74. Sawyer, W.H.: Pharmacological characteristics of the antidiuretic principle in a bronchogenic carcinoma from a patient with hyponatraemia. J. clin. Endocr. 27, 1497-1499 (1967).

75. Lipscomb, H.S., Wilson, C., Retienne, K., Matsen, F., Ward, D.N.: The syndrome of inappropriate secretion of antidiuretic hormone: a case report and characterisation of an antidiuretic hormone-like material isolated from an oat cell carcinoma of the lung. Cancer Res. 28, 378-383 (1968).

76. Utiger, R.D.: Inappropriate antidiuresis and carcinoma of the lung: detection of arginine vasopressin in tumour extracts by immunoassay. J. clin. Endocr. 26, 970-974 (1966).

77. Marks, L.J., Berde, B., Klein, L.A., Roth, J., Goonan, S.R., Blumen, D., Nabseth, D.C.: Inappropriate vasopressin secretion and carcinoma of the pancreas. Am. J. Med. 45, 967-974 (1968).

78. Azzopardi, J.G., Freeman, E., Poole, G.: Endocrine and metabolic disorders in bronchial carcinoma. Brit. med. J. 4, 528-530 (1970).

79. Rees, L.H., Ratcliffe, J.G.: Ectopic hormone production by non-endocrine tumours. Clin. Endocr. 3, 263-299 (1974).

80. Bloomfield, G.A., Holdaway, I.M., Corrin, B., Ratcliffe, J.G., Rees, G.M., Ellison, M., Rees, L.H.: Lung tumours and ACTH production. Clin. Endocr. 6, 95-104 (1977).

81. Whitelaw, A.G.L.: Ultrastructure of an oat cell carcinoma of the bronchus producing an antidiuretic hormone. Brit. J. Cancer 23, 69-72 (1969).

82. Ellison, M.L., Neville, A.M.: In: Modern Trends in Oncology Ed. Raven, R.W., London, p. 163-181(1973).

83. Pearse, A.G.E.: Common cytochemical and ultrastructural characteristics of cells producing polypeptide hormones (the APUD series) and their relevance to thyroid and ultimobronchial cells and calcitonin. Proc. R. Soc. B, 170, 71 (1968).

84. Feyrter, F.: In: Endocrinology, Ed. Taylor, S., London, p. 134-139(1972).

85. Padfield, P.L., Brown, J.J., Larkin, H., Lever, A.F., Morton, J.J., Robertson, J.I.S.: Antidiuretic hormone as a marker for bronchial carcinoma. Scottish Medical Journal 22, 331 (1977).

86. Bower, B.F., Mason, D.M., Forsham, P.H.: Bronchogenic carcinoma with inappropriate antidiuretic activity in plasma and tumor. New Engl. J. Med. 271, 934-938 (1964).

87. Lee, J., Jones, J.J., Barraclough, M.A.: Inappropriate secretion of vasopressin. Lancet, ii, 792-793 (1964).

88. De Sousa, R.C., Delaere, J., Berde, B.: Inappropriate secretion of vasopressin. Lancet i, 436-437 (1965).

89. Barraclough, M.A., Jones, J.J., Lee, J.: Production of vasopressin by anaplastic oat cell carcinoma of the bronchus. Clin. Sci. 31, 135-144 (1966).

90. Mornex, R., Gharib, U., Veyrat, A., Dutruge, Mlle., Byron, P.A., Maguin, J.M.: Syndrome de Schwartz-Bartter par tumeur mediastino-pulmonaire. Annls Endocr. 28, 391-399 (1967).

91. Vorherr, H., Massry, S.G., Utiger, R.D., Kleeman, C.R.: Antidiuretic principle in malignant tumor extracts from patients with inappropriate ADH syndrome. J. clin. Endocr. 28, 162-168 (1968).

92. Cullen, D.R., Tomlinson, B.E.: Carcinoma with multiple ectopic hormone secretion and associated myopathy. Postgrad. Med. J. 44, 472-491 (1968).

93. Segar, W.E., Moore, W.W.: Increased antidiuretic hormone and inappropriate thirst in a patient with bronchogenic carcinoma. Minerva med. 51, 625-629 (1968).

94. Hamilton, B.P.M., Upton, G.V., Amatruda, T.T.: Peptides with ADH-like activity in tumours producing the syndrome of inappropriate antidiuresis. Programme of the Fifty-Third Meeting of the Endocrine Society, A 205 (1971).

95. David, G.S.: Solid state lactoperoxidase: a highly stable enzyme for simple, gentle iodination. Biochem. biophys. Res. Commun. 48, 464-471 (1972).

96. Burford, G.D., Pickering, B.T.: Intra-axonal transport and turnover of neurophysins in the rat: a proposal for the possible origin of the minor neurophysin component. Biochem. J. 136, 1047-1052 (1973).

97. Morton, J.J., Waite, M.A.: The possible relationship between the affinity of arginine vasopressin antibodies and the degree of polyuria and polydipsia in actively immunized rabbits. J. Endocr. 54, 523-524 (1972).

HUMAN SEX STEROID BINDING PLASMA PROTEIN

Christine Mercier-Bodard, J. M. Renoir, E.-E. Baulieu
Unité de Recherches sur le Métabolisme Moléculaire et la Physio-Pathologie des Stéroides de l'Institut National de la Recherche Médicale, Hôpital de Bicêtre, 78, rue du Général Leclerc, 94270 - Bicêtre, France

R. Emiliozzi, Danièle Duval
Biochimie PCEM, Université de Nice, Petit Valrose, Avenue J. Vallot, 06034 - Nice Cedex, France

Summary

The human sex steroid binding plasma protein (h-Sbp) from late pregnancy plasma was purified by a three-step procedure including ammonium sulfate precipitation, affinity chromatography and preparative electrophoresis. The biospecific adsorbent was prepared by coupling 1α-carboxymethyl-5α-dihydrotestosterone to AH-Sepharose 4B. Homogeneity of Sbp was shown in polyacrylamide gel electrophoresis in the presence or absence of sodium dodecyl sulfate and in immunoelectrophoresis.

The mean molecular radius of 2.99 nm and an apparent molecular weight of 92,000 daltons were obtained for the native pure Sbp using polyacrylamide gel electrophoresis, whereas in the presence of sodium dodecyl sulfate, a value of 67,000 daltons for the molecular weight of denatured Sbp was determined.

A highly specific and precise radioimmunoassay for human Sbp has been developed using a monospecific rabbit anti-human Sbp antiserum. No cross-reactivity was observed with transferrin, IgG or α-fetoprotein and with any mammalian plasma except primate plasma. The sensitivity was 0.3 ng of pure Sbp at the highest antiserum dilution of 1/122,000. The concentration of Sbp (mean ± s.e.m.) in the plasma of normal men, normal, pregnant (9th month) and hirsute (non pregnant) women were measured as 1.3 ± 0.2, 2.6 ± 0.2, 25 ± 16 and 2.0 ± 0.1 mg/l respectively.

The human and monkeys' Sbps were compared. Detailed studies of steroid binding specificity gave the same results in all primates, with the exception of the human and the chimpanzee where estrone did not compete for dihydrotestosterone binding. Immunoelectrophoretic experiments performed with a monospecific antiserum against h-Sbp indicated variable cross-reactivities with Sbps of primates, from complete in chimpanzee and gorilla to weak in prosimii.

Introduction

In the plasma of humans and many other mammalian species, a β-glycoprotein that occurs in low concentration, binds dihydrotestosterone (DHT)[1], testosterone and estradiol with high affinity ($K_d \sim 0.5$, 1 and 2 nM respectively) and has been called sex steroid binding plasma protein (Sbp) (1), testosterone-estradiol binding globulin (Tebg) (2) or sex hormone binding globulin (Shbg) (3).

Sbp possibly functions as reservoir/buffer, influencing free (active) hormone concentration in the plasma (4), but as in the case for other high affinity hormone plasma binding proteins such as thyroxine binding globulin or corticosteroid binding globulin, its physiological role is poorly understood.

The Sbp concentration is not constant during life and consequently the free fraction of the sex hormones shows important variations. However, at 37°C and in adult subjects, the free fraction of testosterone represents about 2.5% in normal men and 1.4% in women of its total concentration (5) (total testosterone concentration in men : ∿8 ng/ml, in women: ∿0.5 ng/ml). The majority of plasma 17β-hydroxysteroids is bound to proteins, 35% in men and 66% in women to Sbp, and 62% in men and 33% in women to serum albumin with a weaker affinity. Estradiol binds less well than testosterone to Sbp and better to serum albumin.

Several purifications of Sbp from human late pregnancy plasma/serum and from Cohn's fraction IV have already been published (6, 7, 8, 9, 10). We report here on a new biospecific adsorbent to purify Sbp whose stability and capacity seem satisfactory and on physiochemical properties determined on pure Sbp. Monospecific antibodies have been raised (11, 12) and a highly specific and precise radioimmunoassay for Sbp has been developed. Finally these antibodies have been used, together with binding studies, to investigate some phylogenic aspects of Sbp.

Results

1. Purification

Since the Sbp concentration increases markedly during pregnancy, human late pregnancy plasma was used as a suitable starting material. After sequential precipitations of total plasma, the pellet obtained in a 25 to 50% range ammonium sulfate saturation, was further purified by affinity chromatography.

The first affinity resin used (Fig. 1A) was a 3-0-succinyl-estradiol-ethylenediamino acrylamide (8) synthesized by R. Bucourt (Roussel Uclaf). This ligand was very labile and continually released from the matrix during the fixation step. Therefore the capacity was very low and the resin could only be used once.

---

[1]The abbreviations used are : Sbp, Sex steroid binding plasma protein; Tebg, Testosterone-estradiol binding globulin ; Shbg, Sex hormone binding globulin ; DHT, 5α-androstanolone or dihydrotestosterone ; T, testosterone ; E_2, estradiol ; IEA, immunoelectrophoresis analysis ; PAGE, polyacrylamide gel electrophoresis ; SDS-PAGE, sodium dodecyl sulfate polyacrylamide gel electrophoresis ; RIA, radioimmunoassay.

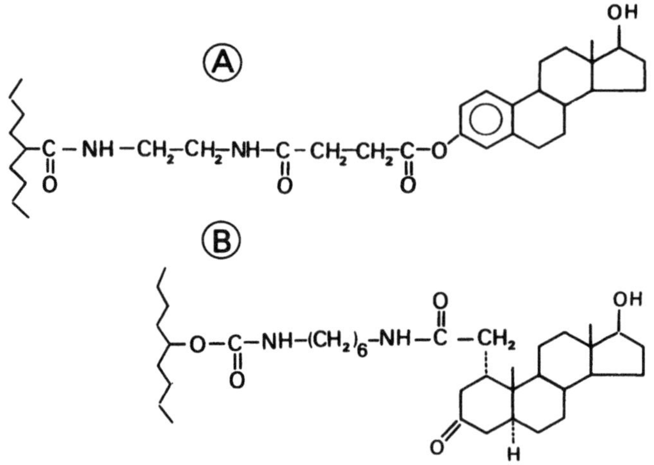

Fig. 1. Structure of the biospecific adsorbents used in the purification of Sbp.
A. 17β-estradiol 3-0-succinate-ethylenediamino-acrylamide;
B. 1α-carboxymethyl 5α-dihydrotestosterone-1,6-diaminohexan-AH Sepharose 4B

A second biospecific adsorbent was synthesized (Fig. 1B) using 1α-carboxymethyl-DHT as ligand, the inhibition constant K_i (of DHT binding) was about 10 nM. The steroid was covalently linked by a one-step carbodiimide coupling reaction to AH-Sepharose 4B which has a six-carbon long "spacer arm". This affinity resin has been used many times without any loss of capacity. Sbp was eluted at 4 °C by an exchange procedure using a buffer containing 0.5 µM [^{3}H]-DHT. Finally, pure Sbp was obtained after preparative electrophoresis according to Mickelson et al. (9). The total yield (Table 1) obtained was 28% instead of 5% as previously reported (8).

Homogeneity of pure Sbp was checked by polyacrylamide gel electrophoresis (PAGE) in the presence or absence of sodium dodecyl sulfate. In both cases, Sbp gave one stained band at five different acrylamide concentrations. Moreover, using immunoelectrophoresis analysis (IEA), one precipitin line could

TABLE 1

h-Sbp purification scheme.

Step	Protein (mg)	nM of DHT bound	Cumulative purification	Cumulative yield (%)
Late pregnancy plasma (250 ml)	13,440	41.35	1	100
$(NH_4)_2SO_4$ ppt (25-50%)	2,688	26.88	3.6	65
Affinity chromatography (resin B)	3.84	13.29	1,252	32
Preparative PAGE	0.95	11.5	4,368	28

be detected when pure Sbp was applied against crude anti-Sbp rabbit antiserum, whereas when human plasma was used instead of Sbp, four lines were visualized (8).

2. Physicochemical parameters of pure Sbp

a) Molecular radius and molecular weight of native Sbp. As originally proposed by Ferguson (13) a linear relationship between the logarithm of electrophoretic mobility and gel concentration in PAGE has been validated over molecular weight range 450 to 670,000 daltons and pH range 3.6 to 10.2 (14), in gels of 3 to 30% in total acrylamide gel concentration (% T)[2] and in 1 to 5% cross-linking (% C). The slope of the Ferguson plot (K_R or retardation coefficient) could be

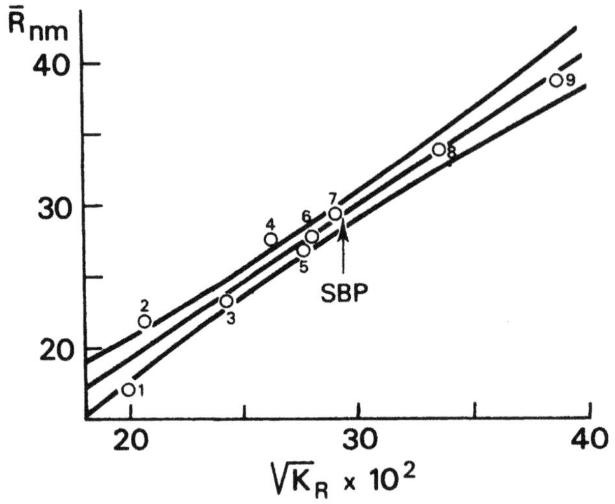

Fig. 2. Standard curve of $\bar{R}$ vs. $\sqrt{K_R}$ for Sbp and nine proteins in PAGE.
Standard proteins used are : 1, myoglobin; 2, pepsin-monomer; 3, ovalbumin-monomer; 4, pepsin-dimer; 5, BSA-monomer; 6, transferrin; 7, ovalbumin-dimer; 8, BSA-dimer; 9, BSA-trimer. Regression line and 95% confidence limits are indicated.

considered as a constant characteristic of a protein in any one system. Moreover, there is a linear relation between $\sqrt{K_R}$ and molecular radius $\bar{R}$, calculated from the known molecular weight (MW) with the relationship :

$$\bar{R} = (3(MW)\bar{\nu}/4\pi N)^{1/3}$$

where N is Avogadro's number, $\bar{\nu}$ is partial specific volume and assuming no hydration of the molecules. The geometric mean radius of pure Sbp was determined by PAGE as previously reported by Corvol et al. (15) in a multiphasic buffer system operative at pH 10.2 which allowed a good separation of Sbp and transferrin. These two proteins exhibited similar molecular size and net charge in the buffer systems usually

---

[2]Total acrylamide gel concentration is defined as % T = acrylamide + methylene-bis-acrylamide; percent cross-linking, % C = 100 (methylene-bis-acrylamide/T).

described. The Ferguson plots for standard proteins and pure Sbp were drawn and the slopes K_R were then plotted versus the geometric mean radii; the regression line and its 95% confidence limits were drawn (Fig.2). The molecular radius of pure Sbp was obtained from this curve. Therefore, the molecular weight of the native Sbp was calculated by assuming sphericity, no hydration and a partial specific volume of 0.735 ml/g. Mean values of 2.99 ± 0.12 nm for $\bar{R}_{Sbp}$ and 92,000 ± 7,000 daltons for the molecular weight have been thus determined.

b) Stokes radius, R_s, and friction coefficient, f/f_o. A mean value of 38 ± 1.6 Å for the Stokes radius of Sbp has been obtained from similar linear regression of R_s vs $\sqrt{K_R}$ of the standard proteins. The frictional ratio, i.e. $R_s/\bar{R}$ was 1.26 ± 0.01.

c) Molecular weight in SDS-PAGE. After denaturation of pure Sbp by heating at 95°C for 5 min in the presence of 1% SDS and 1% 2-mercaptoethanol, the molecular weight of denatured Sbp was determined in SDS-PAGE as previously reported (8). The mean molecular weight was obtained from the plot of K_R vs. MW as suggested by Banker and Cotman (16) and was found to be 67,000 ± 2,500 daltons (Fig. 3).

3. Radioimmunoassay of pure Sbp (17).

a) Anti-Sbp antiserum. Antibodies against highly purified human Sbp were elicited in rabbits after primary and booster injections and assessed further for specificity by IEA (11). Actually, without any more purification, anti-human Sbp antisera produced a single monospecific precipitin line when reacted against either highly purified Sbp or total human late pregnancy plasma, whereas with the first crude antisera, four precipitin lines were obtained against total human late pregnancy plasma.

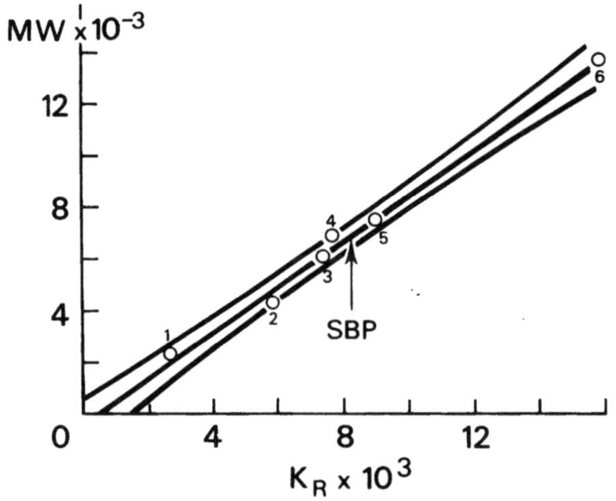

Fig. 3. Relationship between molecular weight (MW) and retardation coefficient (K_R) in SDS-PAGE, for Sbp and six proteins.
Standard proteins used are : 1, soyabean trypsin inhibitor; 2, ovalbumin; 3, catalase; 4, BSA-monomer; 5, transferrin; 6, BSA-dimer. Regression line and 95% confidence limits are indicated.

b) Iodination of Sbp. Pure Sbp was labelled with ^{125}I by the chloramine T method of Hunter and Greenwood (18) and purified by filtration on Sephadex G-50. The specific activity of the labelled protein was 40 to 60 µCi/µg. Antigen-antibody complexes were separated from the free Sbp by adsorption onto a cellulose powder which had been covalently linked to sheep anti-rabbit IgG; the non-specific precipitation by this immuno-adsorbent was approximately 2% and the maximum of precipitated complexes was 53 to 56%.
Control experiments showed that iodination had not destroyed the antigenic sites of Sbp molecules.

c) Standard curve. The displacement of ^{125}I-Sbp by unlabelled Sbp described a sigmoid curve on a semilogarithmic plot (Fig. 4) and the steep portion of the curves was effected

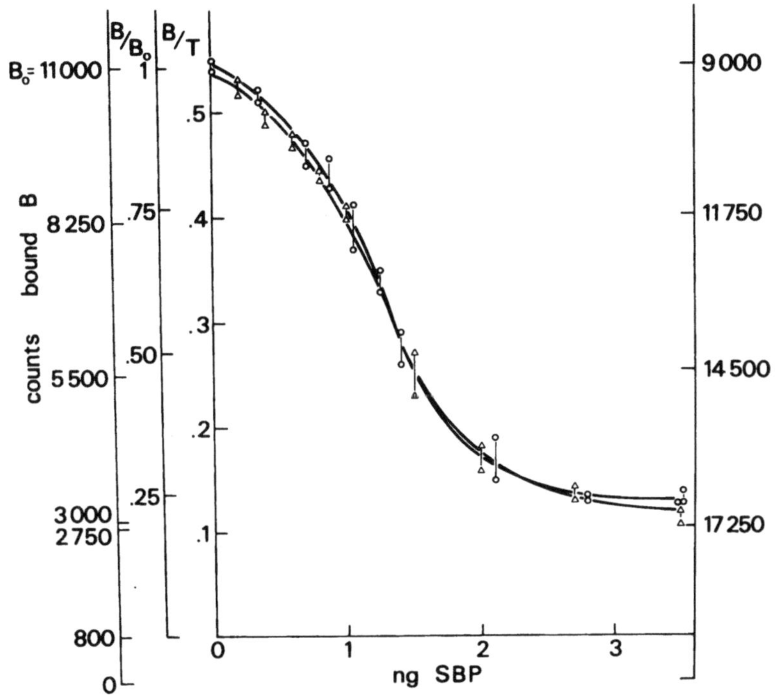

Fig. 4. Sbp radioimmunoassay dose/response curves. ^{125}I-Sbp was displaced from anti-Sbp antibody by pure Sbp (o——o) or by standard late pregnancy plasma (Δ——Δ); the final dilution of antiserum was 1/55,000.

by 0.5 to 2 ng of unlabelled Sbp with a final dilution of anti-Sbp antiserum of 1/55,000. When total human late pregnancy plasma was assayed concurrently with pure Sbp, no significant differences were observed between the two curves; therefore, pregnancy plasma may conveniently be used as a standard.

d) Accuracy and sensitivity. The best dilution of anti-Sbp antiserum was determined for each batch of antiserum and chosen according to the mean slope of the standard curves. Sbp quantities as small as 0.3 ng could be detected with the highest

antiserum dilution of 1/122,000.
The coefficient variation was 3% for within-run variance and 8% for between-run variance.

e) Stability of labelled Sbp. When the specific activity does not exceed 70 µCi/µg, the immunological activity is stable for 5 weeks. No significant difference was observed when the dose/response curves were measured just after iodination, one week or five weeks later (Fig. 5).

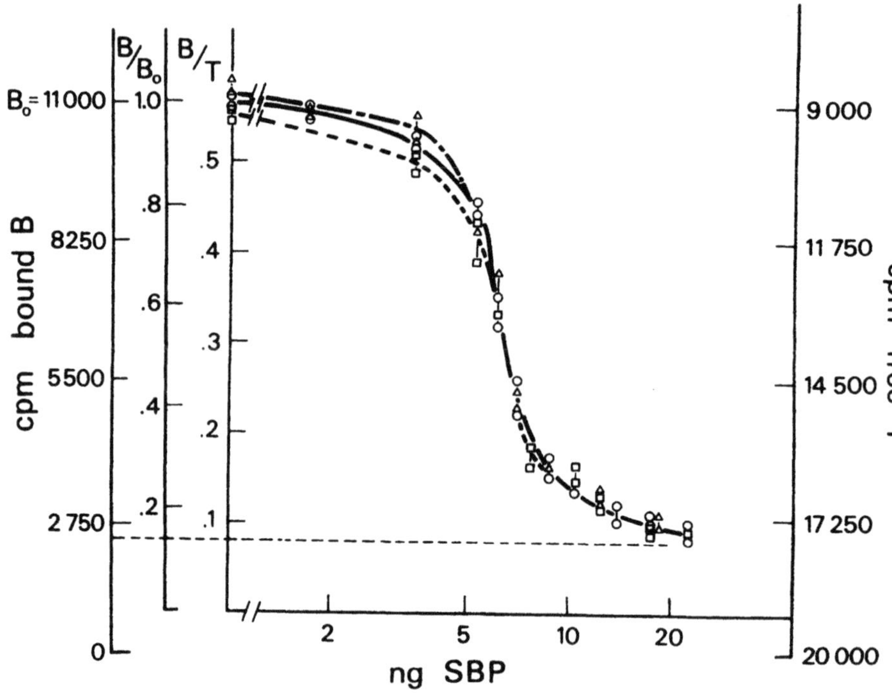

Fig. 5. Stability of ^{125}I-Sbp.
Dose/response curves obtained just after iodination of pure Sbp (Δ——Δ), one week later (o——o) and five weeks later (□——□). The final dilution of antiserum was 1/11,000.

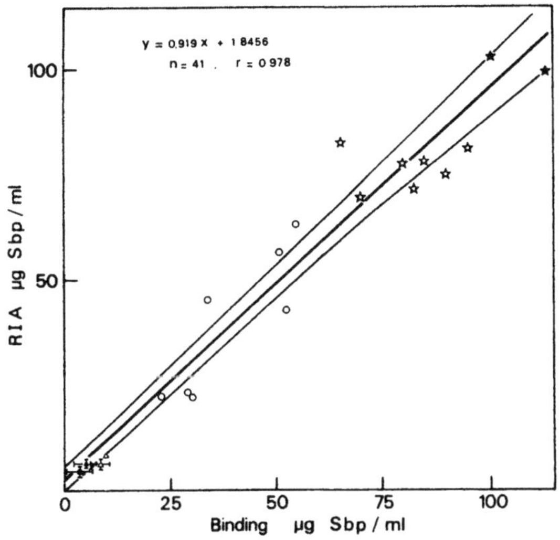

Fig. 6. Correlation of plasma Sbp concentrations determined by RIA and by radioligand binding measurements. 84 Human plasmas were assayed from normal men (●), normal (Δ), pregnant (2nd trimester o, 9th month ⋆) and hirsute (▲) women. In radioligand binding measurements, Sbp concentrations were calculated assuming 1 binding site/molecule.

f) Correlation with radioligand assay. The Sbp concentrations were measured in 84 human plasmas from normal men, normal and pregnant women, and from hirsute non-pregnant subjects, either by radioimmunoassay (RIA) or by [^{3}H]-DHT binding determination using equilibrium dialysis and Scatchard plot (19) as corrected according to Rosenthal (20). Equilibrium dialysis measurements were then plotted against the values determined by RIA and the results were compared (Fig. 6). The correlation (r) was 0.978 indicating a good agreement.

g) Plasma Sbp concentrations. The mean plasma Sbp concentrations as measured in RIA were significantly different, according to the Student's t test, in men (1.3 $\pm$ 0.2 mg/l, n = 30) and in women (2.6 $\pm$ 0.2 mg/l, n = 30) ($p < 0.001$), in hirsute (2.0 $\pm$ 0.1 mg/l, n = 8) and in normal women ($p < 0.01$). As measured by radioligand assay, the results

TABLE 2

h-Sbp plasma concentrations determined by RIA and [^{3}H] -DHT binding measurements.

Plasma source	Number of samples	h-Sbp [^{3}H] -DHT binding (nM)	h-Sbp RIA (mg/l)
Normal men	30	28.8 ± 12.6	1.3 ± 0.2
Normal women	30	60.3 ± 9.3 p<0.01(1)	2.6 ± 0.2 p<0.001(1)
Hirsute women	8	47.1 ± 3.4 p<0.2(2)	2.0 ± 0.1 p<0.02(2)
Pregnancy (2nd trimester)	8	354 ± 70	12.4 ± 0.2
Pregnancy (9th month)	8	724 ± 90	25 ± 1.6

Sbp concentrations in plasmas from normal men, normal, hirsute and pregnant women were determined either by equilibrium dialysis and expressed in nM [^{3}H] -DHT bound per liter or by radioimmunoassay using pure Sbp as standard. The 95% confidence limits and probability of significance (Student's t test) were reported, compared to normal men (1) and to normal women (2).

obtained are significantly different in normal men (28.8 ± 12.6 nM) and in normal women (60.3 ± 9.3 nM) ($p < 0.01$) whereas there is no significant difference between hirsute (47.1 ± 3.4 nM) and normal women ($0.1 < p < 0.2$) (Table 2).

4. Immunological cross-reactivity of primate Sbp

We were able to obtain sera from chimpanzee, gorilla, 4 baboon subspecies (Papio papio, Papio anubis, Papio cynocephalus and Hamadryas), 2 subspecies of macaca (Macaca mulata or Rhesus and Macaca fascicularis or Cynomolgus), 2 subspecies of new world monkeys cebidae (Ateles paniscus or Spider monkey and

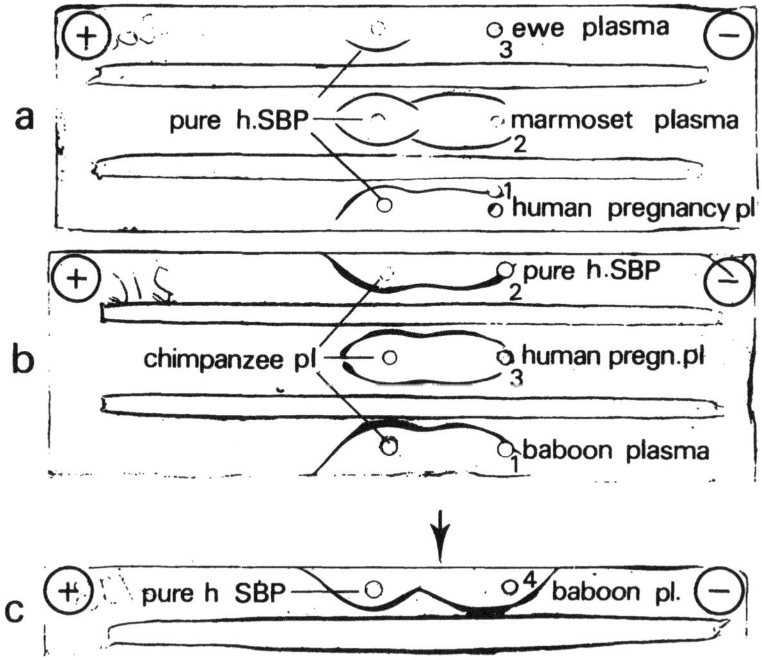

Fig. 7. Immunoelectrophoresis studies in 1.3% agar gel. Antigen samples (right wells), were first submitted to electrophoresis (11). Then the troughs and the left wells were cut off and filled with the monospecific anti-h-Sbp antiserum, pure h-Sbp (600 µg/ml) respectively (7a and c), and with chimpanzee plasma (7b). Precipitin lines were allowed to develop during 48 h at 25°.

Figure 7a: human late pregnancy plasma ①, marmoset plasma ② and ewe plasma ③ show total, partial and no immunological cross-reactivity with pure h-Sbp, respectively.

Figure 7b and c: papio-papio plasma ①, pure h-Sbp ② and human late pregnancy plasma ③ show total immunological cross-reactivity with chimpanzee Sbp, while a weak and partial immunological identity occurs between papio-papio Sbp ④ and pure h-Sbp (note the spur ↓).

Lagothrix or Wooley monkey), one other cebidae (Saimiri sciureus or Squirrel monkey), one species of callithricidae (Callithrix jacchus or Marmoset) and one prosimii (Microcebus murinus).

In order to demonstrate the immunological cross-reactivity of Sbp, samples of plasma/serum were submitted to electrophoresis. Pure h-Sbp was secondarily introduced into a second well (Fig. 7). The anti-h-Sbp antiserum was then deposited in the trough and immunodiffusion allowed to take place at room temperature for 48 h. Total immunological identity was observed with the corresponding protein of human late pregnancy plasma (Fig. 7a), which demonstrated that the purification had not altered the immunological determinants of the molecule.

When the monkey plasmas were studied, precipitin lines were obtained, as opposed to what was observed using plasmas of other animals (Fig. 7a). However, only the chimpanzee and the gorilla (data not shown) Sbps gave identical cross-reaction with anti-h-Sbp antiserum (Fig. 7b). Furthermore, although immunological cross-reactivity with baboons (Fig. 7c) was partial, it was strong and with other monkeys, the partial immunological identity essentially followed the primate phylogeny (Fig. 7 and Tables 3 and 4). Finally, the number of common antigenic determinants with h-Sbp was the smallest with Prosimii.

5. Hormone binding specificity

Equilibrium dialysis experiments were performed on diluted plasma/serum samples from which endogenous steroids had been removed with charcoal (5 mg/ml for 10 min at 37°C). Samples (1 ml) were dialyzed against 15 ml Tris 0.05 M, $CaCl_2$ 0.05M, NaCl 0.2 M HCl buffer pH 7.4 containing 0.1 to 50 nM [^{3}H]-hormone. After 24 h at 4°C under constant stirring, bound and unbound hormones were calculated by counting aliquots of both internal and external solutions. The equilibrium dissociation constant (K_d) and concentration of binding sites were determined (19, 20).

TABLE 3

	ANTHROPOIDAE								PROSIMII
			Old World Monkeys				New World Monkeys		
	Hominidae	Pongidae	Cercopithecidae		Cebidae	Callithrichidae	(Cebidae)		Cherogaleidae
	Homo	Chimpanzee	Baboon	Macaca	Squirrel M	Marmoset	Wooly M	Spider M	Microcebus
Homo		T	P****	P***	P**	P**	P**	P**	P*
Chimpanzee	T		T	T	P**	P**	P***	-	-
Baboon	P****	T		T	P***	P***	P***	P***	-
Macaca	P***	T	T		T	P****	P****	P****	P*
Squirrel M	P**	P**	P***	T		T	T	T	-
Marmoset	P**	P**	P***	P****	T		T	P****	-
Wooly M	P***	P***	P***	P****	T	T		T	P*
Spider M	P***	-	P***	P****	T	P****	T		-
Microcebus	P*	-	-	P*	-	-	P*	-	

Immunological cross-reactivity of monkey Sbp with anti-h-Sbp antibody (see also Fig. 7).
T = total identity; P = partial identity with gradation from rather strong (****) to very weak and partial (*) cross-reactivity.

TABLE 4

Binding of androgens and estradiol to primates Sbp

	Immunoreactivity with anti-h Sbp antibodies	K_d (nM)		
		Dht	T	E_2
Human	T	0.4	0.8	2.0
Chimpanzee	T	0.5	0.8	2.2
Gorilla	T	0.4	0.9	1.7
Baboon (Papio papio)	P	0.5	1.0	2.5
Macaca mulata	P	0.8	2.4	4.2

K_d measured at 4°C by equilibrium dialysis. Immunoreactivity determined by immunoelectrophoresis.

The K_d of Sbp for dihydrotestosterone, testosterone and estradiol (Table 4) are quite similar in the various primates whereas the concentration of binding sites is lower in human and chimpanzee as opposed to other monkeys where it was 2-5 times greater (Table 5). The mean (± 95% confidence limits) of K_d and of the number of sites are reported in Table 5.

The binding specificity of monkeys' Sbp was further investigated by adding 10 nM of the competitive steroid to 0.1 nM [^{3}H]-DHT and performing dialysis at 4°C for 13-20 h.

TABLE 5

Steroids	Man	Chimpanzee	Baboon	Macaca mulata	Squirrel monkey	Marmoset
DHT	100	100	100	100	100	100
Testosterone	79	92	83	87	81	77
Oestradiol	33	57	38	55	60	79
5α-androstane-3α, 17β-diol	101	104	98	97	96	97
5α-androstane-3β, 17β-diol	104	101	96	100	91	99
Diethylstilbestrol	0	0	0	0	0	0
Oestrone	0	0	30	20	42	52
Oestriol	0	0	4	0	0	16
Cortisol	0	3	0	0	0	0
Progesterone	0	0	0	0	0	3
K_d 4° (nM)	(M) 0.43±0.06 (F-G) 0.43±0.06	(F) 0.48±0.05	(F) 0.50±0.06	(F) 0.8±0.1	(F) 1.1±0.1	(F) 1.1±0.1
Plasma concentration (nM)	(M) 29±13 (F) 60±9 (F-G) 700±185	(M) 30±11 (F) 60±15	(F) 200±67	(F) 155±75	(F) 259±133	(F) 108±81

Binding of steroid hormones by Sbp in primates.
The competitive binding test was performed with 0.1 nM [^{3}H] -DHT and 10 nM of non radioactive competitors. The decrease of bound radioactivity measured after addition of competitors was expressed relative to that measured after DHT addition ("100"). M = males, F = females, F-G = pregnant females.

All primates showed no specific binding for progesterone, cortisol, estriol (a natural steroidal estrogen metabolite) and diethylstilbestrol (a synthetic non steroidal estrogen) (Table 5). Estradiol binding was identical, weaker than that for testosterone. Curiously, estrone was a good competitor for [^{3}H]-DHT binding in tested monkeys, including gorilla (data not shown), but not in man and in chimpanzee. In addition to binding DHT, primate Sbp bound testosterone and 3α/3β-5α-androstanediols with high affinity.

Discussion

1. Purification

The new biospecific adsorbent, 1α-carboxymethyl-DHT-AH-Sepharose 4B used has increased the cumulative yield from 5 to 28%. This affinity chromatography could be improved either by using a longer spacer arm or by varying the capacity of the resin. However, it is quite difficult to calculate the amount of bound steroid per ml of gel since the tritiated ligand was not readily available. The new three-step purification procedure has yielded 1 mg of pure Sbp starting from 250 ml of human late pregnancy plasma and a monospecific antiserum has been obtained in rabbits without further purification (Table 1).

2. Molecular weight of native and denatured Sbp

The molecular weight of the native plasma Sbp as determined by PAGE is 92,000 ± 7,000 daltons and is very similar to the value of 89,000 daltons found by the same method in our laboratory for the pure serum Sbp isolated by Mickelson et al. (Table 6); the slight discrepancy could be explained by the fact that only two experiments have been performed on the latter. The results

TABLE 6

Some physicochemical properties of h-Sbp.

Property		Method	h-Sbp Isolated by	h-Sbp Tested by
Molecular weight of:				
- Native h-Sbp	: 89,000	PAGE	Petra	Mercier-Bodard (17)
	: 92,000	PAGE	Mercier-Bodard	Mercier-Bodard (17)
	: 120,000	Filtration	Petra	Petra (9)
- Denatured h-Sbp	: 94,000	SDS-PAGE	Rosner	Rosner (7)
	: 52,000	SDS-PAGE	Petra	Petra (9)
	: 48,000	SDS-PAGE	Petra	Mercier-Bodard (17)
	: 67,000	SDS-PAGE	Mercier-Bodard	Mercier-Bodard (17)
	: 36,000	Guanidine-HCl ultracentrifugation	Petra	Petra (9)
Stokes radius	: 55.5	calculated	Rosner	Rosner (7)
R_s (Å)	: 37.4	PAGE	Petra	Mercier-Bodard (17)
	: 38.0	PAGE	Mercier-Bodard	Mercier-Bodard (17)
Molecular radius	: 2.95	calculated	Rosner	Rosner (7)
$\bar{R}$ (nm)	: 2.96	PAGE	Petra	Mercier-Bodard (17)
	: 2.99	PAGE	Mercier-Bodard	Mercier-Bodard (17)
Frictional ratio	: 1.87	calculated	Rosner	Rosner (7)
f/f_o	: 1.26	calculated	Petra	Mercier-Bodard (17)
	: 1.27	calculated	Mercier-Bodard	Mercier-Bodard (17)

should be considered to be only an approximation and sedimentation equilibrium still remains the method of choice for accurate molecular weight determinations but both native plasma and serum Sbp seem to be denatured during such an experiment.

An apparent molecular weight of 120,000 daltons has recently been reported by Michelson et al. (9) for the native serum Sbp using gel filtration on agarose; this significantly higher value is probably due to the carbohydrate moiety of Sbp which results on a more expanded structure than those of typical globular proteins. In solution, carbohydrate chains would have a greater hydration as compared with polypeptide chains.

There is a marked discrepancy about the molecular weight of Sbp as determined in SDS-PAGE. Rosner obtained a value of 95,000 daltons but he did not use a Ferguson plot since electrophoresis was performed with only one acrylamide concentration. Mickelson et al. (9) reported a molecular weight of 52,000 daltons. Using a Ferguson plot and the representation of MW vs K_R, we found a value of 48,000 daltons for their Sbp instead of 67,000 for our protein. This difference could be due to the fact that Ca^{++} ions, which are known to stabilize Sbp, were not present in Sbp from Mickelson. Further investigations are in progress to explain this discrepancy and the possible role of Ca^{++} ions in the maintainance of a stable configuration. The most reliable value could be 36,000 daltons as obtained by Mickelson et al. in 6 M guanidine hydrochloride ultracentrifugation, but it is important to note that the protein in the SDS complex is not a random coil as in 6 M guanidine hydrochloride and contains a high degree of order. However, this would mean that Sbp consists of subunits of very similar size but it is not possible to decide now if there are two as suggested for human (21) and canine Sbp (22) or three as reported for bovine Sbp (23).

3. Radioimmunoassay

The RIA offers a precise and highly specific determination of Sbp in human plasma and is the method of choice in routine clinical assays of Sbp. It is superior to radioligand binding determinations not only because it is a direct measurement of protein concentration but also in rapidity, efficiency and reproducibility.

The sensitivity may be improved using higher antiserum dilutions and therefore should allow Sbp assays in other biological fluids or in cells where the Sbp concentrations may be very low. Cross-reaction studies with other plasma proteins (transferrin, IgG, α-fetoprotein) show that the assay is specific for human and primate Sbp.

The iodinated protein stability over a long period of time is indicated by a high reproducibility of the standard curve. Moreover, the dose/response curves are identical using either pure Sbp or late human pregnancy plasma, the Sbp concentration of which has been previously determined by radioligand assay; therefore only very small amounts of pure Sbp are required for iodination. The potential importance of a better understanding of the free and h-Sbp bound androgens and estrogens in the plasma warrant the use of Sbp radioimmunoassay systematically with the measurement of T and E_2.

4. h-Sbp and monkey Sbp

Detailed studies with monkey sera strongly implied that the human and chimpanzee Sbp have the same immunological and hormone-binding properties. These two proteins have no affinity for estrone contrary to other primates' Sbp including gorilla Sbp, the latter appearing immunologically identical to h-Sbp. Moreover, the concentrations in human and chimpanzee plasmas are similar and, as previously reported in the human, there is a two-fold larger concentration in the chimpanzee female than in the male. Sbp measurements during gestation have not yet been performed on the chimpanzee.

It is remarkable that high affinity estradiol binding is found only in primates (24) whose Sbp react with the anti-h-Sbp antibody suggesting that a specific role for plasma proteins emerged with evolution, possibly related to a fine regulatory function of androgen/estrogen imbalance in the blood (25). However, the physiological significance of such a precise mechanism for binding sex steroids is not known.

Acknowledgements

We would like to acknowledge P.H. Petra for valuable discussion and helpful collaboration. We wish to thank J. Barry, M. Courot, J. Dorst, J.J. Petter and A. Psychoyos who provided us with monkey blood samples; F. Bayard for the supply of late pregnancy human plasma; R. Mortel and A. Wolfson for writing the manuscript and F. Boussac for secretarial assistance.

Partial support was obtained from Inserm Grant AT 49 7781 and Faculté de Médecine Paris-Sud, Contract n° 726.

References

1. Mercier-Bodard, C., Alfsen, A., Baulieu, E.E.: Sex steroid binding plasma protein (Sbp). Acta Endocrinol. 147, 204-224 (1970).

2. Corvol, P.: Testosterone-estradiol binding globulin (Tebg): Physical properties, binding capacity and species distribution : 52nd Meeting of Endocrine Society, June 1970. Abst. 73.

3. Murphy, B.E.P.: Protein binding and hormone assay. Recent Progr. Hormone Res. 25, 563-601 (1969).

4. Tait, J.F., Burstein, S.: In vivo studies of steroid dynamics in man. In: "The Hormones", Eds. Pincus, G., Thimann, K.V., Astwood, E.B., Academic Press, New York, Vol. V, pp. 441-557 (1964).

5. Moll, G.W., Rosenfield, R.L.: Testosterone binding and free plasma androgen concentrations under physiological conditions : characterization by flow dialysis technique. J. clin. Endocrinol. Metab. 49, 730-736 (1979).

6. Mickelson, K.E., Petra, P.H.: Purification of the Sex steroid binding protein from human serum. Biochemistry 14, 957-963 (1975).

7. Rosner, W., Smith, R.N.: Isolation and characterization of the Testosterone-estradiol binding globulin from human plasma. Use of a novel affinity column. Biochemistry 14, 4813-4820 (1975).

8. Mercier-Bodard, C., Renoir, J.M., Fox, L.L., Baulieu, E.E.: Physicochemical properties of Sex steroid binding plasma protein (Sbp). In: "Proceedings of the V International Congress of Endocrinology", Hamburg, Vol. 1, pp. 446-451 (1976).

9. Mickelson, K.E., Teller, D.C., Petra, P.H.: Characterization of the Sex steroid binding protein of human pregnancy serum. Improvements in the purification procedure. Biochemistry 17, 1409-1415 (1978).

10. Iqbal, M.J., Johnson, M.W.: Purification and characterization of human sex hormone binding globulin. J. Steroid Biochem. 10, 535-540 (1979).

11. Renoir, J.M., Fox, L.L., Baulieu, E.E., Mercier-Bodard, C.: An antiserum specific for human sex steroid binding plasma protein (Sbp). Febs Letters 75, 83-88 (1977).

12. Bordin, S., Lewis, J., Petra, P.H.: Monospecific antibodies to the sex steroid-binding protein (Sbp) of human and rabbit sera : cross-reactivity with other species. Biochem. biophys. Res. Commun. 85, 391-401 (1978).

13. Ferguson, K.A.: Starch gel electrophoresis. Application to the classification of pituitary proteins and polypeptides. Metabolism 13, 985-1002 (1964).

14. Rodbard, D., Chrambach, A.: Estimation of molecular radius, free mobility and valence using polyacrylamide gel electrophoresis. Anal. Biochem. 40, 95-134 (1971).

15. Corvol, P.L., Chrambach, A., Rodbard, D., Bardin, C.W.: Physical properties and binding capacity of Testosterone-estradiol binding globulin in human plasma, determined by polyacrylamide gel electrophoresis. J. biol. Chem. 246, 3435-3443 (1971).

16. Banker, G.A., Cotman, C.W.: Measurement of free electrophoretic mobility and retardation coefficient of protein-sodium dodecyl sulfate complexes by gel electrophoresis. J. biol. Chem. 247, 5856-5861 (1972).

17. Mercier-Bodard, C., Renoir, J.M., Baulieu, E.E.: Further characterization and immunological studies of human sex steroid binding plasma protein. J. Steroid Biochem. 11, 253-259 (1979).

18. Hunter, W.M., Greenwood, F.C.: Preparation of ^{125}I-labelled human growth hormone of high specificity. Nature 194, 495-496 (1962).

19. Scatchard, G.: The attraction of proteins for small ions and molecules. Ann. N.Y. Acad. Sci. 51, 660-672 (1949).

20. Rosenthal, H.E.: A graphic method for the determination and presentation of binding parameters in a complex system. Anal. Biochem. 20, 525-532 (1967).

21. Petra, P.H.: The serum sex steroid binding protein. Purification, characterization and immunological properties of the human and rabbit proteins. J. Steroid Biochem. 11, 245-252 (1979).

22. Suzuki, Y., Okumura, Y., Sinohara, H.: Purification and characterization of testosterone-binding globulin of canine serum. J. Biochem., Tokyo, 85, 1195-1203 (1979).

23. Suzuki, Y., Itagaki, E., Mori, H., Hosoya, T.: Isolation of testosterone binding globulin from bovine serum by affinity chromatography and its molecular characterization. J. Biochem., Tokyo, 81, 1721-1731 (1977).

24. Renoir, J.M., Mercier-Bodard, C., Baulieu, E.E.: Hormonal and immunological aspects of the phylogeny of sex steroid binding plasma protein. In preparation.

25. Burke, C.W., Anderson, D.C.: Sex hormone binding globulin is an oestrogen amplifier. Nature 240, 38-40 (1972).

ROLE OF THE INSULIN RECEPTOR IN HUMAN PHYSIOLOGY AND DISEASE

V. R. Soman
Department of Medicine, Yale University School of Medicine,
New Haven, Connecticut 06510, U.S.A.

The first step in the action of insulin as in the case of other polypeptide hormones is its binding to a specific cell surface receptor on the target organ (1). Insulin receptors serve two important functions i) specific recognition of insulin molecules amongst other circulating hormones and chemicals and ii) the triggering of a chain of intracellular biologic events resulting in increased transport of substrates or altered enzyme activity. Insulin binding sites have been identified not only in the conventional target tissues (liver, adipocyte and muscle) but also in a wide variety of other organs such as brain, kidney and placenta (2). The effects of various pathologic and physiologic perturbations on insulin receptors have been studied by examining the specific binding of ^{125}I-insulin to membranes from various target tissues. However, such tissues, and in particular liver cells, are generally not easily accessible for human studies. Therefore, most of the information in man is derived from the studies employing monocytes (3) and more recently erythrocytes (4) as the models for examining insulin receptor function. Although the monocyte is not a conventional target tissue for insulin, changes in insulin binding to monocytes generally mirror alterations in insulin receptors in target organs (2). In addition, insulin binding to monocytes has been shown to correlate well with _in vivo_ sensitivity to insulin in healthy men (5). For these reasons, the circulating monocyte has been used extensively in human investigations examining the role of insulin receptors in altered insulin action. These studies have underscored the role of insulin receptors in modula-

Hormones in Normal and Abnormal Human Tissues, Vol. II

ting tissue sensitivity to insulin in various physiologic and pathologic conditions in man.

I. Role of Insulin Receptors in Physiologic States

Recent studies have provided evidence that insulin receptors undergo dynamic changes during various physiologic changes in man and have been implicated in the pathogenesis of altered tissue sensitivity to insulin (Table 1).

Table I

PHYSIOLOGIC STATES CHARACTERIZED BY ALTERATIONS IN INSULIN RECEPTORS

	Insulin Binding	Insulin Sensitivity
1. Exercise	↑	↑
2. Diet		
a. High CHO Diet	↓	↑
b. Total Starvation	↑	↓
c. Low Calorie Diet	↑	↑
3. Pregnancy (late)	↓, N, ↑	↓
4. Newborn State	↑	—

1. Exercise

Physical exercise is associated with a variety of alterations in hormonal regulation and body fuel homeostasis (6). Exercise results in a marked increase in glucose uptake by exercising muscle tissue, a 3-5 fold increase in hepatic glucose production, and a moderate decline in plasma glucose concentration. If exercise is prolonged, fat is mobilized from the adipose tissue resulting in elevations in free fatty acids (FFA) and increased utilization of FFA as the oxidative fuel. These changes in substrate metabolism, glucose and FFA, are regulated by alterations in plasma insulin levels as well as anti-insulin hormones (glucagon, catecholamines and growth hormone) (7). During exercise glucose uptake by muscle tissue increases markedly despite a fall in plasma insulin levels, thus suggesting a state of increased sensitivity to insulin. In addition, in diabetics exercise is known to improve glucose tolerance and to decrease requirements for exogenous insulin (7). Recently we have examined the possibility that changes in insulin receptors may play a role in exercise-induced augmentation in insulin sensitivity.

a) Effect of acute exercise in normal man. In initial studies we examined ^{125}I-insulin binding to monocytes and changes in plasma glucose and insulin levels in ten healthy males before and after acute exercise (3 h bicycle ergometer) and on the day after exercise with the subjects in the post-absorptive state (8). In all subjects a similar relative work intensity (absolute intensity: 632 ± 40 kpm/min) was achieved by maintaining the heart rate at 120 beats/min during exercise. At the end of 3 h exercise plasma glucose concentration declined significantly (88 ± 3 mg/dl before and 77 ± 4 mg/dl after exercise, $P < 0.02$) in the face of a 35% reduction in plasma insulin levels suggesting increased body sensitivity to insulin.

Insulin binding to monocytes rose by 36% at the end of exercise (6.6 ± 0.4% before and 9.0 ± 0.9% after exercise, $P < 0.02$). When subjects were restudied 24 h after exercise, insulin binding had returned to pre-exercise levels (7.2 ± 0.7%). The analysis of insulin binding data revealed an increase in insulin binding affinity (Fig. 1) as reflected by $\bar{K}e$ (average affinity profile plot), whereas the concentration of insulin receptors remained unaltered (14,000 ± 1,000 sites/cell before and after exercise). Thus in normal men acute exercise leads to augmentation in insulin receptor affinity which may contribute at least in part, to increased *in vivo* sensitivity to insulin.

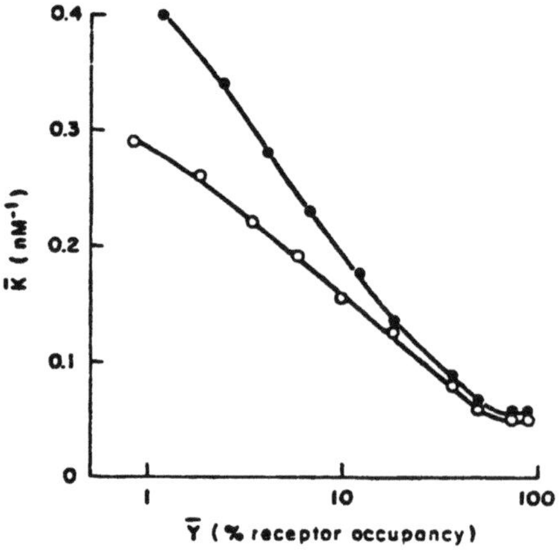

Fig. 1. Average affinity profile plots of ^{125}I-insulin binding from basal (o) and 3 h post-exercise (●) studies in 10 normal men. From Soman et al (8).

b) Effect of acute exercise in obesity. In obese subjects acute exercise enhanced insulin sensitivity as reflected by a reduction in glucose-mediated insulin secretion without impairment in glucose utilization (9). In recent studies we examined the possibility that exercise-induced enhanced insulin sensitivity in obesity may be mediated via changes in insulin receptors such as observed in non-obese humans. This is of particular interest, since obesity is characterized by insulin resistance and decreased insulin receptors (5). During exercise plasma glucose concentration decreased from 98 ± 3 mg/dl to 90 ± 3 mg/dl ($P < 0.05$) in the face of a 50% fall in plasma insulin levels suggesting increased *in vivo* insulin sensitivity (10). As expected, in obese subjects insulin binding to monocytes in the basal state was 27% lower than in non-obese controls. After acute exercise there was a small but significant increase in insulin binding from 4.8 ± 0.3% to 5.4 ± 0.2% ($P < 0.05$) mainly due to an increase in insulin receptor affinity (10). It is noteworthy that increase in insulin binding induced by acute exercise in obese subjects was significantly lower than that observed in the non-obese group (13 ± 1% vs 36 ± 3%, $P < 0.01$). The factor(s) responsible for the difference in the insulin binding response to acute exercise in obese and non-obese subjects remain to be explored. Nevertheless, the results suggest that increased insulin binding may contribute to the augmented insulin sensitivity following acute exercise in obese subjects. However, the small magnitude of the changes in insulin binding make it likely that changes in post-receptor events may also play an important role in augmenting insulin sensitivity after acute exercise.

c) Athletes vs untrained subjects: changes during resting state and after acute exercise. Physical training has been shown to markedly diminish the insulin response to glucose administration (11). Since glucose tolerance remains unimpaired, augmentation in *in vivo* sensitivity to insulin characterizes the well-trained athletes. On the other hand, physical inactivity is reported to impair glucose tolerance despite hyperinsulinemia, thus suggesting the development of insulin resistance. To examine the cellular mechanism of increased insulin sensitivity in athletes, we studied insulin binding to monocytes in ten well-trained male long distance runners and in fifteen untrained, age-and weight-matched male control subjects (12).

As shown in Table 2, the maximal aerobic power (VO_2 max) was 55% greater in athletes as compared to untrained controls. In the basal state ^{125}I-insulin binding to monocytes was 70% higher in athletes than in controls. Scatchard analysis of insulin binding data revealed that the increased insulin binding in athletes was due mainly to an increase in the number of insulin receptors (22,600 ± 1,800 vs 14,500 ± 900 sites/monocyte, $P < 0.001$). In athletes there was a positive correlation between insulin binding and VO_2 max ($r = 0.63$, $P < 0.001$) and insulin binding correlated inversely with

Table 2*

	ATHLETES (N=10)		UNTRAINED CONTROLS (N=15)	
	Basal State	After 3 hr Exercise	Basal State	After 3 hr Exercise
1. Age (y)	29±2	-	26±1	-
2. Wt. (Kg)	68±2	-	72±2	-
3. $\dot{V}O_2$ max (ml/kg/min)	66±1**	-	43±1	-
4. Plasma Glucose (mg/dl)	85±2**	73±3	93±2	73±2
5. Plasma Insulin (μU/ml)	12.0±1.0	7.2±1.4§	16.0±2.0	8.6±1.4§
6. Respiratory Exchange Ratio	0.86±0.03	0.79±0.02§	0.86±0.02	0.85±0.01
7. ^{125}I-Insulin Binding to Monocytes (%)	14.0±1.4†	9.7±2.1	8.3±0.5	11.2±1.4

* From Koivisto et al (12)
** P <0.005 as compared to control subjects
† P <0.01 as compared to control subjects
§ P <0.05 as compared to basal state.

fasting plasma insulin levels (r = -0.62, P <0.02). These results indicate that in athletes insulin binding to monocytes is increased in direct proportion to their physical fitness and plasma insulin levels are decreased which may contribute in part to augmented insulin sensitivity.

With respect to the effect of acute exercise, athletes differ from untrained controls in that the fall in plasma glucose during exercise in athletes was 40% less than in controls and the respiratory exchange ratio at the end of exercise was lower in athletes as compared to controls (Table 2). Based on the respiratory exchange ratio, during submaximal exercise, athletes appear to derive more energy from fat and less from carbohydrates than do sedentary subjects. To examine the mechanism of their paradoxical metabolic pattern, the effect of acute exercise on insulin binding was compared in athletes and in untrained controls. In sedentary controls insulin binding to monocytes rose by 35%, whereas in well-trained athletes insulin binding decreased by 31% after 3 h of acute exercise (Table 2). Changes in insulin binding in both groups were due to alterations in insulin binding affinity rather than a change in insulin binding capacity (12). These results suggest that directionally opposite changes in insulin binding affinity in athletes and sedentary controls may play a role in the lesser dependence on carbohydrate and the greater utilization of fat observed in athletes as compared to the sedentary subjects.

d) Effect of physical training in untrained subjects. To investigate whether a short-term physical training program in previously untrained subjects could augment insulin binding and insulin sensitivity, the effect of a 6 week training program on insulin binding to monocytes and *in vivo* insulin sensitivity (as determined by the euglycemic insulin clamp technique) was studied in six, healthy sedentary male subjects (13). The training program consisted of cycle ergometer exercise at 70% of each subjects VO_2 max for 1 h, four times a week for 6 weeks. Physical training resulted in about 20% increase in VO_2 max (42.6 ± 0.9 ml/kg/min before and 50.8 ± 2.3 ml/kg/min after training, $P < 0.02$) without affecting body weight (74.1 ± 4.3 kg before and 73.3 ± 4.3 kg after training), fasting plasma glucose levels (92 ± 1 mg/dl vs 94 ± 2 mg/dl) and plasma insulin levels (15.5 ± 3μU/ml vs 15.5 ± 1.6 μU/ml).

At the end of the training program, insulin-mediated glucose uptake was 30% higher and ^{125}I-insulin binding to monocytes was 35% higher compared to the pre-training period (Fig. 2). We found a direct correlation between the rise in VO_2 and insulin-mediated glucose uptake ($r = 0.81$, $P < 0.05$) induced by physical training. The increase in insulin binding after training was mainly due to an increase in the concentration

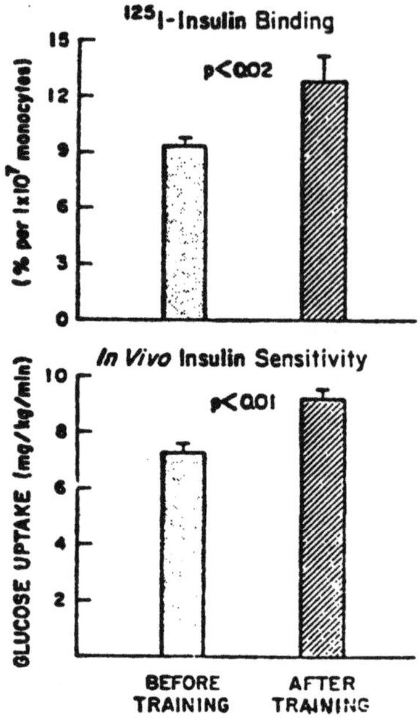

Fig. 2. Effect of physical training (6 wks) on insulin binding and insulin-mediated glucose uptake in six untrained, healthy subjects. From Soman et al (13).

of insulin receptors (15,600 ± 850 vs 24,120 ± 1,080 sites/ monocyte, P <0.01). These findings thus provide direct evidence that short-term physical training in previously untrained, healthy subjects augments in vivo insulin sensitivity in direct proportion to the improvement in their physical fitness and independent of changes in body weight. Furthermore, increased insulin binding may play a role in enhanced tissue sensitivity to insulin after physical training.

To investigate whether physical training will lead to changes in insulin binding in target tissues (e.g. muscle) similar to that observed in the monocyte, we examined the effect of a training program (forced swimming twice a day for ten days) in healthy rats on insulin binding and insulin action in soleus muscle. The preliminary results indicate that trained animals exhibit increased insulin binding and enhanced insulin-mediated 2-deoxy-D-glucose uptake in soleus muscle compared to untrained controls.

The above findings suggest that physical exercise may provide a physiologic means of increasing insulin sensitivity and augmenting insulin binding in disease states such as obesity and maturity-onset diabetes which are characterized by insulin resistance and impaired insulin binding.

2. Effect of diet

The carbohydrate content of the diet as well as the total caloric intake have been shown to be important determinants of *in vivo* sensitivity to insulin (14). In normal men, high carbohydrate, isocaloric diets are reported to improve insulin-mediated glucose metabolism despite causing a decrease in insulin binding to adipocytes (15). The latter appears to result from the hyperinsulinemia induced by high carbohydrate feeding. Similarly, a dissociation between insulin binding and insulin sensitivity is observed following total starvation in obese subjects (5). After starvation (3-14 days) insulin binding to monocytes increases markedly, whereas there is a decrease in insulin-mediated glucose metabolism (5). On the other hand, weight loss achieved on a hypocaloric diet results in augmented insulin binding as well as increased insulin sensitivity (16). Whether insulin-resistant maturity onset diabetics respond similarly to various dietary manipulations has not been established.

3. Pregnancy

Pregnancy is associated with a variety of changes in fuel homeostasis and hormonal regulation (17). The second half of pregnancy is recognized to have a diabetogenic effect on the mother. Glucose intolerance during the third trimester of pregnancy is characterized by hyperinsulinemia and insulin resistance (17). Insulin receptor studies have shown that ^{125}I-insulin binding to monocytes is increased during late pregnancy, despite significant hyperinsulinemia (18). On the other hand, animal studies reveal that in 18-21 day pregnant rats, insulin binding to liver is normal, whereas insulin binding to soleus muscle is markedly decreased (19). The latter is accompanied by a significant decline in insulin-stimulated glucose uptake (19). These results indicate that insulin binding to monocytes may not always mirror changes in other tissues and that the pregnancy is characterized by heterogeneity of changes in insulin receptors. Since the muscle tissue is a major site of insulin-mediated glucose disposal, it is likely that insulin resistance of late pregnancy may at least in part, result from decreased insulin binding to this target tissue.

II. Role of Insulin Receptors in Disease States

As shown in Table 3, changes in insulin receptors have been demonstrated in a variety of disease states characterized by increased as well as decreased tissue sensitivity to insulin. It should, however, be pointed out that in addition to alterations in insulin receptors, changes in post-receptor events may also contribute significantly to the overall insulin sensitivity in many of these pathologic conditions.

A) Insulin receptors in disease states characterized by increased insulin sensitivity

1. Growth hormone deficiency. Growth hormone is known to modulate tissue sensitivity to insulin. Patients with isolated growth hormone deficiency have tendency to fasting hypogly-

Table 3

PATHOLOGIC CONDITIONS ASSOCIATED WITH CHANGES IN INSULIN RECEPTORS

		Insulin Binding	Insulin Sensitivity
1.	Growth Hormone Deficiency	↑	↑
2.	Glucocorticoid Deficiency	↑	↑
3.	Anorexia Nervosa	↑	↑
4.	Obesity	↓	↓
5	Maturity Onset Diabetes	↓	↓
6.	Acromegaly	↓	↓
7.	Glucocorticoid Excess	↓	↓
8.	Uremia	↓	↓
9.	Myotonia Dystrophica	N, ↓	↓
10.	Lipoatrophic Diabetes	N, ↓	↓
11.	Diabetes with Acanthosis Nigricans (Type A and B)	↓	↓
12.	Ataxia Telangiectasia	↓	↓

cemia and are believed to have increased insulin sensitivity (20), whereas acromegaly is characterized by insulin resistance and glucose intolerance (21). To examine whether changes in insulin receptors play a role in altered insulin sensitivity induced by growth hormone, we examined insulin binding and insulin sensitivity in 5 children and 1 adult with isolated growth hormone deficiency before and after growth hormone treatment (0.1 U/kg three times a week for 3-12 weeks).

In untreated growth hormone deficient patients, fasting plasma glucose and insulin levels were 20% and 40% lower respectively than in age-matched controls suggesting increased insulin sensitivity (22). In addition, in the adult with growth hormone deficiency, insulin-mediated glucose uptake was 25% higher than that observed in age-matched controls (Fig. 3).

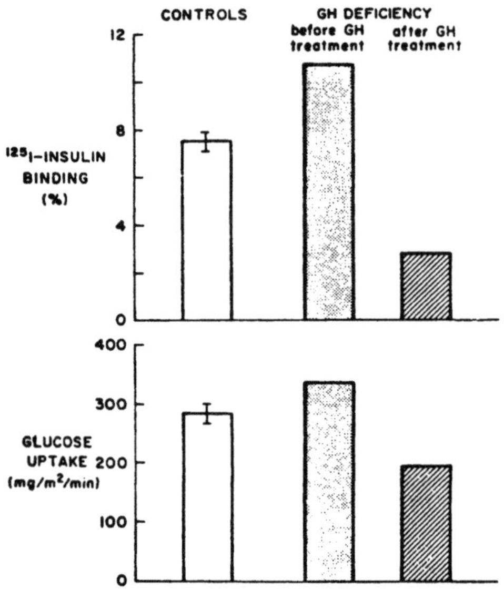

Fig. 3. ^{125}I-insulin binding to monocytes and insulin-mediated glucose uptake in control subjects and in patients with isolated growth hormone deficiency before and after growth hormone treatment. From Soman et al (22).

^{125}I-Insulin binding to monocytes in untreated patients was significantly higher than controls (Fig. 3). After growth hormone treatment fasting plasma glucose levels returned to normal, whereas fasting plasma insulin levels rose significantly to values 75% above controls ($P < 0.005$). Plasma growth hormone levels were significantly higher (6.2 ± 0.4 ng/ml) after growth hormone treatment than before treatment (1.0 ± 0.1, $P < 0.01$) and in controls (2.1 ± 0.1, $P < 0.01$). As shown in Fig. 3, ^{125}I-insulin binding to monocytes decreased significantly after growth hormone treatment to values 50% below control levels ($P < 0.01$) (22). Thus changes in insulin binding may contribute to alterations in insulin sensitivity accompanying growth hormone deficiency and excess. In keeping with this, patients with acromegaly have been reported to have decreased insulin binding to monocytes.

2. Anorexia nervosa. Studies of Wachslicht-Rodbard et al. (23) indicate that patients with anorexia nervosa have increased insulin binding to erythrocytes in the untreated state and that after weight gain insulin binding returned to control values. Data from our laboratory are consistent with those observations (24); prior to treatment patients with anorexia nervosa exhibited hypoinsulinemia, increased insulin binding to monocytes and enhanced insulin sensitivity. After weight gain all parameters returned to normal levels. Changes in insulin binding in these patients correlated directly with insulin sensitivity and inversely with fasting plasma insulin levels suggesting that hypoinsulinemia may lead to increased insulin binding, which in turn may contribute to augmented insulin sensitivity (24). It is of interest that in obese subjects fasted for 3-10 days, there is an increase in insulin binding to monocytes which is accompanied by a decline in insulin sensitivity (5). These data suggest that mechanisms regulating insulin-mediated glucose metabolism in anorexia nervosa may differ from the regulatory factors in starvation.

B) Insulin receptors in disease states characterized by decreased insulin sensitivity

1. Obesity. Obesity is the most commonly encountered insulin resistant state in man. A decrease in the concentration of insulin receptors has been reported in obese humans as well as in animal models of obesity (5, 26, 27, 30, 31, 32). The defect in the insulin receptor in obesity has been observed in monocytes (5, 26, 30) and adipocytes (30) in humans and in liver, adipocyte, muscle and other tissues (26, 27, 31, 32) in animals. Since decreased insulin binding in obesity has been shown to correlate inversely with the elevated fasting plasma insulin levels (5, 26, 32), it has been proposed that the decrease in the concentration of insulin

receptors in obesity may be secondary to hyperinsulinemia (26). Studies of Gavin et al (28) demonstrating downregulation of insulin receptors in IM-9 lymphocyte culture line on *in vitro* incubation with insulin (>10^{-9}M) are in support of this notion. Recent *in vivo* studies from our laboratory demonstrate that in normal men physiological hyperinsulinemia decreases insulin binding to monocytes (29). In these studies when the plasma insulin concentration was raised to 102 ± 6 and 31 ± 2 µU/ml, while maintaining plasma glucose at the fasting level by the euglycemic insulin clamp technique, insulin binding to monocytes decreased significantly by 3 and 5 hours respectively (29). These results thus provide direct support for the hypothesis that decreased insulin binding in obesity may be secondary to elevated plasma insulin concentration.

With respect to the significance of the insulin receptor defect in the pathogenesis of insulin resistance in obesity, decreased insulin binding to monocytes in obese humans has been shown to correlate directly with impairment in tissue sensitivity to insulin. As shown in Fig. 4, this correlation is observed over a wide range of insulin sensitivity in obese and in non-obese humans (5). These findings suggest an important role for insulin binding in modulating insulin sensitivity in human obesity. In contrast, animal studies employing isolated adipocytes have indicated that impairment in intracellular glucose metabolism rather than decreased insulin binding is a major determinant of insulin resistance (31, 32). However, recent studies demonstrate that in obese humans the dose-response curve relating plasma insulin concentration to insulin-mediated glucose metabolism is shifted to the right as evidenced by resistance to the action of insulin at low plasma insulin concentrations with normalization at higher levels (33). These observations are consistent with the interpretation that decreased sensitivity to insulin in human obesity is a receptor-mediated defect.

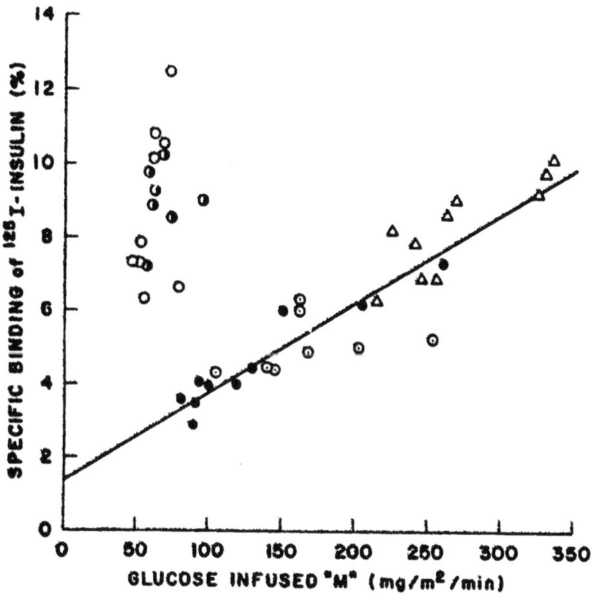

Fig. 4. Correlation between ^{125}I-insulin binding to monocytes and <u>in vivo</u> insulin sensitivity as reflected by insulin-mediated glucose uptake in non-obese controls (Δ) and in obese subjects in the basal state (●) and after 3 day (o) and 14 day (◑) fast and after refeeding (◑). From DeFronzo et al (5).

2. <u>Maturity-onset diabetes</u>. While juvenile-onset diabetes is characteristically associated with a failure of insulin secretion, patients with maturity-onset diabetes may exhibit decreased, normal or increased insulin secretion (34, 35). Impaired glucose tolerance in the presence of normal or increased insulin levels suggests a defect in tissue responsiveness to insulin in some patients with maturity-onset diabetes.

Studies by Reaven and Olefsky have shown that non-obese, chemical as well as maturity-onset diabetics have decreased insulin binding in association with diminished sensitivity

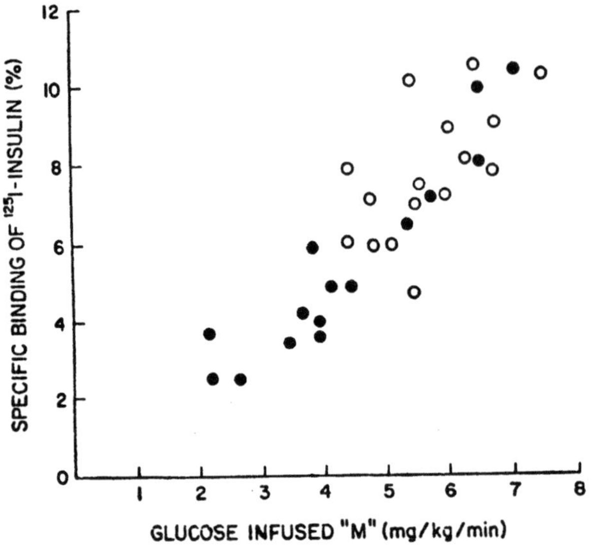

Fig. 5. Correlation between insulin binding to monocytes and insulin-mediated glucose uptake in control subjects (o) and in patients with maturity-onset diabetes (•). From DeFronzo et al (37).

to insulin as reflected by increased steady-state plasma glucose levels observed with their quadruple infusion technique (32, 35, 36). Our results are in keeping with those observations (37); patients with maturity-onset diabetes were heterogeneous with respect to both insulin binding and insulin sensitivity. While some patients have normal insulin binding and <u>in vivo</u> sensitivity to insulin, a significant proportion of patients (66%) exhibited decreased insulin binding to monocytes as well as diminished tissue responsiveness to insulin (Fig. 5). More importantly, there was a direct correlation between insulin binding and insulin-mediated glucose uptake in these patients (Fig. 5) and an inverse correlation between insulin binding and fasting plasma insulin levels (37) suggesting that decreased concentration of insulin receptors may be secondary to higher ambient insulin levels. In summary, it appears that decreased insulin binding may play an important pathogenetic role in most but not all patients with maturity-onset diabetes.

3. Uremia. Chronic renal failure is associated with an increased incidence of diabetes. Carbohydrate intolerance in uremia is characterized by hyperinsulinemia suggesting resistance to the action of insulin (38). In an animal model of chronic uremia (partially nephrectomized rats), ^{125}I-insulin binding to liver membranes was decreased in association with increased plasma glucose and insulin levels (39). These findings thus suggest a role for insulin receptors in insulin resistance in uremia. Whether insulin receptors in other tissues such as muscle and adipocytes exhibit similar changes is not known. There is paucity of insulin binding data in humans with chronic renal failure.

4. Insulin resistance induced by counterregulatory hormones. Growth hormone, glucocorticoids and epinephrine, when present in excess, lead to diminished tissue responsiveness to insulin. Changes in insulin receptors have been implicated in insulin resistance induced by growth hormone and glucocorticoids (22, 25, 40). It should, however, be emphasized that these counterregulatory hormones, in addition to altering insulin binding, affect membrane (e.g. glucose transport) and intracellular processes (e.g. enzymes regulating glucose metabolism) which may also contribute to the overall change in tissue sensitivity to insulin.

5. Insulin resistance in miscellaneous conditions. A rare, but an interesting cause of insulin resistance is a syndrome of diabetes with acanthosis nigricans which consists of two subtypes (41). Patients with type A syndrome exhibit ovarian dysfunction and insulin resistance which is associated with a decrease in insulin binding to monocytes. In type B syndrome extreme insulin resistance is often accompanied by

autoimmune disorders such as systemic lupus erythematosus. The insulin resistance in these patients appears to be secondary to circulating anti-insulin receptor antibodies resulting in decreased insulin binding (41). Some of these patients have been successfully treated by therapeutic modalities used in autoimmune disorders such as steroids and plasmapheresis.

Lipo-atrophic diabetes is a rare disease characterized by a paucity of subcutaneous adipose tissue and insulin-resistant diabetes. Insulin binding to monocytes in these patients has been reported to be decreased mainly due to a decrease in insulin receptor affinity (42). On the other hand, insulin binding to cultured fibroblasts from patients with lipo-atrophic diabetes has been reported to be normal (43) suggesting that the insulin receptor defect in this syndrome is likely to be acquired rather than genetic in origin. Alterations in insulin receptors have also been implicated in the insulin resistance observed in patients with myotonia dystrophica and ataxia telangiectasia.

Acknowledgements

The author would like to thank Mrs. Phyllis Strumpf for her excellent secretarial assistance. This work was supported by a Clinical Investigator Award (AM 00356) and grants (AM 21158 and RR 125) from the National Institutes of Health, Bethesda, MD.

References

1. Roth, J.: Peptide hormone binding to receptors: a review of direct studies in vitro. Metabolism 22, 1059-1073 (1973).
2. Kahn, C.R.: Membrane receptors for hormones and neurotransmitters. J. Cell Biol. 70, 261-286 (1976).

3. Archer, J.A., Gorden, P., Gavin, J.R., Lesniak, M., Roth, J.: Insulin receptors in human circulating lymphocytes: application to the study of insulin resistance in man. J. clin. Endocrinol. Metab. 36, 627-633 (1973).

4. Gambhir, K.K., Archer, J.A., Carter, L.: Insulin radio-receptor assay for human erythrocytes. Clin. Chem. 23, 1590-1595 (1977).

5. DeFronzo, R.A., Soman, V., Sherwin, R.S., Hendler, R., Felig, P.: Insulin binding to monocytes and insulin action in human obesity, starvation and refeeding. J. clin. Invest. 62, 204-213 (1978).

6. Felig, P., Wahren, J.: Fuel homeostasis in exercise. New Engl. J. Med. 293, 1078-1084 (1975).

7. Vranic, M., Berger, M.: Exercise and diabetes mellitus. Diabetes 28, 147-167 (1979).

8. Soman, V.R., Koivisto, V.A., Grantham, P., Felig, P.: Increased insulin binding to monocytes after acute exercise in normal man. J. clin. Endocrinol. Metab. 47, 216-219 (1978).

9. Bjorntorp, P., DeJounge, K., Sjostrom, L., Sullivan, L.: The effect of physical training on insulin production in obesity. Metabolism 19, 631-638 (1970).

10. Koivisto, V.A., Soman, V.R., Felig, P.: Effect of acute exercise on insulin binding to monocytes in obesity. Metabolism (in press).

11. Lohman, D., Liebold, F., Heilman, W., Senger, H., Pohl, A.: Diminished insulin response in highly trained athletes. Metabolism 27, 521-524 (1978).

12. Koivisto, V.A., Soman, V., Conrad, P., Hendler, R., Nadel, E., Felig, P.: Insulin binding to monocytes in trained athletes. Changes in the resting state and after exercise. J. clin. Invest. 64, 1011-1015 (1979).

13. Soman, V.R., Koivisto, V.A., Deibert, D., Felig, P., DeFronzo, R.A.: Increased insulin sensitivity and insulin binding to monocytes after physical training. New Engl. J. Med. 301, 1200-1204 (1979).

14. Brunzell, J.D., Lerner, R.L., Hazzard, W.R., Porte, D. Jr., Bierman, E.L.: Improved glucose tolerance with high carbohydrate feeding in mild diabetes. New Engl. J. Med. 284, 521-524 (1971).

15. Kolterman, O.G., Greenfield, M., Reaven, G.M., Saekow, M., Olefsky, J.M.: Effect of high carbohydrate diet on insulin binding to adipocytes and on insulin action in vivo in man. Diabetes 28, 731-736 (1979).

16. Bar, R.S., Gorden, P., Roth, J., Kahn, C.R., DeMeyts, P.: Fluctuations in the affinity and concentrations of insulin receptors on circulating monocytes of obese patients. J. clin. Invest. 58, 1123-1135 (1976).

17. Felig, P.: Body fuel metabolism and diabetes mellitus in pregnancy. Med. Clin. N. Amer. 61, 43-66 (1977).

18. Soman, V., Coustan, D., Felig, P.: Dissociation between insulin binding to monocytes and insulin sensitivity in normal pregnancy. In: Program of 61st Annual Meeting of The Endocrine Society, Anaheim, Ca. p. 118 (1979).

19. Soman, V.: Heterogeneity of insulin receptor changes in pregnancy. Diabetes 28, 393 (1979).

20. Marimee, T.J., Rabinowitz, D., Rimoin, D.L., McKusick, V.A.: Isolated growth hormone deficiency. II. Insulin secretion in sexual ateliotic dwarfism. Metabolism 17, 1005-1011 (1968).

21. Beck, P., Schalch, P.S., Parker, M.L., Kipnis, D.M., Daughaday, W.H.: Correlative studies of growth hormone and insulin plasma concentrations with metabolic responses in acromegaly. J. Lab. clin. Med. 66, 366-379 (1965).

22. Soman, V., Tamborlane, W., DeFronzo, R., Genel, M., Felig, P.: Insulin binding and insulin sensitivity in isolated growth hormone deficiency. New Engl. J. Med. 299, 1025-1030 (1978).

23. Wachslicht-Rodbard, H., Gross, H.A., Rodbard, D., Ebert, M.H., Roth, J.: Increased insulin binding to erythrocytes in anorexia nervosa. New Engl. J. Med. 300, 882-887 (1979).

24. Soman, V.R., Felig, P.: Insulin binding to monocytes and insulin sensitivity in anorexia nervosa. Am. J. Med. (in press).

25. Kahn, C.R., Goldfine, I.D., Neville, D.M. Jr., DeMeyts, P.: Alterations in insulin binding induced by changes in vivo in the levels of glucocorticoids and growth hormone. Endocrinology 103, 1054-1066 (1978).

26. Roth, J., Kahn, C.R., Lesniak, M.A., Gorden, P., DeMeyts, P., Megyesi, K., Neville, D.M. Jr., Gavin, J.R., Soll, A.H., Freychet, P., Goldfine, I.D., Bar, R.S., Archer, J.A.: Receptors for insulin, NSILA-S and growth hormone: applications to disease states in man. Recent Prog. Horm. Res. 31, 95-139 (1976).

27. Kahn, C.R., Neville, D.M., Roth, J.: Insulin-receptor interaction in obese-hyperglycemic mouse. A model of insulin resistance. J. biol. Chem. 248, 244-250 (1973).

28. Gavin, J.R., Roth, J., Neville, D.M., DeMeyts, P., Buell, D.M.: Insulin dependent regulation of insulin receptor concentrations: a direct demonstration in cell culture. Proc. natn. Acad. Sci. U.S.A. 71, 84-88 (1974).

29. Soman, V.R., DeFronzo, R.A.: Direct evidence for downregulation of insulin receptors by physiologic hyperinsulinemia in man. Diabetes (in press).

30. Olefsky, J.M.: Decreased insulin binding to adipocytes and circulating monocytes in obesity. J. clin. Invest. 57, 1165-1172 (1976).

31. Czech, M.P.: Cellular basis of insulin insensitivity in large rat adipocytes. J. clin. Invest. 57, 1523-1532 (1976).

32. Olefsky, J.M.: The insulin receptor: its role in insulin resistance of obesity and diabetes. Diabetes 25, 1154-1162 (1976).

33. DeFronzo, R., Deibert, D., Sherwin, R.S., Hendler, R., Soman, V.: Insulin resistance in obesity: evidence for a receptor defect as the rate limiting step. Clin. Res. 27, 483A (1979).

34. Felig, P., Soman, V.: Insulin receptors in diabetes and other conditions. Am. J. Med. (in press).

35. Reaven, G.M., Bernstein, R., Davis, B., Olefsky, J.M.: Nonketotic diabetes mellitus: insulin deficiency or insulin resistance. Am. J. Med. 60, 80-88 (1976).

36. Olefsky, J.M., Reaven, G.M.: Insulin binding in diabetes. Relationships with plasma insulin levels and insulin sensitivity. Diabetes 26, 680-688 (1977).

37. DeFronzo, R., Deibert, D., Hendler, R., Felig, P., Soman, V.: Insulin sensitivity and insulin binding to monocytes in maturity-onset diabetes. J. clin. Invest. 63, 939-946 (1979).

38. DeFronzo, R.A., Andres, R., Edgar, P., Walker, W.G.: Carbohydrate metabolism in uremia: a review. Medicine (Baltimore) 52, 469-481 (1973).

39. Soman, V., Felig, P.: Glucagon and insulin binding to liver membranes in a partially nephrectomized uremic rat model. J. clin. Invest. 60, 224-232 (1977).

40. Olefsky, J.M., Johnson, J., Liu, F., Jen, P., Reaven, G.M.: The effects of acute and chronic dexamethasone administration on insulin binding to isolated rat hepatocytes and adipocytes. Metabolism 24, 517-527 (1975).

41. Flier, J.S., Kahn, C.R., Roth, J.: Receptors, antireceptor antibodies and mechanisms of insulin resistance. New Engl. J. Med. 300, 413-419 (1979).

42. Oseid, S., Beck-Nielsen, H., Pedersen, O., Sovik, O.: Decreased binding of insulin to its receptor in patients with congenital generalized lipodystrophy. New Engl. J. Med. 296, 245-248 (1977).

43. Rosenbloom, A.L., Goldstein, S., Yip, C.C.: Normal insulin binding to cultured fibroblasts from patients with lipoatrophic diabetes. J. clin. Endocrinol. Metab. 44, 803-806 (1977).

DISTRIBUTION AND METABOLISM OF ALDOSTERONE

D. J. Morris and R. P. Davis
Department of Laboratory Medicine, The Miriam Hospital, and Division of Biological and Medical Sciences, Brown University, Providence, Rhode Island, U.S.A.

Introduction

After the isolation and chemical characterization of aldosterone (1), its metabolism was studied extensively. Several reviews describe the history and development of methods used to characterize and quantify the metabolism and distribution of aldosterone (2-7). The isolation and identification of aldosterone metabolites and conjugates enabled the development of analytical methods to study the secretion of aldosterone and its metabolites in normal and pathophysiological conditions.

In the initial studies, difficulty was encountered in obtaining pure labeled d-aldosterone separate from the l-isomer and 17α-iso-aldosterone. The chemical instability of small quantities of aldosterone and its metabolites and their ability to isomerize or react with organic solvents also made their isolation a formidable task. The wide range of polarities and physicochemical properties of the various metabolites and conjugates of aldosterone made their separation, identification, and quantification even more difficult.

In this review, recent findings related to the metabolism and distribution of aldosterone in man are discussed. Since little work has been performed on the distribution of aldosterone and its metabolites in tissues of man, animal investigations will also be included. Limited comparative studies of aldosterone metabolism and action suggest that cautious extra-

Hormones in Normal and Abnormal Human Tissues, Vol. II

polation to man from other experimental animals is not unreasonable.

Plasma Clearance Studies of Aldosterone

Aldosterone is rapidly metabolized in both human and other mammalian species and has a much smaller half-life than cortisol or corticosterone. After rapid intravenous administration of tracer amounts of ^{3}H-aldosterone, its clearance from plasma of normal human subjects appears to be at least biexponential. The half-life of aldosterone in the initial component is approximately 15 min. The half-life in the slower second component has been calculated to be 30-35 min (2-4, 8-13), significantly shorter than that for cortisol and corticosterone (approximately 80-90 min). It has generally been concluded (2, 4, 8-13) that binding of aldosterone to albumin and other plasma binding proteins is weaker than cortisol, so that it diffuses more rapidly into tissues, particularly liver. Thus, the turnover and metabolism of aldosterone is much faster than that of cortisol.

Mathematical analysis of disappearance rates of ^{3}H-aldosterone from plasma is best represented by a two-compartment model (2, 8-13). Aldosterone is first distributed rapidly into an inner pool with a volume of approximately 25 l in man and then re-equilibrates more slowly into a second pool with a volume of approximately 40 l (2-8).

Because of the complexity of the metabolism, distribution, excretion and internal circulation of aldosterone and its metabolites, this characterization may well be an oversimplification. Using both analog and digital computers, Luetscher et al (13) successfully applied a more complex, multicompartmental analysis of aldosterone distribution and metabolism to experimental data. Some of the compartments accessible to plasma aldosterone have so far not been described anatomically but the hormone has been shown to be ultimately distributed in man approximately 80% to liver and 15% to kidney. The hormone is rapidly extracted by the kidney at a clearance rate proportional to renal plasma flow (12). In congestive heart failure in man, both hepatic clearance and renal clearance of aldosterone decrease (12), the latter proportionately to the decline in renal blood flow. The decline in hepatic extraction of aldosterone is proportionate to the severity of congestive heart failure, perhaps contributing to the higher plasma hormone levels seen in that disorder. Decreased hepatic clearance of aldosterone is also seen in cirrhosis of the liver (13).

The clearance of ^{3}H-aldosterone from plasma is also rapid in both dog (14, 15) and rat (16, 17). The plasma half-life for the second component of aldosterone disappearance is 40 min in the dog (14, 15) 32 min in Holtzman rats (16) and 12 min in Sprague-Dawley rats (17). The differences in the rat could be due to the different strains of animals used. The clearance of ^{3}H-aldosterone from plasma in adrenalectomized rats (30-33 min) was significantly slower than in intact rats (18). The rates of distribution, metabolism, and excretion of aldosterone are also much slower in adrenalectomized rats. Adrenalectomy has been reported (19) to decrease also the clearance of corticosterone from plasma of rats.

3α, 5β-Tetrahydroaldosterone and conjugates of aldosterone and tetrahydroaldosterone have been identified in human plasma (20). After administration of ^{3}H-aldosterone, a peak of tetrahydroaldosterone and also of polar metabolites appeared in plasma within the first 60 min post-injection (17, 18, 21) in dogs and rats. In the dog, polar metabolites of aldosterone appear on Sephadex DEAP-LH-20 chromatography (21, 22) to consist principally of neutral metabolites and glucuronide and sulfate conjugates (Table 1). Small quantities of "acidic" metabolites are also present. In male rats, the polar metabolites in plasma (Table 1) also consist principally of "neutral" compounds and "monosulfate" conjugates. Of interest, in both dog and rat, the majority of the polar metabolites of aldosterone in plasma are "neutral", highly polar and non-conjugated. With high-pressure liquid chromatography, these highly polar

Table 1

Sephadex DEAP-LH-20 column chromatography of non-extractable polar metabolites (NEDP) of aldosterone in rat and dog tissues

	Metabolic fractions (percent of NEDP)				
	Neutral	Acidic	Glucuronide	Monosulfate	Disulfate
Male Rat					
Liver	88	3	3	6	0
Kidney	50	23	7	18	2
Plasma	61	5	3	29	2
Bile	11	2	27	47	13
Male Dog					
Liver	17	3	69	8	3
Kidney	36	14	41	7	2
Plasma	56	5	18	20	1

Male rats were injected s.c. with 0.1 µg ^{3}H-aldosterone (10 µCI) and tissues obtained 30 minutes post-injection. Male dogs were injected s.c. with 2.5 µg ^{3}H-aldosterone (250 µCI) and tissues obtained 40 minutes post-injection.

"neutral" metabolites resolve into several peaks. As yet, the chemical structures of these metabolites of aldosterone are unknown. Nor is it known whether similar metabolites are present in human plasma. So far, in both human and other experimental animals, only the fate of unmodified ^{3}H-aldosterone has been described; very little attention has been paid to the reduced metabolites of aldosterone or to the polar, water-soluble metabolites of aldosterone which are not extractable with organic solvents conventionally used for the separation of aldosterone.

Tissue Distribution Studies of Aldosterone

In dogs (15, 22), intravenously administered ^{3}H-aldosterone rapidly disappears from plasma with concomitant uptake of labeled aldosterone in tissues. Hollander et al (15) demonstrated that ^{3}H-aldosterone reached maximal levels in the kidney, liver, heart, and aorta within 5-15 min. During and after the peak of tissue radioactivity, levels of ^{3}H-aldosterone were greater in these tissues than in plasma. The majority of the ^{3}H-aldosterone appeared in supernatant fractions of kidney, heart and aorta. Only small quantities were present in subcellular particles.

Radioautography of kidney (15) showed that ^{3}H-aldosterone was localized along walls of convoluted tubular epithelial cells and glomerular capillaries, arterioles and Bowman's capsule but was not present in the walls of collecting duct epithelium. In heart, ^{3}H-aldosterone was localized along cell walls of heart muscle cells,in aorta in cytoplasm of smooth muscle cells.

Surprisingly, uptake and subcellular distribution of ^{3}H-aldosterone in arteries, heart, kidney and liver was not different in dogs pretreated with the aldosterone antagonist, spironolactone (15). Radioautographic experiments confirmed these findings. These _in vivo_ studies in dogs (15) as well as distribution studies with rat tissues (23, 24) do not support the preferential localization of aldosterone in nuclei of cells. However, Hollander et al (15) did not examine the large quantities of radioactivity which remained in tissue fractions after ^{3}H-aldosterone was extracted with organic solvents. This remaining radioactivity represents polar, non-extractable metabolites of aldosterone which are rapidly synthesized and distributed in tissues.

Recently the tissue distribution of ^{3}H-aldosterone and its metabolites in dogs within the first 40 min after injection was studied (21, 22). Substantial quantities of polar metabolites of aldosterone were present, together with aldosterone and 3α-5β-tetrahydroaldosterone, in liver, kidney and plasma. Sephadex

DEAP-LH-20 column chromatography showed that polar metabolites present in liver and kidney consisted principally (Table 1) of "neutral" metabolites of aldosterone and glucuronide conjugates. However, in liver and particularly in kidney, substantial quantities of "acidic" metabolites of aldosterone were also present (Table 1). Only small quantities of "sulfate" conjugates were present. High pressure liquid chromatography (HPLC) resolved the polar "neutral" metabolites of aldosterone in liver and kidney into several metabolite peaks. The majority of these polar "neutral" metabolites of aldosterone present in the plasma of the dog are more polar than the metabolites present in liver and kidney.

In rats, Read, McCaa and Sulya (16) found ^{3}H-aldosterone to be rapidly distributed in tissues particularly in liver. Within 5-15 min of injection, ^{3}H-aldosterone was concentrated in kidney, heart and lung relative to blood. Radioautographically (23) ^{3}H-aldosterone was in tubular epithelial cells of the kidney and along fibers of skeletal and cardiac muscle. In these experiments with dogs and rats (15, 16, 23), only the distribution and fate of unmodified aldosterone was studied; the distribution of the various metabolites and conjugates of aldosterone was not investigated. It is difficult to interpret radioautographic results since it is impossible to distinguish between unmodified hormone and its metabolites. In other in vivo studies in rats (25, 26), ^{3}H-aldosterone was also distributed in the brain.

In our earlier studies in male rats (27), ^{3}H-aldosterone was rapidly taken up by liver and kidney. In both tissues the majority of ^{3}H-radioactivity was present in cytosol, with smaller amounts in subcellular particles. Aldosterone and tetrahydroaldosterone are present in subcellular fractions of kidney but only tetrahydroaldosterone is found in subcellular fractions of liver. Moreover, the majority of the radioactivity was highly polar and non-extractable with CH_2Cl_2, representing polar radiometabolites of aldosterone present in these tissues. In gel filtration studies, ^{3}H-radioactivity appears to bind in these tissues to proteins similar to the binding proteins for cortisol and corticosterone metabolites (28, 29). However, further work is necessary to confirm this.

These polar metabolites of aldosterone are present in liver, kidney, and plasma in very large quantities in male rats and, 30 min post-injection (halfway through the latent period of hormone action) they represent 40%, 2.4% and 4%, respectively, of total injected radioactivity. Importantly, the majority of these polar metabolites of aldosterone are "neutral" polar metabolites and are non-conjugated (Table 1). Of the polar metabolites in kidney, 23% are "acidic" metabolites of aldosterone. These "acidic" metabolites on further purification with HPLC and methylation with diazomethane appear to be carboxylic acid metabolites (21, 30). The percentages of "acidic" metabolites were smaller in liver and plasma, 3% and 5% respectively (Table 1). Also, substantial percentages of the polar metabolites in both the kidney and plasma are "monosulfate" conjugates; only small quantities are in the "glucuronide" fraction. The synthesis and distribution of these "neutral" polar metabolites of aldosterone and the other families of polar metabolites are altered by treatment of male rats with the aldosterone antagonist, spironolactone (31).

The "neutral" metabolite fractions obtained from liver, kidney and plasma of male rats were resolved with HPLC into at least nine peaks of metabolites (Figure 1). Two of the major peaks of metabolites in both liver and kidney, on GC-mass spectrographic analysis appear to be hydroxylated metabolites of aldosterone (21). Furthermore, several of the "neutral" polar metabolites of aldosterone present in tissues and plasma of the male dog possess identical retention times on HPLC to those present in tissues and plasma of the male rat. At this time, the chemical structures of the several metabolites isolated in these fractions cannot be determined with certainty.

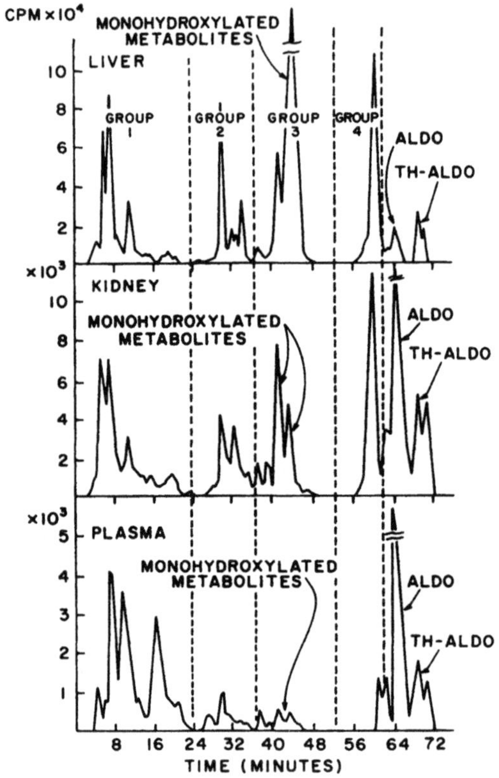

Fig. 1. High pressure liquid chromatogram showing separation of the polar neutral metabolites of [^{3}H]-aldosterone present in the liver, kidney and plasma of male rats (21).

Routes of Metabolism of Aldosterone

Several metabolites of aldosterone have so far been isolated from human urine and chemically identified. The majority of these metabolites are rapidly synthesized in the liver; it has been estimated (2-4, 8, 11) that 90 to 95% of aldosterone may be removed from the blood in one passage through the liver. The kidney is the major extrahepatic site of metabolism of aldosterone.

The principal metabolites of aldosterone synthesized in the liver are reduced in ring A and are excreted in the urine as glucuronides (Figure 2). Sulfates of aldosterone have also been isolated from human urine (32, 33). Sulfation appears to be an important route of aldosterone metabolism in the human fetus. The principal reduced metabolite of aldosterone has been isolated from human urine (34, 35) and identified to be 3α, 5β-tetrahydroaldosterone. This metabolite, excreted as a 3 - glucuronide (36) accounts for 30-40% of the metabolites excreted in the urine after intravenous administration of ^{3}H-aldosterone (2, 6, 10, 35). From *in vitro* experiments with tissue slices, it appears to be synthesized principally in the liver (37). Of the 3α, 5β-tetrahydroaldosterone-3-glucuronide in the urine, 90% is excreted within 24 h of administration of the hormone.

Three additional reduced metabolites of aldosterone, 3α, 5α- and 3β, 5β-tetrahydroaldosterone and 5β-dihydroaldosterone are excreted in urine as glucuronides (38, 40) and account for smaller percentages of administered aldosterone. A 21-deoxy-tetrahydroaldosterone metabolite and a 21-deoxybicyclic acetal metabolite have also been identified (39, 40) and represent up to 10% of administered aldosterone. A 21-hydroxy-bicyclic acetal metabolite has also been identified (39). In all these metabolites, the 11, 18-hemiacetal system appears to remain intact. Only about 1% of secreted aldosterone is excreted in human urine unmetabolised. It should be noted that metabolites have been isolated from human urine after the administration of varying and sometimes large quantities of aldosterone. Routes of administration have also varied. Some uncertainty, therefore, remains as to the fraction of endogenous aldosterone which is excreted as these metabolites under physiological conditions.

The reduced metabolites of aldosterone including 3β, 5α-tetrahydroaldosterone and 5α-dihydroaldosterone have also been synthesized *in vitro* by rat liver and their structures confirmed (41). In earlier work, these reduced metabolites of aldosterone were considered to be biologically inactive. In recent experiments (42-45), both 5α-dihydroaldosterone and 3α, 5β-

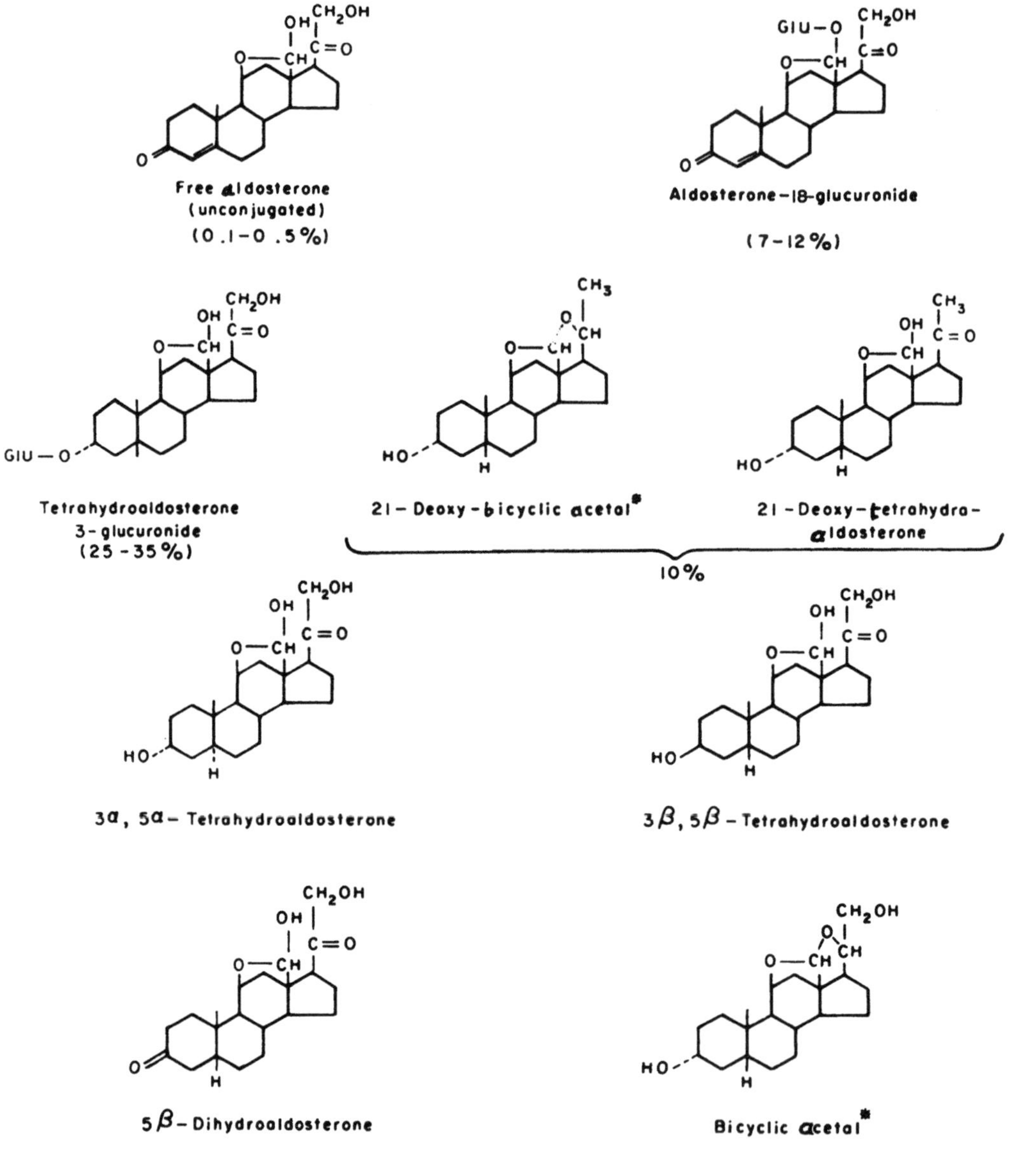

Fig. 2. Principal Metabolites of Aldosterone in Human Urine. Percentage of total metabolites excreted in urine are shown in parentheses (3, 6).
*21-Deoxybicyclic acetal = 3α-Hydroxy-5β-pregnane-11β, 18S:18S, 20α-Diepoxide. Bicyclic acetal = 3α, 21-Dihydroxy-5β-pregnane-11β, 18S:18S, 20α-Diepoxide.

tetrahydroaldosterone show 1/30th and 1/50th respectively of the mineralocorticoid activity of aldosterone. Two other isomers of tetrahydroaldosterone, 3β, 5β- and 3β, 5α-tetrahydroaldosterone were considerably less active, having relative mineralocorticoid activities in the range of 1/300 to 1/500 that of aldosterone (43, 44).

Of the metabolites of aldosterone excreted in the urine of man, 20-35% has not yet been accounted for nor chemically identified (6, 46). We have recently described several, previously unidentified metabolites of aldosterone present in tissues and plasma of both rat and dog (21). Two of these are hydroxylated metabolites of aldosterone (21, 47). It is interesting to speculate whether similar polar metabolites of aldosterone may be present in plasma and tissues of man. In preliminary experiments with incubation of microsomal preparations from human and dog liver, several "neutral" polar metabolites of aldosterone have now been synthesized (21). Their identification is currently being pursued.

The other major aldosterone metabolite found in human urine is an acid labile (pH 1) conjugate of aldosterone (48) and has been identified as aldosterone - 18 - glucuronide (50-52). It was earlier referred to as the 3-oxo-conjugate of aldosterone (49) since the conjugated 4-en-3-one system in ring A remains intact. Whereas 3α, 5β-tetrahydroaldosterone-3-glucuronide can be synthesized only by liver preparations, aldosterone - 18 - glucuronide can be synthesized by both human liver and kidney (37). The ability of kidney to conjugate aldosterone has been studied intensively (2-7, 37, 50-53). Not only is this conjugate synthesized in kidney but it is actively secreted by renal tubules (53, 51). Approximately 10% of the metabolites of aldosterone excreted in urine may be accounted for as the 18-glucuronide, at least 50% of it synthesized in the kidney (50, 53, 51). Unlike 3α, 5β-tetrahydroaldosterone-3-glucuronide, aldosterone-18-glucuronide is rapidly excreted, 80-90% appearing in urine within 6 h of injection of aldosterone.

Historically, the isomer 17α-isoaldosterone, commonly present as a contaminant in aldosterone, presents problems in the study of aldosterone metabolism. The metabolism of 17-isoaldosterone in man is different from that of aldosterone (54). After an intravenous dose of 17-isoaldosterone 35% is converted to the labile 17-isoaldosterone-18-glucuronide. Very little 17-isoaldosterone is converted to the tetrahydro-17-isoaldosterone-3-glucuronide. In earlier experiments, it was not always possible to rapidly separate or detect the presence of isomers of aldosterone. Recently, however, a high pressure liquid chromatography technique was developed which readily separates these isomers of aldosterone within 20 min (21) and will permit further studies of the biological properties of 17α-iso-aldosterone.

Pathways of Excretion of Aldosterone

In man, the major route of excretion of aldosterone is the urine, 90% of intravenously injected ^{3}H-aldosterone appearing in urine within 48 h of injection (2-4, 6, 10). Approximately 80% of the radioactivity in urine was excreted within 24 h of injection. In dog, although urine is also the main excretory pathway for aldosterone, recovery of injected hormone in urine is smaller (14). Aldosterone is mainly excreted in urine of both man and dog as polar conjugates of aldosterone and its reduced metabolites; very little free, unmetabolized aldosterone appears in urine.

Unlike corticosterone, only very small quantities (0-5%) of ^{3}H-aldosterone are excreted in bile in both man and dog (2, 14). 21-Deoxymetabolites of aldosterone are found in human urine, possibly a result of metabolism of tetrahydroaldosterone by intestinal microflora (55). Therefore, biliary secretion of aldosterone in man may be greater than previously suspected. The routes of administration and quantities of aldosterone have also varied in these experiments (56). Aldosterone or its metabolites secreted in the bile may undergo biochemical transformation in the gut. Metabolic products would then be reabsorbed into the enterohepatic circulation and ultimately excreted in urine. Further studies are necessary to clarify the role of these processes in man.

The biliary route is the major pathway for excretion of aldosterone in rat (57, 58) as with corticosterone and other steroids (59, 60). The majority of radiometabolites of aldosterone are rapidly excreted in bile and pass slowly through the intestinal tract into faeces (50-65%) (57, 58, 61). The enterohepatic circulation of aldosterone and its metabolites is important in male rats (62) and contributes to the 10-20% of administered hormones which is excreted in urine within 48 h of injection. Only small quantities of free, unmetabolized aldosterone and tetrahydroaldosterone are present in rat urine (21, 63). Our studies (21) show that the majority of the radiometabolites of aldosterone excreted in urine of male rats consists of several "neutral" polar metabolites, which are nonconjugated and have not yet been chemically identified.

Plasma Binding Proteins

Plasma binding proteins play an important role in regulating the levels of unbound ("free"), physiologically active steroid hormones. Binding of steroid hormones to plasma proteins in normal and disease states determines not only their biological half-lives but also their routes and rates of metabolism. Similarly, binding affects the interaction of steroid hormones with their target tissues and, hence, their resultant biological activity.

Earlier studies, particularly those with double equilibrium dialysis have shown that, unlike cortisol, binding of aldosterone to plasma proteins is not strong, the majority of aldosterone being bound to albumin (64, 65). However, it has now been suggested that aldosterone may be bound to other plasma proteins and such binding may be physiologically important in normal and pathological states (65, 66).

Using Sephadex G-75 column chromatography, aldosterone binding proteins were found in plasma of both adrenalectomized and intact rats (17, 18). These same proteins also bind the reduced metabolite, 3α, 5β-tetrahydroaldosterone, as well as other, as yet unidentified polar metabolites of aldosterone. Nowaczynski et al (67) found aldosterone to bind in human plasma to proteins other than albumin or corticosteroid binding globulin (transcortin). Using our column chromatographic techniques, two other peaks of aldosterone binding proteins were detected in human plasma (67). One of these aldosterone binding proteins is heat stable at 60°C and has a molecular weight of 36,000 daltons; the other is heat labile and has a molecular weight of 26,000 daltons. Binding of aldosterone to these proteins is reversible and their binding properties appear specific for aldosterone. The heat-labile protein has a very high affinity and a low binding capacity for aldosterone. At both 25°C and 37°C, both cortisol and progesterone do not bind to either of these aldosterone binding proteins. 17-isoaldosterone does not bind to the high affinity, low capacity plasma binding proteins, but does bind to albumin. The heat-labile protein appears identical to the previously identified "transcortin-like plasma fraction" which has earlier been shown to be increased in essential hypertension (68, 69).

The clearance of aldosterone from plasma has been reviewed in detail by Melby (6). The MCR is increased by ACTH administration to healthy adult male subjects and to patients with essential hypertension (70). ACTH leads to a decrease in the fraction of aldosterone bound to plasma proteins and to an alteration in the routes of metabolism and conjugation of aldosterone. The ratio and quantities of urinary aldosterone-18-glucuronide (synthesized in kidney) and tetrahydroaldosterone-3-glucuronide (synthesized in liver) are altered by ACTH infusion (71). Further experiments are necessary to clarify how aldosterone-protein interactions affect the routes and rates of metabolism of aldosterone as well as the physiological activity of this hormone.

Uptake of Aldosterone into Target Tissues

The regulation of adrenal biosynthesis, transport in extracellular fluid and peripheral target tissue uptake and action of aldosterone is complex. Studies in animals provide models that appear relevant to the action of aldosterone in humans. The notion that aldosterone may be preferentially taken up into some particular tissue or subcellular fraction was suggested by the finding in human subjects (8) that the volume of distribution of aldosterone was greater than the volume of total body water. A recent review by Pasqualini and Sumida (46) lists colon, skin and kidney as human tissues investigated *in vitro* for aldosterone receptors. In radioautographic studies of skin, ^{3}H-aldosterone entered the eccrine sweat gland (72) after loading of tissue slices with physiological doses of aldosterone (1×10^{-10} *M*). Human colon exposed to 100-1000 fold more aldosterone took up hormone into cell nuclei (73), perhaps reflecting a mode of action of the hormone.

Aldosterone uptake into various tissues has been studied principally in rats, guinea pigs, mice and toads, the latter because of the specificity of aldosterone action on toad urinary bladder. After injection of ^{3}H-aldosterone into rats (23), the hormone was taken up within 5 min by kidney to a concentration over 3-fold that of blood. At 30 min the kidney concentration was 5-fold that of blood, duodenum nearly 3 times, while liver had a 3.5 fold concentration. Renal uptake was principally in tubular epithelium throughout the nephron proximal to the collecting tubule (24). In fetal guinea pig, Pasqualini et al (46) found a wider distribution of ^{3}H-aldosterone into virtually all tissues, liver and placenta showing the highest concentration of hormone, largely converted to tetrahydroaldosterone. Nearly 9% of administered aldosterone was found in fetal liver, the highest concentration observed. Uptake into guinea pig fetal kidney was maximal in about 1 h (46). Mice showed rapid uptake of ^{14}C-aldosterone into the renal system, but this was cleared within 1 h (74). Uptake was less transient in mouse liver.

In urinary bladder of the toad (75), uptake of aldosterone was slower and required about 1000-fold more ^3H-aldosterone to achieve the most rapid uptake (75, 76), principally in the form of unmetabolized ^3H-aldosterone. This uptake was mainly into mucosal epithelium (77).

Using differential centrifugation of cell homogenates, Fanestil and Edelman (78) found early uptake of aldosterone in rat kidney cytosol, microsomes and mitochondria, with later nuclear uptake; plasma hormone concentrations achieved in these experiments may have been many times physiological levels. At more nearly physiological levels, nuclei of duodenal mucosa and kidney showed twice the uptake of nuclei of non-target tissues such as brain, liver and spleen (79). The quantity of aldosterone taken up by liver in similar experiments by Morris and Davis (27) was about 10 times that taken up by kidney. In kidney, 70% of the radioactivity appeared in cytosol while only 3% was found in nuclei. Adrenalectomy was associated with an increase in the free aldosterone or tetrahydroaldosterone fractions in kidney cytosol and nuclei. In cytosol the major metabolites were non-extractable polar derivatives of aldosterone, while in the nucleus free aldosterone and tetrahydroaldosterone were mainly present. These distributions were sex-dependent (80) with no nuclear uptake of aldosterone in kidney or liver of female rats with intact adrenals. In subcellular fractions of kidney from female rats, there were less aldosterone metabolites, both polar and non-polar, than in kidney from male rats.

In fetal guinea pig, 17 times as much ^3H-aldosterone was taken up into kidney cytosol as into kidney nuclei (46). Over half of the nuclear fraction was associated with the chromatin fraction; the remainder was distributed in several other nuclear fractions.

With intact explanted toad bladder, incubation with 10^{-7} M ^3H-aldosterone resulted in nuclear uptake (81). To achieve nuclear concentration of aldosterone in toad bladder required higher gradients of aldosterone than in comparable studies in mammalian tissues. Cytosol and nuclei of normal human kidney took up aldosterone when slices of kidney were incubated in medium containing labeled hormone. Human renal adenocarcinoma showed an affinity for aldosterone 2-3 times normal for cytosol and 7-8 fold less than normal for nuclei (82).

Specific Receptors for Aldosterone

By a variety of techniques aldosterone appeared to bind to macromolecular components of subcellular organelles. These include displacement studies of bound-labeled hormone with unlabeled hormone (72, 76), Sephadex column chromatography (27, 46, 83-85) and ammonium sulfate precipitation (83). It has been possible to examine the binding affinity of subcellular macromolecules for aldosterone in target and non-target tissues and to determine both affinity constants, stoichiometry of binding and, by estimation from affinity constants, free energy of binding. So far, decisive proof has not been forthcoming of a direct relationship between the physicochemical properties of macromolecular - steroid interaction and the physiological functions of the hormone in regulating both sodium and potassium transport.

For aldosterone action it has been hypothesized, as for steroid hormones generally (86), that:

a) the steroid hormone gains access to the cell by permeating the cell membrane;
b) the hormone associates with both steroid-specific and non-specific receptors within the cytoplasm;
c) the hormone, with or without its receptors is transferred to the cell nucleus and binds to nuclear receptors which undergo a transformation;
d) under hormonal influence upon chromatin, DNA dependent nucleic acid synthesis and consequently specific protein synthesis are initiated;
e) newly synthesized protein initiates the physiological actions of the hormone.

The relationship between hormone-receptor complexes and nucleic acid and protein synthesis and between specific protein synthesis and physiological hormone function have yet to be fully described. Crabbé has reviewed these issues critically (86). An important further consideration is the possibility of species variation in aldosterone action and function between toad bladder and mammalian kidney. For example, in mammalian renal systems, aldosterone has at least two separable functions, antinatriuretic and kaliuretic, while in toad bladder only the antinatriuretic function has been demonstrated (87).

The macromolecular interaction of aldosterone in target tissues is of two types: the first, a specific receptor(s) relating to physiological function, and a second physiologically non-specific receptor(s). Specific hormone receptor sites in this sense tend to have high affinity and low capacity for hormone binding, while less specific receptor sites have low affinity and high capacity. Generally, use of the term "receptor" is reserved for the first type of macromolecular hormone interaction. In toad bladder cytosol (88, 89) macromolecular binding of aldosterone is of very low affinity ($K_A \sim 10^4\ M^{-1}$). However, in the cytosol of other tissues and in the nuclei of toad bladder and renal epithelium, receptors of more specificity are the rule.

Aldosterone Receptors in Kidney

As noted earlier, kidney and duodenum of the rat concentrate aldosterone from blood. The hormone is found in cytosol and nuclear fractions of epithelial cells (23, 79). From earlier studies (83) cytosol binding is 80 times that of the nucleus per gram of kidney, but the specificity of binding is greater for nucleus than for cytosol in adrenalectomized rats. From later <u>in vitro</u> studies in kidney from adrenalectomized rats, three binding sites have been postulated: two with high affinities and one with low affinity (90, 91). Of the two sites with higher affinity, $K_A \sim 10^8\ M^{-1}$, the second is considered to be a glucocorticoid receptor while the highest affinity site may be a specific aldosterone binding receptor (84). The capacities of these higher affinity binding sites differ by less than an order of magnitude, suggesting that their specificity might be modified by the macromolecular microenvironment, particularly the presence of competing, less specific adrenal steroids generally present in higher concentrations.

Many studies of receptors for aldosterone in rat kidney have been carried out in adrenalectomized animals on the principle that adrenalectomy removes the sole source of endogenous aldosterone. This may enhance the availability of binding sites to exogenous labeled hormone. Adrenalectomy enhances the recognition of aldosterone receptors resulting in higher specific activity of ^{3}H-aldosterone complexes per unit protein in cytosol and nuclei (85). However, change in receptor availability is not the only consequence of adrenalectomy to aldosterone handling. Morris and Davis (27, 87), in comparing adrenalectomized and intact rats, found that adrenalectomy was associated with not only enhanced protein binding of aldosterone in kidney cytosol but also with a decrease in appearance of unbound polar derivatives of aldosterone. Thus, adrenalectomy produces qualitative differences in handling of aldosterone by rat kidney cytosol and in aldosterone metabolism as well as quantitative differences in receptor binding.

Moreover, other adrenal steroids of varying mineralocorticoid activity can compete with aldosterone for higher affinity cytosol binding sites (84). Aldosterone itself appears more effective than corticosterone and deoxycorticosterone in displacing ^{3}H-aldosterone from cytosol receptors in rat cortex and renal papilla (84) supporting specificity of the cytosol receptor for aldosterone.

In nuclei of kidney from adrenalectomized rats, aldosterone was associated with soluble proteins of nucleus and with proteins derived from the chromatin fraction (83, 92). Complexes of macromolecule and steroid derived from kidney cytosol and nucleus resisted attack by deoxyribonuclease and ribonuclease and were susceptible to proteolytic digestion with pronase, chymotrypsin and trypsin, suggesting that the receptors were protein, free of nucleic acid (83, 92). Furthermore, there is evidence that nuclear receptors are non-histone proteins (92). It has been estimated that about 600 molecules of aldosterone can be bound by the kidney cell nucleus in adrenalectomized rat (46, 92). Electron microscopic radioautography has shown that aldosterone can be localized in plasma membranes and mitochondria of rat kidney (24). In adrenalectomized rats, the kidney plasma membrane binding of ^{3}H-aldosterone appears specific, for it can be competitively displaced by d-aldosterone and 9α-fluorohydrocortisone, but not by testosterone or estradiol (93).

Sedimentation coefficients of the several aldosterone-macromolecular complexes have been measured by density-gradient centrifugation (94). A complex of 8.5S appeared natively in kidney cytosol and was dissociated by KCl to a 4.5S complex and further dissociated by calcium ion to a 3.5S complex. A nuclear complex of 3S size could not be further dissociated. The nuclear receptor associated with non-histone chromatin derived protein of kidney had a sedimentation coefficient of 4S and a tendency to form aggregates (92, 94). In these respects, aldosterone-protein complexes are similar to cytosol and nuclear receptors for estradiol in rat uterus (46).

Aldosterone receptors have also been shown to be present in cytosol of rat duodenal mucosa and liver (79). In liver aldosterone may bind to receptors more specific for glucocorticoid than for aldosterone (95). Other studies demonstrate specific aldosterone receptors in cytosol (96) and nuclei (97) of brain.

In kidney of fetal guinea pig, aldosterone receptors are present in cytosol and nuclei, in the latter as part of soluble nuclear protein and in protein extractable from nuclear chromatin (46). Approximately 1500 molecules of aldosterone are bound per nucleus, about 2.5 times the number in adult rat kidney (46). In rabbit kidney, cytosol receptors for aldosterone are present in both renal cortex and medulla but not in the renal papilla (98). Similar cytosolic receptors for aldosterone are found in human kidney (99, 100). In their capacities and specificities for aldosterone binding, human kidney receptors are similar to those found in other, more extensively studied experimental animals.

Aldosterone Receptors in Toad Bladder

On incubation of toad bladder with ^{3}H-aldosterone there was saturable uptake of aldosterone into the tissue at physiological hormone concentrations (76). Two principal receptors were present with association constants of 4.4×10^{10} M^{-1} and 3×10^8 M^{-1}. The latter lower affinity site had a capacity for aldosterone binding 35 times that of the higher affinity site. These results were confirmed by Snart using other techniques (88), who also found a very low affinity non-specific binding ($K_A = 10^4$ M^{-1}) for aldosterone. Since the highest affinity site was already saturated at concentrations of aldosterone which began to show physiological effects, the lower of the two higher affinity sites probably represents physiologically important receptors (76).

About 60% of aldosterone bound in toad bladder is taken up into epithelial cell nuclei (81). Nuclear binding is complex, comprising at least 3 components, none of which is extractable with chromatin (89). Binding of aldosterone in cytosol of toad bladder is of low affinity and non-specific and is absent from mitochondria and microsomes.

Spironolactone and progesterone, which antagonize the physiological effects of aldosterone, competed with ^{3}H-aldosterone for nuclear binding in toad bladder (76, 101). Functional mineralocorticoids such as d-aldosterone, deoxycorticosterone and 9α-fluorohydrocortisone, displaced ^{3}H-aldosterone from its nuclear receptor in toad bladder (81, 102) but physiologically inactive steroids, including androgens, estrogens, and isoaldosterone, did not (102). Inhibitors of protein and nucleic acid synthesis, such as puromycin and actinomycin, also inhibited the physiological action of aldosterone on sodium transport (75, 103) but did not alter the affinity of aldosterone for its receptor nor does ouabain, the classical inhibitor of sodium transport (76).

After purification by column chromatography, the receptor hormone complex is labile and has a molecular weight of 1-2 x 10^5 daltons (101). From enzyme digestive studies, Alberti and Sharp (101) conclude that the aldosterone receptor is a protein.

Implications of Receptors for Hormone Action

The presence of several aldosterone binding receptors in plasma membrane, cytosol and nucleus of renal epithelium has led to a model of aldosterone action analogous to that for estrogens and other steroid hormones. Circulating aldosterone interacts with a cytosolic receptor and then moves onto soluble nuclear proteins and thence onto chromatin-related proteins, where physiological function may be mediated by altered rates of protein synthesis. There is substantial experimental support for the general outlines of this hormone pathway. However, more complex hypotheses for hormonal transformation in the nucleus require some restraint in interpretation since:

a) the specificity of the receptors is only relative;
b) complete description is lacking of free and bound hormone levels in plasma, cytosol and nucleus under circumstances of physiological hormone action;
c) aldosterone concentration is several orders of magnitude less than the concentration of competing hormones in blood and possibly also in subcellular compartments;
d) there is no detailed connection yet demonstrated directly between hormone availability in the several subcellular compartments and any specific role for aldosterone in nucleic acid function and protein synthesis;

e) evidence is lacking of a direct connection between nuclear events and physiological function.

While these are <u>ad hoc</u> criticisms in the face of tempting data and a sense of symmetry with other steroidal hormones, they are meant simply to introduce a note of caution in model building for aldosterone action. Much more information is needed before a meaningful and directly testable theory of aldosterone action can be constructed.

Acknowledgements

The authors are grateful to Kathy Moos for expert secretarial assistance in the preparation of this manuscript. Our studies reported in this review were supported by The Miriam Hospital Research Fund and a Research Grant from the U.S.P.H.S. AM 19179.

References

1. Simpson, S.A.S., Tait, J.F., Wettstein, A., Neher, R., Von Euw, J., Reichstein, T.: Isolierung eines neuen Kristallisierten Hormons aus Nebennieren mit besonders hoher Wirksamkeit auf den Mineralstoffwechsel. Experientia 9, 333-335 (1953).
2. Peterson, R.E.: Studies of radioactive aldosterone in man. In: "Isotopes in Experimental Pharmacology", Ed. Roth, L.J., University of Chicago Press, Chicago, pp. 177-190 (1965).
3. Coghlan, J.P., Blair-West, J.R.: Aldosterone. In: "Hormones in Blood", Ed. Gray, C.H., Academic Press, New York, pp. 391-488 (1967).
4. Peterson, R.E.: Metabolism of adrenocortical steroids. In: "The Human Adrenal Cortex", Ed. Christy, M.P., Harper and Row, New York, pp. 87-189 (1971).
5. Gláz, E., Vecsei, P.: In: "Aldosterone", Eds. Gláz, E., Vecsei, P., Pergamon Press, Oxford, pp. 76-89 (1971).
6. Melby, J.C.: Intermediatry metabolism of aldosterone. In: "Handbook of Experimental Pharmacology" vol. 37, Eds. Page, I.H., Bumpus, F.N., Springer Verlag, New York, pp. 298-321 (1973).

7. Ross, E.J.: In: "Aldosterone and Aldosteronism", Ed. Ross, E.J., Lloyd-Duke, London, pp. 10-52 (1975).

8. Tait, J.F., Tait, S.A.S., Little, B., Laumas, K.R.: The disappearance of 7-^{3}H-d-aldosterone in the plasma of normal subjects. J. clin. Invest. 40, 72-80 (1961).

9. Tait, J.F., Little, B., Tait, S.A.S., Flood, C.: The metabolic clearance rate of aldosterone in pregnant and non-pregnant subjects estimated by both single injection and constant-infusion methods. J. clin. Invest. 41, 2093-2100 (1961).

10. Flood, C., Layne, D.S., Ramcharan, S., Rossipal, E., Tait, J.F., Tait, S.A.S.: An investigation of the urinary metabolites and secretion rates of aldosterone and cortisol in man and a description of methods for their measurement. Acta Endocrinol. 36, 237-264 (1961).

11. Coppage, W.S., Island, D.P., Cooner, A.E., Liddle, G.W.: The metabolism of aldosterone in normal subjects and in patients with hepatic cirrhosis. J. clin. Invest. 41, 1672-1680 (1962).

12. Cheville, R.A., Luetscher, J.A., Hancock, E.W., Dowdy, A.J., Nokes, G.W.: Distribution, conjugation and excretion of labeled aldosterone in congestive heart failure and in controls with normal circulation: development and testing of a model with an analogue computer. J. clin. Invest. 45, 1302-1316 (1966).

13. Luetscher, J.A., Camargo, C.A., Cheville, R.A., Hancock, E.W., Dowdy, A.J., Nokes, G.W.: Conjugation and excretion of aldosterone: testing of models with an analogue computer. In: "Steroid Dynamics", Ed. Pincus, G., Academic Press, New York, pp. 341-356 (1966).

14. Ayers, C.R., Davis, J.O., Lieberman, F., Carpenter, C.C.J., Berman, M., Casper, A.: The effects of chronic, hepatic venous congestion on the metabolism of d, 1-aldosterone and d-aldosterone. J. clin. Invest. 41, 884-895 (1962).

15. Hollander, W.D., Kramsch, D.M., Chobanian, A.V., Melby, J.C.: Metabolism and distribution of intravenously administered d-aldosterone-1, 2-^{3}H in the arteries, kidneys and heart of dog. Circulat. Res. (Suppl. 1) 18, 35-47 (1966).

16. Read, V.H., McCaa, C.S., Sulya, L.L.: Effect of sodium on the tissue uptake and metabolism of ^{3}H-1, 2-d-aldosterone in rats. Endocrinology 85, 1079-1083 (1969).

17. Morris, D.J., Caron, P.C., Graham, W.C., Silverman, J.A., DeConti, G.A.: Sex dependence of clearance rates of aldosterone in plasma and its metabolites from plasma of intact rats. Steroids 25, 763-771 (1975).

18. Morris, D.J., Graham, W.C., Davis, R.P.: The metabolism and binding properties of ^{3}H-aldosterone in plasma and its sex dependence in adrenalectomized rats. Endocrinology 96, 178-184 (1975).

19. Colby, H.D., Kitay, J.I.: Sex and substrate effects on hepatic corticosteroid metabolism in the rat. Endocrinology 90, 473-478 (1972).

20. Pasqualini, J.R., Jayle, M.F.: Conjugation of plasma aldosterone and tetrahydroaldosterone after administration of 1,2-tritiated-d-aldosterone. Nature 198, 1095-1096 (1963).

21. Morris, D.J., Tsai, R.: Chromatographic separation of aldosterone and its metabolites. Advances in Chromatography, vol. 19 (in press).

22. Morris, D.J., Rosen, M., McEnany, T.M.: Manuscript in preparation.

23. Sulya, L.L., McCaa, C.S., Read, V.H., Bonner, D.: Uptake of tritiated aldosterone by rat tissues. Nature 200, 788-789 (1963).

24. Williams, M.A., Baba, W.I.: The localization of ^{3}H-aldosterone and ^{3}H-cortisol within renal tubular cells by electron microscope autoradiography. J. Endocr. 39, 543-554 (1967).

25. McEwen, B.S., Davis, P.G., Parsons, B., Pfaff, D.W.: The brain as a target for steroid hormone action. Ann. Rev. Neurosci. 2, 65-112 (1979).

26. Anderson, N.S., Fanestil, D.D.: Corticoid receptors in rat brain: evidence for an aldosterone receptor. Endocrinology 98, 676-684 (1976).

27. Morris, D.J., Davis, R.P.: Complex formation of ^{3}H-aldosterone in rat kidney and liver. Steroids 21, 383-396 (1973).

28. Singer, S., Morey, K.S., Litwack, G.: Properties of the cortisol metabolite binding system in liver cytosol. Physiol. Chem. Phys. 2, 117-126 (1970).

29. Morris, D.J., Sarma, M.H., Barnes, F.W.: Labeled complexes in liver cytosol after administration of 4-^{14}C-corticosterone and 4-^{14}C-cortisol. Endocrinology 87, 486-493 (1970).

30. Monder, C., Bradlow, H.L.: General review of carboxylic acid metabolites of steroids. J. Steroid Biochem. 8, 897-908 (1977).

31. Tsai, R., Davis, R.P., Morris, D.J.: The effects of spironolactone on the synthesis of polar metabolites of aldosterone in the liver of male rats. J. Steroid Biochem. (in press, April 1980).

32. Pasqualini, J.R.: Modes de conjugation de la corticostérone et de la 11-déhydrocorticostérone. C.r. hebd. Séanc. Acad. Sci., Paris, 246, 2945-2946 (1958).

33. Grose, J.H., Nowaczynski, W., Kuchel, O., Genest, J.: Isolation of aldosterone urinary metabolites, glucuronides and sulfate. J. Steroid Biochem. 4, 551-566 (1973).

34. Ulick, S., Lieberman, S.: Evidence for the occurrence of a metabolite of aldosterone in urine. J. Amer. chem. Soc. 79, 6567-6568 (1957).

35. Ulick, S., Kusch, K., August, J.T.: Correction of the structure of a urinary metabolite of aldosterone. J. Amer. chem. Soc. 83, 4482-4483 (1961).

36. Pasqualini, J.R.: Aldosterone and tetrahydroaldosterone conjugation in human urine and plasma. In: "Aldosterone", Eds. Baulieu, E.E., Robel, P., Blackwell, Oxford, pp. 131-143 (1964).

37. Sandor, T., Lanthier, A.: The metabolism of aldosterone. Studies in vitro and in vivo in man. Acta Endocrinol. 39, 87-102 (1962).

38. Kelly, W.G., Bandi, L., Lieberman, S.: Isolation and characterization of human urinary metabolites of aldosterone. Three isomeric tetrahydrometabolites. Biochemistry 1, 792-803 (1962).

39. Kelly, W.G., Bandi, L., Shoolery, J.N., Lieberman, S.: Isolation and characterization of aldosterone metabolites from human urine: metabolites bearing a bicyclic acetal structure. Biochemistry 1, 172-181 (1963).

40. Kelly, W.G., Bandi, L., Lieberman, S.: Isolation and characterization of human urinary metabolites of aldosterone. Dihydroaldosterone and 21-deoxytetrahydroaldosterone. Biochemistry 2, 1249-1254 (1963).

41. Kohler, H., Hesse, R.H., Pechet, M.M.: The metabolism of aldosterone. Metabolic pathway, isolation, characterization and synthesis of metabolites. J. biol. Chem. 239, 4117-4123 (1964).

42. Möhring, J., Möhring, B., Siegenthaler, W.: Die biologische Aktivität von Tetrahydroaldosteron, Tetrahydroaldosteronglucuronid und 18-Aldosteronglucuronid im Vergleich mit Aldosteron. Klin. Wschr. 46, 22-24 (1968).

43. Morris, D.J., DeConti, G.A., Latif, S.A.: The mineralocorticoid activity of reduced metabolites of aldosterone in rats. J. Steroid Biochem. 9, 821, Abstract No. 43 (1978).

44. Morris, D.J.: The biological significance of reduced metabolites of aldosterone. Human Pathology 10, 128-131 (1979).

45. Sekihara, H., Island, D.P., Liddle, G.W.: New mineralocorticoids: 5α-dihydroaldosterone and 5α-dihydro-11-deoxycorticosterone. Endocrinology 103, 1450-1452 (1978).

46. Pasqualini, J.R., Sumida, C.: Mineralocorticoid receptors and target tissues. In: "Receptors and Mechanism of Action of Steroid Hormones", Ed. Pasqualini, J.R., Marcel Decker Inc., New York, pp. 399-511 (1977).

47. Latif, S.A., Tsai, R., Reinhold, V., Morris, D.J.: Isolation and partial identification of several polar metabolites of aldosterone synthesized in the liver of male rats. 5th International Congress on Hormonal Steroids (1978), J. Steroid Biochem. 9, 828 (1978).

48. Axelrod, B.J., Cates, J.E., Johnson, B.B., Luetscher, J.A.: Aldosterone in urine of normal man and of patients with edema. Its increased recovery after acid and β-glucuronidase. Brit. med. J. 1, 196-199 (1955).

49. Ayres, P.J., Barlow, J., Garrod, O., Kellie, A.E., Tait, S.A.S., Tait, J.F., Walker, G.: The metabolism of (16-^{3}H)-aldosterone in man. In: "An International Symposium on Aldosterone", Eds. Muller, A.F., O'Connor, C.M., Churchill Ltd., London, pp. 73-99 (1958).

50. Underwood, R.H., Tait, J.F.: Purification, partial characterization and metabolism of an acid labile conjugate of aldosterone. J. clin. Endocrinol. Metab. 24, 1110-1124 (1964).

51. Luetscher, J.A., Hancock, E.W., Camargo, C.A., Dowdy, E.J., Nokes, G.W.: Conjugation of 1,2, ^{3}H-aldosterone in human liver and kidneys and renal extraction of aldosterone and labeled conjugates from blood plasma. J. clin. Endocrinol. Metab. 25, 628-638 (1965).

52. Pasqualini, J.R., Uhrich, F., Jayle, M.F.: Contribution to the study of the structure of the aldosterone conjugate isolated from human urine. Biochim. biophys. Acta 104, 513-523 (1965).

53. Siegenthaler, W.E., Peterson, R.E., Frimpter, G.W.: The renal clearance of aldosterone and its major metabolites. In: "Aldosterone", Eds. Baulieu, E.E., Robel, P., Blackwell, Oxford, pp. 51-72 (1964).

54. Flood, C., Pincus, G., Tait, J.F., Tait, S.A.S., Willoughby, S.: A comparison of the metabolism of radioactive 17-iso-aldosterone administered intravenously and orally in normal human subjects. J. clin. Invest. 46, 717-727 (1967).

55. Bokkenheuser, V.D., Winter, J., Honour, J.W., Shackleton, C.H.L.: Reduction of aldosterone by anaerobic bacteria: origin of urinary 21-deoxy metabolites in man. J. Steroid Biochem. 11, 1145-1149 (1979).

56. Bledsoe, T., Liddle, G.W., Riondel, A., Island, D.P., Bloomfield, D., Sinclair-Smith, B.: Comparative fates of intravenously and orally administered aldosterone: evidence of extrahepatic formation of acid hydrolizable conjugates in man. J. clin. Invest. 45, 264-269 (1966).

57. McCaa, C.S., Sulya, L.L.: Pathways of excretion of ^{3}H-1,2-d-aldosterone radiometabolites in the rat. Endocrinology 79, 815-818 (1966).

58. Morris, D.J., Silverman, J.A.: Biliary excretion of ^{3}H-aldosterone and its sex dependence in adrenalectomized rats. Endocrinology 96, 1386-1391 (1975).

59. Lowy, J., Albepart, T., Pasqualini, J.R.: ^{3}H-corticosterone metabolism in the rat. Acta Endocrinol. 61, 483-493 (1969).

60. Taylor, W.: Excretion of steroid hormone metabolites in bile and faeces. Vitam. and Horm. 29, 201-285 (1971).

61. Morris, D.J., Silverman, J.A., Tsai, R.: Fecal and urinary excretion of ^{3}H-aldosterone and its sex dependence in rats. J. Steroid Biochem. 7, 561-564 (1976).

62. Morris, D.J., Hantoot, M.S., DeConti, G.A.: The enterohepatic circulation of aldosterone metabolites and its sex dependence in rats. Endocrinology 101, 1776-1783 (1977).

63. Guelpa-Decorzant, C., Riondel, A.M., Chabert, P.R., Vallotton, M.B.: Comparison of the urinary excretion of free aldosterone and its acid-labile conjugate in rats during experimental hyperaldosteronism. J. Steroid Biochem. 10, 365-369 (1979).

64. Meyer, C.J., Layne, D.S., Tait, J.F., Pincus, G.: The binding of aldosterone to plasma proteins in normal, pregnant and steroid-treated women. J. clin. Invest. 40, 1663-1671 (1961).

65. Daughaday, W.H., Holloszy, J., Mariz, I.K.: Binding of corticosteroids by plasma proteins. VI. The binding of cortisol by corticosteroid binding globulin and by the estrogen induced binding system of plasma. J. clin. Endocrinol. Metab. 21, 53-61 (1961).

66. Davidson, F.T., DeVenuto, F., Westphal, U.: Steroid-protein interactions. IX. Interaction of aldosterone with human serum proteins in competition with spironolactone and other steroids. Endocrinology 71, 893-900 (1962).

67. Richardson, K.S.C., Nowaczynski, W., Genest, J.: Specific aldosterone binding proteins in human plasma: partial characterization. J. Steroid Biochem. 8, 951-957 (1977).

68. Nowaczynski, W., Kuchel, O., Genest, J., Messerli, F.H., Honda, M., Tolis, G., Seth, K., Parvin-Pande, R., Kubo, S., Grose, J., Ledoux, F., Lebel, M.: Dynamic aldosterone and 18-hydroxydeoxycorticosterone studies in labile and stable benign essential hypertension. J. Steroid Biochem. 6, 767-778 (1975).

69. Nowaczynski, W., Genest, J., Kuchel, O., Messerli, F.H., Guthrie, G.P., Richardson, K., Grose, J.: Age- and posture-related changes in plasma protein binding and metabolism of aldosterone in essential and secondary hypertension. J. Lab. clin. Med. 90, 475-489 (1977).

70. Pratt, J.H., Melby, J.C.: Alterations in aldosterone metabolism induced by adenocorticotropin (ACTH). J. clin. Invest. 53, 62A (1974).

71. Messerli, F.H., Nowaczynski, W., Honda, M., Genest, J., Kuchel, O.: Effects of ACTH on steroid metabolism. J. clin. Endocrinol. Metab. 42, 1074-1079 (1976).

72. Dixon, K., Schwartz, V.: Uptake of aldosterone by human gland in vitro. J. Endocr. 45, 231-244 (1969).

73. Alberti, K.G., Sharp, G.W.: The isolation of bound aldosterone from the nuclei of human, toad and rat colon. Ann. Endocrinol. 31 Suppl. 4: 777 (1970).

74. Appelgren, L.E., Marrero, E.: The distribution of labeled aldosterone in mice using whole body autoradiography. Acta Pharmacol. Toxicol. 31, 86-96 (1972).

75. Edelman, I.S., Bogoroch, R., Porter, G.A.: On the mechanism of action of aldosterone on sodium transport: the role of protein synthesis. Proc. natn. Acad. Sci. U.S.A. 50, 1169-1177 (1963).

76. Sharp, G.W.G., Komack, C.L., Leaf, A.: Studies of the binding of aldosterone in the toad bladder. J. clin. Invest. 45, 450-459 (1966).

77. Bogoroch, R.: In: "Autoradiography of Diffusable Substances", Eds. Roth, L.J., Stumpf, W., Academic Press, New York, pp. 99-112 (1962).

78. Fanestil, D.D., Edelman, I.S.: Characteristics of the renal nuclear receptors for aldosterone. Proc. natn. Acad. Sci. U.S.A. 56, 872-879 (1966).

79. Swaneck, G.E., Highland, E., Edelman, I.S.: Stereospecific nuclear and cytosol aldosterone-binding proteins of various tissues. Nephron 6, 297-317 (1969).

80. Morris, D.J., Berek, J.S., Davis, R.P.: Sex-dependence of the metabolism of aldosterone in adrenalectomized and intact rats. Steroids 21, 397-407 (1973).

81. Ausiello, D.A., Sharp, G.W.G.: Localization of physiological receptor sites for aldosterone in the bladder of the toad, Bufo marinus. Endocrinology 62, 1163-1169 (1968).

82. Fanestil, D.D., Vaughn, D.A., Ludens, J.H.: Steroid hormone receptors in human renal carcinoma. J. Steroid Biochem. 5, 338 (1974).

83. Herman, T.S., Fimognari, G.M., Edelman, I.S.: Studies on renal aldosterone-binding proteins. J. biol. Chem. 243, 3849-3856 (1968).

84. Funder, J.W., Feldman, D., Edelman, I.S.: The roles of plasma binding and receptor specificity in the mineralocorticoid action of aldosterone. Endocrinology 92, 994-1004 (1973).

85. Mills, A.J., Wheldrake, J.F., Feltham, L.A.W.: Aldosterone-binding components in rat kidney: evidence for heterogeneity. Enzymologia 43, 311-323 (1972).

86. Crabbé, J.: The mechanism of action of aldosterone. In: "Receptors and Mechanism of Action of Steroid Hormones", Ed. Pasqualini, J.R., Dekker, New York, pp. 513-568 (1977).

87. Morris, D.J., Davis, R.P.: Progress in endocrinology and metabolism. Aldosterone: Current Concepts. Metabolism 23, 473-494 (1974).

88. Snart, R.S.: Binding of aldosterone in the toad bladder. Biochim. biophys. Acta 135, 1056-1058 (1967).

89. Sharp, G.W.G., Alberti, K.G.M.: In: Advances in the Biosciences. Ed. Raspi, G., vol. 7, Pergamon Press, Oxford, p. 281 (1971).

90. Funder, J.W., Feldman, D., Edelman, I.S.: Specific aldosterone binding in rat kidney and parotid. J. Steroid Biochem. 3, 209-218 (1972).

91. Rousseau, G., Baxter, J.D., Funder, J.W., Edelman, I.S., Tomkins, J.: Glucocorticoid and mineralocorticoid receptors for aldosterone. J. Steroid Biochem. 3, 219-227 (1972).

92. Swaneck, G.E., Chu, L.H., Edelman, I.S.: Stereospecific binding of aldosterone to renal chromatin. J. biol. Chem. 245, 5382-5389 (1970).

93. Forte, L.R.: Effect of mineralocorticoid agonists and antagonists on binding of ^{3}H-aldosterone to adrenalectomized rat kidney plasma membranes. Life Sci. 11, 461-473 (1972).

94. Marver, D., Goodman, D., Edelman, I.S.: Relationships between renal cytoplasmic and nuclear aldosterone receptors. Kidney International 1, 210-223 (1972).

95. Duval, D., Funder, J.W.: The binding of tritiated aldosterone in the rat liver cytosol. Endocrinology 94, 575-579 (1974).

96. Anderson, N.S., Fanestil, D.D., Ludens, J.H.: Study of adrenal corticoid receptors in brain. J. Steroid Biochem. 5, 335 (1974).

97. Kolpakao, M.G., Shulga, V.A., Mertvetsov, N.P., Selyatitskaya, V.G., Salgahik, R.I.: Interaction of aldosterone and corticosterone with cell nuclei of target organs under different function states. J. Steroid Biochem. 5, 917-923 (1974).

98. Marver, D.: Aldosterone receptors in rabbit renal cortex and red medulla. Endocrinology 106, 611-618 (1980).

99. Fuller, P.J., Funder, J.W.: Mineralocorticoid and glucocorticoid receptors in human kidney. Kidney International 10, 154-157 (1976).

100. Matulich, D.T., Spindler, B.J., Shambelan, M., Baxter, J.D.: Mineralocorticoid receptors in human kidney. J. clin. Endocrinol. Metab. 43, 1170-1174 (1976).

101. Alberti, K.G., Sharp, G.W.G.: Macromolecular binding of aldosterone in the toad bladder. Biochim. biophys. Acta 192, 337-346 (1969).

102. Alberti, K.G., Sharp, G.W.G.: Identification of four types of steroids by their interaction with mineralocorticoid receptors in the toad bladder. J. Endocr. 48, 563-574 (1970).

103. Williamson, H.E.: Mechanism of the antinatriuretic action of aldosterone. Biochem. Pharmacol. 12, 1449-1450 (1963).

THE SYNTHESIS, SECRETION AND ASSAY OF INSULIN

K. W. Taylor and I. D. Caterson
The London Hospital Medical College, University of London,
Department of Biochemistry, Turner Street, London E1 2AD,
England, U.K.

Introduction

During the last ten years, knowledge of the biosynthesis, storage and release of insulin has increased to a remarkable extent. Such additional information has now materially altered a number of investigative procedures concerning insulin and its release. This Chapter will begin, therefore, with an account of the general mechanisms by which insulin is made, stored and secreted into the circulation.

Site of origin of insulin

Insulin is found only in the β cells of the islets of Langerhans, which in some species of fish are separated off from the acinar pancreas as Brockman bodies. In most mammals (including man), the β cells constitute approximately 80% of the islet tissue, although in other species, including birds, the A2 glucagon producing cells, predominate.

Structure of insulin

The sequence of human insulin is shown in Figure 1. As with all mammalian insulins it consists of two chains : an A chain containing 21 amino acids with glycine as the N-terminal amino acid, and a B chain containing 30 amino acids in which the N-terminus is phenylalanine (1). The two chains are joined by disulphide

Hormones in Normal and Abnormal Human Tissues, Vol. II

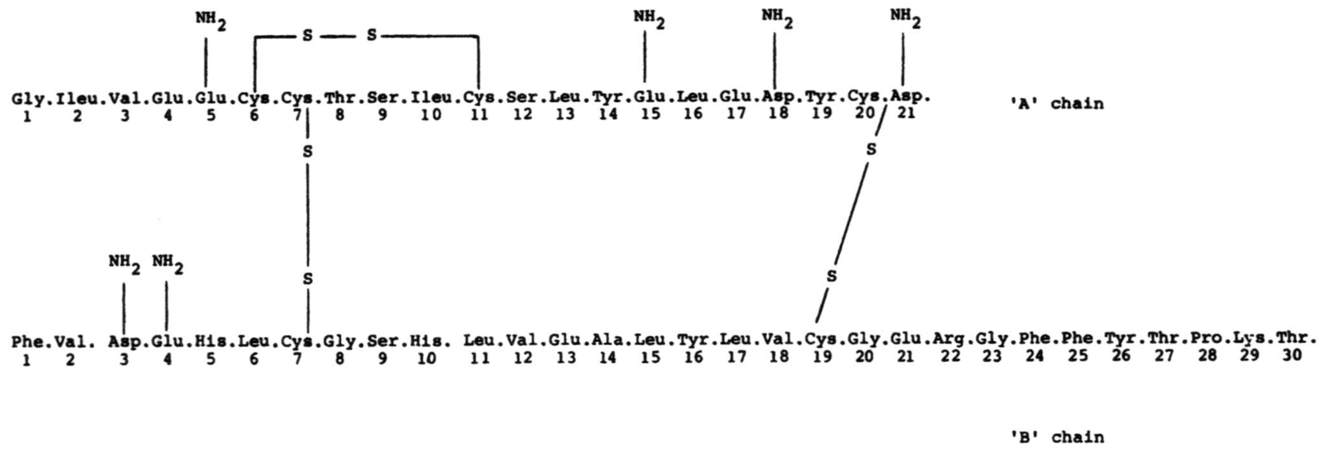

FIGURE 1. Structure of Human Insulin

linkages. The insulin molecule is particularly rich in cysteine residues, there being an additional two present in the A chain where a further intra-chain disulphide ring is situated (2). In mammalian insulins the differences between sequences are relatively slight and may sometimes only involve the substitution of a single amino acid in the intra-chain disulphide ring (3). However, in many other species there may be more complex differences. This is particularly the case in animals such as the guinea-pig and coypu where over 15 residues may be different from those in human insulin. Detailed accounts of the sequence of vertebrate insulins have been given elsewhere (4, 5). Such differences in species structure are important since they may result in the production of antibodies when one species insulin is injected into another animal, and also for the information they give about the residues in insulin which are essential for the maintenance of its three-dimensional structure and for its biological activity (6, 7).

Biosynthesis of Insulin

As is the case for other polypeptide hormones, insulin is made from larger molecular weight precursors which are transformed into insulin within the β cells of the islets of Langerhans.

The first product made in the endoplasmic reticulum of the β cells is termed pre-proinsulin. This is a single chain structure (Fig. 2). It has a molecular weight of about 11,000 and an extra sequence of approximately 20 amino acids has been added to the N-terminus of the phenylalanine chain (i.e. β chain). The production of proteins with an additional sequence of this kind is now thought to be very common at an early stage in the genesis of secretable proteins (8). It has been supposed that this extra length of amino acids in some way facilitates the passage of newly synthesised protein across membranes. This material has a very transitory existence and its half-life may be less than a minute. The extra length of amino acids is then

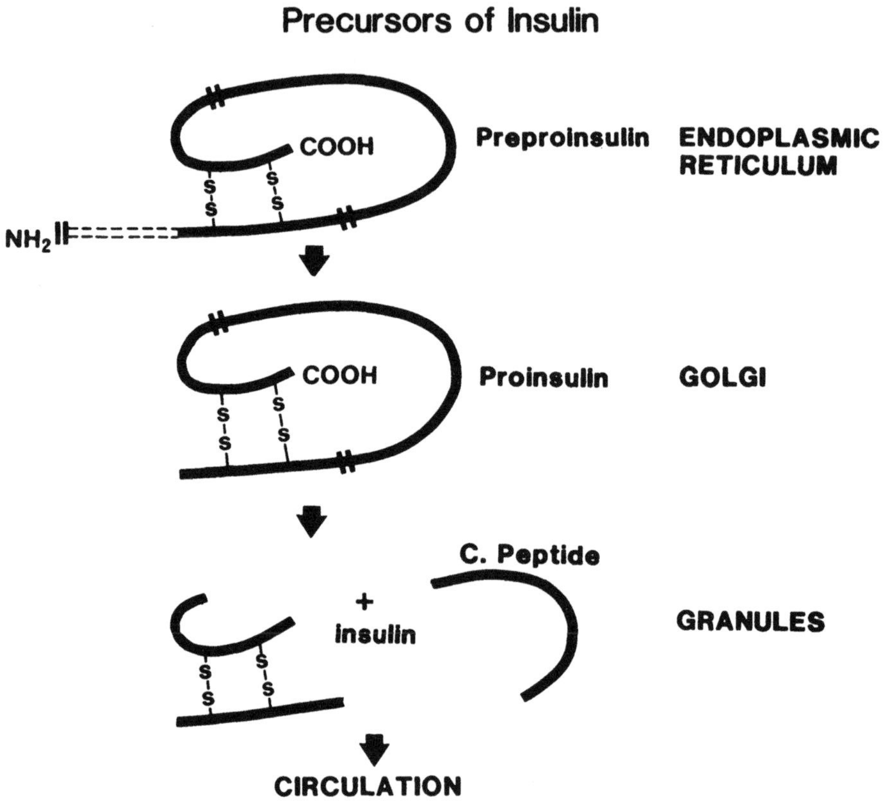

Fig. 2

split off to yield proinsulin (see Figure 2).

<u>Proinsulin</u> is a single chain polypeptide containing the intact insulin molecule but having a bridging peptide - the C or connecting peptide - which extends from the C-terminal amino acid of the B chain to the N-terminus of the A chain. It was first described in normal pancreas by Steiner and his colleagues (9, 10). The extra chain contains 35-40 amino acids. Proinsulin is present as an insulin precursor in all animal islets so far examined. It is usually thought that the synthesis of this

single chain derivative of insulin makes it possible for the correct positioning of cysteine residues so that the appropriate disulphide bonds in insulin can easily be made. Proinsulin is thought to be converted to insulin by enzymatic degradation just before the formation of mature granules. This transformation may take place in the Golgi area of the cell, so that the granules contain both intact insulin and the C-peptide. Insulin is stored in granules in a crytalline form with zinc. When insulin is secreted, the granules discharge both insulin and the C-peptide in an equimolar ratio into the circulation. In mammals the rate of insulin synthesis is increased by glucose (11).

Secretion of Insulin

The histological details of insulin secretion have been reviewed (12). However, the biochemistry of the process is still unclear.

Glucose concentration is the major determinant of the rate of insulin secretion in mammals. To a lesser extent, release of insulin is also controlled by blood amino acid concentrations and perhaps by circulating ketone bodies. Glucose may influence insulin secretion in at least two ways. It may provide the signal for release either acting by itself or through a glucose metabolite. In addition metabolism of glucose is necessary to provide ATP for granule movement and to produce other co-factors necessary in the release process. Cyclic-AMP has a major though as yet not well defined role in the secretory process (13). Secretion is also dependent upon calcium ion movement. This may be either from one organelle to another or it may be due to calcium fluxes across the plasma membranes.

A number of drugs, particularly the sulphonylureas, may also increase the rates of insulin release. Table 1 shows the principal agents which may promote insulin release.

There are also long term physiological adjustments which the islet makes in response to changes in physiological states

Table 1

Substances which promote insulin release

Substance	Remarks
Sugars	
Glucose	
Mannose	
Ribose)	For some animals
Xylulose)	
Xylitol)	
Amino acids especially :	
Arginine	
Leucine	
Lysine	
Fatty acids and ketones	
Octanoate)	Potentiators of release in some species
Palmitate)	
β-Hydroxybutyrate)	
Drugs	
Sulphonylureas	
Diesterase inhibitors (e.g. caffeine, theophylline)	

such as fasting, excessive carbohydrate intake, pregnancy and growth. In fasting, islet activity is depressed whereas, in pregnancy (14), after growth hormone treatment (15), and after excessive carbohydrate intake, islet activity may be greatly increased.

Assay of Insulin

Until the advent of immunoassay procedures insulin was assayed by biological methods. Classically these were dependent upon the depression of blood sugar in animals (e.g. mice or rabbits). Later, methods dependent on the glucose uptake of isolated tissues such as rat diaphragm tissue or rat adipose tissue were used. These later methods were sufficiently sensitive for assaying blood insulin in animals and in man but lacked specificity. Such methods may occasionally be required to confirm values obtained by immunoassay procedures. A full account of these and their history is given elsewhere (16). If a bioassay is to be used, effects of insulin on the oxidation of ^{14}C labelled glucose by adipose tissue to carbon dioxide is the preferred method (17).

Immunoassay of insulin

Insulin is now usually measured by immunoassay methods. The earliest attempts to do this by Berson and Yalow (18) were achieved using paper electrophoretic methods to separate free from bound insulin. Since then a wide variety of other methods (double antibody precipitation (19), charcoal (20, 21) and solid phase techniques (22)), for separating free and bound insulin have been used.

Measurement of C-peptide and proinsulin

Assays of both of these are becoming increasingly important in clinical medicine. The C-peptide assay provides a means of assessing β cell function, since a molecule of C-peptide is released for every molecule of insulin secreted. In insulin treated diabetics, the presence of insulin binding antibodies makes immunoassay of insulin extremely difficult. Therefore measurement of blood levels of the C-peptide is a convenient alternative for the assessment of islet function. It also may be important to assay proinsulin in cases of islet tumour where circulating levels of this precursor are frequently raised.

Problems in the accurate measurement of this peptide have largely been overcome. The lack of antigenicity of the C-peptide molecule has in part been overcome by combining it with larger proteins such as albumin. Another problem lies in the lack of a tyrosyl group in the peptide and a preliminary tyrosylation of the peptide is necessary before iodination can take place. A comprehensive review of the nature, release and clinical significance of C-peptide has been published (23). A convenient assay method for C-peptide in blood has been described by Heding (24).

Since insulin and C-peptide both cross-react with antibodies made against proinsulin, direct immunoassay of proinsulin in the presence of insulin is not often possible. The difficulty was originally overcome by purifying the proinsulin moiety by gel filtration (25). Alternatively, insulin and proinsulin may be extracted by immunoabsorption from the C-peptide and the proinsulin separately measured by a C-peptide assay technique.

Recently, a more sophisticated technique, utilising both the C-peptide binding sites and the insulin binding sites of proinsulin antibodies, has been devised (26). In this method, both insulin and proinsulin are absorbed by insulin antibody coated on to the walls of polyethylene tubes. Antibodies to C-peptide are then bound to the proinsulin and the uptake measured. Such a method, which has been termed an indirect two-site immunoradiometric assay, is extremely sensitive and easy to perform.

Normal Blood Insulin Values

Serum insulin levels are widely affected by such factors as age, pregnancy, body weight, time of day, nutritional status and other hormones, as well as the quantity and content of recent meals. Before a useful appraisal of the significance of serum insulin levels can be made, such factors need to be taken into consideration. In any case serum insulin levels have little meaning without a knowledge of serum glucose levels measured simultaneously.

Fasting insulin levels

After an overnight fast, serum insulin levels in normal weight individuals are low, ranging from 6.5 - 14μunits/ml (27, 28, 29, 30). The same is true after starvation, in which condition the islet cells respond with less insulin secretion than normal, leading to higher blood sugars on glucose tolerance testing (31, 32, 33, 34, 35). After a period of re-feeding insulin secretion returns to normal. In islets isolated from starved animals cyclic-AMP levels are reduced and insulin secretion blunted (36). When cyclic-AMP is artificially elevated in such isolated islets, insulin secretion is increased to the normal value.

Blood insulin during glucose tolerance tests

A more accurate estimate of β cell function is obtained when blood insulin is measured during glucose tolerance tests (37). As starvation reduces the insulin response to glucose (38) and high carbohydrate feeding enhances it, glucose tolerance tests should be performed after 3 days on a 3000 calorie (12,600kj) high carbohydrate diet and with an overnight fast. These conditions will give a standard response to a high glucose load. Typical blood insulin responses to oral glucose are shown in Fig. 3.

INSULIN RESPONSE TO ORAL GLUCOSE [100g]
AND I.V. GLUCOSE [25g] IN NORMAL SUBJECTS

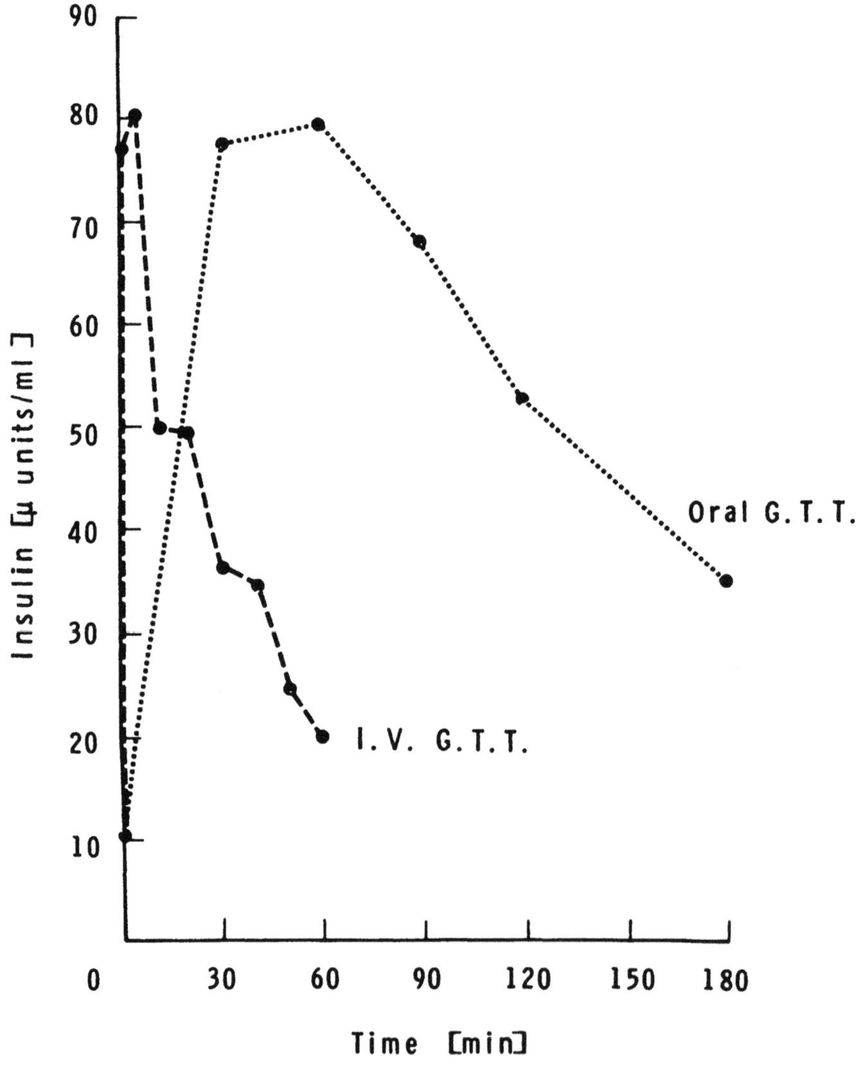

adapted from Santiago et al [1977]

Fig. 3

Oral glucose tolerance tests with varying glucose loads

Various glucose loads have been used (usually 50g, 75g or 100g) although more recently some agreement has been reached on the use of a standard 75g oral glucose load. The levels attained 1 h after 100g load are far greater than those reached with 50g glucose and may range from 100 to 158μunits/ml at 60 min after 100g glucose (19).

Intravenous glucose tolerance tests

Intravenous glucose (e.g. a 25g glucose load given over 2 min) elicits a very rapid insulin response. Peak values of insulin are reached within 5 min. As is well known, the total release of insulin is less when glucose is given intravenously rather than orally (39). This is because oral administration of glucose stimulates the secretion of polypeptide hormones (e.g. gut glucagon and gastric inhibitory peptides) from the wall of the gastro-intestinal tract (40, 41) which, in turn, potentiate insulin secretion.

Diurnal variation in insulin secretion, age/related insulin secretion

It has been suggested that insulin responses to glucose tolerance tests are slightly greater if the tests are undertaken in the morning (42, 43). There is a diurnal variation in serum insulin levels, though this is related to eating rather than any intrinsic variation in secretion. With age, insulin responsiveness to glucose deteriorates.

Blood insulin in obesity

Fasting serum insulin levels are elevated and the insulin response to glucose tolerance testing is exaggerated in this condition (44, 45, 46). The peak insulin response may also be delayed. Obese children, too, have exaggerated insulin responses and the magnitude of the response is related to the degree of obesity, not to its duration (47). The hyperinsulinaemia of obesity may be due either to increased peripheral resistance to the action of insulin, which raises blood glucose, or to changes in the β cells caused by obesity and resulting in increased insulin release. Histological changes and enlargement of the islets in obesity are now well documented (48). In addition, there may be hypersecretion of insulin in experimental obesity (49, 50). Increased insulin synthesis and release from islets has also been recorded in experimental obesity due to goldthioglucose (51, 52). These changes are associated with both increased cyclic-AMP levels and increased oxidation of glucose in the islets of Langerhans. When such animals are dieted by caloric restriction and maintained at normal weight, both increased insulin secretion and synthesis persist for some months. Neither changes in cyclic-AMP levels nor changes in glucose oxidation by themselves adequately account for the altered insulin secretion and synthesis in obesity. There appears to be an effect of obesity directly on the β cell. This may be due to the obesity or to islet sensitivity to increased dietary carbohydrate as has been found in pregnancy. The persistence of these changes on dieting is remarkable.

Other Endocrine Effects

Pregnancy

In pregnant animals, the insulin response to glucose is increased (53), as are the rates both of glucose metabolism (54) and of insulin biosynthesis (55, 56). The same is true in human pregnancy (57). This may be due to a direct effect of placental hormones, human chorionic somatomammotrophin in particular, on the β cells or due to an increased sensitivity of the islets of Langerhans to glucose brought about perhaps by an increase in the dietary intake of carbohydrate (58). Gestational diabetes is not common, and in most cases glucose tolerance returns to normal after delivery.

Growth hormone

The increase in blood insulin levels after growth hormone administration in man or animals (59, 60) are well documented. While some of these effects (as with obesity) may be due to an increased resistance to insulin in peripheral tissues, it is now clear that these may be direct effects of growth hormone on the islets themselves (61). Effects of other hormones such as adrenal steroids and placental lactogen on insulin release (62) have been reviewed elsewhere.

Blood Insulin in Diabetes Mellitus

In insulin-dependent diabetes (the less common form of the disorder), serum insulin levels are often very low (63, 64) and fail to rise to normal levels despite high blood sugar levels and a glucose challenge in the form of a glucose tolerance test. There is also little or no secretory response to other stimuli of insulin release (amino acids, glucagon, sulphonylureas). After treatment with insulin some of these patients may have a remission of the disease with a partial return of cell function lasting weeks or months (65, 66).

In non-insulin-dependent diabetes without obesity the response to glucose is less than normal. The insulin response may show a delayed peak of secretion (67). In mild diabetes, serum insulin may be lowered by a restricted carbohydrate diet before there is any change in blood glucose levels. With adherence to a diet and a reduction in body weight, serum insulin and blood glucose may be kept in the normal range, though on glucose tolerance testing, the defect in insulin secretion remains. In these patients it has been suggested that the β cells may show a defect in glucose recognition, and insulin secretion is not then as great for a given blood glucose as it is in normal subjects (68).

Proinsulin

Basal levels

Proinsulin has been reported to constitute up to 40% of the total immunoactive insulin concentration in the fasting state (69) with values in absolute terms ranging from 0 - 0.4 ng/ml. A recent survey (26) using an immunoradiometric assay for human proinsulin reports fasting levels of 0.009 pmol/ml and a proinsulin to insulin ratio of 0.33.

In non-insulin-dependent diabetes, higher fasting levels of proinsulin are found (0.025 pmol/ml) and also the proinsulin to insulin ratio is higher after glucose (70). Owing to a wide scatter of results the difference is not statistically significant. Similar results have been found in children with chemical diabetes, serum proinsulin being slightly higher than in normal controls (71).

The absolute level of proinsulin is higher in obese subjects, but owing to the higher fasting level of insulin the proportions of each hormone are the same as in non-obese control subjects.

The proportion of proinsulin to insulin found peripherally (approx. 20%) is greater than that in the pancreas, where proinsulin makes up less than 7% of the total immunoreactive insulin. Using portal vein cannulation, it has been found that the ratio of proinsulin to insulin secreted is similar to that present in the pancreas (28). The higher peripheral levels may be explained by the longer half-life of proinsulin in the blood (17.2 min). Insulin appears to be preferentially extracted by the liver from the portal blood.

Proinsulin during glucose tolerance tests

In normal children, the percentage proinsulin falls from 15% to about 9% at 30 mins and then slowly returns to basal levels during oral glucose tolerance tests though the absolute level of proinsulin increases (71). In adults, proinsulin levels increased 8-fold in the peripheral circulation (26) during such tests. The proinsulin/insulin ratio however fell from 0.40 to a minimum of 0.20 at 30 mins. It then increased to 1.0 at 90 mins and fell to the basal level at 120 mins. An earlier study had reported that older normal subjects had a greater proinsulin response than younger subjects (70). Obesity and carbohydrate intolerance were both associated with slightly increased levels of proinsulin (71).

Familial hyperproinsulinaemia

In 1976 Gabbay et al (72) described a family with familial hyperproinsulinaemia, the defect being transmitted as an autosomal dominant. It is asymptomatic. More recently it has been confirmed that in this condition there is an abnormal form of proinsulin which circulates in blood in affected families (73). Proinsulin constituted up to 85% of total immunoreactivity in the blood of propositi. On glucose tolerance testing the proinsulin fraction remained at this level.

C-Peptide Secretion

The connecting peptide is secreted in a molar ratio with insulin from the granules of the β cells. The ratio of C-peptide to insulin is increased in the peripheral blood in comparison with the portal blood. This is on account of the selective removal of insulin by the liver (28). Normal levels of C-peptide in the fasting state are between 0.30 - 0.80 pM (74, 75). Assay of its levels are useful in two situations. The first is in assessing residual β cell function in diabetic patients. If C-peptide levels are measured during a conventional oral glucose tolerance test and if C-peptide rises, then the patients have residual β cell activity. The rise tends to be slower in onset and be more prolonged than in normals. Diabetics with residual C-peptide secretion tend to be more stable (76, 77).

Secondly, the C-peptide assay may be used to investigate factitious hypoglycaemia. Patients with low blood sugar, high insulin levels but low C-peptide levels may have been administering insulin to themselves.

Islet Cell Tumours

In cases of islet cell tumour, insulin secretion is episodic and intermittent so that not all serum insulin samples will be elevated. Serum insulin levels should always be considered with a serum glucose level taken at the same time. Insulin levels may then be seen to be inappropriately high. Multiple blood samples should be taken, especially fasting specimens and samples taken during any symptomatic episode. With insulinomas, proinsulin levels are elevated (78, 79), and proinsulin makes up a greater than normal proportion of total immunoreactive insulin. At least one case of insulinoma with normal serum insulin levels but a high proinsulin level has been reported (80). Generally, both serum insulin and proinsulin are elevated.

Turner and Harris (81) proposed a test involving fish insulin induced hypoglycaemia. Because the fish insulin had a low crossreactivity with the anti-insulin serum used in radioimmunoassay, it allowed assessment of endogenous insulin secretion during hypoglycaemia. With insulinomas this secretion would be inappropriately high. The best methods of investigation rely on simultaneous insulin, proinsulin and glucose determinations followed by CAT-scanning and, if necessary, by arteriography (82).

References

1. Sanger, F.: The Chemistry of Insulin. Brit. med. Bull. 16, 183-188 (1960).

2. Ryle, A.P., Sanger, F., Smith, L.F., Kitai, R.: The disulphide bonds of insulin. Biochem. J. 60, 541-556 (1955).

3. Harris, J.I., Sanger, F., Naughton, M.A.: Species differences in insulins. Arch. Biochem. Biophys. 65, 427-432 (1956).

4. Smith, L.F.: Species variation in the amino acid sequence of insulin. Am. J. Med. 40, 662-666 (1966).

5. Dayhoff, M.O.: Atlas of protein sequence and structure. National Biochemical Research Foundation, Washington D.C. (1972).

6. Blundell, T.L., Dodson, G.C., Dodson, E., Hodgkin, D.C., Vijayan, M.: X-ray analysis of the structure of insulin. Recent Prog. Horm. Res. 27, 1-34 (1971).

7. De Meyts, P., Van Obberghen, E., Roth, J., Wollmer, A., Brandenburg, D.: Mapping of the residues responsible for the negative co-operativity of the receptor binding region of insulin. Nature 273, 504-509 (1979).

8. Blobel, G., Dobberstein, B.: Transfer of proteins across membranes. J. Cell Biol. 67, 835-851 (1975).

9. Steiner, D.F., Clark, J.L., Nolan, C., Rubenstein, A.M., Margoliash, E., Aten, B., Oyer, P.E.: Proinsulin and the Biosynthesis of Insulin. Recent Prog. Horm. Res. 25, 207-282 (1970).

10. Lernmark, A., Chan, S.J., Choy, R., Nathans, A., Carroll, R., Tager, H.S., Rubenstein, A.H., Swift, H.M., Steiner, D.F.: Biosynthesis of insulin and glucagon : a view of the current state of the art. Ciba Found. Symp. 41, 7-28 (1976).

11. Parry, D.G., Taylor, K.W.: Effects of sugars on incorporation of [^{3}H] leucine into insulins in vitro. Biochem. J. 100, 2-4C (1966).

12. Orci, L.T.: Minkowski Lecture - "A portrait of the β cell". Diabetologia 10, 163-187 (1974).

13. Sharp, G.W.G.: The Adenylate-cyclase-cyclic AMP System in Islets of Langerhans and its role in the control of insulin release. Diabetologia 16, 287-296 (1979).

14. Green, I.C., Howell, S.L., Montague, W., Taylor, K.W.: The regulation of insulin release from isolated islets of Langerhans of the rat in pregnancy. Biochem.J. 134, 481-487 (1973).

15. Whittaker, P.G., Taylor, K.W.: Direct effect of rat growth hormone on rat islets of Langerhans in tissue culture. Diabetologia (in press, 1980).

16. Taylor, K.W.: Insulin. In: "Hormones in Blood", 2nd edition Eds. Gray, C.H., Bacharach, A.L., Academic Press, New York and London, pp. 47-81 (1967).

17. Renold, A.E., Martin, D.B., Dagenais, Y.M., Steinke, J., Nickerson, R., Sheps, M.C.: Measurement of small quantities of insulin-like activity using rat adipose tissue. J. clin. Invest. 39, 1487-1498 (1960).

18. Berson, S.A., Yalow, R.S., Assay of plasma insulin in human subjects by immunological methods. Nature 184, 1648-1649 (1959).

19. Hales, C.N., Randle, P.J.: Immunoassay of insulin with insulin antibody precipitate. Biochem. J. 88, 137-146 (1963).

20. Herbert, J., Lau-K-S., Gottlieb, C.W., Bleicher, S.J.: Coated charcoal immunoassay of insulin. J. clin. Endocrinol. Metab. 25, 1375-1384 (1966).

21. Cresto, J.C., Dujovne, I.L., Castellani, P.I., Mitta, E.A., De Majo, S.F., Foglia, V.G.: Insulin radioimmunoassay by charcoal-dextran technique. Diabetologia 8, 292-295 (1972).

22. Wide, L., Porath, J.: Radioimmunoassay of proteins with the use of Sephadex-coupled antibodies. Biochim. biophys. Acta 130, 257-260 (1966).

23. C-Peptide Symposium - Diabetes 27, 145-285 (1978).

24. Heding, L.G.: Radioimmunological determination of human C-peptide in serum. Diabetologia 11, 451-500 (1975).

25. Rubenstein, A.H., Block, M.B., Starr, J., Melani, F., Steiner, D.F.: Proinsulin and C peptide in blood. Diabetes 21, Suppl. 2, 661-672 (1972).

26. Rainbow, S.J., Woodherd, J.S., Yue, D.K., Lazio, S.D., Hales, C.N.: Measurement of human proinsulin by an indirect two site immunoradiometric assay. Diabetologia 17, 229-234 (1979).

27. Pyke, D.A., Cassar, J., Todd, J., Taylor, K.W.: Glucose tolerance and serum insulin in identical twins of diabetics. Br. med. J. 4, 649-651 (1970).

28. Horwitz, D.L., Starr, J.I., Mako, M.E., Blackard, W.G., Rubenstein, A.H.: Proinsulin insulin, and C-peptide concentrations in human portal and peripheral blood. J. clin. Invest. 55, 1278-1283 (1975).

29. Santiago, J.V., Haymond, M.W., Clarke, W.L., Pagliara, A.S.: Glucagon, insulin and glucose responses to physiologic testing in normal and massively obese adults. Metabolism 26, 1115-1122 (1977).

30. Yalow, R.S., Glick, S.M., Roth, J., Berson, S.A.: Plasma insulin and growth hormone in obesity and diabetes. Ann. N.Y. Acad. Sci. 131, 357-373 (1965).

31. Buchanan, K.D., Vance, J.E., Williams, R.H.: Effect of starvation on insulin and glucagon release from isolated islets of Langerhans of the rat. Metabolism 18, 155-162 (1969).

32. Hedeskov, C.J., Capito, K.: The effect of starvation on insulin secretion and glucose metabolism in mouse pancreatic islets. Biochem. J. 140, 423-433 (1974).

33. Wolter, G.H.J., Konijuendijk, W., Bouman, P.R.: Effects of fasting on insulin secretion, islet glucose metabolism and the cyclic adenosine 3'5'-monophosphate content of rat pancreatic islets in vitro. Diabetes 26, 530-537 (1977).

34. Grey, N.J., Goldring, S., Kipnis, D.M.: The effect of fasting, diet and actinomycin D on insulin secretion in the rat. J. clin. Invest. 49, 881-889 (1970).

35. Howell, S.L., Green, I.C., Montague, W.: A possible role of adenylate cyclase in the long-term dietary regulation of insulin secretion from rat islets of Langerhans. Biochem. J. 136, 343-349 (1973).

36. Selawry, H., Gutman, R., Fink, G., Recant, L.: The effect of starvation on tissue adenosine 3'5' monophosphate levels. Biochem. biophys. Res. Commun. 51, 198-204 (1973).

37. Yalow, R.S., Berson, S.A.: Immunoassay of endogenous plasma insulin in man. J. clin. Invest. 39, 1157-1175 (1960).

38. Bagdade, J.D., Bierman, E.I., Porte, D.J.: The significance of basal insulin levels in the evaluation of the insulin response to glucose in diabetic and non diabetic subjects. J. clin. Invest. 46, 1549-1557 (1967).

39. McIntyre, N.I., Holdsworth, D.L., Turner, D.S.: New interpretation of oral glucose tolerance. Lancet 2, 20-22 (1964).

40. Brown, J.: Gastric Inhibitory Peptide (GIP). Gastroenterology 67, 733-734 (1974).

41. Said, S.: Vasoactive intestinal peptide (VIP). Gastroenterology 67, 735-737 (1974).

42. Jarrett, R.J., Keen, H.: Further observations on the diurnal variation in glucose tolerance. Br. med. J. 4, 334-337 (1970).

43. Jarrett, R.J., Baker, I.A., Keen, H., Oakley, N.W.: Diurnal variation in oral glucose tolerance; blood sugar and plasma insulin levels morning, afternoon and evening. Br. med. J. 1, 199-201 (1972).

44. Karam, J.H., Grodsky, G.M., Forsham, P.M.: Excessive insulin response to glucose in obese subjects as measured by immunochemical assay. Diabetes 12, 197-204 (1963).

45. Schultz, R.B., Darra, A.: Relationship between body composition and insulin and growth hormone responses in obese adolescents. Diabetes 19, 492-501 (1970).

46. Young, R.L., Fuchs, R.J., Woltjen, M.J., Cooperman, M.T.: Glucose-insulin responses to oral glucose in healthy obese populations. Diabetes 28, 208-212 (1979).

47. Deschamps, I., Giron, B.J., Lestradet, H.: Blood glucose, insulin and free fatty acid levels during oral glucose tolerance tests in 158 obese children. Diabetes 26, 89-93 (1977).

48. Ogilvie, R.F.: Islets of Langerhans in 19 cases of obesity. J. Path. Bact. 37, 473-481 (1933).

49. Gepts, W., Christophe, J., Major, J.: Pancreatic islets in mice with the obese hyperglycemic syndrome. Lack of effect of carbutamide. Diabetes 9, 63-69 (1960).

50. Malaisse, W.J., Malaisse-Lagae, F., Coleman, D.L.: Insulin secretion in experimental obesity. Metabolism 17, 802-807 (1968).

51. Caterson, I.D.: Insulin secretion in obesity. Proc. 10th International Diabetes Federation Congress Vienna (in press) (1979).

52. Caterson, I.D.: Ph.D. Thesis "Islet cell metabolism in experimental obesity". University of Sydney, 1980.

53. Green, I.C., Taylor, K.W.: Effects of pregnancy in the rat on the size and insulin secretory response of the islets of Langerhans. J. Endocrinol. 54, 317-325 (1972).

54. Green, I.C., Perrin, D., Howell, S.L.: Insulin release in isolated islets of Langerhans of pregnant rats. Relationship between glucose metabolism and cyclic-AMP. Horm. Metab. Res. 10, 32-35 (1978).

55. Bone, A.J., Taylor, K.W.: Metabolic adaptation to pregnancy shown by increased biosynthesis of insulin in islets of Langerhans isolated from pregnant rats. Nature 262, 501-502 (1976).

56. Bone, A.J., Howell, S.L.: Alterations in regulation of insulin biosynthesis in pregnancy and starvation studied in isolated rat islets of Langerhans. Biochem. J. 166, 501-507 (1977).

57. Trayner, I.M., Welborn, T.A., Rubenstein, A.H., Fraser, T.R.: Serum and urine insulin in late pregnancy and in a few pregnant latent diabetics. J. Endocrinol. 37, 443-453 (1967).

58. Green, I.C., Taylor, K.W.: Insulin secretory response of isolated islets of Langerhans in pregnant rats : Effects of dietary restriction. J. Endocrinol. 62, 137-143 (1974).

59. Randle, P.J., Young, F.G.: Plasma insulin in acromegaly. Lancet 1, 441-445 (1954).

60. Randle, P.J., Young, F.G.: The influence of pituitary growth hormone on plasma insulin activity. J. Endocrinol. 13, 335-348 (1956).

61. Whittaker, P.G., Taylor, K.W.: Direct effects of rat growth hormone on rat islets of Langerhans in tissue culture. Diabetologia 18, 323-328 (1980).

62. Taylor, K.W.: Regulation of metabolism by hormones other than insulin. In: "Clinical Diabetes and its Biochemical Basis", Eds. Oakley, W.G., Pyke, D.A., Taylor, K.W., Blackwell Scientific Publications, Oxford, pp. 76-98 (1968).

63. McKiddie, M.T., Buchanan, K.D., Munder, I.A.: Plasma insulin studies in two hundred patients with diabetes mellitus. Quart. J. Med. 38, 445-465 (1969).

64. Parker, M.L., Pildes, R.S., Chao, K.L., Cornblath, M., Kipnis, D.M.: Juvenile diabetes mellitus, a deficiency in insulin. Diabetes 17, 27-32 (1968).

65. Taylor, K.W.: Serum insulin in early cases of severe diabetes. Brit. med. J. 1, 511-513 (1963).

66. Weber, B.: Glucose stimulated insulin secretion during "remission" of juvenile diabetes. Diabetologia 8, 189-195 (1973).

67. Seltzer, H.S., Allen, E.W., Herron, A.L., Brennan, M.J.: Insulin secretion in response to glycaemic stimulus, the relation of delayed initial release to carbohydrate tolerance in diabetes mellitus. J. clin. Invest. 46,323-335 (1967).

68. Perley, M.J., Kipnis, D.M.: Plasma insulin responses to oral and intravenous glucose studies in normal and diabetic subjects. J. clin. Invest. 46, 1954-1962 (1967).

69. Lazarus, N.T.: Insulin and insulin-like substances in the circulation. Clin. Endocr. 1, 623-644 (1972).

70. Duckworth, W.C., Kitabchi, A.B., Heinemann, M.: Direct measurement of plasma proinsulin in normal and diabetic subjects. Am. J. Med. 53, 418-427 (1972).

71. Rosenbloom, A.L., Starr, J.I., John, D., Rubenstein, A.H.: Serum proinsulin in children and adolescents with chemical diabetes. Diabetes 24, 753-757 (1975).

72. Gabbay, K.H., DeLuca, K., Fisher, J.N., Mako, M.E., Rubenstein, A.H.: Familial hyperproinsulinemia - an autosomal dominant defect. New Engl. J. Med. 294, 911-915 (1976).

73. Gabbay, K.H., Bergenstall, R.M., Wolff, J., Mako, M.E., Rubenstein, A.H.: Familial hyperproinsulinemia. Partial characterization of circulating proinsulin-like material. Proc. natn. Acad. Sci. U.S.A. 76, 2881-2885 (1979).

74. Block, M.B., Mako, M.E., Steiner, D.F., Rubenstein, A.H.: Circulating C-peptide immunoreactivity. Studies in normal and diabetic subjects. Diabetes 21, 1013-1026 (1972).

75. Heding, L.G.: Human C-peptide in serum. Diabetologia 11, 541-548 (1975).

76. Yue, D.K., Baxter, R.C., Turtle, J.R.: C-peptide secretion and insulin antibodies as determinants of stability in diabetes mellitus. Metabolism 27, 35-44 (1978).

77. Binder, C., Faber, O.K.: Residual beta-cell function and its metabolic consequences. Diabetes 27, (Suppl. 1) 226-229 (1978).

78. Melani, F., Ryan, W.G., Rubenstein, A.H., Steiner, D.F.: Proinsulin secretion by a pancreatic beta-cell adenoma. New Engl. J. Med. 283, 713-719 (1970).

79. Sherman, B.M., Pek, S., Fajans, S.S., Floyd, J.C. Jr., Conn, J.W.: Plasma proinsulin in patients with functioning pancreatic islet cell tumours. J. clin. Endocrinol. Metab. 35, 271-280 (1972).

80. Alsever, R.N., Roberts, J.P., Gerber, J.G., Mako, M.E., Rubenstein, A.H.: Insulinoma with low circulating insulin levels. The diagnostic value of proinsulin measurements. Ann. intern. Med. 82, 347-350 (1975).

81. Turner, R.C., Harris, E.: Diagnosis of insulinomas by suppression test. Lancet 2, 188-190 (1974).

82. Editorial. Diagnosis and treatment of insulin secreting tumours. Lancet 1, 22-23 (1980).

PITUITARY GONADOTROPHINS

G. Hennen and G. Maghuin-Rogister
Endocrinologie Clinique et Expérimentale, Institut de Médecine,
Université de Liège, Liège, Belgium

Introduction

The vast amount of work devoted to studies of the gonadotrophins is easily explained by their key functional role. This review will deal with recent progress in research on the pituitary gonadotrophins, FSH and LH.

The active forms of these glycoproteins consist of two different subunits, α and β, bound by non-covalent linkages. The isolated subunits exhibit a very limited, if any, biological activity. Thus, pituitary gonadotrophins represent an interesting model for the study of the biosynthesis of secreted glycoproteins and of their structure-function relationships.

LH and the other glycoprotein hormones, FSH, thyrotropin (TSH) and chorionic gonadotrophin (CG) are composed of two different subunits (α and β). The α subunit of the various hormones have a similar amino acid sequence regardless of their site of synthesis and hormonal specificity rests upon structural differences between the β subunits and, probably, the native conformation of the various α-β complexes. Comparison of the amino acid sequences of the various β subunits has additionally revealed large segments of the polypeptide chains exhibiting extensive homology (for reviews, see 1 and 2).

Biosynthesis

Experiments performed to identify the anterior pituitary cell

Hormones in Normal and Abnormal Human Tissues, Vol. II

types responsible for synthesis of the gonadotrophins do not give a clear answer to the question of cellular specialization. Classical histological methods suggested the "one cell-one hormone" concept. Light and electron microscope studies using specific immunoreactions against the β subunits of FSH and LH indicated that one cell could contain secretion granules storing both types of gonadotrophins, the respective abundance of LH or FSH being dependent upon the species studied and the physiological state of the animal (3). This also holds true for the human where 90% of gonadotropic cells contain both LH and FSH (4).

Information concerning biosynthesis of LH and FSH is limited compared to that for hCG and TSH (5-11). Several lines of evidence indicate that the synthesis of the α and β subunits is controlled by two individual genes (8, 11). This contrasts with the mechanism of synthesis of holopeptide hormones, such as insulin where a prohormone, pro-insulin, is first synthesized as a single chain polypeptide which is consequently split to yield the hormone with the A and B chains linked by disulfide bridges. By reoxidation experiments of the fully reduced α subunit, it was demonstrated (12) that formation of the disulfide bridges is made possible by a folding of the polypeptide chain of the α subunit, folding being determined by the specific amino acid sequence of the protein. The control of the genes coding for the α and β subunits is markedly different (11).

Studies of hCG and TSH indicate that the scheme of synthesis for the glycoprotein hormones is similar to that of other glycoproteins (13, 14). The original α subunit chain is synthesized as a preprotein differing from the α subunit of the secreted hormone by an additional hydrophobic N-terminal polypeptide (15). This sequence represents the signal inducing ribosomal binding to the endoplasmic reticulum and permitting the nascent protein to move toward the reticulum lumen. This signal peptide is split by a membrane endopeptidase before completion of the polypeptide chain. Microsomal membranes are responsible for glycosylation of the nascent protein, but this process is not a prerequisite for cleavage of the N-terminal part of the presubunit and its sequestration into membrane vesicles (6). Glycosylation includes as a first step the transfer, to the proper asparagines in the nascent polypeptide, of an oligosaccharide composed of N-acetyl-glucosamine and mannose from a lipid intermediate present into microsomal membranes (16). For hCG α subunit, provided that the medium contained microsomal membranes (17), placental mRNA, in the presence of mouse ascites tumour cell lysate, controlled the synthesis _in vitro_ of a glycosylated molecular form of the subunit, rich in mannose linked to asparagine. The asparagine residues susceptible for glycosylation are determined by the code sequence AsN-X-Ser (Thr) in the nascent protein which, at this stage, has a conformation facilitating the close contact between the oligosaccharide substrate, the transfer enzyme and the polypeptide chain. Processing of the polysaccharide side chains involves removal and addition of various monosaccharide residues. Again, as demonstrated for hCG, carbohydrate processing must occur in another cell compartment than the endoplasmic reticulum as this is accomplished _in vitro_ when ribosome free supernatant fractions are added to the medium (17). Adequate association of the α and β subunits is compulsory for an active hormonal complex. The storage at high concentration of the subunits in the same secretion granule appears to create the most favourable conditions for this last maturation process before secretion (15).

Structure Activity Relationships

Like many polypeptide hormones, the first step in the mechanism of action of the glycoprotein hormones is the binding to a specific receptor located at the external face of the plasma membrane of the target cells. Receptor binding triggers a set of biochemical events involving the activation of the plasma membrane adenylate cyclase and resulting in a specific cellular response.

The integrity of the hormone molecule is important for its recognition by the receptor. Interaction of the isolated α or β subunits with the receptor is very low (19, 20, 21). Reduction and alkylation of disulfide bridges also abolishes the binding activity. Thus, tertiary and quaternary structures of the hormone play an important role in the hormone action. Binding activity of chemically modified glycoprotein hormones is drastically reduced. Chemical modification of the α subunit sometimes leads to loss of ability to combine with the β subunit but almost always to the loss of biological activity *in vivo* and *in vitro*. Conversely, chemically modified β subunits are capable of combining with intact α subunits to give an active hormone derivative (22, 23). Progressive removal of monosaccharide units from carbohydrate side chains of hCG or pregnant mare serum gonadotrophin (PMSG) does not affect binding and *in vitro* biological activity to the same extent as modification of the polypeptide chains (24).

Information about the molecular sites involved in hormone-receptor binding can be obtained by comparative studies of hormones prepared from different species and differing slightly in their amino acid sequence (23, 2) or by comparison of the amino acid sequences of the β subunits of TSH, LH, FSH and CG within the same species (25, 26). Another approach is the chemical modification of amino acid side chains, identification of the modified residues in the sequence and evaluation of the resulting effects on binding to receptors and biological activity (22, 23).

Modification of given amino residues of the hormonal sequence by chemical manipulations can affect the binding of the hormone directly or indirectly. Chemical substitution on an amino acid side chain can induce a destabilization of the three dimensional structure of the protein leading to a change of conformation or to a lowering of the affinity between α and β subunits. This in itself can be sufficient to promote dissociation of the hormone at concentrations used in *in vitro* binding assays (27).

Both chemical and physical methods, sensitive to protein conformation changes, such as circular dichroism (27) and nuclear magnetic resonance (28) spectroscopy, have been used to identify the chemical groups of the hormone which interact with the receptors. Both studies showed the important role played by the carboxy-terminal end of the α subunit of LH in its interaction with receptors. Nuclear magnetic resonance spectroscopy demonstrates a substantial change in the conformation of the core of the α subunit on combination with the β subunit. This change in the conformation involves at least one residue in the core of the molecule (His α87) as well as the carboxy-terminal region (Tyr α92 or α93). Removal of the peptide Tyr-Tyr-His-Lys-Ser at the carboxy-terminal end of LH α yields a subunit able to combine to an intact β subunit but the resulting molecule is not recognized by LH receptors (29). Comparison between NMR spectra of native LH and its biologically inactive derivative reveals that the native and the modified hormone have the same conformation. Thus, the loss of biological activity by shortening the C-terminal portion of the α chain is directly correlated to the absence of α92-96 residues. This suggests that an important site (probably Tyr α92 or α93) for the interaction between the hormone and its receptor is located in the portion of the molecule. The association between the α and β subunits results in a mutual adjustment of conformation (27, 28). This reciprocal control of folding gives to the hormone molecule the appropriate structure for binding to the receptors with high affinity.

The study of the fate of the hormone after initial binding at the plasma membrane receptor site is now a field of increasing interest which could well reveal that fragments of the hormone molecule may play a role as biological messengers inside the cell.

References

1. Ward, D.N., Liu, W.K.: The chemistry of ovine and bovine luteinizing hormone. In: "Structure Activity Relationships of Protein and Polypeptide Hormones", Part 1, Eds. Margoulies M., Greenwood, F.C., Excerpta Medica, Amsterdam, pp. 80-90 (1971).

2. Maghuin-Rogister, G., Closset, J., Hennen, G.: The molecular and functional evolution of glycoprotein hormones in the light of their structural relationships. In: "Peptides 1976", Ed. Loffet, A., Editions de l'Université de Bruxelles pp. 325-338 (1976).

3. Moriarty, G.C.: Immunocytochemistry of the pituitary glycoprotein hormones. J. Histochem. Cytochem. 24, 846-863 (1976).

4. Pelletier, G., Leclerc, R., Labrie, F.: Identification of gonadotropic cells in the human pituitary by immunoperoxidase technique. Mol. Cell. Endocrinol. 6, 123-128 (1976).

5. Landefeld, T.D.: Identification of in vitro synthesized pituitary glycoprotein α subunit. J. biol. Chem. 254, 3685-3688 (1979).

6. Bielinska, M., Grant, G.A., Boime, I.: Processing of placental peptide hormones synthesized in lysates containing membranes derived from tunicamycin-treated ascites tumor cells. J. biol. Chem. 253, 7117-7119 (1978).

7. Bielinska, M., Boima, I.: mRNA-dependent synthesis of a glycosylated subunit of human chorionic gonadotropin in cell-free extracts derived from ascites tumor cells. Proc. natn. Acad. Sci. U.S.A. 75, 1768-1772 (1978).

8. Kourides, I.A., Weintraub, B.D.: mRNA-directed biosynthesis of α subunit of thyrotropin : translation in cell-free and whole-cell systems. Proc. natn. Acad. Sci. U.S.A. 76, 298-302 (1979).

9. Chin, W.W., Habener, J.F., Kieffer, J.D., Maloof, F.: Cell-free translation of the messenger RNA coding for the α subunit of thyroid stimulating hormone. J. biol. Chem. 253, 7985-7988 (1978).

10. Landefeld, T.D., McWilliams, D.R., Boime, I.: The isolation of mRNA encoding the alpha subunit of human chorionic gonadotropin. Biochem. biophys. Res. Commun. 72, 381-390 (1976).

11. Daniels-McQueen, S., McWilliams, D., Birken, S., Canfield, R., Landefeld, T., Boime, I.: Identification of mRNA encoding the α and β subunits of human choriogonadotropin. J. biol. Chem. 253, 7109-7114 (1978).

12. Giudice, L.C., Pierce, J.G.: Studies on the disulfide bonds of glycoprotein hormones. J. biol. Chem. 251, 6392-6399 (1976).

13. Blobel, G., Dobberstein, B.: Transfer of protein across membranes. I. Presence of proteolytically processed and unprocessed nascent immunoglobulin light chains on membrane bound ribosomes of murrine myeloma. J. Cell Biol. 67, 835-851 (1975).

14. Lodish, H.F., Rothman, J.E.: The assembly of cell membranes Scient. Am. 240, 38-53 (1979).

15. Birken, S., Fetherston, J., Desmond, J., Canfield, R., Boime, I.: Partial amino acid sequence of the pre-protein form of the α subunit of human choriogonadotropin and identification of the site of subsequence proteolytic cleavage. Biochem. biophys. Res. Commun. 85, 1247-1253 (1978).

16. Waechter, C.J., Lennarz, W.J.: The role of polyprenol-linked sugars in glycoprotein synthesis. Ann. Rev. Biochem. 45, 95-112 (1976).

17. Bielinska, M., Boime, I.: Glycosylation of human chorionic gonadotropin in mRNA-dependent cell-free extracts : post-translational processing of an asparagine-linked mannose-rich oligosaccharide. Proc. natn. Acad. Sci. U.S.A. 76, 1208-1212 (1979).

18. Salesse, R., Castain, G.M., Pernollet, J.C., Garnier, J.: Association-dependent active folding of α and β subunits of lutropin. J. Mol. Biol. 95, 483-496 (1975).

19. Reichert, L.E., Lawson, G.M. Jr., Leiden, F.L., Trowbridge, C.G.: Influence of α and β subunits on the kinetics of formation and activity of native and hybrid molecules of LH and human chorionic gonadotropin. Endocrinology 93, 938-946 (1973).

20. Catt, K.J., Dufau, M.C., Tsuhuhara, T.: Absence of intrinsic biological activity in LH and hCG subunits. J. clin. Endocrinol. Metab. 36, 73-80 (1973).

21. Maghuin-Rogister, G., Closset, J., Combarnous, Y., Hennen, G., Dechenne, Ch., Ketelslegers, J.M.: Study of follitropin receptors in testis using a homologous system : binding of porcine follitropin to plasma membranes from immature porcine testis and correlation with adenylate cyclase stimulation. Europ. J. Biochem. 86, 121-131 (1978).

22. Ward, D.N.: Chemical approach of the structure-function relationships of luteinizing hormone. In: "The gonadotropins: Structure and Function", Ed. McKerns, K.W., Plenum Press, New York, pp. 31-45 (1979).

23. Pierce, J.G., Faith, M.R., Giudice, L.C., Reeve, J.R.: Structure and structure-function relationships in glycoprotein hormones. Ciba Found. Symp. 225-250 (1976).

24. Bahl, O.P., Moyle, W.R.: Role of carbohydrate in the action of gonadotropins. In: "Receptors and hormone action" vol.III, Eds. Birnbaumer, L., O'Malley, B.W., Academic Press, New York, pp. 261-289 (1978).

25. Stewart, M., Stewart, F.: Constant and variable regions in glycoprotein hormone α subunit sequences: implications for receptor binding specificity. J. Mol. Biol. 116, 175-179 (1977).

26. Ward, D.N., Moore, W.T.: Comparative study of mammalian glycoprotein hormones. In: "Animal models for research on contraception and fertility", Ed. Alexander, Nancy, J., Harper and Row Publishers, New York, pp. 151-164 (1979).

27. Parsons, T.F., Pierce, J.G.: Biologically active covalently cross-linked glycoprotein hormones and the effects of modification of the COOH-terminal region of their α subunits. J. biol. Chem. 254, 6010-6015 (1979).

28. Maghuin-Rogister, G., Degelaen, J., Roberts, G.C.K.: ^{1}H Nuclear Magnetic Resonance studies of porcine lutropin and its α and β subunits. Europ. J. Biochem. 96, 59-68 (1979).

29. Cheng, K.W., Glazer, A.N., Pierce, J.G.: The effects of modification of the COOH-terminal regions of bovine thyrotropin and its subunits. J. biol. Chem. 248, 7930-7937 (1973).

CORTICOSTEROIDS AS HORMONES AND METABOLIC PRECURSORS IN NORMAL AND ABNORMAL TISSUES

C. P. Lantos
Departamento de Quîmica Biológica, Laboratorio de Esteroides and Programa de Regulacîon Hormonal y Metabólica, Buenos Aires, Argentina.

The importance of the cortisol : corticosterone (F:B) ratio throughout vertebrates during embryonic development as well as in health and disease, exceeds the descriptive significance to which they had been relegated. The early suggestions for an enhanced cortisol secretion such as the necessity to produce a different glucocorticoid by higher vertebrates to face new homeostatic requirements may still be valid but they do not account for such phylogenetic curiosities as the lack of a detectable 17-hydroxylase activity in some highly specialized homeotherms or its presence in teleosts or even further down the evolutionary scale.

Although corticosterone has only one third the gluconeogenic activity of cortisol, it is also an intermediate in the biosynthesis of other hormones. Free terpenoid radicals such as geranyl and farnesyl whose pyrophosphates (Fig. 1) may be considered as early sterol precursors are also precursors of open-chain chemical communicants in many invertebrates (1).

Corticosterone and its metabolites such as aldosterone, constitute a unique model for the study of precursor-hormone relationships, their regulation and homeostatic implications.

Corticosterone and Cortisol in Development

Corticosterone is to our present knowledge the only ubiquitous

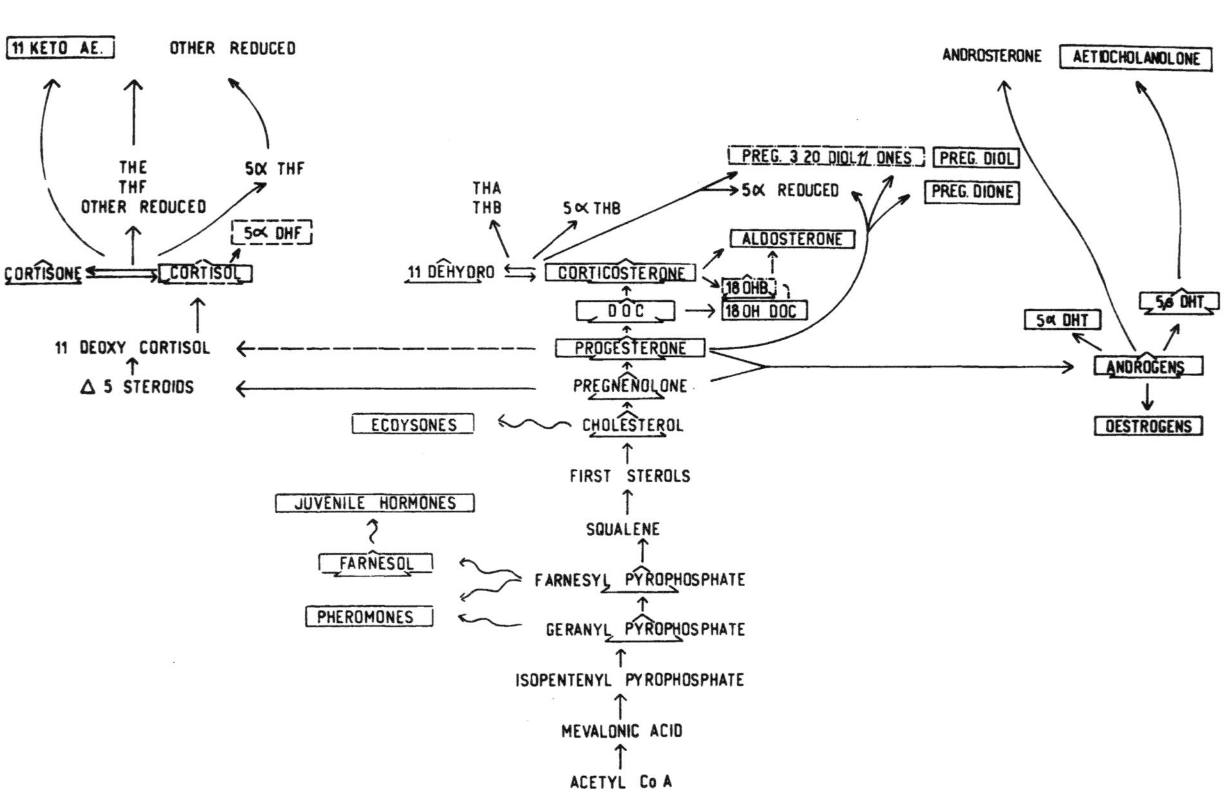

Fig. 1. Metabolic pathways to active steroids and terpenoids. Biologically active compounds are enclosed in rectangles and precursors on cross-roads, in triangles. ———— Important. ------- Secondary. -·-·-·-·-·-·- Postulated. ∿∿→ Invertebrate pathways only.

hormonal corticosteroid throughout the vertebrate scale. Its production is highest among lower, poikilotermic vertebrates: thus in elasmobranchs and reptiles it constitutes the most abundant corticosteroidal hormone and in amphibians its importance is second only to aldosterone (2). Among homeotherms, birds are also predominantly corticosterone secretors, but most normal adult mammals synthesize only minor amounts. Notorious exceptions among mammals are rabbits, secreting less cortisol than corticosterone under basal conditions, and rats as well as most murines which only synthesize the latter.

It is now well established that the _foetal zone_ of early primate adrenals lacks 3 β ol dehydrogenase and that it mainly produces DHEA sulfate. There is no doubt, moreover, that the foetal adrenal's definitive zone is able to produce cortisol (20) and that this production rises before labor. Results regarding foetal corticosterone are less clear-cut. At mid-term, corticosterone secretion by the human foetus is at least as high as the secretion of cortisol and according to several authors (3, 4) even higher. These authors also give clinical and experimental evidence that the foetal adrenal _in toto_ synthesizes more corticosterone than cortisol during this gestational stage.

Cortisol levels increase during gestation but the near-term F:B ratios vary considerably.

Analysis of amniotic fluid provides a method of investigating the offspring's steroid secretion. [^{14}C] Cortisol injected into the maternal circulation reaches the amniotic fluid via foetal urine (5) and the amniotic fluid cortisol level correlates better than maternal cortisol levels with the glucocorticoid concentration in umbilical cord blood. Murphy et al. (7) reported values in the amniotic fluid around 5 ng/ml during weeks 10-15 and around 10 ng/ml at mid-term. Similar values were obtained by Aderjan et al. (8). All studies, however, agree on a rise of cortisol levels starting approximately between the 32nd and the 35th week of gestation. A recent publication (9) describes a high rate of metabolism of cortisol to cortisone by foetal tissues and an increased reduction of cortisone to cortisol by the chorionic membrane during the second half of gestation with a resultant increase in amniotic fluid cortisol before labor. Apparently this sudden increase is elicited by the organism's need for a potent glucocorticoid in response to the stress of labor; but cortisol is also specifically required for parturition as such and for many maturation processes occurring during the last stage of intrauterine life. Thus cortisol seems to have a selective role in pulmonary maturation (10). By contrast, corticosterone maintains constant amniotic fluid levels of 2-20 ng/ml, irrespective of gestational age (8). In plasma of newborns, F:B ratios are around 5.4 and reach values of 10-18 in infant plasmae after delivery (11, 12).

Regulation of F:B Ratios

In most cortisol-producing adrenals the major road of synthesis is the "Δ 5 pathway". Only minor amounts of cortisol originate from progesterone and none at all from DOC or corticosterone. By contrast, the latter is mainly formed via the "Δ 4 pathway". While the variations in both biosyntheses are well established in many species the molecular mechanisms underlying their regulation are complex.

Since the rabbit adrenal produces similar amounts of corticosterone and cortisol, most regulation studies have been carried out on this species. Kass et al. (13) described a decrease in corticosterone and an increase in cortisol secreted by the stimulated rabbit adrenal. Fevold presented evidence that ACTH increased 17-hydroxylase activity <u>in vitro</u> (14) and that the Δ 5 pathway predominated in adrenal tissue from ACTH-stimulated rabbits (15). Yudaev and Morozova reported similar results but suggested that ACTH enhanced 17-hydroxylation of progesterone (16).

Yalow et al. have demonstrated that the pituitaries of corticosterone secretors (rats and mice) contained a molecular species of ACTH approximately twice as large as the 1-39 peptide which predominates in cortisol-producers such as the human, monkey, sheep, pig, dog and cat (17, 18). The rabbit species secretes not only both glucocorticoids but also forms of ACTH. Furthermore, the rabbit responds to stress and to exogenously administered 1-39 ACTH (porcine) with increasing F:B ratios.

In primates, a family of peptides with diverse biological properties stem from a common glycoprotein containing in its molecule the sequences not only of 1-39 ACTH, but also those of β LPH and the short peptides endorphin, α MSH and CLIP, the corticotrophin like-intermediate lobe peptide postulated as the "foetal ACTH", or at least, as the factor on which the foetal adrenal zone depends for its development and persistence (19). In fact, the sequential events described during the development of the foetal adrenal depend greatly, if not exclusively, on a shift in the cleavage pattern of the stem-protein from a CLIP producing, to an ACTH producing, type. In view of the characteristics of glucocorticoid secretions in both zones it is probable that these changes are somehow involved in producing the sudden increase of F:B ratios immediately before delivery. Thus ACTH has been shown to stimulate cortisol production by the human foetus (20) but it has not been demonstrated that CLIP or any other peptide promotes corticosterone secretion.

Adrenal tissue metabolizes the glucocorticoid skeleton to 11-oxo derivatives, with a reduced Ring A and/or a reduced C20 oxo group and, in the particular case of corticosterone, to compounds with an oxidised C18-methyl group. The liver also performs these conversions, the latter excepted, but additionally cleaves the side chain of cortisol thereby giving rise to C11-oxygenated-17-ketosteroids.

Ring A Reduced Derivatives and their Further Metabolism

Vertebrate adrenal or inter-renal tissue, similarly to the liver of vertebrates, contains a particulate and a soluble reductase

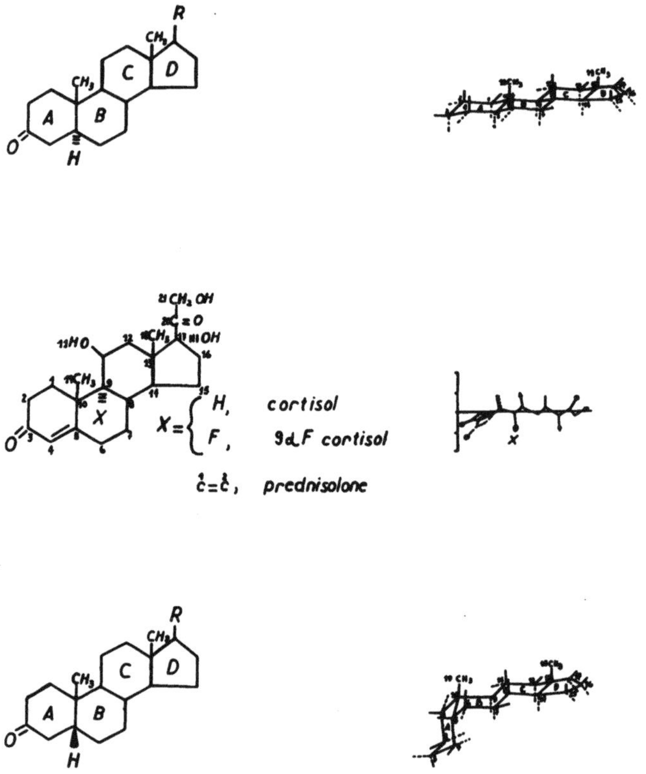

Fig. 2. Conformation of steroids.
Upper: A/B trans or 5α. Middle: Glucocorticoids. Interrupted-line projection corresponds approximately to prednisolone and to 9 F cortisol whereas full-line projection corresponds to cortisol. Lower: A/B cis or 5β, typical of porphyrin inducers if R is not an α ketolic side chain.

system catalysing the biotransformation of 3-oxo-4:5 ene steroids into saturated metabolites (Fig. 2).

We are growing aware, however, that these criteria are by now inadequate, not only for theoretical reasoning - or rationalizations in steroid spectroscopy, but also for explaining most biological or pharmacological effects common to a group of steroidal compounds that apparently do not share structural properties when represented in the classical, planar fashion.

For such correlations, <u>conformational</u> representations, taking into account the tetrahedric distribution of C valences in space, are more appropriate (see Figure 2).

There is evidence for an early appearance of ring A reductase activity in adrenals of mammals and birds while they are still in their embryonic periods. The adrenal of the 15-day old <u>chick-embryo</u>, considered by some authors (21) to represent the species' earliest stage of full endocrine development, synthesizes <u>in vitro</u> 5β-pregnan-3,20-dione from endogenous sources as well as from radioactive progesterone (22). In incubation studies yields were high, indicating the existence of an alternative reductive pathway, at this stage at least as important as corticodiogenesis; 5β-pregnanedione was the most abundant radiometabolite formed and the yields of corticosterone were much lower. Apparently the glucocorticoid was not synthesized in quantities large enough to detect its transformation into reduced compounds. An interesting finding of this work was that no 5α pregnane-3,20-dione could be detected. When radioactive samples from the chromatographic zone were divided into two equal parts and then each aliquot mixed with, respectively, carrier 5α-pregnanedione and 5β-pregnanedione, only the latter could be crystallized to constant specific activity. This was readily achieved, indicating a fair stage of purity of the isolated radioactive fraction even before recrystallizations.

Working with cultures of cortical cells from <u>rat foetuses</u> Salmenperä et al. obtained important yields of "pregnanolone" and "pregnandiols" from ^{14}C progesterone. In some samples they could also detect pregnandiones but unfortunately did not try the separation and characterization of A/B conformers in this mixture nor in other reduced fractions isolated (23).

The adrenal of the <u>near-term human foetus</u> converts labelled progesterone to A/B reduced metabolites. Such metabolites were separated in Villee's laboratory from the adrenal of a foetus 15 cm crown-rump length (24) but could not be detected in glands from younger foetuses (25). In Dorothy Villee's early studies no effort was made to separate epimers.

The corticosteroid composition of human amniotic fluid during the last trimester of pregnancy was studied by means of very specific radioimmunoassays (8). Only THF and THE were found to parallel cortisol and cortisone levels, the four steroids showing a significant correlation with gestational age.

The reductive pathway has been demonstrated in the adult adrenal of almost every mammalian species investigated. A list by no means exhaustive includes the cow (26, 27) the rat (28, 29), mouse (30) and man (25). In birds, the duck adrenal possesses 5α reductase activity but in adults of other avian species the pathway has not been clearly demonstrated. There is evidence that the adult hen has less reductive activity than the 15-day old chick embryo.

Charreau et al. have investigated reduced metabolites originating from [^{3}H] pregnenolone and [^{14}C] progesterone in incubation media of human adult adrenals (25). Tissue samples came from an aldosterone producing tumour, from adrenal tissue adjacent to the tumour and from a case of diffuse nodular adrenal hyperplasia. The authors isolated 5α-pregnanedione but their efforts to isolate the 5β epimer were not successful. The yields of 5α pregnanedione were small: 0.67% for the adrenal adjacent to the aldosterone producing tumour; 0.34% in tissue from nodular hyperplasia. However, comparatively important amounts of reduced metabolites might have been present in the main steroidal fractions isolated, in which crystallizations evidenced a certain degree of contamination of starting material (34).

There can be no doubt, however, that in most adult mammals, especially in the normal human adult, peripheral ring A reduction is quantitatively and functionally more important than the same process in the adrenal. The most important peripheral metabolizing tissue is the liver, but reduction also takes place in the skin, the central nervous system and other sites. Furthermore, target organs of androgens possess strong A/B trans reductive capacity for these hormones.

Fukushima et al. (35) injected [^{14}C] cortisol into five normal men and found after hydrolysis THE and THF, two A/B cis derivatives with unchanged side chains, accounting for almost 50% of radioactivity in urine. Allo-THF, the only A/B trans epimer isolated, accounted only for approximately 10%. Cortols and cortolones having an A/B cis conformation and reduced at C20 correspond to 20-30%, with the 11-ketoderivatives present in much larger proportion. The cleavage of the side chain of cortisol occurred to a limited extent and the authors could isolate 2 to 12% of radioactivity as 11βOH-5α-androstanolone and 11-oxo-5α-androstanolone. All other compounds, including at that time unrevealed steroids (among them, probably, 6β-hydroxycortisol) accounted for less than 10%. The latter group also contained between 0.8 and 2% of unconverted cortisol.

Recent studies on the excretion of human steroid metabolites using high resolution techniques such as gas-chromatography on glass open tubular capillary columns (36) basically confirm Fukushima's results. Unfortunately though, from the comparison of the findings by both groups as well as from numerous other publications, a discrepancy arises as to the quantitative importance of 11-oxo-5α-androstanolone. Pfaffenberger and Horning only detect it in very small amounts, in urine of pregnant women (36). This steroid is the only cortisol metabolite listed above classified as a "strong" porphyrin inducer (see later).

Corticosterone is also metabolized to a high degree in peripheral tissues. Early studies (reviewed in (38)) indicate a greater proportion of A/B trans steroids and a lack of C19 steroids. But Engel et al. (39) showed that corticosterone may be reduced at C-21 during peripheral transformation giving rise to 5β-pregnane-3α 20-diol-11-one and its 5α epimer.

Recently, interesting findings have been made regarding this 21-dehydrogenation. As summarised by Shackleton et al. (40), only compounds that undergo biliary excretion can be reduced at C-21. Cortisol, in contrast to corticosterone and deoxycorticosterone, is not excreted in bile and consequently C-21-reduced metabolites are not found in urine of persons to whom cortisol had been administered. Moreover C-21 reduction in bile is mediated, not by mammalian enzymes but by entero-bacteria.

Shackleton et al. (40) found that 21-deoxycorticoids comprised the major metabolites of [^{14}C] corticosterone injected into an adult woman with 17-hydroxylase deficiency, in urine samples collected on the second and third day after administration. Since in the first 24-hour sample these steroids only account for less than 20% of total radioactivity, the authors conclude that "tetrahydro" and "hexahydro" metabolites of corticosterone may circulate several times between the intestine and the liver before being excreted in the urine and that during circulation these metabolites are increasingly dehydroxylated at C-21 as a consequence of enterobacterial action.

Progesterone and 17-hydroxyprogesterone of adrenal origin constitute minor components of the general progesterone-and 17-hydroxyprogesterone pools which the liver metabolizes to various A/B cis derivatives bearing either carbonyls or hydroxyls at C-3, C-11 and C-20. Most of these derivatives are listed by Granick and Kappas as porphyrin inducers (37).(See also Figures 1 and 2).

Ring A Reduction and Regulation

The importance of ring A reductases in the regulation of rat adrenal function was recognised more than 20 years ago by Yates and collaborators (41) who suggested that hepatic inactivation of corticosterone might be responsible for negative feed-back control of ACTH secretion. Ring A reduction is still considered as one of several factors modulating the hypothalamic-pituitary-adrenal axis.

In fact, in many states of adrenal hypofunction increased ring A reduction occurs <u>in addition to</u> an inhibition of glucocorticoid synthesis and numerous factors stimulating glucocorticoidogenesis inhibit at the same time ring A reduction. This symmetric relationship can be noted in the molecular events occurring during ACTH action. ACTH increases adrenal corticosterone output by making more exogenous cholesterol available to the hydroxylating sites and by activating phosphorylation of proteins leading to specific, precursor hydroxylations (31) in addition to inhibiting further metabolism of corticosterone. An ACTH effect on the reductive pathway in the rat adrenal was first shown by us with quartered glands, ACTH decreased the conversion of labelled corticosterone to a compound with the chemical properties of 3α, 11β, 21-trihydroxy-5α-pregnan-20-one (42, 43). Kitay and his colleagues have found a specific inhibitory effect of administered ACTH on 5α reductase in homogenates of these glands whereas cortisone administration enhanced the activity of the enzyme. Hypophysectomy also resulted in an increased activity of 5α reductase whereas ACTH administration could reverse this effect (44).

The inhibitory action of ACTH is not limited to adrenal tissue; a similar effect was found in rat liver (45). In man, ACTH definitely exerts an extra-adrenal effect on the peripheral metabolism of cortisol. Kornel has reviewed his own clinical studies and those of others, on the role of ACTH in prolonging the biological half-life of cortisol (46). The author gives indirect evidence for decreased 11-hydroxydehydrogenase and ring A reducing activities in ACTH treated patients, but these studies need further confirmation. In the rat, experiments have been reported regarding sex differences (47), effect of gonadectomy (48) and hypothalamic-hypophyseal control (44, 49) of these steroid reductions.

Sex has a definite influence on A/B conformations of metabolites formed by the human liver. It has been known for many years that women excrete larger amounts of A/B cis conformers than men but values for 5α/5β ratios in the former usually showed high dispersions. Only recently could Pfaffenberger and Horning account for this diversity among an otherwise homogeneous female population. The authors established cis/trans ratios in males and in premenopausal, as well as postmenopausal females. Although they could not find any difference between the two latter groups, they were able to divide the total female population, according to the type of their steroid metabolism, into "Pattern A" females, in which these ratios were high, and "Pattern B" females, in which they were indistinguishable from those found in males. This classification was valid for aetiocholanolone/androsterone (0.21 to 0.75 in Pattern B *vs*. 0.92 to 1.83 in Pattern A), as well as for THF/allo-THF (0.70 to 1.59 in Pattern B *vs*. 2.00 to 4.57 in Pattern A). Two thirds of the women analyzed exhibited "Pattern A" ratios (50).

Metabolic differences between rats and humans cast doubts on the existence of similarities in processes regulating specific enzyme reactions in both species. This does not mean, however, that the general mechanisms underlying control of steroid metabolisms in rat liver and adrenal may not operate in the human as well. In the rat, certain enzymes, e.g. adrenal 5α reductase, can be deactivated upon ablation of a regulatory gland (hypophysis) but immediately restored by ACTH (44). Alternatively, alterations may be "programmed" or "imprinted" during a critical period before the onset of puberty, after which replacement becomes inefficient. Most, but not all, sex-linked control mechanisms of hepatic or adrenal steroid-patterns are of this type (48, 66). Imprinting and/or replacement may depend on the presence and/or integrity of the hypothalamic-hypophyseal axis (49), thereby demonstrating that, in some cases, programming (here associated to "maturation") takes place at these central levels while in others it occurs in the metabolizing tissue itself. This complexity and multiplicity of CNS-hypophyseal-gonadal control of hepatic and adrenal ring A reduction in the rat gives an idea of what might be expected in man.

The only clear-cut effect of thyroid hormones on the metabolism of cortisol is a shift from 11β-hydroxyl to 11-oxo steroids. However, androgens, among them 11β-hydroxyandrostenedione, are converted mainly to A/B trans metabolites in the presence of high endogenous thyroxine levels and to A/B cis metabolites when these levels are low (32).

Biological and Pathological Implications of A/B Conformations

Fig. 2 shows that A/B trans steroids, 3-oxo-4,5-ene-steroids and A/B cis derivatives differ in the angles at the union of rings A and B. These angles increase from 0° in A/B trans conformers to about 90° in the latter. Conjugated double bonds of the 3-oxo-4,5-ene type bestow upon ring A a slight torsion that can be augmented by the introduction of a second double bond (1:2) and the substitution of a hydrogen at C9 by a halogen atom (33). Duax et al. have shown that the well known glucocorticoid-potentiating properties of both alterations correlate with angular increments (51), the ability to increase the torsion angle of ring A being, on the other hand, their only common structural characteristic. Based on experiments with steroids and receptor models, the authors postulate an optimal distance between the 3-oxo group and typical functional groups on the α-ketolic side chain for receptor-steroid interactions to take place.

Most probably similar correlations can be applied to A/B cis metabolites of androgens and progesterone, including those of adrenal origin like pregnandione, 11-ketopregnandione, 11-ketoaetiocholanolone and probably some of the 21-dehydro metabolites of corticosterone obtained by enterobacterial action (Figs. 1 and 2). These steroids control haemoglobin formation through the regulation of haemo-(37, 52-56) and globin (57) biosynthesis. The control is characterized by its ubiquitous, as well as its primitive nature. Indeed, the effects have been demonstrated in a surprisingly extensive group of cells, organs, species and developmental stages ranging from chick blastoderm to adult human bone marrow. With cell cultures of the latter, 5β-derivatives could also stimulate the growth of early and late erythroid precursor cells (56). Both at the cellular and the molecular levels, most effects are early, i.e. maturation processes. These steroids catalyze the first steps of porphyrin synthesis (37, 52-56) and probably the translation of mRNA coding for the globin chains of primitive haemoglobins (57).

As mentioned above, 5β-pregnandione is the most important adrenal steroid found in incubations with chick-embryos (22), but 5β-reductase activity in chicken is present as early as the blastoderm (58). This embryonic formation contains high-affinity binding mechanisms, specific for active 5β-steroids (59) and is stimulated by these steroids to produce foetal haemoglobin (57). Active 5β-steroids, including ecdysones, the molting sterols of insects, may in fact be considered as "protohormones".

The biological action of 5β reduced androgens and gestagens has been associated for more than ten years by Kappas and Granick with the "periodic exacerbations which characterize the natural history of the hereditary form of hepatic porphyria" (54). Clinical observations leading to this association included the high incidence of acute intermittent hepatic porphyri in women, despite its genetic nature as an autosomal dominant trait, the relationship of attacks to certain phases of the menstrual cycle, the frequency of the disease during pregnancy and the exacerbations occasionally evoked by the administration of steroid mixtures, including contraceptives (54). Recently, Anderson et al. have studied the influence of cis/trans conformation patterns on the expression of the disease in women in which it was genetically latent (60).

Another syndrome depending on 5β-steroids is "aetiocholanolone fever". In 1957, Kappas discovered that the administration of this steroid provoked an intense fever, rigor and swelling at the site of injection and that these symptoms subsided when the treatment was interrupted (61). Other steroids with similar pyrogenic effects were 5α-pregnanolone, 11-keto 3α-pregnanolone and lithocholic acid, a coincidence which again suggests that A/B cis conformation is mandatory, although not sufficient, for the expression of the syndrome. The latter is thought to be infrequent but more clinical studies are needed to exclude its presence in fevers of unknown origin that can be related to pregnancy, menstrual episodes or a particular pattern of hepatic or adrenal metabolism.

The use of active 5β steroids has been suggested for aplastic anemia and the stimulation of erythropoiesis in certain forms of bone marrow failure (56) but the authors draw attention to the obvious side-effects of the treatment by these pyrogenic steroids.

Mention should be made of erythropoietic and hematopoietic effects of steroids other than A/B cis compounds, if only to emphasize differences. Testosterone stimulates heme and haemoglobin synthesis in liver cells from foetuses of 10-13 weeks only in the presence of erythropoietin. Glucocorticoids possess effects on erythropoiesis that have been applied in the treatment of congenital erythroid hypoplastic anemia. Golde et al. (62) working with mouse foetal livers, suggest that erythroid progenitor cells may contain a glucocorticoid receptor modulating the response to erythropoietin. Bozzini et al. postulate that dexamethasone would be able to induce differentiation of stem cells into pronormoblasts by a mechanism similar to that proposed for erythropoietin (63). On perfusing rat liver with blood or erythrocites, alanine synthetase, the first enzyme of the porphyrin pathway, diminishes rapidly its activity unless glucocorticoids are added to the medium. This protective effect cannot be obtained by aetiocholanolone or testosterone (64).

Unexpected consequences of an abnormality in the peripheral metabolism of cortisol have been found recently: a patient exhibiting subnormal levels of known mineralocorticoids converted labelled cortisol in more than normal amounts to unconjugated metabolites. The free fraction consisted mainly of ring-A reduced dihydroderivatives of cortisol, among which A/B trans conformers predominated (65). In view of these findings and the report by Marver and Edelman (67), according to which 5α-dihydrocortisol possessed mineralocorticoid properties, Adam et al. (65) investigated this steroid's ability to occupy renal mineralocorticoid receptors and its influence on electrolyte excretion in the adrenalectomized rat. The authors found a low affinity of 5α-dihydrocortisol for mineralocorticoid receptors in the kidney and a very low mineralocorticoid activity when administered alone, but an amplification of the action of aldosterone by physiological quantities of the 5α steroid. These astonishing observations may pave the way to a better understanding of steroidal hypertension, and even to new basic concepts regarding hormone-receptor interactions.

Oxidation of the C-18 Methyl

The angular C-18 methyl of almost all steroid families can be oxidised by adrenal-specific enzymes to primary alcohols and some of these, further to aldehydes. From the biological point of view, C-18 oxidation is most important in pregnane derivatives. However, cortisol cannot undergo C-18 oxidation because its angular methyl is sterically protected from attack. In unhindered C-21-steroids, the formation of C-18 aldehydes and C-18 alcohols in close proximity to C-20 carbonyls and/or C-11 hydroxyls gives rise to equilibria with cyclic ketals and hemiacetals (Figs. 3 and 4) which are more stable than their open-ring tautomers. Tautomeric equilibria are one of several structural peculiarities of C-18-oxidised corticosteroids that seem to be related to their characteristic effects on the composition and maintenance of the milieu intérieur.

Quantitatively, the most abundant C-18-oxidised corticosteroid is 18-hydroxydeoxycorticosterone or "18-OH-DOC". The steroid is a major secretion product of the rat adrenal, second only to corticosterone (68-70). In contrast to aldosterone, it is formed by the zona fasciculata where DOC, as well as progesterone, are efficient substrates for its biosynthesis (71). Birmingham and her colleagues have assayed the steroid in the sodium-retention test in adrenalectomized rats (72). They found that it inhibited the excretion of sodium by the kidney to a degree equal to that of DOC at the lower, but not at the higher doses. However, it did not increase potassium excretion and, in fact, had slight potassium-retaining properties and also caused slight urine retention. Due to high 18-OH-DOC levels in the rat, the steroid may be a "true mineralocorticoid" in this species (73).

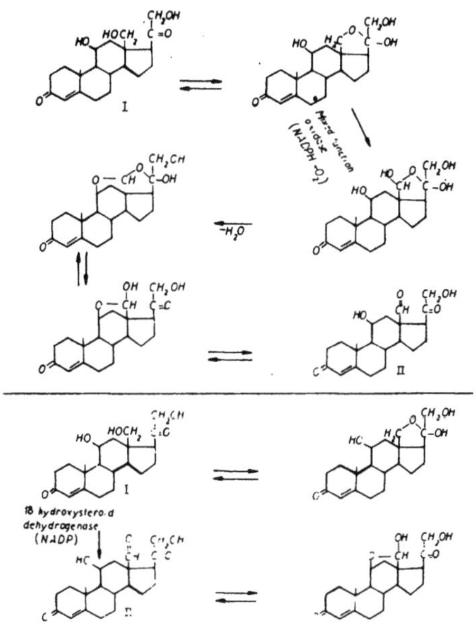

Fig. 3. Two alternatives for the late C18-oxidation step.

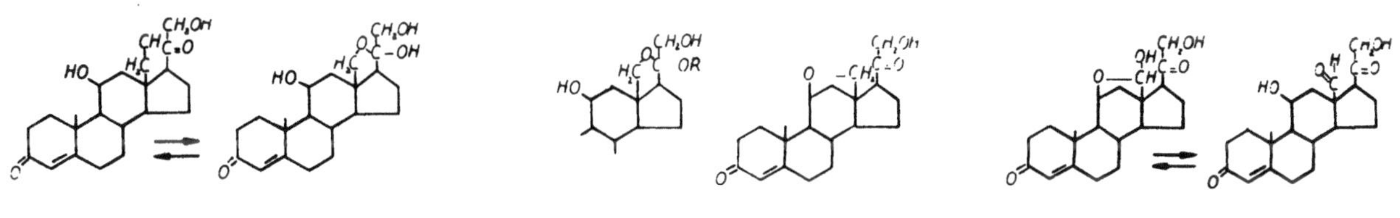

18 OH B

"L" FORMS of 18 OHB

ALDOSTERONE

Fig. 4. 18-OH-B, aldosterone and two "L" forms postulated after mass-spectrometry.
Not shown is a dimeric form whose structure is under discussion.

Other mammals, including Muridae closely related to Rattus, produce 18-OH-DOC in much smaller quantities. De Nicola et al. reported the conversion of radioactive progesterone and DOC to 18-OH-DOC in non-tumorous adrenals obtained from patients with breast carcinoma (74). Moreover, relatively high blood levels are exhibited by some hypertensives whose disease may be ascribed to adrenal abnormalities (75).

It is at the corticosterone level that the biological and clinical importance of C18-oxidation becomes most evident. The formation of aldosterone, mainly via corticosterone, fits into a general scheme of vertebrate adaptations to osmotic challenges of the environment and body fluids. Indeed, aldosterone is absent, or at least undetectable by our present techniques, in ureotelic marine vertebrates but is very important in vertebrates migrating either periodically or once in their life-span, during metamorphosis, from water to dry ground. Thus aldosterone is the main corticosteroid of frogs (2) and its production by dipnoos is among the highest in the animal kingdom (77).

The Biosynthesis of 18-Hydroxycorticosterone and Aldosterone

Theoretically the conversion of corticosterone to aldosterone occurs in two steps: a hydroxylation to 18-hydroxycorticosterone ("18-OH-B") and a dehydrogenation of this diol to aldosterone. The enzymic systems catalyzing these reactions are often collectively referred to as "18 hydroxylase" but this term, appropriate for the first step, has obvious shortcomings when applied to the overall oxidation of the angular methyl to an aldehyde or the biotransformation of 18-OH-B to aldosterone. In fact, many questions on this transformation still remain unanswered. While, for example, corticosterone is an efficient precursor of aldosterone as well as of 18-OH-B, the latter, in spite of its apparent position as a metabolic intermediate, is only poorly converted to the mineralocorticoid. One reason given for this poor conversion was that the 18,20-hemiketal form that predominates in material isolated as 18-OH-B (its "M" form, 78) is not a suitable substrate for aldosterone, whose stable tautomers are bridged between 11 and 18, i.e. in the opposite sense (Figs. 3 and 4). For this hypothesis to be valid, one has to admit that the second step takes place via the open forms of both steroids and hence, that an NADP-dependent hydroxysteroid dehydrogenase catalizes this oxidative reaction.

However, the requirements for NADPH or an NADPH generating system and molecular oxygen (79, 80) are more in agreement with an enzymic hydroxylation. Experimental evidence now points to two consecutive hydroxylations although dehydrogenation as an alternative to the second one cannot be discarded (81). This conversion may even occur spontaneously (82). The alternatives for the second step can be better understood upon inspection of Fig. 3. A more detailed discussion is available (84). As seen in Fig. 3, "opposite-sense" cycling of 18-OH-B vis à vis aldosterone can only be held responsible for the lack of dehydrogenation, but not of hydroxylation of the former. Obviously this complicates the problem of corticosterone being a better precursor of aldosterone than its 18-hydroxylated metabolite.

Prevailing hypotheses generally admit the existence of "active" intermediates that differ structurally from isolated 18-OH-B, but these hypotheses do not agree on the exact role of these intermediates nor that of the latter. The most accepted scheme is that of Ulick (85) who postulates a transient, reactive, metaloenzymebound steroidal intermediate between 18-OH-B and aldosterone. In this scheme, isolated 18-OH-B is biochemically inert and originates from the former, in addition to aldosterone, as an end-product of a secondary reaction. Ulick's hypothesis explains many metabolic, as well as clinical findings (see below) and is in agreement with general ideas proposed for similar conversions (86). But the reactive enzyme-bound intermediate has not been characterized. Whitehouse and Vinson (87) proposed an endogenous chain of protein-bound intermediates .

Another line of investigations emphasizes the structural features of forms and derivatives of 18-OH-B which *in vitro* had a better precursor-capacity for aldosterone. These forms are all less polar than "M" and were therefore denominated "L" forms. They can be obtained upon storage of "M" in alcohols and acidic solutions (88-93). The structures vary greatly according to their origin (91), but most of them result from an interchange of the labile hemiketalic hydrogen. Alkyl ketals have been demonstrated (90, 91) and dimeric structures in which two monomeric molecules of 18-OH-B interact at C-20 have been postulated (89, 92) but need more confirmation. Alternatively, anhydrides have been obtained from acidic solutions (91).

It is not yet quite clear which "L" forms are better aldosterone-substrates (89); at least the anhydride is spontaneously converted with higher yields than other steroids (82) and may also be involved in the second hydroxylation step (95). Moreover, at least one "L" other than the anhydride is efficiently converted to the mineralocorticoid. Until we have a clearer image of these facts, however, we can only speculate on the molecular mechanisms underlying these relative efficiencies. Their less polar nature undoubtedly facilitates solubility in lipids and hence transport through membranes. On the other hand, one possible anhydride-structure (Fig. 4) would make this particular "L" form an appropriate substrate for aldosterone (82, 95, 96).

Corticosterone and 18-OH-B can be synthesized in the fasciculata as well as in the glomerulosa zone. Aldosterone, by contrast, is the only corticosteroid exclusively produced by one zone, the glomerulosa (71). Besides re-emphasizing the importance of a more thorough knowledge of the two-step biosynthesis, this anatomical characteristic is important for a better understanding of clinical syndromes related to the enzymic process.

Clinical Defects in C-18 Oxidation

Ulick (85) reviewed defects in the two steps of aldosterone biosynthesis by the human adrenal, which he denominated "Type 1" and "Type 2" methyl-oxidase deficiencies referring to, respectively, a defective 18-hydroxylation of corticosterone and a defective conversion - by whatever mechanism - of 18-OH-B or the enzyme-bound intermediate to aldosterone.

Type 1 deficiency was described by Visser and Cost (97) in offspring (two girls and one boy) of three families related by consanguinous marriages. Urinary steroid-patterns of these patients revealed high excretions of corticosterone metabolites but very low excretions of tetrahydro-aldosterone and tetrahydro 18-OH-A (85), the main metabolite of 18-OH-B in urine (98). Finkelstein, in a recent review on inborn errors of steroid biosynthesis (95) cites one more report.

Type 2 deficiency was originally described by Ulick et al. in 1964 (98) and this description was complemented (85) with cases reported by David et al. (99). One striking feature of this syndrome is the high urinary TH aldosterone/TH-18-OH-A ratios of affected patients. These ratios are approximately 2 in normal subjects and in Type 1 deficiency but between 80 and 300 in Type 2 variety (85), suggesting that an elevated 18-OH-B secretion is an outstanding feature of this disorder. However, Ulick drew attention to one necessary qualification of the Type 2 methyl oxidase defect, i.e. that the excess 18-OH-B must originate from the zona glomerulosa. "Abnormally high 18-hydroxycorticosterone of fasciculata zone origin does occur in another condition, the 17-hydroxylase defect (96) where accentuation of pathways leading to corticosterone and 18-OH-DOC also results in increased secretion of 18-OH-B from that zone, while the glomerulosa zone secretion is suppressed by the high levels of circulating DOC characteristic of this disorder. Fasciculata zone 18-OH-B is readily distinguished from the glomerulosa zone steroid by the ease with which it can be suppressed be dexamethasone" (85).

Symptoms such as hyperkalaemia, hiponatraemia, occasional dehydration and failure to gain weight are common to both types (95). Interestingly enough, Type 1 patients present with intermittent fever (95) but for the time being one cannot decide whether these temperatures are of steroidal aetiology.

Biological Consequences of C-18 Oxidation

Corticosterone loses its glucocorticoidal properties upon oxidation of the angular C-18 methyl. If, however, C-18 oxidation is only partial, then the angular methyl is converted to a primary alcohol whose hydroxyl cyclises with the C-20 carbonyl of the side chain, the C-11 hydroxyl remaining free. The resulting steroid, 18-OH-B, is neither a glucocorticoid nor has it sodium retaining effects.

Has 18-OH-B a biological role at all, other than that of a possible aldosterone precursor ? Recently, Damasco et al. (108) administered the steroid to adrenalectomized rats and found an increased excretion of buffered hydrogen ions in urine, as well as a seven-fold decrease in the elimination of CO_3H^- ions. In view of the highly complex nature of acid-base regulation in mammals, nothing can be said about the mechanism(s) of the observed steroidal effect nor its anatomical site of action.

Regulation of C-18 Oxidation by ACTH

C-18 oxidation is regulated by a much more complex mechanism than either ring A reduction, C-11-OH dehydrogenation or any other metabolic reaction affecting corticosteroids. The regulation of the various factors affecting ionic changes must be precise.(For excellent reviews see 100-103). From a technical point of view, research on such a complicated feed-back system depends on the model employed. Different effects are obtained with the same regulator if one changes species, dietary condi-

tions or regulator-dose and if in vivo results are compared to in vitro incubations with whole tissue or glomerulosa or with isolated cells of multizonal or unizonal origin.
Two main regulatory loci in the steroidal pathway to aldosterone have been postulated. The first is generally referred to as an "early" locus or as one "prior to corticosterone". It consists mainly of the rate-limiting step at the cleavage of cholesterol side chain, but none of the other "molecular" and "cellular" events known to participate in ACTH control of the common corticoidogenic pathway can here validly be discarded. The second site of regulation is situated between corticosterone and aldosterone. Since the "late oxidation step" of this biotransformation is probably much slower than the first one, it is tempting, in spite of our poor knowledge, to ascribe to the conversion of 18-OH-B to aldosterone a rate-limiting, and hence a regulatory, character (109).

When quartered rat adrenals were incubated with a variety of radioactive precursors, ACTH added to the medium not only inhibited the conversion of corticosterone to a ring A-reduced metabolite but also to aldosterone (43). Likewise, De Nicola demonstrated a decreased aldosterone production by adrenals of rats bearing an ACTH secreting tumour (104) and Müller showed that ACTH administered to rats under various experimental conditions suppressed aldosterone output and decreased radioactive conversions to aldosterone and 18-OH-B by capsular adrenal tissue (105). None of these results are in agreement with publications in which ACTH, in addition to its predominant action on an early locus in the steroidogenic pathway, also stimulates the conversion of corticosterone to aldosterone by the rat adrenal (106-107). It is extremely difficult to correlate the conditions employed by each group with apparently contradictory results. Common features of the experiments in which ACTH had an inhibitory effect were the relatively high quantities of hormone either added in vitro or administered chronically (secreted pathologically) and the more complex nature of the enzyme source in in vitro studies. In contrast, ACTH stimulation of aldosterone biosynthesis in the rat was obtained in isolated glomerulosa cells and at lower ACTH levels. On the other hand, in *in vivo* results in rats, ACTH consistently *lowered* the aldosterone:corticosterone ratio (6). ACTH had no aldosterone-inhibiting effects on normal primate adrenals but in many cortisol-producing species, including man, ACTH administration first stimulates aldosterone secretion acutely and the effect is reversed upon continued treatment.

ACTH action on human adrenal tissue is being studied under conditions similar to those used for a similar study with rat adrenals (83). So far we have analyzed an adrenocortical adenoma and its collateral adrenal in a case of primary aldosteronism, two adrenocarcinomas, one hypernephroma with corticosterone-C-18 methyl-oxidase activity and two "normal" adrenals. Aldosterone secretion rates before and after surgery in the aldosteroma case were similar to the ratios between the tumour's and the collateral adrenal's aldosterone content. These findings validate to a certain extent the *in vitro* results obtained. ACTH inhibited aldosterone formation by the tumour but not by control adrenal tissue (83). Of the more recent cases, only tumours exhibiting a strong C-18 oxidase activity were sensitive to the inhibitory effect of ACTH.

Based on experiments of the last 15 years, we postulate the following ideas on sites and directions of ACTH action: The trophin acts on the biosynthesis of glucocorticoids (site 1) and on their further metabolism (site 2). Site 1 is more important than site 2 which comprise ring A reduction, C-18 oxidation and probably C-11-OH-dehydrogenation (76). While consistently inhibiting ring A reduction, ACTH stimulates or inhibits aldosterone formation depending on the conditions. Stimulation requires low ("physiological" ?) ACTH levels while inhibition requires higher ("pathological" ?) levels and/or chronical secretion. The rat, an exclusive corticosterone producer, is more sensitive than are cortisol producers to the inhibitory effect and this may be due to homeostatic reasons; the organism increasing its glucocorticoid in response to stress but not wanting to raise mineralocorticoid levels at the same time. There are human aldosteromas that behave biosynthetically and from a regulatory viewpoint like rat adrenals whereas normal human adrenals behave consistently like those of other cortisol producers.

Future studies in the field are directed towards the genetic bases of this tumoral "regression" and towards molecular mechanisms underlying bidirectional trophin effects. (Fig. 5).

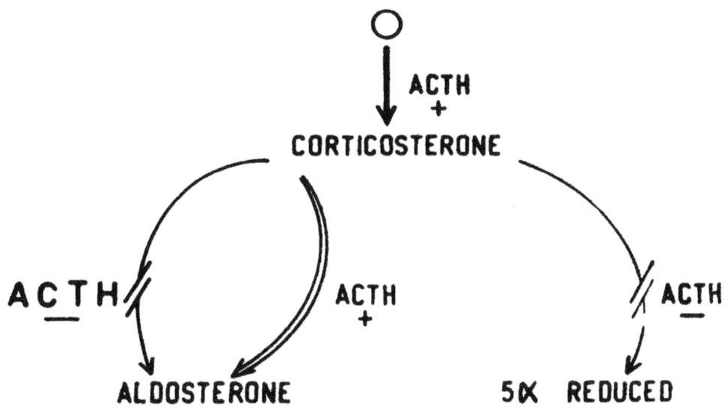

Fig. 5. Multisite and bidirectional effects of ACTH Sites 1 are above corticosterone and sites 2 below corticosterone.

References

1. Pennock, J.F.: Terpenoids in marine vertebrates. In:"International Review of Biochemistry",Biochemistry of Lipids II, vol. 14, Ed. Goodwin, T.W., University Park Press, Baltimore, pp. 153-213 (1977).

2. Carstensen, H., Burgers, A.C.J., Li, C.H.: Demonstration of aldosterone and corticosterone as the principal steroids formed in incubates of adrenals of the American Bullfrog and stimulation of their production by mammalian ACTH. Gen. comp. Endocr. 1, 37-50 (1961).

3. Oakey, R.E., Cawood, M.L., Isherwood, D.M., Heys, R.F., Shahwan, M.M.: Corticosteroid biosynthesis by the human fetal adrenal. J. Steroid Biochem. 8, 505-513 (1977).

4. Cawood, M., Heys, R.F., Oakey, R.E.: Corticosteroid production by the human foetus: evidence from analysis of urine from women pregnant with a normal or an anencephalic foetus. J. Endocrinol. 70, 117-126 (1976).

5. Abramovich, D.R., Wade, A.P.: (quoted in 7).

6. Lantos, C.P., Dahl, V., Cordero Funes, J.R., de Nicola, A.F.: A correlation study between adrenal function and the duration of sustained ACTH treatment in the rat. Acta physiol. lat.-amer. 23, 277-287 (1973).

7. Murphy, B.E.P., Patrick, J., Denton, R.L., Clarks, J., Marvin, M., Haidar, R.: Cortisol in amniotic fluid during human gestation. J. clin. Endocr. Metab. 40, 164-167 (1975).

8. Aderjan, R., Rauh, W., Vecsei, P., Lorentz, U., Rüttgers, H.: Determination of cortisol tetrahydrocortisol, tetrahydrocortisone, corticosterone and aldosterone in human amniotic fluid. J. Steroid Biochem. 8, 525-528 (1977).

9. Murphy, B.E.P.: Cortisol and cortisone in human fetal development. J. Steroid Biochem. 11, 509-513 (1979).

10. Farrell, P.M.: Fetal lung development and the influence of glucocorticoids on pulmonary surfactant. J. Steroid Biochem. 8, 463-470 (1977).

11. Homoki, J., Teller, W.: Studies on cortisol/corticosterone ratios in plasma as indirect measure of 17α-hydroxylase activity during childhood. Acta endocr. 69 (Suppl. 159), 74 (1972).

12. Villee, D.B.: The development of steroidogenesis. Amer. J. Med. 53, 533-544 (1972).

13. Kass, E.H., Hechter, O., Macchi, I.A., Mou, T.W.: Changes in patterns of secretion of corticosteroids in rabbits after prolonged treatment with ACTH. Proc. Soc. exp. Biol. Med. 85, 583-587 (1954).

14. Fevold, R.H.: The pathways of corticosteroid biosynthesis by homogenates of adrenal tissue from rabbits stimulated with adrenocorticotropin. Biochemistry 8, 3433-3439 (1969).

15. Fevold, H.R.: Regulation of the adrenal cortex secretory pattern by adrenocorticotropin. Science 156, 1753-1755 (1967).

16. Yudaev, N.A., Morozova, M.S.: (quoted in 14).

17. Coslovsky, R., Yalow, R.S.: Influence of the hormonal forms of ACTH on the pattern of corticosteroid secretion. Biochem. biophys. Res. Commun. 60, 1351-1356 (1974).

18. Boiti, C., Yalow, R.S.: Corticosteroid response of rabbits and rats to exogenous ACTH. Endocrine Res. Commun. 5, 21-33 (1978).

19. Silman, R.E., Chard, T., Lowry, P.J., Mullen, P.E., Smith, I., Young, I.M.: Human fetal corticotrophin and related pituitary peptides. J. Steroid Biochem. 8, 553-557 (1977).

20. Jaffe, R.B., Serón-Ferré, M., Mitchell, B.F.: Perinatal regulation of cortisol in the primate. J. Steroid Biochem. 11, 549-555 (1979).

21. Willier, B.H.: Phases in embryonic development. J. cell. comp. Physiol. 43, 307-317 (1954).

22. Pedernera, E.A., Lantos, C.P.: The biosynthesis of adrenal steroids by the 15-day old chick embryo. Gen. comp. Endocrinol. 20, 331-341 (1973).

23. Salmenperä, M., Kahri, A.I., Saure, A.: Effects of corticosterone on adrenocorticotrophin induced mitochondrial differentiation with special reference to 11β and 18-hydroxylation. J. Endocrinol. 70, 215-222 (1976).

24. Villee, D.B., Engel, L.L., Villee, C.A.: Steroid hydroxylation in human fetal adrenals. Endocrinology 65, 465-474 (1959).

25. Charreau, E.H., Dufau, M.L., Villee, D.B., Villee, C.A.: Synthesis of 5α-pregnane-3,20-dione by fetal and adult human adrenals. J. clin. Endocr. Metab. 28, 629-632 (1968).

26. Levy, H., Cagill, D.I., Cha, C.H., Hood, B., Carlo, J.J.: The isolation of 18-hydroxy-3-oxo-androst-4-ene-17α-carboxylic acid-20, 18-lactone, its 11β-hydroxy analog and other substances from bovine adrenal perfusions of deoxycorticosterone. Steroids 5, 131-146 (1965).

27. Lantos, C.P., Raman, P.B., Graves, J.M.H., Dorfman, R.I., Forchielli, E.: The biosynthesis of 5α-pregnane-3,20-dione by cow adrenal preparations. Steroids 6, 69-79 (1965).

28. Brown-Grant, K., Forchielli, E., Dorfman, R.I.: The Δ4 hydrogenases of guinea-pig adrenal gland. J. biol. Chem. 235, 1317-1320 (1960).

29. Schneider, J.J., Horstman, P.M.: Effects of incubating desoxycorticosterone with various rat tissues. J. biol. Chem. 191, 327-338 (1951).

30. Ertel, R.J., Ungar, F.: In vitro effect of 2 methyl 1,2 bis (3-pyridil) 1-propanone (SU4885) and NADPH in the mouse adrenal. Endocrinology 75, 949-956 (1964).

31. Garren, L.D., Gill, G.N., Masvi, H., Walton, G.: On the mechanism of action of ACTH. Recent Progr. Hormone Res. 27, 433-478 (1971).

32. Bradlow, H.L., Zumoff, B., Fukushima, D.K., Hellman, L., Gallagher, T.F.: Metabolism of 11β hydroxy Δ^4 androstene dione: effect of thyroid hormone. J. clin. Endocr. Metab. 26, 949-955 (1966).

33. Duax, W.L., Weeks, C.M., Rohrer, D.: Crystal structure of steroids: Molecular conformation and biological function. Recent Progr. Hormone Res. 32, 81-116 (1976).

34. Charreau, E.H.: Personal communication.

35. Fukushima, D.K., Bradlow, H.L., Hellman, L., Zumoff, B., Gallagher, T.F.: Metabolic transformation of hydrocortisone-4-^{14}C in normal men. J. biol. Chem. 235, 2246-2255 (1960).

36. Pfaffenberger, C.D., Horning, E.C.: Determination of human urinary steroid metabolites by glass open tubular capillary columns. J. Chromatogr. 112, 581-594 (1975).

37. Granick, S., Kappas, A.: Steroid induction of porphyrin synthesis in liver cell culture I. structural basis and possible physiological role in the control of heme formation. J. biol. Chem. 242, 4587-4593 (1967).

38. Pasqualini, J.R.: Contribution à l'étude des corticostéroides. Foulon Impr., Paris, p. 13 (1962).

39. Engel, L.L., Carter, P., Fielding, L.: Urinary metabolites of administered corticosterone steroids liberated by glucoronidase hydrolysis. J. biol. Chem. 213, 99-106 (1955).

40. Shackleton, C.H.L., Biglieri, E.C., Rotiman, E., Honour, J.W.: Metabolism of radiolabeled corticosterone in an adult with a 17α hydroxylase deficiency syndrome. J. clin. Endocr. Metab. 48, 976-982 (1979).

41. Yates, A.L., Herbst, A., Urquhart, J.: Sex difference in rate of ring A reduction of Δ4 3-ketosteroids in vitro by rat liver. Endocrinology 63, 887-902 (1958).

42. Lantos, C.P., Birmingham, M.K., Traikov, H.: ACTH action on a reductive pathway in the quartered rat adrenal. Acta physiol. lat.-amer. 16, 278-281 (1966).

43. Lantos, C.P., Birmingham, M.K., Traikov, H.: Effect of ACTH on the metabolism of radioactive C21 steroids by quartered rat adrenals. Acta physiol. lat.-amer. 17, 42-54 (1967).

44. Kitay, J.I., Coyne, M., Swygert, N.H.: Effects of hypophysectomy and administration of cortisone or ACTH on adrenal 5α reductase activity and steroid production. Endocrinology 89, 432-438 (1971).

45. Deckx, R., De Moor, P., Denef, C., Rauss, J.: Effect of adrenalectomy, sham operation or ACTH on the cortisol metabolizing enzymes of rat liver homogenate. Metabolism 14, 264-270 (1965).

46. Kornel, L.: Corticosteroids in human blood. V. Extra-adrenal effect of ACTH upon metabolism of cortisol. Steroidologia 1, 225-245 (1970).

47. Eriksson, H., Gustaffson, J.A.: Metabolism of corticosterone in the isolated perfused rat liver. Europ. J. Biochem. 20, 231-236 (1971).

48. Kitay, J.I., Coyne, M.D., Swygert, N.H.: Influence of gonadectomy and replacement with estradiol or testosterone on formation of 5α reduced metabolites of corticosterone by the adrenal gland of the rat. Endocrinology 87, 1257-1265 (1970).

49. Gustaffson, J.A., Eneroth, P., Pousette, A., Skett, P., Sonnenschein, C., Steinberg, A., Ahlen, A.: Programming and differentiation of rat liver enzymes. J. Steroid Biochem. 8, 429-443 (1977).

50. Pfaffenberger, C.D., Horning, E.C.: Additional data supporting sex differences in human urinary steroid metabolic profiles. Anal. Biochem. 88, 689-694 (1978).

51. Weeks, C.M., Duax, W.L., Wolff, M.E.: A comparison of the molecular structures of six corticosteroids. J. Am. chem. Soc. 95, 2865-2868 (1973).

52. Granick, S.: The induction of δ-aminolevulinic acid synthetase in vivo in chick embryo liver by natural steroids. Proc. natn. Acad. Sci. 61, 509-513 (1968).

53. Congote, L.F., Stern, M.D., Solomon, S.: Hormone control of heme synthesis in cultures of human fetal liver. Biochemistry 13, 4255-4263 (1974).

54. Kappas, A., Granick, S.: Experimental hepatic porphyria: studies with steroids of physiological origin in man. Ann. N.Y. Acad. Sci. 151, 842-849 (1968).

55. Levere, R.D., Kappas, A., Granick, S.: Stimulation of hemoglobin synthesis in chick blastoderm by certain 5β-androstane and 5β-pregnane steroids. Proc. natn. Acad. Sci. 58,985-990 (1967).

56. Urabe, A., Sassa, S., Kappas, A.: The influence of steroid hormone metabolites on the in vitro development of erythroid colonies derived from human bone marrow. J. exp. Med. 149, 1314-1325 (1979).

57. Irving, R.A., Mainwaring, I.P., Spooner, P.M.: The regulation of hemoglobin synthesis in cultured chick blastoderm by steroids related to 5β-androstans. Biochem. J. 154, 81-93 (1976).

58. Parsons, I.C.: The metabolism of testosterone by early chick embryonic blastoderm. Steroids 16, 59-65 (1970).

59. Spooner, P.M. Mainwaring, I.P.: Possible relevance of the formation of 5β-reduced steroids to hematopoesis in chick blastoderm. Acta Endocrinol. Suppl. 177, 181 (1973).

60. Anderson, K.A., Bradlow, H.L., Sassa, S., Kappas, A.: Relationship of the 5α reductive metabolism of steroid hormones to clinical expression of the genetic defect in acute intermittent porphyria. Am. J. Med. 66, 644-650 (1979).

61. Kappas, A., Hellman, L., Fukushima, D.K., Gallagher, T.F.: The pyrogenic effect of etiocholanolone. J. clin. Endocr. Metab. 17, 451-453 (1957).

62. Golde, D.W., Bersch, N., Cline, M.J.: Potentiation of erythropoiesis in vitro by dexamethasone. J. clin. Invest. 57, 57-62 (1976).

63. Bozzini, C.E., Alippi, R.M.: Erythropoietin-like activity of dexamethasone on the time-course of radioiron incorporation into red blood cells of erythremic mice. Acta physiol. lat.-amer. 21, 21-24 (1971).

64. Bock, K.W., Krauss, E., Fröhling, W.: Regulation of δ-aminolevulinic acid synthesis by drugs and steroids in vivo in isolated perfused rat liver. Europ. J. Biochem. 23, 366-371 (1971).

65. Adam, W.R., Funder, J.W., Mercer, J., Ulick, S.: Amplification of the action of aldosterone by 5α-dihydrocortisol. Endocrinology 103, 465-471 (1978).

66. De Moor, P., Denef, C.: The "puberty" of the rat liver. Feminine patterns of cortisol metabolism in male rats castrated at birth. Endocrinology 82, 480-492 (1968).

67. Marver, D., Edelman, I.S.: 5α-dihydroxycortisol: a potential mineralocorticoid. J. Steroid Biochem. 9, 1-8 (1977).

68. Birmingham, M.K., Ward, P.: The identification of the Porter-Silber chromogen secreted by the rat adrenal. J. biol. Chem. 236, 1661-1667 (1961).

69. Péron, F.G.: Isolation of 18-hydroxydeoxycorticosterone from rat adrenals. Endocrinology 69, 39-45 (1961).

70. Lantos, C.P.: Área preóptica y equilibrio endócrino en la rata. Thesis, Doct. Pharmacy and Biochemistry, University of Buenos Aires (1962).

71. Sheppard, H., Swenson, R., Mowles, T.F.: Steroid biosynthesis by rat adrenal. Endocrinology 73, 819-824 (1963).

72. Birmingham, M.K., MacDonald, M.L., Rochefort, J.G.: Adrenal function in normal rats and in rats bearing regenerated adrenal glands. In: "Functions of the Adrenal Cortex", Ed. McKerns., C.C. Appleton, New York, pp. 647-689 (1968).

73. Nicholls, M.G., Brown, W.C.B., Hay, G.D., Mason, P.A., Fraser, R.: Arterial levels and mineralocorticoid activity of 18-hydroxy-11-deoxycorticosterone in the rat. J. Steroid Biochem. 10, 67-70 (1979).

74. de Nicola, A.F., Traikov, H., Birmingham, M.K., Palmer, J.D., Ruddick, D.W.: 18-Hydroxylation by human adrenal tissue in vitro. J. clin. Endocr. Metab. 30, 402-405 (1970).

75. Genest, J., Nowaczynski, W., Kuchel, O., Boucher, R., Rojo Ortega, J., Constantopoulos, G., Ganten, D., Messerli, F.: The adrenal cortex and essential hypertension. Recent Progr. Horm. Res. 32, 377-427 (1976).

76. Devalle, J.J., Lantos, C.P.: An effect of ACTH on the metabolism of 1,2 ^{3}H-corticosterone by a cell free rat adrenal preparation. Acta physiol. lat.-amer. 21, 356-259 (1971).

77. Idler, D.R., Sangalang, G.B., Truscott, B.: Corticosteroids in the South American lungfish. Gen. comp. Endocr. Suppl.3 238-244 (1972).

78. Dominguez, O.V.: The presence of two interconvertible forms of 18-hydroxy-11-deoxycorticosterone. Steroids Suppl. 2, 29-49 (1965).

79. Raman, P.B., Sharma, D., Dorfman, R.I.: Studies on aldosterone biosynthesis in vitro. Biochemistry 5, 1795-1804 (1966).

80. Marusic, E.T., White, A., Haedo, A.R.: Oxidative reactions in the formation of an aldehyde group in the biosynthesis of aldosterone. Archs Biochem. Biophys. 157, 320-321 (1973).

81. Kahnt, F.W., Neher, R.: Über die Adrenale Steroid Biosynthese in vitro. I. Umwandlung endogener und exogener Vorstuffen im Nebennieren Homogenat des Rindes. Helv. chim. Acta 48, 1457-1476 (1965).

82. Aragonés, A., Lantos, C.P., Locascio, G.A.: Spontaneous conversions to aldosterone. Acta physiol. lat.-amer. 26, 277-282 (1976).

83. Dahl, V., Scattini, C.M., Lantos, C.P.: Comparative biosynthesis studies in a case of primary aldosteronism. J. Steroid Biochem. 7, 715-717 (1976).

84. Fraser, R., Lantos, C.P.: 18-Hydroxycorticosterone: a review. J. Steroid Biochem. 9, 273-286 (1978).

85. Ulick, S.: Diagnosis and nomenclature of the disorders of the terminal portion of the aldosterone biosynthetic pathway. J. clin. Endocr. Metab. 43, 92-96 (1976).

86. Hochberg, R.B., McDonald, P.D., Lieberman, S.: Transient, reactive intermediates in the biosynthesis of pregnenolone from cholesterol. In: Proc. Fourth Int. Congr. Endocrinol. Washington 1972, American Elsevier Publishing Co., N.Y. p. 801 (1973).

87. Vinson, G.P., Whitehouse, B.: The biosynthesis and secretion of aldosterone by the rat adrenal zona glomerulosa and the significance of the compartmental arrangement of steroids. Acta endocr. 72, 52-76 (1973).

88. Kondo, E., Mitsugi, T., Tori, K.: Microbiological synthesis of aldosterone from corticosterone. J. Am. chem. Soc. 87, 4655-4656 (1965).

89. Damasco, M.C., Lantos, C.P.: The existence of two interconvertible forms of 18-hydroxycorticosterone. Is one of them an active precursor of aldosterone. J. Steroid Biochem. 6, 69-74 (1975).

90. Roy, A.K., Ramîrez, L.C., Ulick, S.: Structure and mechanism of formation of the two forms of 18 hydroxy 11-deoxycorticosterone. J. Steroid Biochem. 7, 81-87 (1976).

91. Aragonés, A., Gros, E.G., Lantos, C.P., Locascio, G.: Less polar forms and derivatives of 18-hydroxycorticosterone. J. Steroid Biochem. 9, 175-180 (1978).

92. Pappo, R. (quoted in 26).

93. Prost, M., Maume, B.F.: Hormones stéroides de la surrénale de rat: analyse des 18-hydroxycorticostéroides par chromatographie gaz-liquide couplée à la spectrométrie de masse. J. Steroid Biochem. 5, 133-144 (1974).

94. Finkelstein, M., Schaefer, M.: Inborn errors of steroid biosynthesis. Physiol. Rev. 59, 353-406 (1979).

95. Ulick, S.: Normal and alternate pathways in aldosterone biosynthesis. In: Proc. Fourth Int. Congress Endocrin., Washington 1972, American Elsevier Publishing Co., New York, pp. 761-767 (1973).

96. Visser, H.K.A., Cost, W.S.: A new hereditary defect in the biosynthesis of aldosterone. Urinary C21-corticosteroid pattern in three related patients with a salt-loosing syndrome suggesting an 18-oxidation defect. Acta endocr. 47, 589-612 (1964).

97. Ulick, S., Gautier, K.K., Vetter, J.R., Markello, R., Yaffe, S., Lowe, C.: An aldosterone biosynthetic defect in salt-losing disorder. J. clin. Endocr. 24, 669-672 (1964)

98. David, R., Golan, S., Drucker, W.: Familiar aldosterone deficiency. Pediatrics 41, 403-412 (1968).

99. Laragh, J.H., Sealey, J., Brunner, H.: The control of aldosterone secretion in normal and hypertensive man. Am. J. Med. 53, 649-663 (1972).

100. Williams, G.H., Dluhy, R.: Aldosterone biosynthesis. Am. J. Med. 53, 595-605 (1972).

101. Müller, J.: Regulation of aldosterone biosynthesis. Springer Verlag, Heidelberg (1971).

102. Fraser, R., Mason, P.A., Buckingham, J., Gordon, R., Morton, J.J., Nichols, M.G., Semple, P.F., Tree, M.: The interaction of sodium and potassium status, of ACTH and of angiotensin II in the control of corticosteroid secretion. J. Steroid Biochem. 11, 1039-1042 (1979).

103. de Nicola, A.F., Dahl, V., Kaplan, S.: Transformation of ^{14}C-pregnenolone and production of corticosteroids by adrenal glands from rats bearing a transplantable mammotropic pituitary tumor. J. Steroid Biochem. 4, 205-215 (1973).

104. Müller, J.: Suppression of aldosterone biosynthesis by treatment of rats with adrenocorticotrophin: comparison with glucocorticoid effects. Endocrinology 103, 2061-2068 (1978).

105. Aguilera, G., Catt, K.J.: Loci of action of regulators of aldosterone biosynthesis in isolated glomerulosa cells. Endocrinology 104, 1046-1052 (1979).

106. Haning, R., Tait, S.A.S., Tait, J.F.: Effect of ACTH, angiotensin, serotonin and potassium on steroid output and conversion of corticosterone to aldosterone by isolated adrenal cells. Endocrinology 87, 1147 (1970).

107. Damasco, M.C., Diaz, F., Cenal, J.P., Lantos, C.P.: Acute effects of three natural corticosteroids on the acid-base composition of urine in adrenalectomized rats. Acta physiol. lat.-amer. (in press).

108. Aupetit, B., Aubry-Marais, F., Legrand, J.C.: Comportement comparé de la 18 hydroxy-corticostérone de synthèses et de la 18 hydroxycorticostérone "endogène" dans la synthèse de l'aldostérone. Biochimie 59, 311-321 (1977).

ARGININE VASOTOCIN : IDENTIFICATION AND BIOLOGICAL ACTIONS IN MAMMALS

R. L. Zerbe and G. L. Robertson
Veterans Administration Medical Center and Indiana University School of Medicine, Indianapolis, Indiana, U.S.A.

Arginine vasotocin is a phylogenetically ancient hormone which is thought to be the ancestor of all known neurohypophyseal hormones of vertebrates (1-3). In non-mammalian vertebrates, it appears to have an important function in reproduction (4-6) and body fluid balance (7-9). Recent evidence suggests that it is also present and biologically active in mammals but its role in mammalian physiology is unknown. Here we will critically review the evidence for the presence of vasotocin in mammals and review some of its biological actions.

Structural Characteristics of Vasotocin

Arginine vasotocin shares many molecular characteristics with the other eight known neurohypophyseal hormones, all of which are composed of nine amino acids, linked in a pentapeptide ring by a disulfide bond connecting positions 1 and 6. It differs by only one amino acid from the two mammalian neurohypophyseal hormones, oxytocin and arginine vasopressin (Fig. 1). Substitution of leucine for arginine in position 8 yields oxytocin while replacing isoleucine with phenylalanine in position 3 yields arginine vasopressin. Each of these amino acid substitutions could result from a single base change in the respective DNA codon (2). This factor plus its presence in primitive vertebrates which lack oxytocin and vasopressin (10) suggests that vasotocin was the common precursor from which the known neurohypophyseal hormones evolved.

Hormones in Normal and Abnormal Human Tissues, Vol. II

	1		2		3		4		5		6		7		8		9		
ARGININE VASOTOCIN	CYS	-	TYR	-	ILE	-	GLN	-	ASN	-	CYS	-	PRO	-	ARG	-	GLY	-	NH_2
ARGININE VASOPRESSIN	CYS	-	TYR	-	PHE	-	GLN	-	ASN	-	CYS	-	PRO	-	ARG	-	GLY	-	NH_2
OXYTOCIN	CYS	-	TYR	-	ILE	-	GLN	-	ASN	-	CYS	-	PRO	-	LEU	-	GLY	-	NH_2

Fig. 1. Structural characteristics of vasotocin compared to those of vasopressin and oxytocin. The amino acid differences are underlined.

Identification of Vasotocin in Animal Tissues

Historical background

Vasotocin was not identified in animal tissues until well after the structure and biological characteristics of other neurohypophyseal hormones were known. Based on structure activity relationships, it was hypothesized that vasotocin, a molecule containing the ring of oxytocin and the side chain of arginine vasopressin, would share biological properties of both (11). Studies of synthetic vasotocin not only confirmed this hypothesis but also demonstrated a uniquely potent natriferic effect of vasotocin on frog bladders (12, 13). These observations led to the recognition that the natriferic activity of a frog neurohypophyseal extract which had been described previously by Heller (14) was due to vasotocin (12). The hormone has subsequently been identified in all vertebrates (2). While it is most readily detectable in the neurohypophysis of lower vertebrates (15), vasotocin has also been found in the tissues of mammals (16-26), including man (27-29).

Bioassay of Vasotocin

Vasotocin has a number of biological actions in common with both oxytocin and arginine vasopressin (Table 1), but its most characteristic effect is the capacity to stimulate the transport of sodium across frog bladder or skin. Recognition of this natriferic activity led to the original identification of vasotocin in tissue extracts and has since served as the basis for a number of bioassay systems (16, 23, 30-32). The natriferic activity of vasotocin can be detected by crude methods such as increases in body weight in frogs after injection of tissue extracts (14) or by more sophisticated methods involving the measurement of short circuit currents across isolated frog bladders (31). Since oxytocin (33), vasopressin (33) as well as some pharmacologic agents (34) also have natriferic effects on the frog bladder assay, detection of such activity alone is insufficient to conclude that vasotocin is present. To make this distinction additional studies are necessary. Most commonly, bioassay systems rely on ratios of natriferic to oxytocic or antidiuretic activities for the identification of vasotocin (23, 30, 32). Paper (13, 16) or gel column (23) chromatography can be used to separate vasotocin from oxytocin, but the separation of vasotocin from arginine vasopressin generally requires ion exchange chromatography (35). Inhibitory agents such as trypsin, which cleaves peptide bonds involving lysine or arginine (36), can also be used to distinguish vasotocin from oxytocin but not from vasopressin.

Whether by bioassay ratios, chromatography or the use of inhibitors, the techniques which must be employed to achieve specificity in the bioassay of vasotocin are relatively complex. The multiple measurements required by these assay systems make them very cumbersome to perform, subject to increased error and difficult to quantitate. The sensitivity of the bioassay is relatively low and quite variable, depending on the type of animal used (32) and the season of the year (31). Thus, though useful to identify the hormone in tissue extracts of non-mammalian vertebrates, the bioassay of vasotocin is less satisfactory for routine quantitation in other biologic fluids which contain relatively lower concentrations of the hormone.

Table 1

Biological Activities of Neurohypophyseal Hormones

	Rat Uterus (Oxytocic) IU/mg	Rat Antidiuresis (Antidiuretic) IU/mg	Frog Bladder (Natriferic) IU/mg
Arginine Vasotocin	240	195	34,000
Arginine Vasopressin	20	400	90
Oxytocin	500	1	500

Radioimmunoassay of vasotocin

In contrast to bioassays, radioimmunoassays tend to be more sensitive and simpler to perform. Unfortunately, most antibodies to vasotocin cross-react with either vasopressin (25, 37) or oxytocin (38). This cross-reactivity is generally not a problem in studies of lower vertebrates in which oxytocin and/or vasopressin are not present, but significantly complicates the measurement of vasotocin in mammals. To achieve the specificity necessary for mammalian studies, some laboratories have found it necessary to simultaneously measure unknown samples in other radioimmunoassays specific for oxytocin or vasopressin and use the difference between the results as a measure of vasotocin (37). Such multiple assays decrease the sensitivity and accuracy while increasing the complexity of the procedure.

However, it has also been possible to develop some antibodies with sufficient specificity to measure vasotocin directly without interference from vasopressin or oxytocin. One such antibody provided by Dr. Jack George cross-reacts by less than 5% with either hormone (Fig. 2). When used at a dilution of 1:20,000 at 1,000 counts per minute of ^{125}I-vasotocin as tracer, this assay can detect a minimum of 3 pg of unlabeled standard vasotocin. This sensitivity is equal to that of the best bio-

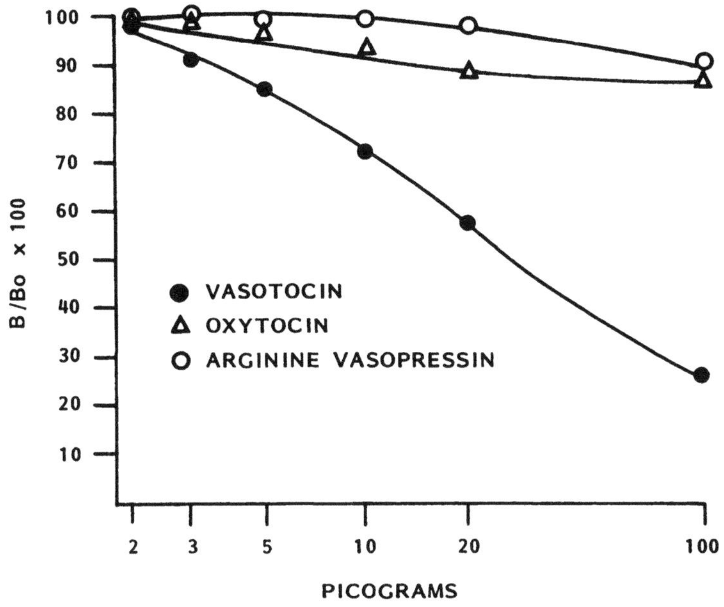

Fig. 2. Curves for standard vasotocin, oxytocin and arginine vasopressin in the vasotocin radioimmunoassay system. Antibody provided by Dr. Jack George is used in a dilution of 1:20,000 with 1000 c.p.m. of ^{125}I vasotocin. Buffers, incubation time and separation procedure identical to those used in our radioimmunoassay for arginine vasopressin (79).

assay and has simplified the measurement of the hormone in man.

Vasotocin in the mammalian central nervous system

Early studies failed to identify vasotocin-like biological activity in mammalian neurohypophyseal tissue (39). Subsequent studies, however, using more sensitive assay procedures have identified the hormone in the pineal (16-19, 23, 22, 24, 26, 28), neurohypophyseal (23, 25, 27, 29), and other neural tissues (20) of mammals.

The pineal gland has been the focus of most studies of vasotocin in mammals. Milcu, Pavel and Neacsu first proposed the existence of vasotocin in bovine pineal tissue when they extracted a partially purified polypeptide which had the biologic, chromatographic and enzymatic inactivation properties of arginine vasotocin (16). The presence of vasotocin in mammalian pineal was subsequently confirmed by radioimmunoassay (19, 28), immunocytochemical staining (22), and peptide sequencing (18). While the latter procedures leaves little question that vasotocin exists in the area of the pineal, evidence is accumulating that vasotocin is not in the pinealocytes per se (40). Instead it appears to be present in and secreted by ependymal cells which are found primarily in the stalk of the adult pineal (41). Thus, extracts of the stalk contain most of the vasotocic activity recoverable from the pineal (42), pineal ependymal cells in culture synthesize vasotocin (43) and immunocytochemical stains for vasotocin in fetal mammals identify cells which are not pinealocytes (22).

The ependymeal origin of vasotocin may explain the relatively low vasotocin content of the adult mammalian pineal (21), since the primitive secretory ependymal cells regress markedly after birth (41). It may also explain the detection of vasotocin in fetal neurohypophyseal tissue (23, 25, 29) since similar ependymal structures are found in the fetal pineal and neurohypophysis (27). The vasotocin content of the neurohypophysis, like that of the pineal, decreases with increasing gestational age (29), and the hormone has not been detected by radioimmunoassay (37) or bioassay (23) in the neurohypophysis of adult mammals. Whether this indicates complete regression of secretory cells or is due to difficulty detecting smaller amounts of vasotocin in the presence of other neurohypophyseal hormones is not clear.

An adult neural structure which does contain vasotocin is the subcommissural organ (20). This primitive ependymal structure projects into the third ventricle at the border between the diencephalon and mesencephalon just below the posterior commissure (44). Early studies suggested histologic and histochemical similarities of the subcommissural organ of both the neurohypophysis and pineal (45). This led to the detection of vasotocin in the subcommissural organ of adult and fetal animals by both bioassay (43) and radioimmunoassay (20).

Vasotocin in human cerebrospinal fluid

The detection of vasotocin in the pineal gland and subcommissural organ of adult mammals led to studies of vasotocin in cerebrospinal fluid since, by virtue of their location, both these organs have direct contact with the third ventricle. In two such studies vasotocin was not detected by bioassay in normal unanesthetized adult humans (46, 47). However, samples of cerebrospinal fluid from the lumbar cistern of nine patients with diabetes insipidus were reported to have vasotocin-like bioactivity averaging 3,855 USP/IU/ml frog bladder activity (= 110 pg/ml) (46). Vasotocin has also been reported in spinal fluid of healthy adults under thiopental anesthesia (47). Levels detected in these subjects were the equivalent of 60-90 pg/ml (47). In both studies the frog bladder activity was destroyed by trypsin which excluded oxytocin as the responsible hormone. Arginine vasopressin is present in the cerebrospinal fluid of patients with diabetes insipidus (48), but the concentrations reported (1.4 to 3.3 pg/ml) could have accounted for only a very small portion of the total activity in the frog bladder assay.

In our studies vasotocin was measured by radioimmunoassay in samples of cerebrospinal fluid obtained from 14 patients during diagnostic lumbar puncture. Three of the patients had diabetes insipidus. We were unable to detect any significant vasotocin like immunoreactivity (<15 pg/ml) in patients either with or without diabetes insipidus. Our results are therefore consistent with previously reported failures to detect the hormone in cerebrospinal fluid of healthy adults, but do not support the observation of very high levels in patients with diabetes insipidus. This difference may be explained in one of four ways. First, quantitation errors related to differences in purity of the vasotocin standards used in the two assay systems. This, however, seems unlikely when we consider that the values previously reported are seven times the lower limit of detectability for our radioimmunoassay. Second, the patient populations may not be comparable. This possibility cannot be excluded since the patients reported in the previous study were not well described as to the origin, severity or chronicity of the underlying illness (46). Third, unlike previous studies, our samples of cerebrospinal fluid were extracted with acetone prior to assay. Such an extraction eliminates nonspecific immunoreactivity due to high molecular weight proteins. Fourth, our cerebrospinal fluid samples were stored for weeks to months at -4°C prior to assay. The stability of vasotocin in cerebrospinal fluid under such conditions is unknown but under similar circumstances vasopressin is completely stable (48). None of these possibilities can be conclusively excluded at this time. Hence, we believe it is premature to draw any conclusions about the presence or absence of vasotocin in the spinal fluid of adult man.

Vasotocin in amniotic fluid

Vasotocin, being a predominantly fetal hormone has been implicated in normal parturition (49) and fetal fluid balance (50). However, in thirteen amniotic fluid samples obtained during diagnostic amniocenteses in 21-41 week pregnancies, vasotocin was found to be uniformly undetectable (< 15 pg/ml). For the reasons previously cited during discussion of spinal fluid, these findings do not necessarily exclude the presence of AVT in amniotic fluid. The failure to detect the hormone in amniotic fluid could also have been due to sampling too late in the gestational period, or to rapid destruction of vasotocin by aminopeptidases present in maternal plasma (51).

Vasotocin in urine

Fetal peptides like α-fetoprotein and carcinoembryonic antigen have proved useful as markers for certain types of neoplasia. Their utility derives from the fact that they are not produced appreciably by healthy adult cells but are sometimes synthesized and released in large amounts by dedifferentiated malignant tissue. Since vasotocin has been reported to be present in the neurohypophysis of fetal but not adult mammals (23, 37), we hypothesized that it too might be useful as a marker for certain malignancies. Oat cell carcinoma of the lung have been shown to produce other peptide hormones including vasopressin (52), and one has been reported tentatively to contain vasotocin (53). We examined urine of 21 patients with various types of lung cancer by our radioimmunoassay for vasotocin. All assays were performed on unextracted urine which had been adjusted to isotonicity by appropriate amounts of distilled water. We found easily detectable levels of immunoactivity in all urine samples. The absolute values ranged from 739 to 8,194 (mean 2,747)pg/mg creatinine (Table 2).

Because a search of the literature revealed no previous attempts to identify vasotocin in urine of healthy adults, we also assayed samples from four normal controls. To our surprise, we found readily detectable levels of vasotocin-like immunoreactivity in all four samples (Table 2). The absolute values ranged from 485 to 4,500 (mean 1,544)pg/mg creatinine. Though slightly lower, the normal values did not differ significantly from those found in the cancer patients.

The unexpected finding of relatively large amounts of vasotocin-like immunoreactivity in the urine of normals as well as cancer patients prompted us to undertake additional studies to more thoroughly characterize the nature of this activity. Several lines of evidence indicated that it was not due to cross-reaction with vasopressin or oxytocin. First, given its low cross-reactivity in the vasotocin assay (Fig. 2), the amounts of vasopressin present in the urine (Table 2) were too low to

Table 2

Urinary Measurement of Vasotocin and Vasopressin

	Vasotocin Immunoreactivity pg/mg creatinine mean ± SE (range)	Vasopressin Immunoreactivity pg/mg creatinine mean ± SE (range)
Normal	1544 ± 986	490 ± 164
(4)	(485 to 4500)	(17 to 750)
Lung Carcinoma	2747 ± 589	1282 ± 429*
(21)	(739 to 8194)	(229 to 9461)

*$p < .05$ vs vasotocin

Table 2. Measurements of vasotocin and vasopressin determined by separate and specific radioimmunoassay systems in the urine of normal subjects and patients with carcinoma.

have produced any appreciable interference. Oxytocin levels were not measured in any of our samples but if they were similar to levels found by others in normal human urine (54) they would also have been too low to significantly cross-react. Second, 10-fold serial dilutions of the urine samples from both normal and cancer patients produced displacement curves which parallel completely that of standard vasotocin (Fig. 3). Vasopressin and oxytocin, on the other hand, produced much shallower displacement curves (Fig. 2), clearly indicating that they contributed virtually nothing to the immunoreactivity detected in urine with the vasotocin assay. Third and most important, gel filtration of the urine samples resulted in a single peak of immunoreactivity which eluted in a position well before that of standard vasopressin (Fig. 4). On the same column standard vasotocin eluted in a position close if not identical to the unknown

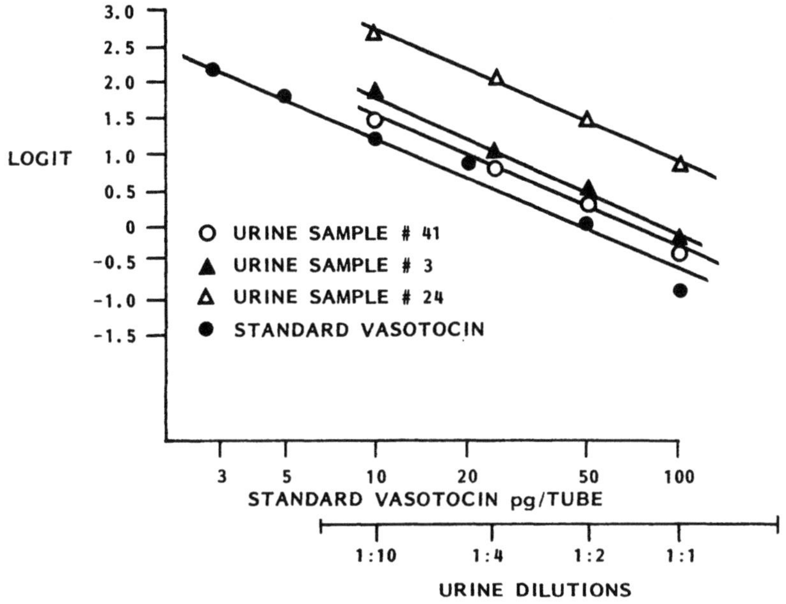

Fig. 3. Immunoreactivity of 10-fold serial dilutions of urines from two patients with carcinoma (3 and 41) and one normal subject (24) compared to the standard curve for synthetic vasotocin.

immunoreactivity.

The foregoing results strongly suggest that vasotocin is present in the urine of healthy adults as well as patients with lung cancer. However, they do not exclude the possibility that at least some of the immunoreactivity detected by the vasotocin assay is due to interference by non-hormonal components of urine. For unknown reasons, antisera to the neurohypophyseal hormones appear to be especially susceptible to such interference (55). Therefore, additional clinical as well as physiochemical studies of the vasotocin-like immunoreactivity in urine are required. For example, we find that incubation with pregnancy plasma

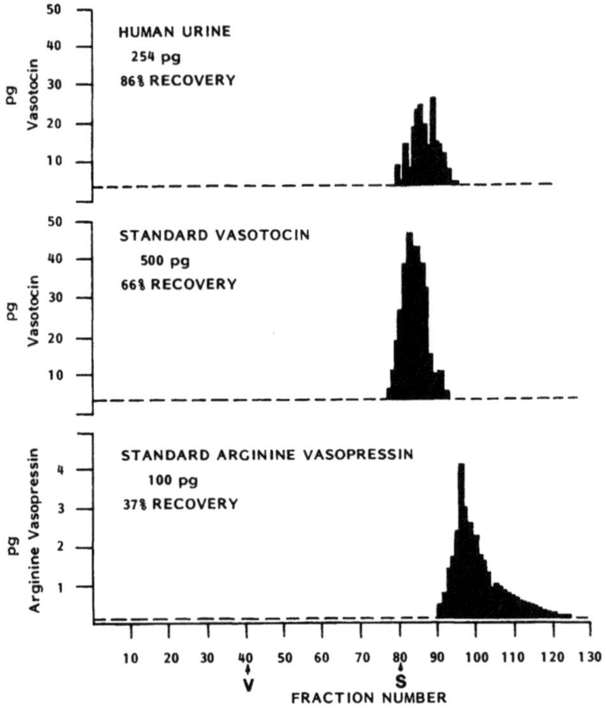

Fig. 4. Chromatograms of urine from a patient with carcinoma and of standard vasotocin and vasopressin. The G-25 Sephadex superfine column was used with a 0.0375 M ammonium acetate buffer. The void volume (V) and salt peak (S) are indicated. Fractions from human urine and standard vasotocin were measured in the vasotocin radioimmunoassay while those for standard vasopressin were measured by a specific vasopressin radioimmunoassay (79).

which contains large amounts of a cystine amino-peptidase destroys virtually all (93%) of the immunoactivity of standard vasotocin in saline solution but only 24 and 43% of the vasotocin-like immunoreactivity from cancer urines. Incomplete degradation of the unknown immunoreactivity by the peptidases does not necessarily mean that factors other than vasotocin are involved. It could be due simply to inhibition of the peptidases by increased pH or other factors present in urine. However, these findings indicate caution in the interpretation of our urinary findings and underline the need for further clinical as well as chemical studies of the nature and origin of the vasotocin-like immunoreactivity in the body fluids of man.

Biological Effects of Vasotocin

In lower animals, the administration of vasotocin affects fertility and fluid balance. The tentative identification of vasotocin in the brain and urine of humans necessitates a careful reevaluation of what is known about its actions in mammals.

Vasotocin is a potent inhibitor of the release (56-63) and action (64-66) of gonadotrophins. It is only one of many pineal hormones believed to have antigonadotrophic effects (60), but its potency is at least as great as melatonin (67) which has long been considered the primary pineal secretory product. Low dose injections given intraventricularly or higher doses given intravenously inhibit the rise in LH which occurs immediately before ovulation (57-59, 61) or after castration (56, 62, 63). Peripherally, vasotocin inhibits the hypertrophy of sexual organs (64, 65) and sometimes ovulation (66) in immature rodents primed with exogenous gonadotrophins. Daily injections may cause abortions in mice (67).

The central and peripheral gonadal inhibitory effects may not be a direct effect of vasotocin since it has no effect on gonadotrophin secretion from _in vitro_ systems (68). Instead, its antigonadotrophic actions may be related to nonspecific effects of intravenous or intraventricular injection, toxic or pharmacologic activity of impurities, or the administration of supraphysiologic doses of the hormone. The first two possibilities seem unlikely since synthetic vasotocin was used and the experiments were appropriately controlled. Most studies, however, were done with pharmacologic and not physiologic doses of vasotocin. The mouse pineal contains only approximately 25 μU of vasotocin, but in many studies intravenous doses ranging from 10 mU to 10 U were given (56). The failure to observe an antigonadotrophic effect at lower intravenous doses may be related to a site of action in the central nervous system (56, 58). When given intraventricularly vasotocin has gonadotrophin inhibiting activity at levels which could be achieved physiologically (56).

The antigonadotrophic effects might also be secondary to other biological actions of vasotocin. The chronic administration of vasotocin systematically could lead to water retention with its nonspecific toxic complications. Such an interpretation is consistent with studies which demonstrate a similar but less potent effect on fertility when vasopressin is given in comparable doses (57). Water intoxication alone, however, cannot account for all antigonadotrophic effects since many of the studies were done over a relatively short period of time. Vasotocin might also act indirectly by stimulation of another antigonadotrophic substance. Prolactin has a complex inhibitory effect on reproduction in mammals (69) and is stimulated by vasotocin both *in vitro* (70) and *in vivo* (71-73). This prolactin stimulatory effect may account, at least in part, for vasotocin's antigonadotrophic actions.

The reported diurnal variation of vasotocin in the pineal (74) suggests that the hormone may play a role in circadian variations of pituitary secretion. Since the synthesis and release of pineal vasotocin is enhanced at night (74) and it stimulates prolactin secretion vasotocin may play some role in the nocturnal increase in prolactin levels. It also stimulates ACTH release when injected directly into the pituitary (75), but suppresses plasma cortisol when given in the third ventricle (76). Thus, the role of vasotocin in the diurnal variation of adrenocortical secretion is very tenuous.

Vasotocin appears to be the major antidiuretic hormone in birds (9) and has been implicated in the control of water balance in amphibians, fish and reptiles (7, 8, 10). It also has an antidiuretic effect in dogs and rats which is reported to be less than arginine vasopressin but roughly equivalent to lysine vasopressin (77). In hydrated dogs (Fig. 5), the antidiuresis produced by vasotocin was comparable in magnitude but more prolonged than that produced by vasopressin. The latter was not due to obvious differences in the rate of disappearance of vasotocin from plasma but may have been due to slightly higher initial hormone levels achieved after injection. Because of this and the different rate of osmolar clearance in the two studies, precise comparison of their relative antidiuretic potencies is not possible. It is evident, however, that the antidiuretic action of vasotocin is sufficiently great that, at the concentration found in human urine, it might be expected to play a role

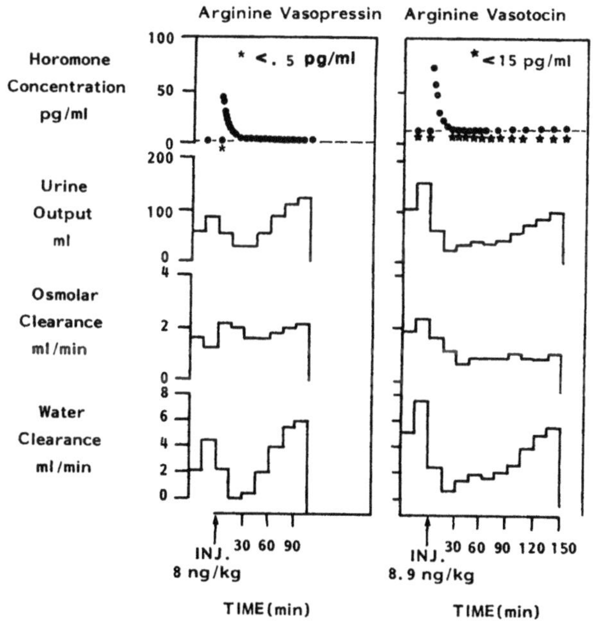

Fig. 5. Plasma hormone concentrations and renal response to injections of vasopressin and vasotocin in the water-loaded dog.

as important as vasopressin in the regulation of water balance. Proof that this second antidiuretic hormone exists in man could explain a number of peculiar observations such as the occurrence of the syndrome of inappropriate antidiuresis in patients who have no demonstrable abnormality in vasopressin secretion (52, 78). It would also revolutionize the diagnostic and/or investigative approach to other disorders of water balance.

Conclusion

Arginine vasotocin which is commonly associated with early stages of both ontogeny and phylogeny, has now been identified in adult mammals. While there remains little question that it is present in certain central nervous system structures of these animals, its presence in the body fluids of humans remains more tentative. Considering its biological action in both the central nervous system and peripheral tissues, it is imperative that its distribution and actions be better defined. At the moment, it is impossible to determine whether vasotocin is merely a vestige of man's development or plays an important, but unrecognized role in human physiology.

Acknowledgements

We wish to thank Dr. Jack George for the vasotocin antibody, Mary Beth Gaskill and Jean Musselman for technical assistance and Chris Goodwin for typing the manuscript. This research was supported by U.S. Public Health Service Grant PHS 50-825-09 and the U.S. Veterans Administration.

References

1. Sawyer, W.H.: Evolution of Antidiuretic Hormones and Their Functions. Am. J. Med. 42, 678-686 (1967).

2. Sawyer, W.H., Pang, P.K.T.: Evolution of Neurohypophyseal Hormones and Their Functions. In: "Neurohypophysis", Eds. Moses, A.M., Share, L., Karger, Basel, pp. 1-8 (1977).

3. Sawyer, W.H.: Evolution of Neurohypophyseal Hormones and Their Receptors. Fed. Proc. 36, 1842-1847 (1977).

4. Pickford, G.E., Strecker, E.L.: The Spawning Reflex Response of the Killfish, Fundulus heteroclitus: Isotocin is Relatively Inactive in Comparison with Arginine Vasotocin. Gen. comp. Endocr. 32, 132-137 (1977).

5. Macey, M.J., Pickford, G.E., Peter, R.E.: Forebrain Localization of the Spawning Reflex Response to Exogenous Neurohypophyseal Hormones in the Killfish. J. exp. Zool. 190, 269-280 (1974).

6. Diakow, C.: Hormonal Basis for Breeding Behavior in Female Frogs: Vasotocin Inhibits the Release of Rana pipiens. Science 199, 1456-1457 (1978).

7. Sawyer, W.H., Pang, P.K.T.: Endocrine Adaptation to Osmotic Requirements of the Environment: Endocrine Factors in Osmoregulation by Lungfishes and Amphibians. Gen. comp. Endocr. 25, 224-229 (1975).

8. Bradshaw, S.D.: Osmoregulation and Pituitary-Adrenal Function in Desert Reptiles. Gen. comp. Endocr. 25, 230-248 (1975).

9. Koike, T.I., Pryor, L.R., Neldon, H.L., Venable, R.S.: Effect of Water Deprivation of Plasma Radioimmunoassayable Arginine Vasotocin in Conscious Chickens. Gen. comp. Endocr. 33, 359-364 (1977).

10. Follett, B.K., Heller, H.: The Neurohypophyseal Hormones of Bony Fishes and Cyclostomes. J. Physiol. 172, 74-91 (1964).

11. Katsoyannis, P.G., du Vigneaud, V.: Arginine Vasotocin. Nature 184, 1465 (1959).

12. Sawyer, W.H.: Evidence for the Identity of Natriferin, the Frog Water-Balance Principle and Arginine Vasotocin. Nature 187, 1030-1031 (1960).

13. Munsick, R.A., Sawyer, W.H., van Dyke, H.B.: Avian Neurohypophyseal Hormones: Pharmacological Properties and Tentative Identification. Endocrinology 66, 860-871 (1960).

14. Heller, H.: Differentiation of an (Amphibian) Water Balance Principle from the Antidiuretic Principle of the Posterior Pituitary Gland. J. Physiol. 100, 125-141 (1941).

15. Heller, H., Pickering, B.T.: Neurohypophyseal Hormones of Non-Mammalian Vertebrates. J. Physiol. 155, 98-114 (1961).

16. Milcu, S.M., Pavel, S., Neacsu, C.: Biological and Chromatographic Characterization of a Polypeptide with Pressor and Oxytocic Activities Isolated from Bovine Pineal Gland. Endocrinology 72, 563-566 (1963).

17. Pavel, S.: Evidence for the Presence of Lysine Vasotocin in the Pig Pineal Gland. Endocrinology 77, 812-817 (1965).

18. Cheesman, D.W., Structural Elucidation of a Gonadotropin-Inhibiting Substance from the Bovine Pineal Gland. Biochim. biophys. Acta 207, 247-253 (1970).

19. Rosenbloom, A.A., Fisher, D.A.: Radioimmunoassayable AVT and AVP in Adult Mammalian Brain Tissue: Comparison of Normal and Brattleboro Rats. Neuroendocr. 17, 354-361 (1975).

20. Rosenbloom, A.A., Fisher, D.A.: Arginine Vasotocin in the Rabbit Subcommissural Organ. Endocrinology 96, 1038-1039 (1975).

21. Pavel, S., Goldstein, R., Calb, M.: Vasotocin Content in the Pineal Gland of Foetal, Newborn and Adult Male Rats. J. Endocr. 66, 283-284 (1975).

22. Bowie, E.P., Herber, D.C.: Immunocytochemical Evidence for the Presence of Arginine Vasotocin in the Rat Pineal Gland. Nature 261, 66 (1976).

23. Vizsolyi, E., Perks, A.M.: Neurohypophyseal Hormones in Fetal Life and Pregnancy II. Chromatographic Studies in the Sheep. Gen. comp. Endocr. 29, 41-50 (1976).

24. Pavel, S., Goldstein, R., Ghinea, E., Calb, M.: Chromatographic Evidence for Vasotocin Biosynthesis by Cultured Pineal Ependymal Cells from Rat Fetuses. Endocrinology 100, 205-208 (1977).

25. Swaab, D.F., Dogterom, J., van Leeuwan, F.W., Boer, K.: Arginine Vasotocin in the Foetal Rat Pituitary Gland. J. Endocr. 72, 4P-5P (1977).

26. Coculescu, M., Matulevicius, V., Goldstein, R., Pavel, S.: Presence and Synthesis of Vasotocin in the Pineal Gland of Brattleboro Rats. J. Endocr. 77, 145-146 (1978).

27. Pavel, S.: Vasotocin Biosynthesis by Neurohypophyseal Cells from Human Fetuses. Evidence for its Ependymal Origin. Neuroendocr. 19, 150-159 (1975).

28. Legros, J.J., Louis, F., Demoulin, A., Franchimont, P.: Immunoreactive Neurophysins and Vasotocin in Human Foetal Pineal Glands. J. Endocr. 69, 289-290 (1976).

29. Skowsky, W.R., Fisher, D.A.: Fetal Neurohypophyseal Arginine Vasopressin and Arginine Vasotocin in Man and Sheep. Pediat. Res. 11, 627-630 (1977).

30. Sawyer, W.H.: Increased Water Permeability of the Bullfrog Bladder In Vitro in Response to Synthetic Oxytocin and to Neurohypophyseal Extracts from Non-Mammalian Vertebrates. Endocrinology 66, 112-120 (1960).

31. Bentley, P.J.: A Method for the Detection and Estimation of Small Amounts of Arginine-Vasotocin. J. Endocr. 26, 295-296 (1963).

32. Dicker, S.E., Elliott, A.B.: Effect of Neurohypophyseal Hormones on Fluid Movement Across Isolated Bladder of Rana Cancrivora, Rana Temporaria and Bufo Melanostictus. J. Physiol. 210, 137-149 (1970).

33. van Dyke, H.B., Sawyer, W.H., Overweg, N.I.A.: Pharmacologic Activities of the 8-Citrulline Analogues of Oxytocin and Vasopressin. Endocrinology 73, 637-639 (1963).

34. Rasmussen, H., Schwartz, I.L., Young, R., Marc-Aurele, J.: Structural Requirements for the Action of Neurohypophyseal Hormones upon the Isolated Amphibian Urinary Bladder. J. gen. Physiol. 46, 1171-1189 (1963).

35. Archer, R., Chauvet, J., Lenci, M.T., Morel, F., Maetz, J.: Présence d'une vasotocine dans la neurohypophyse de la grenouille. Biochim. biophys. Acta 42, 379-380 (1960).

36. Archer, R.: The Comparative Chemistry of Neurohypophyseal Hormones. Symposia of the Zoological Society of London, 9, 83-91 (1963).

37. Rosenbloom, A.A., Fisher, D.A.: Radioimmunoassay of Arginine Vasotocin. Endocrinology 95, 1726-1732 (1974).

38. Legros, J.J., Louis, F., Grötschel-Stewart, U., Franchimont, P.: Presence of Immunoreactive Neurophysin-Like Material in Human Target Organs and Pineal Gland. Ann. N.Y. Acad. Sci. 248, 157-171 (1975).

39. Ferguson, D.R., Heller, H.: Distribution of Neurohypophyseal Hormones in Mammals. J. Physiol. 180, 846-863 (1965).

40. Benson, B.: Current Status of Pineal Peptides. Neuroendocr. 24, 241-258 (1977).

41. Anderson, E.: The Anatomy of Bovine and Ovine Pineals. Light and Electron Microscopic Studies. J. Ultrastruct. Res. Suppl. 8, 5-76 (1965).

42. Benson, B., Matthews, M.J., Hadley, M.E., Powers, S., Hruby, V.J.: Differential Localization of Antigonadotropic and Vasotocic Activities in Bovine and Rat Pineal. Life Sci. 19, 747-754 (1976).

43. Pavel, S.: Evidence for the Ependymal Origin of Arginine Vasotocin in the Bovine Pineal Gland. Endocrinology 89, 613-614 (1971).

44. Gilbert, G.J.: The Subcommissural Organ. Neurology 10, 138-142 (1960).

45. Wislocki, G.B., Leduc, E.H.: The Cytology of the Subcommissural Organ, Reissner's Fiber, Periventricular Glial Cells and Posterior Collicular Recess of the Rat's Brain. J. comp. Neurol. 101, 283-299 (1954).

46. Coculescu, M., Pavel, S.: Arginine Vasotocin-like Activity of Cerebrospinal Fluid in Diabetes Insipidus. J. Clin. Endocr. 36, 1031-1032 (1973).

47. Pavel, S.: Tentative Identification of Arginine Vasotocin in Human Cerebrospinal Fluid. J. Clin. Endocr. 31, 369-371 (1970).

48. Luerssen, T.G., Robertson, G.L.: Arginine Vasopressin in Human Cerebrospinal Fluid. J. Lab. clin. Med. (in press).

49. Swaab, D.F., Boer, K., Honnebier, W.J.: The Influence of the Fetal Hypothalamus and Pituitary on the Onset of Parturition. CIBA Foundation Symposia 47, 379-400 (1977).

50. France, V.M.: Active Sodium Uptake by the Skin of Foetal Sheep and Pigs. J. Physiol. 258, 377-392 (1976).

51. Walter, R., Simmons, W.H.: Metabolism of Neurohypophyseal Hormones: Considerations from a Molecular Viewpoint. In: "Neurohypophysis", Eds. Moses, A.M., Share, L., Karger, Basel, pp. 167-188 (1977).

52. Robertson, G.L.: Cancer and Inappropriate Antidiuresis. In: "Biological Markers of Neoplasia: Basic and Applied Aspects" Ed. Ruddon, R.W., Elsevier North Holland, Inc., Amsterdam, pp. 277-293 (1978).

53. Odell, W., Wolfsen, A., Yoshimoto, Y., Weitzman, R., Fisher, D., Hirose, F.: Ectopic Peptide Synthesis: A Universal Concomitant of Neoplasia. Trans. Assoc. Am. Physio. 90, 204-227 (1977).

54. Zebidi, A., Geelen, G., Allevard, A.M., Sempore, B., Jarsaillon, E., Meunier, C., Gharib, C.: Dosage radioimmunologique de locytocine urinaire chez l'Homme. C. r. Séanc. Soc. Biol. 172, 1155-1161 (1978).

55. Robertson, G.L.: The Regulation of Vasopressin Function in Health and Disease. Recent Prog. Horm. Res. 33, 333-385 (1977).

56. Pavel, S., Petrescu, M., Vicoleanu, N.: Evidence of Central Gonadotropin Inhibiting Activity of Arginine Vasotocin in the Female Mouse. Neuroendocr. 11, 370-374 (1973).

57. Cheesman, D.W., Osland, R.B., Forsham, P.H.: Suppression of the Preovulatory Surge of Luteinizing Hormone and Subsequent Ovulation in the Rat by Arginine Vasotocin. Endocrinology 101, 1194-1202 (1977).

58. Osland, R.B., Cheesman, D.W., Forsham, P.H.: Studies on the Mechanism of the Suppression of the Preovulatory surge of Luteinizing Hormone in the Rat by Arginine Vasotocin. Endocrinology 101, 1203-1209 (1977).

59. Cheesman, D.W., Osland, R.B., Forsham, P.H.: Effects of 8-Arginine Vasotocin on Plasma Prolactin and Follicle-Stimulating Hormone Surges in the Proestrous Rat. Proc. Soc. exp. Biol. Med. 156, 369-372 (1977).

60. Reiter, R.J., Vaughan, M.K.: Pineal Antigonadotrophic Substances: Polypeptides and Indoles. Life Sci. 21, 159-172 (1977).

61. Blask, D.E., Vaughan, M.K., Reiter, R.J., Johnson, L.Y.: Influence of Arginine Vasotocin on the Estrogen-Induced Surge of LH and FSH in Adult Ovariectomized Rats. Life Sci. 23, 1035-1040 (1978).

62. Vaughan, M.K.: Inhibition of the Post-Castration Rise in Luteinizing Hormone (LH) and Follicle-Stimulating Hormone (FSH) by Arginine Vasotocin. Anat. Rec. 2, 571 (1978).

63. Vaughan, M.K., Blask, D.E., Johnson, L.Y., Reiter, R.J.: The Effect of Subcutaneous Injections of Melatonin, Arginine Vasotocin, and Related Peptides on Pituitary and Plasma Levels of Luteinizing Hormone, Follicle-Stimulating Hormone, and Prolactin in Castrated Adult Male Rats. Endocrinology 104, 212-217 (1979).

64. Pavel, S., Petre, S.: Inhibition of Gonadotrophin by a Highly Purified Pineal Peptide and by Synthetic Arginine Vasotocin. Nature 212, 1054 (1966).

65. Vaughan, M.K., Vaughan, G.M., Klein, D.C.: Arginine Vasotocin: Effects on Development of Reproductive Organs. Science 186, 938-939 (1974).

66. Johnson, L.Y., Vaughan, M.K., Reiter, R.J., Blask, D.E., Rudeen, P.K.: The Effects of Arginine Vasotocin on Pregnant Mare's Serum-Induced Ovulation in the Immature Female Rat. Acta endocr. 87, 367-376 (1978).

67. Vaughan, M.K., Reiter, R.J., Vaughan, G.M.: Fertility Patterns in Female Mice Following Treatment with Arginine Vasotocin or Melatonin. Int. J. Fertil. 21, 65-68 (1976).

68. Demoulin, A., Hudson, B., Franchimont, P., Legros, J.J.: Arginine Vasotocin Does Not Affect Gonadotrophin Secretion in Vitro. J. Endocr. 72, 105-106 (1977).

69. Frantz, A.G.: Prolactin. New Engl. J. Med. 298, 201-207 (1978).

70. Vaughan, M.K., Blask, D.E., Johnson, L.Y., Reiter, R.J.: Prolactin-Releasing Activity of Arginine Vasotocin in vitro. Hormone Res. 6, 342-350 (1975).

71. Blask, D.E., Vaughan, M.K., Reiter, R.J., Johnson, L.Y., Vaughan, G.M.: Prolactin-Releasing and Release-Inhibiting Factor Activities in the Bovine, Rat and Human Pineal Gland: In Vitro and in Vivo Studies. Endocrinology 99, 152-162 (1976).

72. Vaughan, M.K., Blask, D.E., Vaughan, G.M., Reiter, R.J.: Dose-Dependent Prolactin Releasing Activity of Arginine Vasotocin in Intact and Pinealectomized Estrogen-Progesterone Treated Adult Male Rats. Endocrinology 99, 1319-1322 (1976).

73. Vaughan, M.K., Little, J.C., Johnson, L.Y., Blask, D.E., Vaughan, G.M., Reiter, R.J.: Effects of Melatonin and Natural and Synthetic Analogues of Arginine Vasotocin on Plasma Prolactin Levels in Adult Male Rats. Hormone Res. 9, 236-246 (1978).

74. Calb, M., Goldstein, R., Pavel, S.: Diurnal Rhythm of Vasotocin in the Pineal of the Male Rat. Acta endocr. 84, 523-526 (1977).

75. Pavel, S.: Opposite Effects of Vasotocin Injected Intrapituitarly and Intraventricularly on Corticotropin Release in Mice. Experientia 31, 1469-1470 (1975).

76. Pavel, S., Cristoveanu, A., Goldstein, R., Calb, M.: Inhibition of Release of Corticotropin Releasing Hormone in Cats by Extremely Small Amounts of Vasotocin Injected into the Third Ventricle of the Brain. Evidence for the Involvement of 5-Hydroxytryptamine-Containing Neurons. Endocrinology 101, 672-678 (1977).

77. Walter, R., Rudinger, J., Schwartz, I.L.: Chemistry and Structure-Activity Relations of the Antidiuretic Hormones. Am. J. Med. 42, 653-677 (1967).

78. Zerbe, R.L., Stropes, L., Robertson, G.L.: Vasopressin Function in the Syndrome of Inappropriate Antidiuresis. Ann. Rev. Med. 31 (in press).

79. Robertson, G.L., Mahr, E.A., Athar, S., Sinha, T.: Development and Clinical Application of a New Method for the Radioimmunoassay of Arginine Vasopressin in Human Plasma. J. clin. Invest. 52, 2340-2352 (1973).

GLUCAGON AND RELATED PEPTIDES

R. F. Murphy*, K. D. Buchanan, R. W. J. Flanagan
Departments of Biochemistry* and Medicine, Queen's University,
Belfast BT9 7BL, Northern Ireland, U.K.

Introduction

The polypeptide hormone glucagon (Fig. 1) has been known as a counterbalancing hyperglycaemic companion of insulin in the pancreas for more than half a century (1).

```
 1              5               10                 15
His-Ser-Gln-Gly-Thr-Phe-Thr-Ser-Asp-Tyr-Ser-Lys-Tyr-Leu-Asp-Ser-

         20             25
Arg-Ala-Gln-Asp-Phe-Val-Gln-Trp-Leu-Met-Asn-Thr
```

Fig. 1. The amino acid sequence of glucagon (2)

While glucagon has not received as much attention as insulin, its history has some unique features. It was one of the first hormones for which there were indications that it might be synthesised in tissues additional to a specialised gland, in this case in cells other than the A cells of pancreatic islets. Sutherland and de Duve (3) reported hyperglycaemic and glycogenolytic activity and Unger and associates (4, 5) found glucagon-like immunoreactivity (GLI) in gut extracts. It subsequently became clear that a variety of molecular forms of polypeptides related to glucagon exist in the gut and pancreas and that the gut can release glucagon-like materials into the circulation. This complexity is a background to all physiological and clinical studies on glucagon.

Hormones in Normal and Abnormal Human Tissues, Vol. II

Detection of Glucagon and Related Peptides

In recent years, most investigators used antibodies to detect glucagon and related peptides by radioimmunoassay (6, 3) of tissue extracts and biological fluids or by immunofluorescent (7) labelling of tissue slices in which the peptides are chemically insolubilized with fixatives. While much valuable information has been provided, there are important limitations (6, 8) to the significance of results obtained with antibodies raised against glucagon since they bind only to a small region and not to the whole structure of the hormone. Assan and Slusher (9) first showed that either of two types of antibody are formed when experimental animals are immunized with glucagon: one which binds the C-terminal region of glucagon and the other a region in the N-terminal to central portion of the hormone. These types of antibody were also encountered in our laboratories (10, 11) and the antibodies, coded YY57 and YY59, which react with the N-terminal to central portion of glucagon bind in the region of Tyr_{10} and Tyr_{13} whereas C-terminal antibody, coded YY89, binds near Trp_{25} and Met_{27}. Antibodies raised in other laboratories which appear to have regional specificity for the C-terminal region of glucagon, include those coded K47, K814 and K964 (12), 30K (13), AGS18 (14), G58 (15), 4304 (16) and an antibody described by Von Schenk (17). Antibodies which appear to bind the N-terminal to central region of glucagon include those coded 4023 (12), G128 (15), AGS10 (14) and 33D (18). The specificity of antibodies obtained when animals are immunized with conjugates of whole glucagon with carrier molecules such as albumin appears to be a function of the method of conjugation, the additives in immunization mixtures and the species of animals used but it is, as yet, difficult to predict the specificity before immunization.

Because of the limited regional specificities of the antibodies currently available for glucagon, it is clearly not possible to distinguish between intact glucagon, partially degraded glucagon or precursor forms of the hormone using one or even both types of antibody in immunoassays or immunohistochemistry. Nevertheless, many research groups erroneously accept that immunoreactivity detected with antibodies specific for the C-terminal region indicates the presence of glucagon, whereas immunoreactivity detected with the antibodies which bind the N-terminal to central portion of the hormone is regarded as evidence for the presence of glucagon and for glucagon-like peptides from the gut. In the light of the multiplicity of pancreatic and gut peptides described below and also because of the extensive homology which exists between glucagon and other gut hormones, simplistic interpretation of immunoassay or immunohistochemical results is no longer justifiable (8). It is unsatisfactory that clinical or physiological studies concerning a hormone as large as glucagon should still be attempted with one antibody which can recognise only a limited structural region, yet this is the rule rather than the exception.

Other problems may be encountered using antibodies. Discrepancies between immunoassay and immunohistochemical data occur because the chemical fixatives modify residues in the immunogenic site so that they no longer bind to the antibodies. Conversely, precursor forms of the hormone in cell extracts may not react with the antibodies in immunoassay because the immunogenic site is buried but the chaotropic fixatives may expose this site by unfolding the precursor tissue sections. In our view, future studies on glucagon should be carried out by simultaneous assay with a variety of antibodies which are specific for selected sequences of the hormone and preferably these sequences should overlap. The antibodies could be raised against peptides produced synthetically, by judicious degradation of glucagon or by immunization with glucagon to which selective chemical modifications had been introduced. The principle should also apply to structures in the extension peptides in precursor forms of glucagon as these become known. Moody and associates (19, 22) have already used an antibody, coded R64 which binds a non-glucagon structure in gut glucagon-like immunoreactivity.

The current deficiencies of immunoassays and immunohistochemical analyses caused by a lack of antibodies and the certain delay before sufficient antibodies become available for fully rational studies should possibly draw attention to the alternative and theoretically more valid assays based on the biological action of glucagon. These include the binding of glucagon to target cells and the activation of adenylate cyclase, discussed below. In the light of the common homology, biological activities and tissue distribution of glucagon with other gut hormones (8) and of the finding that fragments of glucagon may retain partial binding and stimulating activities (see below), it is clear that neither immunochemical nor biological assays alone are likely to suffice for studying glucagon and related peptides. Moreover, because of the multiplicity of glucagon-like peptides, there is a need for constant physiochemical analysis of materials under investigation to support results from other methods.

Distribution of Extrapancreatic Cells which Contain GLI

Since the early (4, 5) reports of GLI in gut extracts, most studies on distribution and characterisation were carried out using animals other than humans. In general (8, 19, 20, 23-32), highest levels of GLI are located in the lower gut, especially in the ileum and colon and lowest amounts are found in the stomach with the exception of dog fundus (16, 33-35). The identification of A cells in canine gastric fundus (16, 36) supports observations with tissue extracts.

While Kenny and Say (37) had initially described glucagon-like biological activity in human jejunum it seems that lack of availability of fresh tissue has restricted the range of studies (38-39) on GLI from human tissues. Extraction was sometimes delayed during autopsy so that partial proteolytic degradation of the glucagon-like materials had already taken place. Nevertheless, results obtained with human tissue extracts are generally supported by immunohistochemical data (7, 41, 42). In summary, the distribution of GLI in human gut appears to reflect that in other non-canine mammals; highest amounts are found in the ileum and colon. Recently, Dawson and co-workers (43), using density gradient centrifugation, were able to isolate storage granules containing GLI from cells in biopsies from human jejunum and rectum. While Monoz-Barragan and associates (44) obtained immunocytochemical evidence for cells which produce GLI in the oxyntic mucosa of human stomach, this observation is not supported by the findings of other workers (7). GLI has also been detected in human and rat submaxilliary gland (45-47), in canine brain (18) and in epithelial cells of the pancreatic duct in rats (48).

Multiplicity of Glucagon-Related Peptides

Soon after the initial detection of GLI in the gut (45) Unger and associates showed that, in addition to material the size of glucagon, GLI larger than glucagon was present in gut (49) and pancreatic extracts. Subsequently, the predominant fraction of ileal GLI, referred to as large GLI, was purified by immunoaffinity chromatography and found to have a molecular weight of about 12000 (23). The material is electrophoretically heterogeneous (23) and apparently, biologically inert (23, 51, 52). Large GLI was found to react with antibodies specific for the N-terminal to central, but not the C-terminal, region of glucagon (10) and this was in agreement with the observations of Assan and Slusher (9) with another purified preparation from the gut. The GLI in extracts from colon (25, 26) was bound noncovalently to a larger protein but otherwise resembled the material from ileum. A minor fraction (<5%) of ileal and colonic GLI included material with the same size as glucagon and which bound both types of antibody. Further extensive multiplicity of GLI species which differ in size, charge and immunoreactive properties was encountered in extracts of small intestine and stomach in these and other laboratories (35, 52-54). In general, the incidence of low molecular weight forms increased with proximity to the upper gut; extracts of dog fundus contained highest amounts of material which resembles glucagon in size and immunoreactivity. Also, biological activity was usually reported only when the GLI preparations had molecular weights close to that of glucagon (35, 54, 55). Large GLI which reacts with antibodies specific for the C-terminal region of glucagon is seldom encountered in tissue extracts; the material from the salivary gland (46) is an exception.

The concept that extrapancreatic forms of GLI are mainly due to proglucagon, in cells which do not possess the enzymic mechanism to generate the biologically active species (8), is supported by the convergence of evidence obtained with gut as well as pancreatic materials. In 1973, Tager and Steiner (56) discovered that GLI, present as a contaminant in preparations of pancreatic glucagon, included a peptide with molecular weight about 4500. This was found to be glucagon extended at the C-terminal end by an octapeptide. The methionyl residue at position 27 of glucagon (Fig. 1) provided a convenient site for cleavage with CNBr. This facilitated the determination of the sequence of the fragments Asn-Thr-Lys-Arg-Asn-Asn-Lys-Ile-Ala which contains the C-terminal dipeptide and the extension peptide. Flanagan et al. (10) in 1974 found that large gut GLI contained a structure which was homologous with the C-terminal region of glucagon in addition to the region which is homologous with the N-terminal region. While the C-terminal structure is buried in native GLI this region was uncovered when the large GLI was subjected to limited proteolysis with serum proteases. This result indicated a possible precursor role for large GLI and was confirmed later by degradative studies using solid-phase trypsin (57). Jacobsen and co-workers (27) however, obtained chemical evidence that a large GLI from gut, glicentin, had strong similarities with the proglucagon described by Tager and Steiner. Using the same chemical degradation as for the pancreatic material, a peptide with the following sequence was detected: Lys-Arg-Asn-Lys-Asn-Asn-Ile-Ala. They also obtained additional structural evidence that other regions of glucagon were present in GLI. Comparison of the methods used (56, 27) to determine the sequence of the extension peptides suggests that the pancreatic material may eventually be shown to have the same structure as that found in the gut.

The proglucagon role for gut GLI is further supported by the finding that large GLI is present as a minor constituent in the pancreas (35). It is similar in size to the material from ileum and binds only to antibodies specific for the N-terminal to central region of glucagon (25). More significantly, Moody and associates, using an antibody binding a non-glucagon portion of glicentin,demonstrated glicentin-like immunoreactivity in foetal and juvenile rat pancreas (19-22), pig pancreas (20-22), human pancreas (58) and canine gastric A cells (58) as well as in the jejunum and ileum of man and other animals (20-22). Using serial semi-thin sections they obtained immunohistochemical evidence that glicentin and glucagon-like immunoreactivities are contained in the same cells (22). Recently, Tager and Markese (32) produced further evidence that intestinal GLI from rabbit contains the C-terminal tryptic peptide of glucagon and that larger fragments of the gut material have counterparts in the pancreas.

While large GLI of gut may be a precursor of glucagon, the GLI in turn may be derived from a big common precursor for hormones additional to glucagon, analogous to the β-lipotropin (59) precursor of ACTH and endorphins. Grube et al (60) found endorphin-like immunoreactivity in the glucagon-producing A cells of the pancreas; the pancreas has no ACTH. Smith et al. (61) claimed that the same cells also contained a GLI-like material and Aluemets et al. (62) report that GLI is present in pancreatic glucagonomas as well as in the glucagon-containing cells of the pancreas and gut in rat, guinea pigs, cats, dogs and pigs.

Release of Glucagon into the Circulation

The biological significance of GLI depends on the molecular species (glucagon or precursors) stored in cells of synthesis, on the molecular form released under physiological stimuli and on the possibility that large inactive molecules, once released, may be converted to active species under the influence of plasma or target tissue proteases. The extensive recent literature on the release of glucagon from the pancreas and extrapancreatic tissue is pervaded with confusion which arises from the above-mentioned assumption that antibodies to glucagon can be "tissue-specific". Nevertheless, general trends are apparent and we attempt to review this topic without further reference to erroneous terminology.

Glucagon is stored in pancreatic A cells in amorphous α granules (63, 64) and released into the circulation apparently by exocytosis (29). The nervous, endocrine and metabolic factors which control the release of glucagon are widely reviewed (28, 29, 65-69) and are in accord with the generally hyperglycaemic effect of the hormone: insulin-induced hypoglycaemia stimulates glucagon release while glucose depresses, though it is possible that the response of the A cells to hyper - or hypoglycaemia is absent in diabetes (70, 71). Somatostatin is a classical inhibitor and it is also possible that endogenous enkephalins and endorphins of the pancreas exert an influence by suppressing pancreatic somatostatin levels (72). In the light of the suggestion (29) that excessive release of glucagon, basal or stimulated, may contribute to diabetic hyperglycaemia, the recently synthesised analogue (73), [des - Ala (1), Gly (2)] His (4, 5)-D - Trp (8) - somatostatin, with prolonged activity in suppressing release of glucagon but not insulin, may have important therapeutic application. Arginine and ornithine rank predominantly among metabolic stimulators of A cells (74). It is proposed (75) that an influx of calcium into the A cell is required for the stimulation by arginine.

It appears that glucagon and not large precursor material is released from the arginine stimulated pancreas (29). This was shown by isolated perfused pancreas from rat (74) and pig (75) and isolated islets from dogs (77). The contribution made by extrapancreatic sources to the circulation is more difficult to assess. Depancreatized humans and experimental animals are an obvious source of information. A major distractant, however, has been the overdependence on dogs for model studies even though the species is unique among mammals in having large quantities of material similar to glucagon in the stomach. The A cells of dog stomach appear to be as classically sensitive to arginine in releasing glucagon-like material as are those of the pancreas (29, 78). Release of glucagon-like material from these A cells is reduced with very low concentrations of insulin though a basal secretion of glucagon-like immunoreactivity is not suppressed (79). Both hypoglycaemia and cytoglycopenia stimulated gastric GLI secretion. The results with islets and isolated stomach are in agreement with observations using depancreatized dogs; in general, there is strong evidence that the A cells of dog stomach have the same stimulators, including arginine and same repressors, including somatostatin, as has the pancreas.

The circulation of depancreatized dogs also contains glucagon-like immunoreactivity which does not appear to have come from A cells but is probably large GLI from other gut cells. This material accounts for most of immunoreactivity which is detected in the circulation of depancreatized humans and other animals and its release does not appear to be influenced by the effectors which control the A cells. Buchanan et al. (83) obtained early evidence that gut GLI is released in depancreatized dogs in response to absorbed glucose. It has since been demonstrated that introduction of the sugar to jejunal pieces (84), everted jejunal sacs (85) and isolated perfused ileum (86) from rat causes release of large GLI. Highest levels of GLI are present in the lower gut but it is possible that dietary sugar might be absorbed before it reaches that region. Sugar evokes a much greater GLI release in gastrectomized patients (87) and patients with shortened jejunum (21). Frame (31) showed that when glucose is placed directly into the ileum and colon of rat, the observed GLI response was the same as when only the duodenum and the jejunum were stimulated by intraluminal glucose but more GLI is released by ileum and colon in other animals. Alexander et al. (88) demonstrated stimulation of GLI release by intraduodenal glucose in sheep foetal gut. Studies with depancreatized humans (52, 89-92) indicate that neither arginine nor insulin-induced hypoglycaemia stimulated release of large GLI and that neither the basal level nor stimulation of release by glucose is altered by somatostatin or insulin. The results with depancreatized humans are in general accord with those obtained using other animals (52, 93). While there is some evidence with rats (93) that somatostatin suppresses the release of large GLI, the effect may be an indirect one by suppressing absorption of glucose in the lower gut (87, 89).

Occasional reports of partial and variable response of GLI levels to arginine in depancreatized humans (92) and other mammals (93), excluding dog, may be due to a small number of A cells in the upper gut which secrete glucagon. It appears unlikely that the gut of man or most other animals secretes enough glucagon to have a significant effect on glucose metabolism additional to that of glucagon from pancreatic A cells. The dog is clearly different with the unusually high incidence of A cells in the upper gut which are under the same control as pancreatic A cells and which release glucagon in sufficient quantities to alter glucose metabolism (82). Dogs should not be used as models to reflect the physiological or clinical significance of glucagon-like materials in man.

Circulating Molecular Species

While A cells appear to synthesise precursors, convert them to glucagon, store glucagon and release the hormone under the control of effectors which include arginine and somatostatin, the extrapancreatic cells which store large GLI may synthesise the same precursors as the pancreas but seem to store polypeptides which vary between and within cells and to release these peptides under the influence of dietary glucose. It is also possible that, in some instances, cells which store large GLI convert it to molecules which more closely resemble pancreatic glucagon in size and immunoreactivity during the secretory process (88). Plasma proteases may contribute to the multiplicity of circulating peptides by partial proteolytic degradation of released GLI and glucagon.

The multiplicity of molecular species of GLI detected in normal human plasma has been reviewed (94, 95, 96). These include immunoreactive materials with molecular weight 3500, presumably glucagon, 9000 intermittently and > 40000 in addition to possible fragments with molecular weight < 2000. In these studies, however, there was an inordinately exclusive reliance on antibodies which bind the C-terminal region of glucagon. The material with molecular weight 9000 could be derived from large gut GLI of molecular weight 12000 which binds only to the antibodies specific for the N-terminal to central region of glucagon and is the predominant form stored in intestinal cells. It must be emphasised, however, that the parent material would not be detected in surveys carried out only with C-terminal antibodies. In these laboratories, studies on circulating glucagon were conducted using both types of antibody. To avoid interference by plasma constituents in gel-filtration and radioimmunoassay, the glucagon and related materials were first purified by immunoaffinity chromatography (24, 97, 98). Plasma from normal fasting subjects was applied to columns of immobilised C-terminal antibodies and the effluent was directed through columns with the N-terminal to central antibodies. The GLI recovered from the C-terminal antibody column reacted with both types of antibody in radioimmunoassay; 30% had molecular weight 3500 and the remainder appeared to be tightly bound to large plasma proteins, in agreement with the observations of Weir (95). Only one fraction, with molecular weight 4500, was recovered from the column of N-terminal to central antibodies and this reacted only with the N-terminal to central antibodies in radioimmunoassay. The material represented about 10% of the total immunoreactivity.

The GLI with molecular weight 3500 is probably glucagon since intravenous arginine caused about two-fold increase. Unexpectedly, however, the material with molecular weight 4500 showed similar response. The GLI associated with plasma proteins was released by treatment with 0.1% sodium dodecyl sulphate and appeared to be a mixture of materials with molecular weight 4500 and 3500.

When the GLI with molecular weight 4500 and reacting with the N-terminal to central antibodies was subjected to limited proteolysis, it was converted to material with the same size (3500) and immunoreactivity (binding both antibodies equally) as glucagon. The parent material may be a precursor of glucagon with a C-terminal extension similar to that described by Tager and Steiner (56) but the extension peptide may mask the C-terminal immunogenic site. It is also possible that the material has biological activity since the N-terminal to central region is exposed; Wright et al. (99) showed that glucagon$_{1-21}$ is a full agonist of the hormone (see below). While arginine stimulates increased levels of the GLI with molecular weight 4500, it is still not possible to speculate on whether it originates in the pancreas or gut. Conlon et al. (77) observed GLI components with molecular weight 150 000 and 200 000 in the effluent from isolated dog pancreas after prolonged stimulation with arginine but were able to dissociate both forms into GLI with molecular weight 3500 and non-immunoreactive protein. In many of the recent studies on circulating GLI, the immunoreactive material was extracted from plasma or serum with ethanol before radioimmunoassay. This procedure, however, prevented the detection of aggregates of glucagon or related peptides with large carrier proteins since these are precipitated by the ethanol.

Pathology

Glucagonomas. Glucagon-producing tumours are the least controversial examples of the involvement of glucagon in a pathological condition and are reviewed by Mallinson and Bloom (100) and by Holst (101). Pancreatic islet cell tumours which appeared to arise from the alpha cells have been described (102, 103). While McGavran and associates (104), in 1966, were the first to report that a tumour secreted glucagon which could be detected by radioimmunoassay, the syndrome was not thoroughly documented until 1974 when Mallinson et al. (105) described nine patients.

The main clinical features are necrolytic migratory erythema, diabetes mellitus, diarrhoea, anaemia, glossitis and vulvovaginitis, mental disturbance, weight loss, venous thrombosis and hypoaminoacidaemia. Of these, the skin rash is the most dramatic and diagnostic. The lower abdomen, perineum and legs are most affected although the rash may be more generalised and involve the face. The earliest abnormality is a reddened oedematous patch, slightly raised, which spreads within 2 or 3 days. The epidermis is denuded exposing a raw surface. The edge of the lesion spreads, taking on a marginate and geographic appearance with an erythematous edge and healed centre. The differential diagnosis is psoriasis, pemphigus or eczema. The picture can be markedly altered by secondary infection. Histology shows that the upper half of the epidermis is necrotic and lytic. The cause of the rash is unknown but it may be due to hypoaminoacidaemia and zinc deficiency. Some patients with glucagonoma do not have a rash and conversely, the rash can appear in the absence of a glucagonoma. Most glucagonoma patients are diabetic with hyperinsulinaemia and so do not require insulin but there is a case report of cure of insulin-dependent diabetes by removal of a glucagonoma (106). Several glucagonoma patients have had disturbed and variable personalities.

The hallmark of the diagnosis of glucagonoma is a markedly elevated level of GLI in the peripheral blood. The immunoreactivity is present variably in multiple fractions (94-96). Three patients were examined in this centre. In two, the circulating GLI bound only to the C-terminal antibodies and was present predominantly in a fraction with molecular weight 12500 while the remainder was detected in fractions with molecular weight 3500 and > 30000. In the third patient, the material with molecular weight 12500 was not detected, but small amounts of the material described above with molecular weight 4500 and bound by the N-terminal to central antibodies were present.

While it is difficult to study the release of GLI from glucagonomas against the background of materials released by the gut and pancreas, it is apparent that in some patients tolbutamide and arginine stimulate glucagonomas to release GLI. Such patients should not be treated with sulphoryl ureas. The tumour has usually metastasied before diagnosis, possibly because the GLI secretions are innocuous, until the circulating levels of GLI have been grossly elevated for several years. Screening patients, in diabetic clinics for increased GLI levels and in dermatology clinics for the rash, may increase the rate of detection. As for apudomas in general, surgical removal is the favoured treatment. When this is not possible, some patients respond to streptozotocin and the rash may be improved with rest, better nutrition and zinc supplements.

While common features of glucagonomas have been described above, the syndrome can vary widely. Gleeson et al. (107) reported a patient with a GLI-secreting tumour in the kidney. The clinical features were mainly intestinal, exhibiting stasis and giant intestinal villi. The present authors (108) have observed a patient with a GLI-secreting tumour in the pancreas but had the typical glucagonoma syndrome in addition to the intestinal features.

Other causes of elevated levels of circulating GLI. The pancreas, alone or in conjunction with the gut, releases increased quantities of GLI in a variety of conditions including diabetic ketoacidosis and in the worsening stages of diabetes mellitus during infections, during the abnormal carbohydrate metabolism in trauma and after severe burns. Elevated GLI levels are also observed in pancreatitis, acromegaly, glucocorticoid excess and hyperlipaemia but the cause is unclear. The marked elevation of circulating GLI in patients with either coeliac disease, intestinal by-pass or the dumping syndrome are probably mainly of intestinal origin.

There is considerable controversy about the role of glucagon in diabetes mellitus as is advocated by Unger (109) in his "Double Trouble" hypothesis and Lefebvre and Luyckx (110) have recently contributed a masterly review. Relative or absolute hyperglucagonaemia develops in diabetes mellitus and this cannot be suppressed with glucose. The reduction of plasma glucagon levels and improvement of the diabetic state by somatostatin infusion indicates that glucagon may be producing many of the abnormal features. It is crucial, however, to determine whether the glucagon changes are secondary to the insulin deficiency. Barnes et al. (111) found that pancreatectomized subjects still developed hyperglycaemia when glucagon was withheld, suggesting that the hormone is not essential for the worsening of the diabetic state.

Circulating GLI levels in patients with renal failure are markedly higher than in normal subjects (94, 96, 98). Most of the immunoreactivity, however, is present in molecular species larger than glucagon (96, 98). While the kidney is regarded as the major site for the normal catabolism of glucagon and of large GLI (94, 111, 112), it seems that glucagon is still degraded outside the kidney in uraemic patients but at a slower rate.

Increased levels of basal and arginine-stimulated glucagon in the circulation of cirrhotic compared with normal human subjects are attributed to increased production rather than altered clearance rate (113). A patient with liver failure was recently reported to have a pseudoglucagonoma syndrome (114).

Deficiency states. There have been several early reports of patients with hypoglycaemia due to glucagon deficiency (115, 116). The first reports of antibodies to islet cells in juvenile onset diabetes (117, 118) paved the way for a potential marker of endocrine deficiency of the islet cells. In 1976, Bottazzo and Lendrum (119) detected specific antibodies to glucagon-producing cells. The significance of these autoantibodies is not yet clear but they may be useful in the future to identify glucagon-deficiency states and to characterise the associated clinical features.

Interaction of Glucagon with Target Cells

Binding to membranes. Glucagon in common with other polypeptide hormones exerts its effect on target cells by elevating the intracellular concentration of cyclic AMP (120) through activation of adenylate cyclase. Firstly, the hormone binds to the receptor on the external surface of target cells which then activates adenylate cyclase located on the inner surface. In accordance with the glycogenolytic and lipolytic effects of glucagon, the targets most commonly studied are liver plasma membranes and to a far lesser extent, adipocytes. The initial interaction of glucagon with the membranes is dependent on the full structural integrity and conformation of the hormone in addition to other factors mentioned below. While glucagon in crystals adopts a predominantly helical conformation stabilized by hydrophobic interactions between trimers, Moran et al. (121) showed that in dilute solution the hormone undergoes a conformational transition to a predominantly pleated sheet structure. They suggest that the latter may bind with greatest affinity to receptors. Dockerill and associates (63, 64) suggest that the complex with receptor is formed through hydrophobic interactions with glucagon side-chains brought together in the α-helical conformation. This conformational fit may be induced in the hydrophobic membrane by analogy with the induction of helical structure in glucagon by a variety of lipids (64, 122). The receptor appears to be an independent dissociable (123) and mobile (124) unit in the membranes.

Houslay and associates (124) suggest that the interaction of the receptor with glucagon on the outside of the membrane may cause a locking interaction with the catalytic unit facing the cytoplasm which is then activated. They recently suggested (125) that lysophosphatidyl cholines can modulate the activity of the catalytic unit, adenylate cyclase, once it is in the 'hormone-stimulated state'. Similarly, Kiss (126) demonstrated the interaction of calcium together with insulin at membrane level and in the presence of adenosine, to cause inhibition of glucagon-stimulated adenylate cyclase activity.

While maximal binding of glucagon to target cells is dependent on the full amino acid sequence including the N-terminal imidazole groups (127-129), tyrosyl residues (130-132) and free α- and ε-amino groups (128, 132), it is now apparent that fragments of the hormone have comparable biological activity at higher concentrations. Wright and co-workers (99) have recently shown that $glucagon_{1-21}$ is a full agonist of glucagon; at the same concentration it has 0.1% of the binding activity with liver plasma membranes and 0.1% of the biological potency. This suggests that the hydrophobic C-terminal region is important for the initial anchoring of the hormone into the membrane but is not involved in the intramembrane reactions with catalytic units. More dramatically, they have shown that $glucagon_{1-6}$ is a partial agonist since, at saturating conditions, it stimulates 75% of the maximal cyclase activity given by the native hormone (123). The binding affinity and potency are 0.001% those of glucagon. None of the antibodies currently used for radioimmunoassays would detect $glucagon_{1-6}$ even if it were to accumulate in conditions of abnormal hormone catabolism.

Activation of adenylate cyclase. Rodbell and associates pioneered much of the early work (120) on the mechanism of activation of adenylate cyclase in plasma membranes of rat liver. They proposed that the glucagon-sensitive system contained at least three components: a specific receptor for glucagon, a regulatory component containing sites specific for GTP and the catalytic component which converts ATP to cAMP in the presence of Mg^{2+} or Mn^{2+}. It seemed, at first, that GTP and glucagon activated the system in a concerted fashion but the molecular basis for this was unclear. Much research is still required to establish the role of GTP[134-139] and its analogue, Gpp(NH)p, which is often used (134, 136-138) because it is not hydrolysed by nucleotide phosphohydrolases. The results of Kimura and Nagata (135) cast some doubt on earlier studies by showing that GTP was present as an impurity in most ATP preparations then available. They also suggest that GDP rather than GTP may be involved in the coupling process. While Welton and associates (137) were able to use detergent to separate glucagon receptors from adenylate cyclase in forms which were each able to interact with guanyl nucleotides, it is not possible yet to cite a definitive model which explains the role of GTP in the interaction between receptor and cyclase and the full regulation of these events. It is still unclear whether the guanyl nucleotide site associated with the catalytic entity is necessary for coupling (139). Some general difficulties in the interpretation of experimental data may arise from the differences in the properties (137, 139) of GTP and Gpp(NH)p. Levitzky and Helmreich (140), in a recent review, discuss several possible models for the role of GTP in coupling receptors to adenylate cyclase.

Down regulation. The concept of receptor regulation in response to changes in the concentration of circulating glucagon, especially in conditions associated with hyperglucagonaemia, is another highly controversial topic. Pilkis and co-workers (141) found that adenylate cyclase in livers from diabetic rats was abnormally responsive to the concentration of the hormone. Subsequently, it was shown that hyperglucagonaemia, produced by injecting glucagon or by streptozotocin, was associated with decreases in glucagon binding to liver cells (142, 143), in glucagon-stimulated adenylate cyclase activity (143) and in cAMP response (142). In general, these results were comparable with the highly significant inverse correlation observed between circulating levels of plasma insulin and insulin binding to specific receptors in the experimental diabetic animal (144) and hyperinsulinaemic diabetic patient (145). The reduction in the binding of insulin to target cells caused by hyperinsulinaemia has been termed "down regulation".

It is unlikely that a single or simple mechanism accounts for the observations with glucagon; there are many anomalies and even contradictions in the results obtained between and within laboratories. The decrease in cAMP response to glucagon observed by Bhathena et al. (142) was inordinately high compared with the decrease in glucagon binding. Also, Soman and Felig (143) note that the decrease in glucagon binding did not take place until after continuous infusion for 5 h whereas plasma glucose levels declined to baseline between 30 min and 3 h. They suggest that while the decrease in the responsiveness of the cAMP system in hyperglucogonaemia is mediated, at least in part, by a reduction in glucagon binding, other mechanisms account for the rapid evanescence which characterises the action of the hormone on hepatic glucose output. Bhathena et al. (142) suggest that the reason for down regulation is a decrease in the number of receptors rather than a change in their affinity. A reduction in the number of binding sites was not observed in insulin-deficient or starved rats until hyperglucagonaemia had proceeded for at least 12 h (146). Even then, the ability of glucagon to stimulate adenylate cyclase was not reduced. These results are in contrast with the above reports and with the observation by Fouchereau et al. (147) that starvation-induced hyperglucagonaemia is associated with decreased glucagon binding.

Bloomgarden et al. (148) studied down regulation in non-obese men by infusing glucagon while suppressing pancreatic hormone production with somatostatin. Glucose production peaked at 1.5 h but returned to basal levels at 2.5 h. They also showed, however, that subsequent glucagon withdrawal, at 5 h, produced an immediate decline in glucose production, indicating that, even after down regulation, the maintenance of basal glucose production is dependent on circulating glucagon. Some of the unexplained effects of glucagon may now be accounted for in the light of the recent work of Cote and Epand (149) who produced fresh and convincing evidence that the hormone can also activate glycogenolysis by a cAMP-independent process. Having synthesised N^{α}-trinitrophenyl glucagon they found that the derivative had no ability to activate adenylate cyclase, to increase the levels of cAMP in isolated hepatocytes or to stimulate protein kinase activity (see below). Nevertheless, it activated glycogenolysis and augmented the effect of glucagon on glycogenolysis.

While it is obvious that there is still no satisfactory explanation for down regulation, it is possible that a peptide which inhibits glucagon-sensitive adenylate cyclase, analogous to that observed in hypocalcaemic liver cells (150), is involved. Alternatively, glucagon-receptor complexes may enter target cells to be degraded inside (151). The increased basal and arginine-stimulated levels of glucagon in cirrhotic patients would support the concept of degradation in liver cells were it not for the views of Sherwin and associates (113) that there is increased production of glucagon in this condition. Since the kidney is regarded as a major site of degradation of glucagon (see above) accumulation of intact glucagon in uraemia could be expected to induce responses in liver cells similar to the down regulation caused by other "hyperglucagonaemic" conditions. The contrary appears to pertain. Sherwin et al. (152) showed that the hyperglycaemic effects of physiological increments of glucagon are increased in uraemia. The results indicate that glucagon levels cannot be constantly elevated in uraemia. While the levels of the other GLI species are raised, they appear to have no effect on the liver cells.

Biochemical Consequences of Cyclic AMP Formation

Glucagon-induced changes in levels of cAMP affect metabolism of target cells by causing changes in the levels of protein kinases (153-155). These kinases in turn have an intermediary role in regulating the activity of key enzymes in metabolism by phosphorylation of other proteins including enzymes of glycogenolysis and gluconeogenesis. The duration between activation of adenylate cyclase and manifestation of consequential biochemical events appears to depend on whether the protein kinases modify cytoplasmic enzymes immediately or must first be translocated to particulate fractions. Schwoch and Hilz (156) showed that while maximal elevation of cAMP levels and of protein kinase activation occurred in the liver 2 min after presentation of glucagon, a significant transfer of kinase to sub-cellular particles was seen after 90 to 120 min when the cAMP levels had already fallen. In cytoplasm, however, a cAMP-dependent kinase catalysed the phosphorylation of inactive glycogen phosphorylase to form the active phosphorylase (157, 158) and this effect was maximal within 1 min of presenting glucagon to hepatocytes *in vitro*. It has also been suggested that glucagon and cAMP control the proportions of glucose and glycogen by causing the conversion of active glycogen synthetase I to the inactive synthetase D or to control the activity of the phosphatase which catalyses the activation of the synthetase (159).

There seems to be no doubt that glucagon can cause the inactivation of cytoplasmic pyruvate kinase with the intervention of a protein kinase (160-165). The phosphorylated inactive form has a decreased affinity for the positive modulator, fructose 1,6-diphosphate, as well as for the substrate phosphoenolpyruvate. Glucagon is now known to influence fatty acid metabolism in adipose tissue and liver with the demonstration that acetyl coenzyme A carboxylase is a substrate for a cAMP-dependent kinase; phosphorylation results in inactivation (166). Phenylalanine hydroxylase is also activated by phosphorylation apparently as a result of the interaction of glucagon with liver cells (167).

Increased *de novo* synthesis of enzymes which include phenylalanine pyruvate transaminase (168) and phosphoenolpyruvate carboxykinase (169) and altered mitochondrial metabolism are longer-term consequences of the binding of glucagon to cells. Effects on the mitochondrion include increased respiration (170), manifested by elevated succinate dehydrogenase activity and stimulation of electron transport between cytochromes c_1 and c[171] and increased retention of Ca^{2+} (172, 173). Glucagon also influenced the uptake of calcium by the microsomes (172) while insulin had the opposite effect (174); ion distribution may be an integral part of the mechanism by which hormones influence liver metabolism. It has been proposed that Ca^{++} mediates the action of glucagon on triacyl glycerol synthesis and ketogenesis in liver cells (175) but a molecular basis for the role of calcium is not yet clear (173).

It is likely that further research on the biochemical mechanisms of glucagon action, with particular regard to the differentiation between short- and long-term effects of the hormone will make useful contributions to understanding its physiological and clinical roles.

References

1. Kimball, C.P., Murlin, J.R.: Aqueous extracts of pancreas. III. Some precipitation reactions of insulin. J. biol. Chem. 58, 337-346 (1924).
2. Bromer, W.W., Sinn, L.G., Behrens, O.K.: The amino acid sequence of glucagon. J. Am. chem. Soc. 79, 2807-2810 (1957).
3. Sutherland, E.W., De Duve, C.: Origin and distribution of the hyperglycaemic-glycogenolytic factor of the pancreas. J. biol. Chem. 175, 663-674 (1948).
4. Unger, R.H., Ketterer, H., Eisentraut, A.M.: Distribution of immunoassayable glucagon in gastrointestinal tissues. Metabolism 15, 865-867 (1966).
5. Valverde, I., Rigopoulou, D., Marco, J., Faloona, G.R., Unger, R.H.: Characterisation of glucagon-like immunoreactivity (GLI). Diabetes 19, 614-623 (1970).

6. Murphy, R.F., Conlon, J.M., Buchanan, K.D.: The use of antibodies in the characterisation of glucagon-like polypeptides. In: "Gut Hormones", Ed. Bloom, S.R., Churchill-Livingstone, Edinburgh, pp. 379-382 (1978).

7. Grimelius, L., Polak, J.M., Solcia, E., Pearse, A.G.E.: The enteroglucagon cell. In: "Gut Hormones", Ed. Bloom, S.R., Churchill-Livingstone, Edinburgh, pp. 365-368 (1978).

8. Murphy, R.F.: The chemical characterisation of gastrointestinal hormones. Clinics in Endocrinology and Metabolism 8, 281-298 (1979).

9. Assan, R.A., Slusher, N.: Structure/function and structure/immunoreactivity relationships of the glucagon molecule and related synthetic peptides. Diabetes 21, 843-855 (1972).

10. Flanagan, R.W.J., Buchanan, K.D., Murphy, R.F.: Specificity of antibodies in radioimmunoassay of glucagon. Diabetologia 10, 365 (1974).

11. Murphy, R.F., Imam, A., Hughes, A., McGucken, M.J., Buchanan, K.D., Conlon, J.M., Elmore, D.T.: Avoidance of strongly chaotropic eluents for immunoaffinity chromatography by clinical modification of the immobilized ligand. Biochim. biophys. Acta 420, 87-96 (1976).

12. Heding, L.G., Fransden, E.K., Jacobsen, H.: Structure - function relationship : immunologic. Metabolism 25, 1327-1329 (1976).

13. Eisentraut, A.M., Ohneda, A., Parada, E., Unger, R.H.: Immunological discrimination between pancreatic and enteric glucagon-like immunoreactivity (GLI) in tissues and plasma. Diabetes 17, 321-322 (1968).

14. Foa, P.P., Matsuyama, T., Foa, N.L.: Radioimmunoassay of glucagon. In: "Handbook of Radioimmunoassay", Ed. Abraham, G.E., Marcel Dekker Inc., New York, pp. 299-318 (1977).

15. Valverde, I., Lemon, H.M., Kessinger, A., Unger, R.H.: Heterogeneity of plasma glucagon immunoreactivity in normal, depancreatized and alloxan diabetic dogs. Metabolism 24, 1021-1028 (1975).

16. Larsson, L.I., Holst, J., Hakanson, R., Sundler, F.: Distribution and properties of glucagon immunoreactivity in the digestive tract of various mammals : an immunohistochemical and immunocytochemical study. Histochemistry 44, 281-290 (1975).

17. Von Schenk, H.: Production and characterisation of an antiserum against pancreatic glucagon. Clin. chim. Acta. 80, 455-463 (1977).

18. Conlon, J.M., Samson, W.K., Dobbs, R.E., Orci, L., Unger, R.H.: Glucagon-like peptides in canine brain. Diabetes 28, 700-702 (1979).

19. Moody, A.J., Jacobsen, H., Sundby, F., Frandsen, E.K., Baetens, D., Orci, L.: Heterogeneity of gut glucagon-like immunoreactivity. In: "Glucagon : Its Role in Physiology and Clinical Medicine", Eds. Foa, P.P., Bajaj, J.S., Foa, N.L., Springer-Verlag, New York, pp. 129-135 (1977).

20. Moody, A.J., Jacobsen, H., Sundby, F.: Gastric glucagon and gut glucagon-like immunoreactants. In: "Gut Hormones", Ed. Bloom, S.R., Churchill-Livingstone, Edinburgh, pp. 369-378 (1978).

21. Moody, A.J., Sundby, F., Jacobsen, H., Lauritsen, K.B.: The tissue distribution and plasma levels of glicentin (gut GLI-I). Scand. J. Gastroenterol. 13, Suppl. 49, 127 (1978).

22. Garaud, J.C., Eloy, R., Moody, A.J., Grenier, J.F.: Cells immunoreactive to glucagon and gut GLI-I antisera. A light and electron microscopic study. Scand. J. Gastroenterol. 13, Suppl. 49, 65 (1978).

23. Murphy, R.F., Buchanan, K.D., Elmore, R.F.: Isolation of glucagon-like immunoreactivity of gut by affinity chromatography on antiglucagon antibodies coupled to Sepharose 4B. Biochim. biophys. Acta 303, 118-127 (1973).

24. Conlon, J.M., Flanagan, R.W.J., Murphy, R.F.: An improved affinity chromatographic system for the purification of glucagon-like immunoreactivity. Diabetologia II, 336 (1975).

25. Conlon, J.M., Buchanan, K.D., Murphy, R.F.: Glucagon-like materials in porcine and rat intestinal mucosa. In: "Glucagon: Its Role in Physiology and Clinical Medicine", Eds. Foa, P.P., Bajaj, J.S., Foa, N.L., Springer-Verlag, New York, pp. 137-141 (1977).

26. Conlon, J.M., Murphy, R.F., Buchanan, K.D.: Physiochemical and biological properties of glucagon-like polypeptides from porcine colon. Biochim. biophys. Acta 577, 229-240 (1979).

27. Jacobsen, A., Demandt, A., Moody, A.J., Sundby, F.: Sequence analysis of porcine gut GLI-I. Biochim. biophys. Acta 493, 452-459 (1977).

28. Holst, J.J.: Extrapancreatic glucagons. Digestion 17, 168-190 (1978).

29. Unger, R.H., Dobbs, R.E., Orci, L.: Insulin, glucagon and somatostatin secretion in the regulation of metabolism. Ann. Rev. Physiol. 40, 307-343 (1978).

30. Basset, J.M., Madill, D.: Glucagon-like immunoreactivity in the gut and plasma of foetal and post-natal lambs. J. Physiol. (Lond.), 278, 22P-23P (1978).

31. Frame, C.: The contribution of the distal gastrointestinal tract to glucagon-like immunoreactivity secretion in the rat. Proc. Soc. exp. Biol. Med. 152, 667-670 (1976).

32. Tager, H.S., Markese, J.: Intestinal and pancreatic glucagon-like peptides. Evidence for identity of higher molecular weight forms. J. biol. Chem. 254, 2229-2233 (1979).

33. Baetens, D., Rufener, C., Srikant, C.B., Dobbs, R.E., Unger, R.H., Orci, L.: Identification of glucagon-producing cells in dog gastric mucosa. J. Cell Biol. 69, 455-464 (1976).

34. Morita, S., Doi, K., Yip, C.C., Vranic, M.: Measurement and partial characterisation of immunoreactive glucagon in gastrointestinal tissues of dogs. Diabetes 25, 1018-1025 (1976).

35. Srikant, C.B., McCorkle, K., Unger, R.H.: Properties of immunoreactive glucagon fractions of canine stomach and pancreas. J. biol. Chem. 252, 1847-1851 (1977).

36. Sasaki, H., Rubalcava, B., Baetens, D., Blasquez, E., Srikant, C.B., Orci, L., Unger, R.H.: Identification of glucagon in the gastrointestinal tract. J. clin. Invest. 56, 135-145 (1975).

37. Kenny, A.J., Say, R.R.: Glucagon-like activity extractable from the gastrointestinal tract of man and other animals. J. Endocrinol. 25, 1-17 (1962).

38. Valverde, I., Villanueva, M.L., Lozano, I., Roman, D., Diaz-Fierros, M., Marco, J.: Chromatographic pattern of human intestinal glucagon-like immunoreactivity. J. clin. Endocrinol. Metab. 36, 185-187 (1973).

39. Samols, E., Tyler, J., Megyesi, C., Marks, V.: Immunochemical glucagon in human pancreas, gut and plasma. Lancet ii, 727-729 (1966).

40. Makman, M.H., Sutherland, E.W.: Use of liver adenyl cyclase for assay of glucagon in human gastrointestinal tract and pancreas. Endocrinology 75, 127-134 (1964).

41. Bryant, M.G., Bloom, S.R.: Characterisation of the new gastrointestinal hormones. Gut 16, 840 (1975).

42. Knudsen, J.B., Holst, J.J., Asnaes, S., Johansen, A.: Identification of cells with pancreatic-type and gut-type glucagon immunoreactivity in the human colon. Acta Pathol. microbiol. scand. A83, 741-743 (1975).

43. Dawson, J., Bryant, M.G., Gregor, M., Bloom, S.R., Peters, T.J.: Isolation and characterisation of gut hormone storage granules from human stomach, jejunum and rectum. Clin. Sci. 57, 12p (1979).

44. Munoz-Barragan, L., Rufener, C., Srikant, C.B., Dobbs, R.E., Shannon, W.A., Baetons, D., Unger, R.H.: Immunocytochemical evidence for glucagon-containing cells in the human stomach. Horm. Metab. Res. 9, 37-39 (1977).

45. Lawrence, A.M., Tan, S., Hojvat, S., Kirsteins, L., Mitton, J.: Salivary gland glucagon in man and animals. Metabolism 25, 1405-1408 (1976).

46. Hjovat, S., Kirsteins, L., Kisla, J., Paloyan, V., Lawrence, A.M.: Immunoreactive glucagon in the salivary glands of man and animal. In: "Glucagon: Its Role in Physiology and Clinical Medicine", Eds. Foa, P.P., Bajaj, J.S., Foa, N.L., Springer-Verlag, New York, pp. 143-156 (1977).

47. Smith, S., Mazur, A., Voyles, N., Bhathena, S., Recant, L.: Is submaxillary gland immunoreactive glucagon important in carbohydrate homeostasis. Metabolism 28, 343-347 (1979).

48. Dorn, V.A., Lorenz, D., Koch, G.: Immunohistochemical evidence of insulin and glucagon in the epithelium of the pancreatic duct. Acta Histochem. Bd. 58, s. 346-367 (1977).

49. Valverde, I., Rigopoulou, D., Marco, J., Faloona, G., Unger, R.H.: Molecular size of extractable glucagon and glucagon-like immunoreactivity (GLI) in plasma. Diabetes 19, 624-629 (1970).

50. Rigopoulou, D., Valverde, I., Marco, J., Faloona, G.F., Unger, R.H.: Large glucagon-like immunoreactivity in extracts of pancreas. J. biol. Chem. 245, 496-501 (1970).

51. Langslow, D.R.: The action of gut glucagon-like immunoreactivity and other intestinal hormones on lipolysis in chicken adipocytes. Horm. Metab. Res. 5, 428-432 (1973).

52. Holst, J.J.: Extraction, gel-filtration pattern and receptor binding of porcine gastrointestinal glucagon-like immunoreactivity. Diabetologia 13, 159-169 (1977).

53. Sundby, F., Jacobsen, H., Moody, A.J.: Purification and characterisation of a protein from porcine gut with glucagon-like immunoreactivity. Horm. Metab. Res. 8, 366-371 (1976).

54. Horigome, K., Ohneda, A., Mapuhana, Y., Abe, R., Kai, Y.: Heterogeneity of extractable gut glucagon-like immunoreactivity and its lipolytic activity. Horm. Metab. Res. 9, 370-374 (1977).

55. Bataille, D.P., Freychet, P., Kitabgi, P.E., Rosselin, G.E.: Gut glucagon: a common receptor site with pancreatic glucagon in liver plasma membranes. FEBS Letters 30, 215-218 (1973).

56. Tager, H.S., Steiner, D.F.: Isolation of a glucagon-like containing peptide, primary structure of a possible fragment. Proc. natn. Acad. Sci. U.S.A. 70, 2321-2325 (1973).

57. Conlon, J.M., Murphy, R.F., Buchanan, K.D.: Possible precursor relationship between gut glucagon-like immunoreactivity and glucagon. Gut 18, A401 (1977).

58. Ravazzola, M., Siperstein, A., Moody, A.J., Sundby, F., Jacobsen, H., Orci, L.: Glicentin-immunoreactive cells: Their relationship to glucagon-producing cells. Endocrinology 105, 499-508 (1979).

59. Mains, R.E., Eipper, B.A.: Coordinate synthesis of corticotropins and endorphins by mouse pituitary tumour cells. J. biol. Chem. 253, 651-655 (1978).

60. Grube, D., Voight, K.H., Weber, E.: Pancreatic glucagon cells contain endorphin-like immunoreactivity. Histochemistry 59, 75-79 (1978).

61. Smith, P.H., Marchant, F.W., Johnson, D.G., Fujimoto, W.Y., Williams, R.H.: Immunocytochemical localization of a gastric inhibitory polypeptide-like material within A cells of the endocrine pancreas. Am. J. Anat. 149, 585-590 (1977).

62. Aluemets, J., Hakanson, R., Dorisit, T.O., Sjöland, K., Sundler, F.: Is GIP a glucagon cell constituent? Histochemistry 58, 253-257 (1978).

63. Blundell, T.L., Dockerill, K., Sasaki, K., Tickle, I.J., Wood, S.P.: The relation of structure to storage and receptor binding of glucagon. Metabolism 25, 1331-1338 (1976).

64. Dockerill, S., Blundell, T.L., Sasaki, K., Tickle, I.J., Wood, S.P.: The relation of structure to storage and receptor binding of glucagon. Biochem. Soc. Trans. 5, 1121-1122 (1977).

65. Bloom, S.R.: Signals for glucagon secretion. Ciba Found. Symp. 55, 161-172 (1977).

66. Kaneto, A.: The role of the autonomic nervous system in glucagon secretion. In: "Glucagon: Its Role in Physiology and Clinical Medicine", Eds. Foa, P.P., Bajaj, J.S., Foa, N.L., Springer-Verlag, New York, pp. 272-286 (1977).

67. Edwards, A.V., Bloom, S.R.: Nervous control of pancreatic hormones. In: "Gut Hormones", Ed. Bloom, S.R., Churchill-Livingstone, Edinburgh, pp. 394-405 (1978).

68. Foa, P.P.: Glucagon. In:"Glucagon: Its Role in Physiology and Clinical Medicine", Eds. Foa, P.P., Bajaj, J.S., Foa, N.L., Springer-Verlag, New York, pp. xvii-x1 (1977).

69. Gerich, J.E.: Control of pancreatic IRG secretion in vivo. Metabolism 25, 1437-1442 (1976).

70. Gerich, J.E.: On the causes and consequences of abnormal glucagon secretion in human diabetes mellitus. In: "Glucagon: Its Role in Physiology and Clinical Medicine", Eds. Foa, P.P., Bajaj, J.S., Foa, N.L., Springer-Verlag, pp. 617-641 (1977).

71. Ohneda, A., Watanabe, K., Horigome, K., Sakai, T., Kai, Y., Oikawa, S.-I.: Abnormal response of pancreatic glucagon to glycaemic changes in diabetes mellitus. J. clin. Endocrinol. Metab. 46, 504-510 (1978).

72. Ipp, E., Dobbs, E., Unger, R.H.: Morphine and β-endorphin influence the secretion of the endocrine pancreas. Nature 276, 190-191 (1978).

73. Sarantakis, D., Teichman, J., Fenichel, R., Lien, R.: [des-Ala^1, Gly^2] $His^{4,5}$ D-Trp^8 -somatostatin. A glucagon specific and long-acting somatostatin analog. FEBS Lett. 92, 153-155 (1978).

74. Assan, R.A., Attali, J.R., Ballerio, G., Boillot, J., Girard, J.R.: Glucagon secretion induced by natural and artificial amino acids in the perfused rat pancreas. Diabetes 26, 300-307 (1977).

75. Leclercq-Meyer, V., Marchand, J., Malaisse, W.J.: The Role of calcium in glucagon release. Diabetes 27, 996-1004 (1978).

76. Holst, J.J., Von Schenk, H., Lindkaer, S.: Gel-filtration of immunoreactive glucagon secreted by the isolated, perfused, porcine pancreas. Scand. J. clin. Lab. Invest. 39, 47-52 (1979).

77. Conlon, J.M., Ipp, E., Unger, R.H.: The molecular forms of immunoreactive glucagon secreted by the isolated perfused dog pancreas. Life Sci. 23, 1655-1658 (1978).

78. Lefebvre, P.J., Luyckx, A.S., Brassinne, A.H., Nizet, A.H.: Glucagon and gastrin release by the isolated perfused dog stomach in response to arginine. Metabolism 25, 1477-1480 (1976).

79. Lefebvre, P.J., Luyckx, A.S.: Glucose and insulin in the regulation of glucagon release from the isolated perfused dog stomach. Endocrinology 103, 1579-1582 (1978).

80. Blazquez, E., Munoz-Barragan, L., Patton, G.S., Orci, L., Dobbs, R.E., Unger, R.H.: Gastric A-cell function in insulin-deprived depancreatised dogs. Endocrinology 99, 1182-1188 (1976).

81. Matsuyama, T., Tanaka, R., Shima, K., Tarui, S.: Failure of somatostatin to decrease blood glucose by suppression of extrapancreatic glucagon in severely diabetic depancreatised dogs. Endocrinol jap. 25, 529-532 (1978).

82. Ross, G., Lickley, L., Vranic, M.: Extrapancreatic glucagon in control of glucose turnover in depancreatised dogs. Am. J. Physiol. 234, E213-E219 (1978).

83. Buchanan, K.D., Vance, J.E., Teruaki, A., Williams, R.H.: Rise in serum glucagon after intrajejunal glucose in pancreatectomised dogs. Proc. Soc. exp. Biol. Med. 126, 813-815 (1967).

84. Buchanan, K.D., Zandomeneghi, R., Murphy, R.F., Teale, J.D.: Glucagon and the gut. Gut 12, 861 (1971).

85. Murphy, R.F., Teale, J.D., Buchanan, K.D.: Use of antibody-Sepharose complexes to study the release of glucagon-like immunoreactivity from rat small intestine. Diabetologia 8, 60 (1972).

86. O'Connor, F.A., Conlon, J.M., Buchanan, K.D., Murphy, R.F.: The use of perfused rat intestine to characterise the glucagon-like immunoreactivity released into serosal secretions following stimulation by glucose. Horm. Metab. Res. 11, 19-24 (1979).

87. Marco, J., Hedo, J.A., Villanueva, M.L.: Inhibition of intestinal glucagon-like immunoreactivity secretion by somatostatin in men. J. clin. Endocrinol. Metab. 44, 695-698 (1977).

88. Alexander, D.P., Assan, R., Britton, H.G., Fenton, E., Forsling, M.L.: The effect of intraduodenal glucose on plasma glucagon and glucagon-like activity in the foetal sheep. J. Physiol. (Lond.) 265, 52p-53p (1977).

89. Botha, J.L., Vinik, A.I., Child, P.T., Paul, M., Jackson, W.P.M.: Pancreatic glucagon-like immunoreactivity in a pancreatectomised patient. Horm. Metab. Res. 9, 199-205 (1977).

90. Werner, P.L., Palmer, J.P.: Immunoreactive glucagon responses to oral glucose, insulin infusion and deprivation and somatostatin in pancreatectomised man. Diabetes 27, 1007-1012 (1978).

91. Barnes, A.J., Bloom, S.R.: Pancreatectomised man: A model for diabetes without glucagon. Lancet i, 219-221 (1976).

92. Palmer, J.P., Werner, P.L., Benson, J.W., Ensinck, J.W.: Immunoreactive glucagon responses to arginine in three pancreatectomised humans. Metabolism 25, 1483-1485 (1976).

93. Chisholm, D.J., Alford, F.P., Harewood, M.S., Findlay, D.M., Gray, B.N.: Nature and biologic activity of extrapancreatic glucagon: Studies in pancreatectomised cats. Metabolism 27, 261-273 (1978).

94. Valverde, I.: Quantification of plasma glucagon immunoreactive components in normal and hyperglucagonaemic states. In: "Glucagon: Its Role in Physiology and Clinical Medicine", Eds. Foa, P.P., Bajaj, J.S., Foa, N.L., Springer-Verlag, New York, pp. 77-92 (1977).

95. Weir, G.C.: Assessment of glucagon-like immunoreactivity in plasma. In: "Glucagon: Its Role in Physiology and Clinical Medicine", Eds. Foa, P.P., Bajaj, J.S., Foa, N.L., Springer-Verlag, New York, pp. 65-76 (1977).

96. Jaspan, B.J., Rubenstein, A.H.: Circulating glucagon. Diabetes 26, 887-889 (1977).

97. Flanagan, R.W.J., Trimble, E.R., Conlon, J.M., Murphy, R.F.: Purification and characterisation of plasma glucagon-like immunoreactivity. Diabetologia 11, 342 (1975).

98. Flanagan, R.W.J., Murphy, R.F., Buchanan, K.D.: Circulating forms of glucagon and related peptides in normal subjects and uremic patients. Biochem. Soc. Trans. (1980) (in press).

99. Wright, D.E., Hornby, V.J., Rodbell, M.: A reassessment of structure - function relationships in glucagon. J. biol. Chem. 253, 6338-6340 (1978).

100. Mallinson, C., Bloom, S.R.: The hyperglycaemic cutaneous syndrome: Pancreatic glucagonoma. In:"Surgical Endocrinology", 13, Ed. Friesen, S.R., J.B. Lippincott, Philadelphia pp. 171-202 (1978).

101. Holst, J.J.: Gut endocrine tumour syndromes. Clinics in Endocrinology and Metabolism 8, 413-432 (1979).

102. Hess, W.: Über ein endokrin inaktives Carcinom der langerhansschen Inseln. Schweiz. med. Wochenschr. 76, 802-804 (1946).

103. Unger, R.H., Eisentraut, A.M., Lochner, J.R.: Glucagon producing tumours of the islets of Langerhans. J. clin. Invest. 42, 987-988 (1963).

104. McGavran, M.H., Unger, R.H., Recant, L., Polk, H., Kilo, C., Levin, M.E.: A glucagon secreting alpha-cell carcinoma of the pancreas. New Engl. J. Med. 274, 1408-1413 (1966).

105. Mallinson, C.N., Bloom, S.R., Warin, A.P., Salmon, P.R., Cox, B.: A glucagonoma syndrome. Lancet ii, 1-5 (1974).

106. Lightman, S.L., Bloom, S.R.: Cure of insulin-dependent diabetes mellitus by removal of a glucagonoma. Br. med. J. 1, 367-368 (1974).

107. Gleeson, M.H., Bloom, S.R., Polak, J.M., Henry, K., Dowling, R.H., Pearse, A.G.E.: Endocrine tumour in kidney affecting small bowel structure, motility and absorptive function. Gut 12, 773-786 (1971).

108. Stevens, F.M., Flanagan, R.W.J., Buchanan, K.D., O'Gorman, D.J.: The first Irish glucagonoma. Ir. J. med. Sci. 146, 350 (1977).

109. Unger, R.H.: Role of glucagon in the pathogenesis of diabetes: the status of the controversy. Metabolism 27, 1691-1709 (1978).

110. Lefebvre, P.J., Luyckx, A.S.: Glucagon and the kidney. In: "Glucagon: Its Role in Physiology and Clinical Medicine", Eds. Foa, P.P., Bajaj, J.S., Foa, N.L., Springer-Verlag, New York, pp. 167-176 (1977).

111. Barnes, A.J., Bloom, S.R., Alberti, K.G.M.M., Smythe, P., Alford, A.P., Chisholm, D.J.: Ketoacidosis in pancreatectomised patients. New Engl. J. Med. 296, 1250-1253 (1977).

112. Kuku, S.F., Ziedler, A., Emmanuel, D.S., Katz, A.I., Rubenstein, A.N., Levin, N.W., Teller, A.: Heterogeneity of plasma glucagon: patterns in patients with chronic renal failure and diabetes. J. clin. Endocrinol. Metab. 42, 173-176 (1976).

113. Sherwin, R.S., Fisher, M., Bessoff, J., Snyder, N., Hendler, R., Conn, H.O., Felig, P.: Hyperglucagonaemia in cirrhosis; altered secretion and sensitivity to glucagon. Gastroenterology 74, 1224-1228 (1978).

114. Doyle, J.A., Schroeter, L.S., Rogers, R.S.: Hyperglucagonaemia and necrolytic migratory erythemia in cirrhosis-possible pseudoglucagonoma syndrome. Br. J. Derm. 101, 581-587 (1979).

115. Grollman, A., McCaleb, W.E., White, F.N.: Glucagon deficiency as a cause of hypoglycaemia. Metabolism 13, 686-690 (1964).

116. Bleicher, S.T., Spengel, G., Levy, L., Zarowitz, H.: Glucagon-deficiency hypoglycaemia: a new syndrome. Clin. Res. 18, 355 (1970).

117. Bottazzo, G.F., Flonn-Christensen, A., Doniach, D.: Islet antibodies in diabetes mellitus with autoimmune polyendocrine deficiency. Lancet ii, 1279-1282 (1974).

118. MacCuish, A.C., Barnes, E.W., Irvine, W.J., Duncan, L.: Antibodies to pancreatic islet cells in insulin-dependent diabetics with coexistent autoimmune disease. Lancet ii, 1529-1531 (1974).

119. Bottazzo, G.F., Lendrum, R.: Separate autoantibodies to human pancreatic glucagon and somatostatin cells. Lancet ii, 2873-2876 (1976).

120. Rodbell, M., Landos, C.: Regulation of hepatic adenylate cyclase by glucagon, GTP, divalent cations and adenosine. Metabolism 25, 1347-1349 (1976).

121. Moran, E.C., Clou, P.Y., Fasman, G.D.: Conformational transitions of glucagon in solution; the $\alpha \rightarrow \beta$ transition. Biochem. biophys. Res. Commun. 77, 1300-1306 (1977).

122. Epand, R.M., Jones, A.J.S., Seyer, B.: Molecular interactions in the model lipoprotein complex formed between glucagon and dimyristoylglycerophosphocholine. Biochemistry 16, 4360-4368 (1977).

123. Schramm, M.: Transfer of glucagon receptor from liver membranes to a foreign adenylate cyclase by a membrane fusion procedure. Proc. natn. Acad. Sci. U.S.A. 76, 1174-1178 (1979).

124. Houslay, M.D., Ellory, J.C., Smith, G.A., Hesketh, T.R., Stein, J.M., Warren, G.B., Metcalfe, J.C.: Exchange of partners in glucagon receptor-adenylate cyclase complexes. Biochim. biophys. Acta 467, 208-219 (1977).

125. Houslay, M.D., Palmer, R.W.: Lysophosphatidyl cholines can modulate the activity of the glucagon-stimulated adenylate cyclase from rat liver plasma membranes. Biochem. J. 178, 217-221 (1979).

126. Kiss, Z.: Involvement of calcium in the inhibition by insulin of the glucagon-stimulated adenylate cyclase activity. Europ. J. Biochem. 95, 607-611 (1979).

127. Epand, R.M., Epand, R.F., Grey, V.: The essential role of the imidazole group of glucagon in its biological function. Arch. Biochem. Biophys. 154, 132-136 (1973).

128. Lande, S., Gorman, R., Bitensky, M.: Selectively blocked and des-histidine-glucagons; preparation and effects on hepatic adenylate cyclase activity. Endocrinology 90, 597-604 (1972).

129. Sonne, O., Gliemann, J.: Receptor binding of glucagon and adenosine 3', 5'- monophosphate accumulation in isolated rat fat cells. Biochim. biophys. Acta 499, 259-272 (1977).

130. Lin, M.C., Nicosia, S., Rodbell, M.: The effects of iodination on the binding action of glucagon at its receptor. Biochemistry 15, 4537-4540 (1976).

131. Desbuquois, B.: Acetylglucagon; preparation and characterisation. Europ. J. Biochem. 60, 335-347 (1975).

132. Desbuquois, B.: Iodoglucagon; preparation and characterisation. Europ. J. Biochem. 53, 569-580 (1975).

133. Wright, D.E., Rodbell, M.: Glucagon $_{1-6}$ binds to the glucagon receptor and activates adenylate cyclase. J. biol. Chem. 254, 268-269 (1979).

134. Birnbaumer, L., Swartz, T.L.: Guanyl nucleotide regulation of the liver glucagon-sensitive adenylate cyclase system. In: "Glucagon: Its Role in Physiology and Clinical Medicine" Eds. Foa, P.P., Bajaj, J.S., Foa, N.L., Springer-Verlag, New York, pp. 349-372 (1977).

135. Kimura, N., Nagate, N.: The requirement of guanine nucleotides for glucagon stimulation of adenylate cyclase in rat liver plasma membranes. J. biol. Chem. 252, 3829-3835 (1977).

136. Lin, M.C., Nicosia, S., Lad, P.M., Rodbell, M.: Effects of GTP on binding of [^{3}H] glucagon to receptors in rat hepatic plasma membranes. J. biol. Chem. 252, 2790-2792 (1977).

137. Lad, P.M., Welton, A.F., Rodbell, M.: Evidence for distinct guanine nucleotide sites in the regulation of the glucagon receptor and of adenylate cyclase activity. J. biol. Chem. 252, 5942-5946 (1977).

138. Welton, A.F., Lad, P.M., Newby, A., Yamamura, H., Nicosia, S., Rodbell, M.: Solubilisation and separation of the glucagon receptor and adenylate cyclase in guanine nucleotide-sensitive states. J. biol. Chem. 252, 5947-5950 (1977).

139. Iyengar, R., Swartz, T.L., Birnbaumer, L.: Coupling of glucagon receptor to adenylate cyclase; requirement of a receptor-related guanyl nucleotide binding site for coupling of the receptor to the enzyme. J. biol. Chem. 254, 1119-1123 (1979).

140. Levitzky, A., Helmreich, J.M.: Hormone-receptor - adenylate cyclase interactions. FEBS Lett. 101, 213-219 (1979).

141. Pilkis, S.J., Exton, J.H., Johnson, R.A., Park, C.R.: Effects of glucagon on cyclic AMP and carbohydrate metabolism in livers from diabetic rats. Biochim. biophys. Acta 343, 250-267 (1974).

142. Bhathena, S.J., Voyles, N.R., Smith, S., Recant, L.: Decreased glucagon receptors in diabetic rat hepatocytes; evidence for regulation of glucagon receptors by hyperglucagonaemia. J. clin. Invest. 61, 1488-1497 (1978).

143. Soman, V., Felig, P.: Regulation of the glucagon receptor by physiological hyperglucagonaemia. Nature 272, 829-832 (1978).

144. Davidson, M.B., Kaplan, S.A.: Increased insulin binding by hepatic plasma membranes from diabetic rats. Normalisation by insulin therapy. J. clin. Invest. 59, 22-30 (1977).

145. Olefsky, J.M., Reaven, G.M.: Decreased insulin binding to lymphocytes from diabetic patients. J. clin. Invest. 54, 1323-1329 (1974).

146. Srikant, C.B., Freeman, D., McCorkle, K., Unger, R.H.: Binding and biological activity of glucagon in liver cell membranes of chronically hyperglucagonaemic rats. J. biol. Chem. 252, 7434-7436 (1977).

147. Fouchereau-Peron, M., Pancon, F., Freychet, P., Rosselin, G.: The effect of feeding and fasting on the early steps of glucagon action in isolated rat liver cells. Endocrinology 98, 755-760 (1976).

148. Bloomgarden, Z.T., Liljenquist, A.D., Cherrington, A.D., Rabinowitz, D.: Persistent stimulatory effect of glucagon on glucose production despite down regulation. J. clin. Endocrinol. Metab. 47, 1152-1155 (1978).

149. Cote, T.E., Epand, R.M.: N^{α}-Trinitrophenyl glucagon; an inhibitor of glucagon-stimulated cyclic AMP production and its effects on glycogenolysis. Biochim. biophys. Acta 582, 295-306 (1979).

150. Lehotay, D.C., Levey, G.S., Canterbury, J.M., Bricker, L.A., Ruiz, E.: A peptide inhibitor of glucagon-responsive adenylate cyclase in liver. In: "Glucagon: Its Role in Physiology and Clinical Medicine", Eds. Foa, P.P., Bajaj, J.S., Foa, N.L., Springer-Verlag, New York, pp. 373-378 (1977).

151. Kolata, G.B.: Polypeptide hormones; what are they doing in cells ? Science 201, 895-897 (1978).

152. Sherwin, R.S., Bastl, C., Finkelstein, F.O., Fisher, M., Black, H., Hendler, R., Felig, P.: Influence of uraemia and haemodialysis on the turnover and metabolic effects of glucagon. J. clin. Invest. 57, 722-731 (1976).

153. Schwoch, G.: Differential activation of type-1 and type-11 adenosine 3': 5'- cyclic monophosphate-dependent protein kinases in liver of glucagon-treated rats. Biochem. J. 170, 469-477 (1977).

154. Garrison, J.C.: The effects of glucagon, catecholamines and the calcium ionophore A23187 on the phosphorylation of rat hepatocyte cytosolic proteins. J. biol. Chem. 253, 7091-7100 (1978).

155. Avruch, J., Witters, L.A., Alexander, M.C., Bush, M.A.: Effects of glucagon and insulin on cytoplasmic protein phosphorylation in hepatocytes. J. biol. Chem. 253, 4754-4761 (1978).

156. Schwoch, G., Hilz, H.: Time dependent translocation of protein kinase in liver of glucagon-treated rats. FEBS Lett. 90, 127-131 (1978).

157. Vandenheede, J.R., Keppens, S., De Wulf, H.: The activation of liver phosphorylase β kinase by glucagon. FEBS Lett 61, 213-217 (1976).

158. Birnbaum, M.J., Fain, J.N.: Activation of protein kinase and glycogen phosphorylase in isolated rat liver cells by glucagon and catecholamines. J. biol. Chem. 252, 528-535 (1977).

159. Gilboe, D.P., Nuttall, F.Q.: In vivo glucose -, glucagon - and cAMP - induced changes in liver glycogen synthase phosphatase. J. biol. Chem. 253, 4078-4081 (1978).

160. Blair, J.B., Cimbale, M.A., Foster, J.L., Morgan, R.A.: Hepatic pyruvate kinase: regulation by glucagon, cyclic adenosine 3' : 5'-monophosphate and insulin in the perfused rat liver. J. biol. Chem. 251, 3756-3762 (1976).

161. Riou, J.P., Claus, T.H., Pilkis, S.J.: Control of pyruvate kinase by glucagon in isolated hepatocytes. Biochem. biophys. Res. Commun. 73, 591-599 (1976).

162. Riou, J.P., Claus, T.H., Pilkis, S.J.: Stimulation by glucagon of in vivo phosphorylation of rat hepatic pyruvate kinase. J. biol. Chem. 253, 656-659 (1978).

163. Ishibashi, H., Cottam, G.L.: Glucagon-stimulated phosphorylation of pyruvate kinase in hepatocytes. J. biol. Chem. 253, 8767-8771 (1978).

164. Van Berkel, T.J.C., Kruÿt, J.K., Koster, J.F.: Hormone-induced changes in pyruvate kinase. Effects of glucagon and starvation. Europ. J. Biochem. 81, 423-432 (1977).

165. Van Berkel, T.J.C., Kruÿt, J.K., Van Den Berg, G.B., Koster, J.F.: Difference in the effect of glucagon and starvation upon L-type pyruvate kinase from rat liver. Europ. J. Biochem. 92, 553-561 (1978).

166. Witters, L.A., Kowaloff, E.M., Avruch, J.: Glucagon regulation of protein phosphorylation. Identification of acetyl coenzyme A carboxylase as a substrate. J. biol. Chem. 254, 245-248 (1979).

167. Donlon, J., Kaufman, S.: Glucagon stimulation of rat hepatic phenylalanine hydroxylase through phosphorylation in vivo. J. biol. Chem. 253, 6657-6659 (1978).

168. Shih, J.C., Chan, Y.-L.: Direct evidence for de novo synthesis of rat liver phenylalanine: Pyruvate transaminase after glucagon treatment. Arch. Biochem. Biophys. 192, 414-420 (1979).

169. Oliver, T., Edwards, M., Pitot, H.C.: Hormonal regulation of phosphoenol-pyruvate carboxykinase in primary cultures of adult-rat liver parenchymal cells. Europ. J. Biochem. 87, 221-227 (1978).

170. Siess, E.A., Wieland, O.H.: Isolated hepatocytes as a model for the study of stable glucagon effects on mitochondrial respiratory functions. FEBS Lett. 101, 277-281 (1979).

171. Halestrap, A.P.: Stimulation of the respiratory chain of rat liver mitochondria between cytochrome c, and cytochrome c by glucagon treatment of rats. Biochem. J. 172, 399-405 (1978).

172. Hughes, B.P., Barritt, G.J.: Effects of glucagon and $N^6O^{2'}$-dibutyryl-adenosine 3' : 5" - cyclic monophosphate on calcium transport in isolated rat liver mitochondria. Biochem. J. 176, 295-304 (1978).

173. Prpić, V., Spencer, T.L., Bygrave, F.L.: Stable enhancement of calcium retention in mitochondria isolated from rat liver after the administration of glucagon to the intact animal. Biochem. J. 176, 705-714 (1978).

174. Waltenbaugh, A.-M.A., Friedman, N.: Hormone sensitive calcium uptake by liver microsomes. Biochem. biophys. Res. Commun. 82, 603-608 (1978).

175. Soler-Argilaga, C., Russell, R.L., Werner, H.W., Heimberg, M.: A possible role of calcium in the activation of glucagon, cAMP and dibutyryl cAMP on the metabolism of free fatty acids by rat hepatocytes. Biochem. biophys. Res. Commun. 85, 249-256 (1978).

PHOTOBIOLOGY, METABOLISM, AND CLINICAL ASPECTS OF VITAMIN D

M. F. Holick
Endocrine Unit, Massachusetts General Hospital, Boston, MA 02114
U.S.A.

Historical Aspects of Rickets

Rickets was reported as early as the second century A.D., but, until people began to congregate in the cities of northern Europe during the fifteenth and sixteenth centuries, the disease was not considered a significant health problem (1). By the mid-seventeenth century, Whistler and DeBoot and Glisson each independently recognized many of the diagnostic signs of this disease and established rickets as a clinical entity (2, 3). Before the advent of x-rays, rickets was seldom recognized until several months after birth, and it most commonly attracted attention at the end of the first year of life. The symptoms and diagnostic features included great tenderness of the bones, gradual changes in the shape of the bones, at first chiefly noticed at the ends of the long bones, causing enlargement of the wrists, knees, and ribs, curvature of the spine, enlargement of the head, and bowing of the lower limbs. The incidence of this debilitating bone disease increased dramatically during the industrial revolution, especially in northern Europe and North America, and, by the end of the nineteenth century, autopsy studies of infants suggested that as many as 90% of all the infants born in these crowded cities had the disease (4).

As early as 1822 the Polish physician Sniadecki realized the importance of exposure to the sun for the prevention and cure of rickets (5). In 1890, Palm (6) collated clinical observations from the British Empire and the Orient and also concluded that exposure to sunlight was most important for the preven-

Hormones in Normal and Abnormal Human Tissues, Vol. II

tion and cure of this debilitating disease. In 1919 Huldschinsky reported 4 patients with severe rickets who were cured, based upon x-ray examination, after being treated with exposures to a mercury-vapor quartz lamp (7). Soon after, Hess and co-workers demonstrated that children in New York City exposed to varying amounts of sunlight could also be cured of this disease (8).

During this same period, Mellanby announced successful production of rickets in puppies as a result of feeding them a diet that lacked a fat-soluble nutritional factor (9). This observation prompted extensive investigations into food substances that could prevent and cure rickets. Using this model, it was demonstrated that cod-liver oil had the highest antirachitic activity (10). Soon after, McCollum and co-workers demonstrated that the antirachitic factor present in cod-liver oil was not vitamin A but a new fat-soluble factor that was called vitamin D (11). The great confusion that arose over whether rickets was cured solely by ultraviolet irradiation or a dietary factor was resolved when Powers et al. (12) reported that radiations from a mercury-vapor quartz lamp had identical healing effects in rachitic rats when compared with those brought about by administration of cod-liver oil. Steenbock and Black (13) and Hess and Weinstock (14) independently demonstrated that ultraviolet irradiation of the diet also imparted antirachitic properties. These observations paved the way for the isolation and structural characterization of vitamin D a decade later and provided the basis for the supplementing of dairy products with vitamin D, which was essentially responsible for the eradication of the disease

Photobiology of Vitamin D_3

It has been generally accepted that during sunlight exposure, cutaneous stores of 7-dehydrocholesterol are partly converted to vitamin D_3. However, when 7-dehydrocholesterol is dissolved in an organic solvent and exposed to ultraviolet radiation in a quartz vessel, it absorbs a photon of radiation energy, causing cleavage of the C_9-C_{10} bond to form a 9,10-secosteroid, previtamin D_3 (15). Vitamin D_3 is not formed during this photochemical reaction. Vitamin D_3 is derived solely from previtamin D_3, which is thermally labile and undergoes a temperature-dependent rearrangement of its double bonds and a [1-7] sigmatropic shift of the hydrogen from C_9 to C_{19} (15) to form a thermally-stable 9,10-secosteroid, vitamin D_3 (Figure 1). Previtamin D_3 can also absorb radiation energy, which causes rearrangements of its double bonds to form lumisterol and tachysterol (Figure 1). Until recently, however, little was known regarding the mechanism for vitamin D_3 synthesis in skin _in vivo_ on exposure to

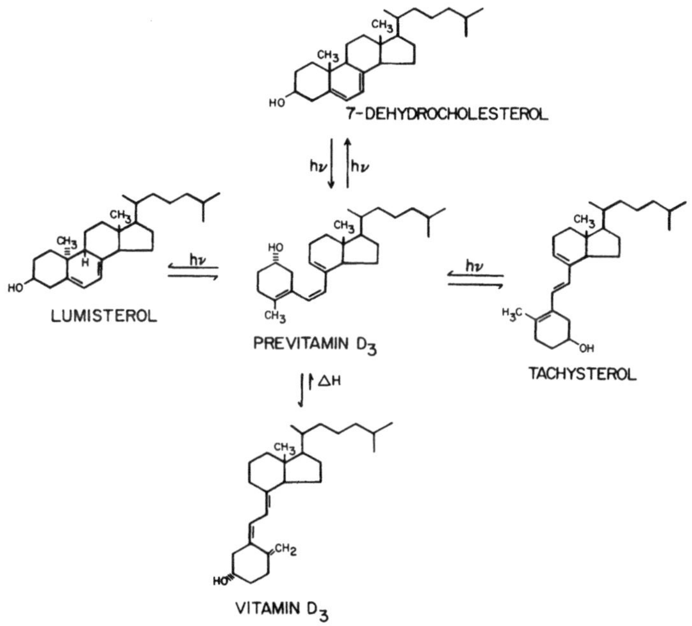

Fig. 1. Structures for 7-dehydrocholesterol, previtamin D_3, lumisterol$_3$, tachysterol$_3$, and vitamin D_3 (reproduced from Holick et al. (21) with permission).

sunlight. A number of investigators demonstrated vitamin D_3 in the skin as a result of exposure to artificial ultraviolet radiation, but did not determine the steps involved in its production (16-18). It was established that the endogenous product formed in the skin during exposure to ultraviolet radiation was previtamin D_3 (19, 20). Furthermore, because careful analysis of lipid extracts of skin showed no detectable amounts of vitamin D_3, it was concluded that, during exposure to physiologic amounts of ultraviolet radiation, previtamin D_3 is the principal if not sole photo-product generated in the skin (20). Similar investigations using human skin specimens also revealed that previtamin D_3 was the major photoproduct formed during exposure to simulated solar radiation (21).

These observations prompted an investigation to determine whether there were any biologic advantages to making previtamin D_3 in the skin. The thermal isomerization of previtamin D_3 to vitamin D_3 was studied <u>in vitro</u> to determine the time course of this thermal equilibrium reaction at various temperatures, including those that approximate the temperature of the epidermis. At 25°C, previtamin D_3 slowly equilibrates to vitamin D_3, with 50% conversion in about 48 h and equilibrium in about 14 days with 83% conversion (Figure 2). In comparison, at 37°C, 50% of previtamin D_3 was converted to vitamin D_3 by 28 h, and equilibrium was reached after 4 days. At -20°C less than 2% of previtamin D_3 is converted to vitamin D_3 even after 7 days' incubation (21).

There appears to be a transport system that preferentially translocates vitamin D_3 from the skin into the circulation as it is being made from its previtamin, since the vitamin-D-binding protein has essentially no affinity for previtamin D_3 compared to its affinity for vitamin D_3 (21, 22). To determine where vitamin D_3 is synthesized in the epidermis, two techniques were used that separate the epidermis and dermis without altering either the integrity of the cells or the stratum corneum barrier. Surgically-obtained skin was incubated with staphylococcal exfoliatin, a toxin that was found to cleave the epider-

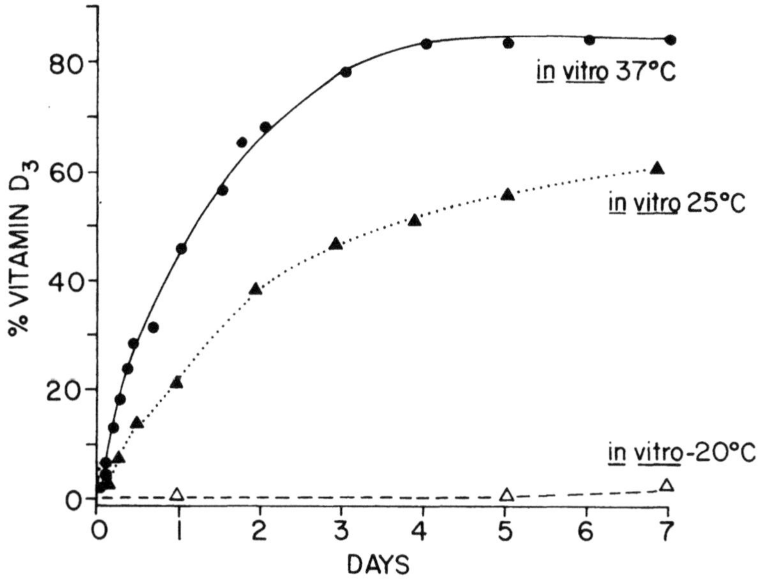

Fig. 2. Thermal conversion of previtamin D_3 to vitamin D_3 as a function of time at 37°C (—●), 25°C (···▲), and -20°C (--Δ) (reproduced from Holick et al. (21) with permission)

mis between the stratum granulosum and stratum Malpighian without altering cellular integrity (23). After incubation, the skin was either exposed to ultraviolet radiation or kept in the dark. High-pressure liquid chromatographic analyses of the lipid extracts of the skin layers demonstrated that 7-dehydrocholesterol and previtamin D_3 concentrations were the highest in the Malpighian layer and dermis, whereas there was very little 7-dehydrocholesterol or previtamin D_3 in the stratum corneum and stratum granulosum layers (21). Other human skin samples obtained at surgery were immersed in hot water at 60°C for 45 minutes and then either exposed to ultraviolet radiation or kept in the dark. (The water-immersion technique makes it possible to separate skin samples into two sections: the upper section contains the entire epidermis minus the basal layer, and the bottom section contains the entire dermis plus the basal layer (24)). The basal layer was mechanically scraped off from the bottom section, and the three isolated layers were extracted and subjected to high-pressure liquid chromatography. Chromatograms of these lipid extracts demonstrated that although previtamin D_3 synthesis occurred throughout the entire epidermis, the basal layer of the Malpighian layer had the highest concentrations of both 7-dehydrocholesterol and previtamin D_3 (25). Furthermore, there was also a small amount of previtamin D_3 produced in the dermis. The physiologic advantage of forming previtamin D_3 in the skin during exposure to the sun and the role of the vitamin-D-binding protein in the processing of the thermal product of the previtamin are illustrated schematically in Figure 3. During exposure to sunlight, the UV-B portion of the solar spectrum produces the photochemical conversion of epidermal 7-dehydrocholesterol to previtamin D_3. As soon as previtamin D_3 is made in the skin, it begins to isomerize to vitamin D_3, the rate of the reaction being controlled by the temperature of the skin. Once vitamin D_3 is formed from its precursor, it is preferentially bound to a vitamin-D-binding protein in the capillaries and transported into the circulation. Thus the skin is the site for the synthesis of 7-dehydrocholesterol, a reservoir for the storage of the primary photoproduct, previtamin D_3, and the site for the slow thermal conversion to vitamin D_3. The slow thermal conversion of previtamin D_3 to vitamin D_3, which occurs over several days at physiologic temperatures and the selective removal of vitamin D_3 by the vitamin-D-binding protein permit the efficient use of small quantities of previtamin D_3 that are generated in the skin during exposure to the sun (21, 22, 25).

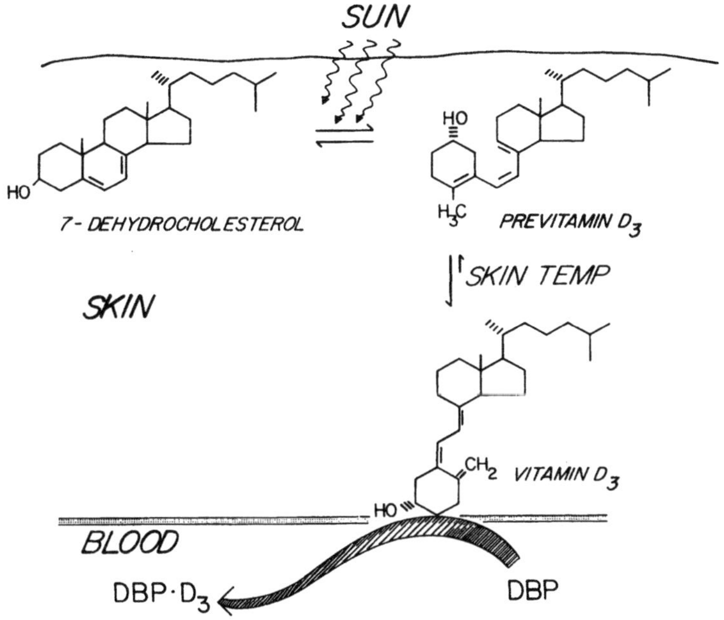

Fig. 3. The photochemical and thermal events that lead to the formation of vitamin D_3 in the skin. During exposure to sunlight 7-dehydrocholesterol in the epidermis partly converts to previtamin D_3 . Previtamin D_3 undergoes a temperature-dependent [1-7] hydrogen shift from C_9 to C_{19} and a rearrangement of its triene system to form vitamin D_3 . The vitamin-D-binding protein preferentially translocates vitamin D_3 from the skin into the circulation, leaving the previtamin in the skin for further conversion to vitamin D_3 (reproduced from Holick et al. (21) with permission).

Metabolism of Vitamin D

Once vitamin D_3 is made in the skin or ingested in the diet (Figure 4), it, along with dietary vitamin D_2, enters the circulation bound to vitamin-D-binding protein and both are transported to the liver where they are hydroxylated at C_{25} to generate the major circulating vitamin-D metabolite, 25-hydroxyvitamine D (25-OH-D) (26-28). Like vitamin D (vitamin D and vitamin-D metabolites without a subscript denote vitamin D_3 or vitamin D_2, or both, and their metabolites interchangeably), 25-OH-D at physiologic concentrations is incapable of stimulating either intestinal calcium transport or bone calcium mobilization (26, 27). The liver is the major site for C_{25}-hydroxylation of vitamin D (26-28). The hepatic vitamin-D-25-hydroxylase(s) is located both in mitochondria and in microsomes. The enzymatic reaction is supported by reduced NADP and molecular oxygen (26-28). This enzyme(s) does not appear to be tightly regulated, inasmuch as the circulating serum 25-OH-D levels correlate with dietary intake (26) and environmental conditions that allow the cutaneous synthesis of vitamin D_3 (29).

The importance of the liver in maintaining calcium homeostasis through its ability to generate 25-OH-D remains an open question. Although there are extrahepatic 25-hydroxylases in the rat and chicken that can utilize vitamin D as a substrate, there is no evidence to suggest that such enzymes are operative in man (30). Serum 25-OH-D levels are reduced in severe parenchymal and cholestatic liver disease, but there is poor correlation between low serum 25-OH-D levels and osteomalacia and osteopenia in these diseases (31). Patients with nephrotic syndrome who have significant proteinuria (>4g/24h) may also have decreased serum 25-OH-D levels due to loss in the urine of vitamin-D-binding protein, which is similar in size to albumin, carrying tightly bound 25-OH-D (32, 33).

The association between osteomalacia or rickets and anticonvulsant drug therapy in epileptic patients has been amply demonstrated. Initially, it was believed that phenytoin and phenobarbital induced liver microsomal enzymes that rapidly inactivated vitamin D and its metabolites (34). It appears, however, that these drugs disrupt calcium homeostasis by other mechanisms as well. When phenobarbital is given acutely to rats, it stimulates the vitamin-D-25-hydroxylase and, at least initially, there is an elevation of 25-OH-D levels in serum (35).

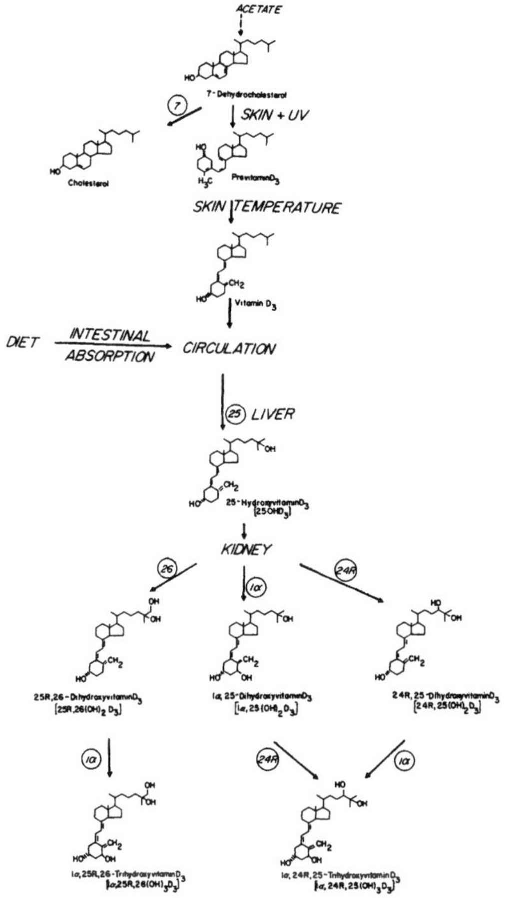

Fig. 4. The photochemical, thermal, and metabolic pathways for vitamin D_3 . Circled letters and numbers denote specific enzymes: 7= 7-dehydrocholesterol reductase; 25= vitamin-D-25-hydroxylase; 1α= 25-OH-D-1α-hydroxylase; 24R= 25-OH-D-24R-hydroxylase; 26= 25-OH-D-26-hydroxylase. The 1α-hydroxylation of 25R,26-$(OH)_2$-D_3 to 1α, 25R,26-$(OH)_2$ -D_3 is presumed to occur based upon biological experiments in anephric rats (reproduced from Holick and Potts (70) with permission).

Chronic ingestion of phenobarbital inhibits vitamin-D-25-hydroxylase and stimulates bile excretion with a resultant decrease in serum 25-OH-D levels (36). Phenytoin and phenobarbital also inhibit intestinal calcium-transport through a specific inhibitory effect on the energy-dependent calcium-transport system in the intestinal mucosa or by an inhibition of calcium-binding-protein synthesis, or both (37-39). Phenytoin also has a direct inhibitory effect on parathyroid-hormone-mediated bone resorption and this effect may also be a factor in the relation of this drug with osteopenia (40). However, Wark et al. (41) analyzed serum 25-OH-D levels in patients after myocardial infarction randomized to a control group or a treatment group (400 mg diphenylhydantoin a day for two years). No differences were noticed in serum 25-OH-D levels in either group at the end of the two-year study. The clinical problem however, appears to be worse in patients receiving multiple drugs and whose vitamin-D intake or exposure to the sun is minimal.

There is a strong correlation between high-dose glucocorticoid therapy and bone disease, most notably osteopenia. Initially, it was believed that glucocorticoids induced liver microsomal enzymes which utilize vitamin D as a substrate (42). However, like the anticonvulsant drugs, their action on vitamin-D-mediated calcium metabolism is complicated. Glucocorticoids have been reported to decrease bone formation (43), to inhibit collagen synthesis by osteoblasts (44) and to decrease turnover of bone cytosol 1,25-$(OH)_2$-D_3 receptors (45). Patients receiving chronic glucocorticoid therapy are reported to have low serum 1α,25-dihydroxyvitamin D (1,25-$(OH)_2$-D) levels (46) and a decrease in the fractional absorption of calcium by the small intestine.

Metabolism of 25-OH-D to 1,25-$(OH)_2$-D

Once 25-OH-D is formed in the liver, it is transported to the kidney (Figure 4) on a vitamin-D-binding protein where it is hydroxylated at either C_1 or C_{24} (26-28). Hypocalcemia enhances renal mitochondrial 25-OH-D-1α-hydroxylase activity so that the rate of conversion of 25-OH-D to 1α,25-$(OH)_2$-D increases (26-28). However, hypocalcemia does not appear to directly control this hydroxylation. Any decrease in the serum calcium level below normal is a stimulus for increased secretion of parathyroid hormone (PTH). PTH in addition to acting upon mineral metabolism in the bone and kidney, also acts physiologically as a trophic hormone to increase the renal synthesis of 1,25-$(OH)_2$-D (26-28). The mechanism by which this peptide hormone exerts its influence on renal metabolism of 25-OH-D is not yet established. It has been suggested, based upon studies in thyroparathyroidectomized rats, that the effect of PTH on phosphate metabolism is the more immediate mediator regulating the production of 1,25-$(OH)_2$-D (26-28). In thyroparathyroidectomized rats, 25-OH-D is metabolized to 1,25-$(OH)_2$-D when serum phosphate levels are kept below normal, even if hypercalcemia is present. When hyperphosphatemia is produced in these animals by increasing dietary phosphate, the renal production of 1,25-$(OH)_2$-D is diminished, and, in turn, 25-OH-D is metabolized to 24R,25-dihydroxyvitamin D (24,25-$(OH)_2$-D). Some investigators have questioned, on the basis of studies in chicks, whether the serum or renal tissue phosphorus levels, exclusively or even principally, regulate renal 25-OH-D-1α-hydroxylase (47). However, the bulk of available data in humans and animals suggests that the renal production of 1,25-$(OH)_2$-D is closely correlated with serum phosphorus concentrations (26-28, 48).

Other hormones have also been implicated in regulating the renal 25-OH-D-1α-hydroxylase. Kenny (49) suggested, on the basis of a laying chicken's need to increase intestinal calcium absorption for the production of eggshell, that gonadal hormones, which are elevated during gestation, may play a critical role in the control of vitamin D metabolism. Their experiments have demonstrated that ovariectomy and antiestrogen therapy inhibit the renal metabolism of 25-OH-D_3 to 1,25-$(OH)_2$-D_3 in Japanese quail and that estradiol and progesterone replacement in immature quail increase the renal production of 1,25-$(OH)_2$-D_3. It is well established in humans as well as other mammals that there is adaptation to increased calcium requirements during growth, pregnancy, and lactation by increasing the efficiency of intestinal calcium absorption. Using either a hypophysectomized rat model or a chick kidney-tubule preparation, a number of investigators have demonstrated that both growth hormone and prolactin will stimulate the renal 25-OH-D-1α-hydroxylase (26, 28). However, when this is put in physiologic perspective, there has been no clear demonstration, in disease states of excess pituitary-hormone production of either growth hormone or prolactin, that there are excessively high levels of circulating 1,25-$(OH)_2$-D. Calcitonin has also been reported to enhance the renal metabolism of 25-OH-D to 1,25-$(OH)_2$-D in vitamin-D-deficient rats (26). It was concluded that this increase in enzyme activity was due to the increased secretion of PTH in response to the hypocalcemia produced by calcitonin. However, Horiuchi et al. (50) recently reported that salmon calcitonin infusion in vitamin-D-deficient thyroparathyroidectomized rats caused a dose-dependent increase in the plasma 1,25-$(OH)_2$-D_3 levels (50).

Metabolism of 25-OH-D to 24R,25-$(OH)_2$-D

When the body's calcium and phosphorus requirements are satisfied, and there is little need for either enhanced intestinal calcium or phosphate transport or bone mineral mobilization, the kidney regulatory system decreases the 25-OH-D-1α-hydroxylase and increases the activity of the 25-OH-D-24R-hydroxylase (26-28). Normocalcemia, hypercalcemia, normophosphatemia, and hyperphosphatemia, as well as vitamin-D supplementation and 1,25-$(OH)_2$-D_3 itself, all have a stimulatory influence on renal 25-OH-D-24R-hydroxylase activity. 25-OH-D-24R-hydroxylase activity has also been demonstrated in the small intestine of rats (27) and in cultured chondrocytes isolated from rabbit growth plate (51). The physiologic significance of these observations is unclear at this time.

Ornoy et al (52) reported that in chicks, treatment with 1α-hydroxy-vitamin D_3 cannot prevent rachitic changes in bones despite normal levels of plasma calcium and phosphate, whereas treatment with 24,25-$(OH)_2$-D_3 is sufficient to prevent rickets. Norman and Henry (53) reported that fertile eggs from hens treated with either 24,25-$(OH)_2$-D_3 or 1,25-$(OH)_2$-D_3 were either incapable of hatching or resulted in fewer hatchings compared with eggs from hens treated with a combination of 1,25-$(OH)_2$-D_3 and 24,25-$(OH)_2$-D_3. Bordier et al. (54) made a comparison of the biochemical and osseous effects of 1,25-$(OH)_2$-D_3, 24,25-$(OH)_2$-D_3, and a combination of 1,25-$(OH)_2$-D_3 plus 24,25-$(OH)_2$-D_3 in adult vitamin-D-deficient men and concluded that only those receiving a combination of these metabolites had the return of a normal mineralization front. Kanis et al. (55) also reported that short-term oral administration of 24,25-$(OH)_2$-D_3 daily to patients with chronic renal failure stimulated intestinal calcium absorption and reduced serum alkaline phosphatase, suggesting a role of this metabolite in bone mineralization. 24, 25-$(OH)_2$-D_3 is more potent, on a weight basis, than 1,25-$(OH)_2$-D_3 in promoting proteoglycan synthesis in cultured rabbit chondrocytes (56). Collectively, these data would seem to suggest that 24,25-$(OH)_2$-D_3 has a unique biologic action that is independent of its metabolism in the kidney to 1α,24R,25-trihydroxyvitamin D_3 (1,24,25-$(OH)_3$-D). However, an analog of 25-OH-D_3, 24,24-difluoro-25-OH-D_3 (an analog of 25-OH-D_3 that has two fluorine molecules on C-24, which presumably prevent any C-24 hydroxylation), heals rachitic lesions in rats equally as well as 25-OH-D_3, suggesting that C-24 hydroxylation is not absolutely required for bone mineralization (27). Therefore, controversy remains regarding any unique role for 24,25-$(OH)_2$-D in either bone or calcium metabolism.

Metabolism of Vitamin D in Pregnancy

Recently, much interest has focused on the metabolism of vitamin D during pregnancy. Unlike the chicken, which appears to require both 24,25-$(OH)_2$-D_3 and 1,25-$(OH)_2$-D_3 for hatchability, pregnant rats can be brought to term when fed a diet that is deficient in vitamin D (57, 58). An analysis of the distribution of metabolic products of radioactive 25-OH-D_3 in pregnant rats has demonstrated that there are differences in the distribution of the various vitamin D_3 metabolites in the maternal and fetal small intestine, blood and bone. 24,25-$(OH)_2$-D_3 is the predominant dihydroxy metabolite in fetal bone and blood, whereas 1,25-$(OH)_2$-D_3 is the predominant dihydroxy metabolite in maternal blood (59). When maternal kidneys are removed, 25-OH-D_3 is still metabolized to 1,25-$(OH)_2$-D_3, suggesting either an extrarenal 25-OH-D-1α-hydroxylase or the fetal synthesis of 1,25-$(OH)_2$-D_3 (57, 60). It has now been demonstrated that rat placental tissue is capable of converting 25-OH-D_3 to 1,25-$(OH)_2$-D_3 and that human placental tissue is able to convert 25-OH-D_3 to either 1,25-$(OH)_2$-D_3 or 24,25-$(OH)_2$-D_3 (61, 62). The role of these extrarenal enzymes in controlling calcium and phosphorus metabolism and the hormonal factors responsible for modulating vitamin D metabolism in the placenta are presently being investigated.

Metabolism of 24,25-$(OH)_2$-D and 1,25-$(OH)_2$-D

Since the identification of 1,25-$(OH)_2$-D_3 and 24,25-$(OH)_2$-D_3 and the introduction of a simple method for making these two metabolites from tritiated 25-OH-D with chick kidney homogenates, much has been learned regarding the biologic response, target-tissue appearance, and metabolism of both 1,25-$(OH)_2$-D and 24,25-$(OH)_2$-D. Frolik et al. (63), using vitamin-D-deficient rats and chicks, were able to correlate the presence of unaltered 1,25-$(OH)_2$-D_3 in the intestine and bone (which accounted for

98% and 80% of the total radioactivity in the respective target tissues) with the induction of intestinal calcium transport and bone calcium mobilization. These results strongly support the idea that 1,25-$(OH)_2$-D_3 is the biologically active form of vitamin D_3 that is responsible for intestinal calcium transport and bone mineral mobilization and that no further metabolism is required for biologic activity. 1,25-$(OH)_2$-D is recognized as a substrate for the renal 25-OH-D-24R-hydroxylase, and 24, 25$(OH)_2$-D is a substrate for the renal 25-OH-D-1α-hydroxylase (Figure 4). The resultant product is 1,24,25-$(OH)_3$-D_3, which is biologically less active in stimulating intestinal calcium transport and bone mineral mobilization in the rat when compared with 1,25-$(OH)_2$-D_3 (26). The physiologic function of this trihydroxy metabolite remains to be defined. Harden et al. (64) showed, using [26,27-^{14}C]1,25-$(OH)_2$-D_3, that up to 30% of the intravenous dose of this isotope is expired as CO_2 in 24 hours. This conversion appears to be specific for 1,25-$(OH)_2$-D_3 and occurs principally in the intestine and liver and is not dependent upon bacterial metabolism. Recently, a metabolite of 1,25-$(OH)_2$-D_3 was isolated and identified as a 23-acid derivative of 1,25-$(OH)_2$-D_3 (1α-hydroxytetranor-vitamin-D-23-carboxylic acid (27)). Two additional metabolites recently were isolated from chick blood and identified as 25-hydroxyvitamin-D_3-26,23-lactone and 25,26,27-trinor-vitamin-D-carboxylic acid (65). The biological activity and physiologic actions of these three new metabolites remain to be determined.

Metabolism of 25-OH-D to 25R,26-Dihydroxyvitamin D (25,26-$(OH)_2$-D_3)

25,26-$(OH)_2$-D_3 was first isolated from the blood of pigs and chicks that had received pharmacologic doses of vitamin D_3 and then was found to be a circulating metabolite in man. It was synthesized chemically, and an analysis of its biologic activity in vitamin-D-deficient rats and their nephrectomized counterparts suggested that, like 24,25-$(OH)_2$-D_3, it required renal 1α-hydroxylation (Figure 4) before it could stimulate intestinal calcium transport (26, 27).

Vitamin-D and Vitamin-D-Metabolite Levels in Health and Disease

Before 1970, vitamin-D assays were principally bioassays, e.g. antirachitic activity by the rat line test, in vitro and in situ intestinal calcium absorption, bone mineral mobilization and bone ash. These assays were useful in determining the biologic potency of synthetic vitamin D and its analogs but were not very useful for quantitative determinations of vitamin-D levels in serum. The current knowledge that vitamin D requires successive hydroxylations before it is active has prompted the development of specific assays for vitamin D and its metabolites. The two principal assay methods used today are competitive-binding-protein assays and direct analysis of vitamin D and its metabolite by high-pressure liquid chromatography (hpcl) using an ultraviolet-absorption detector system (28, 66). In the former case, 25-OH-D, 24,25-$(OH)_2$-D, and 25,26-$(OH)_2$-D are measured using either a rat plasma vitamin-D-binding protein (67) or a chick binding protein (68) as the radioreceptor protein. 1,25-$(OH)_2$-D is measured with either a chick cytosol receptor or chick chromatin receptor (27, 28). Vitamin D as well as some of the vitamin-D metabolites, including 25-OH-D and 24,25-$(OH)_2$-D, which are present in ng quantities in the serum, are measured by direct detection of the metabolite with UV monitoring. This method requires a lipid extraction of the serum and a preparative chromatography step that eliminates most of the contaminating lipids. The fraction of interest is then chromatographed on hplc and the UV absorbance of the vitamin-D metabolite measured. Recently, a number of laboratories reported the development of a radioimmunoassay for 1,25-$(OH)_2$-D (69). However, this assay is not specific for 1,25-$(OH)_2$-D, thus making it necessary to isolate the individual metabolites by chromatography before the assay is performed. The normal ranges for circulating levels of vitamin D and its metabolites using the methods described above are: vitamin D, 1-5 ng/ml; 25-OH-D, 5-80 ng/ml; 24,25-$(OH)_2$-D, 0.5-5 ng/ml; and 1,25-$(OH)_2$D, 15-50 pg/ml.

It is generally believed that the 25-OH-D level in the serum directly reflects the vitamin-D status, and it is routinely used as a screening test to determine whether vitamin-D deficiency is present in patients with metabolic bone disease and hypocalcemic disorders and to rule out vitamin-D toxicity in patients with hypercalcemia. Serum 25-OH-D levels are low in vitamin-D deficiency, and may be low in severe chronic liver disease, nephrotic syndrome, and malabsorption syndromes, and in institutionalized patients receiving multiple anticonvulsant drugs (26). Serum 1,25-$(OH)_2$-D levels are reported to be low in patients with severe renal disease (GFR <30 ml/min). Patients with hypoparathyroidism and pseudohypoparathyroidism have mean serum levels of 1,25-$(OH)_2$-D that are lower than normal, although there is considerable overlap with the normal range (28, 33). Patients receiving high doses of a corticosteroid may have decreased levels of 1,25-$(OH)_2$-D, but whether this is related to steroid-induced osteopenia remains to be determined. Attention has been directed to serum 1,25-$(OH)_2$-D levels in patients with vitamin-D-dependent rickets Type I and X-linked familial hypophosphatemic rickets. It was suggested that children with vitamin-D-dependent rickets type I have an inborn error of metabolism that causes a deficiency in 1,25-$(OH)_2$-D and that patients with X-linked familial hypophosphatemic rickets have a defect in the control mechanism for the synthesis of 1,25-$(OH)_2$-D, inasmuch as normal or low-normal 1,25-$(OH)_2$-D levels in these patients are inappropriate for the degree of hypophosphatemia present. In addition, there have been a few reports of patients with familial vitamin-D-dependent rickets Type II whose serum 1,25-$(OH)_2$-D levels are normal or high. It has been postulated that these patients have a hyporesponsiveness at the receptor for 1,25-$(OH)_2$-D (28, 33, 70).

Serum 1,25-$(OH)_2$-D levels were found to be elevated in a subgroup of patients with idiopathic hypercalcuria and in a few patients with sarcoidosis but were either normal or low in patients with hypervitaminosis D (28, 71).

Therapeutic Uses for Vitamin D Metabolites and Analogs

Since the discovery of vitamin D almost a half-century ago, numerous analogs of vitamin D have been synthesized in an attempt to develop therapeutic agents that would be superior to vitamin D. Vitamin D_2 when given orally or parenterally is effective in preventing or curing rickets and osteomalacia. However, a few calcium-metabolism disorders that are resistant to the action of physiological doses of vitamin D - namely, severe chronic renal failure, hypoparathyroidism, and vitamin-D-dependent rickets Type I. In the late 1940's, dihydrotachysterol (a reduction product of either vitamin D or tachysterol, Figure 5) was synthesized (72) and found to be less biologically active on a weight basis compared to vitamin D, although it had the unique property of being more effective on a weight basis than vitamin D in stimulating intestinal calcium transport in hypoparathyroid rats (72). This analog proved to be useful in the treatment of vitamin-D-resistant syndromes such as renal osteodystrophy and hypoparathyroidism. Our recent knowledge of the absolute requirement for vitamin D to be hydroxylated on C_1 and C_{25} now explains why this analog is so effective. As illustrated in Figure 5, the structure of dihydrotachysterol, which is similar to that of 5,6-trans-vitamin D_3, shows that ring A of the vitamin D molecule is rotated 180° as a result of the reduction reaction, placing the $C_{3\beta}$-OH in a position that mimics the critical $C_{1\alpha}$-OH of the active form of vitamin D. Furthermore, because dihydrotachysterol and 5,6-transvitamin D_3 are metabolized to 25-hydroxydihydrotachysterol and 5,6-trans-25-OH-D_3 (72), the resulting metabolites are pseudo-1α-hydroxy analogs of the natural metabolite 1,25-$(OH)_2$-D_3 (Figure 5). Another analog

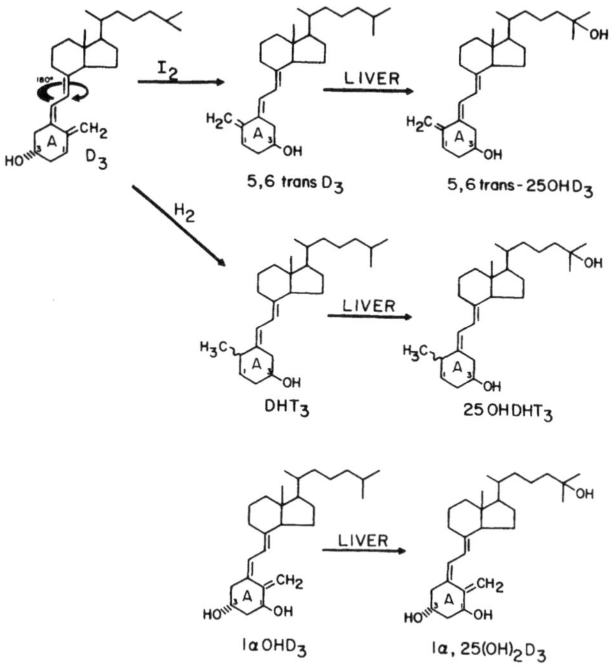

Fig. 5. When vitamin D is treated with I_2 or reduced with H_2 ring A of the vitamin D molecule rotates 180° to spatially reorient the 3β-OH in a pseudo-1α-OH position. These analogs, 5,6-trans-vitamin D_3 and dihydrotachysterol$_3$ (DHT_3) are called pseudo-1α-hydroxy analogs. 1α-OH-D_3 is a synthetic analog of 1α,25$(OH)_2D_3$ that lacks a C_{25} -OH. 1α-OH-D_3 , 5,6-trans-vitamin D_3 and DHT_3 all undergo a hepatic C_{25}-hydroxylation before they are biologically active (reproduced from Holick and Potts (70) with permission).

that has been widely used for treatment of vitamin-D-resistant syndromes is 1α-hydroxyvitamin D_3 (Figure 5). This analog is identical in structure with the natural hormone except that it lacks a C_{25}-OH. This analog which must be metabolized at C_{25}

before it is biologically active, is rapidly and efficiently metabolized by the liver in rats and man (26, 30) to 1,25-$(OH)_2$-D_3 and has been effective in the treatment of renal osteodystrophy, hypoparathyroidism, and vitamin-D-dependent rickets.

In the late 1960's, the first metabolite to be isolated and chemically synthesized was 25-OH-D_3 (26, 27). This metabolite is effective in curing vitamin-D-deficiency rickets and has been used in relatively high doses (up to 200 μg three times a week) for treating renal osteodystrophy (33). This metabolite is not yet available for use in the U.S. but is available in Europe.

At present the most effective vitamin-D metabolite for the treatment of vitamin-D-resistant syndrome is 1,25-$(OH)_2$-D_3. This metabolite is effective for the treatment of many disorders of calcium metabolism that are related to a derangement in the synthesis of this hormone. Patients with mild to moderate renal failure (GFR >30 cc/min) still have the reserve capacity to synthesize enough 1,25-$(OH)_2$-D for body needs. However, in order to take advantage of this reserve capacity, the serum phosphate should be maintained within the normal range because the hyperphosphatemia that accompanies renal failure is believed to be a potent inhibitor of the 25-OH-D-1α-hydroxylase (26-28). When the renal 25-OH-D-1α-hydroxylase reserve is depleted due to marked destruction of the renal cortex (GFR < 30 cc/ml), the kidney is unable to synthesize enough 1,25-$(OH)_2$-D to maintain adequate intestinal calcium absorption. There is a decrease in the serum calcium that causes the parathyroid glands to increase the secretion of PTH. PTH stimulates the renal synthesis of 1,25-$(OH)_2$-D and, combined with 1,25-$(OH)_2$-D, mobilizes calcium from bone (26-28). In the absence of 1,25-$(OH)_2$-D, higher circulating levels of PTH are required for bone mineral mobilization and, in the face of decreased calcium absorption and the resultant hypocalcemia, PTH synthesis and secretion steadily rise. Thus, the blood calcium pool is maintained principally by the mobilization of the bone calcium stores by high circulating levels of PTH. A majority of patients who receive hemodialysis have benefited greatly from oral 1,25-$(OH)_2$-D_3. The dose schedule begins with 0.25 µg/d, with frequent monitoring of serum calcium and phosphorus. The dose is gradually increased in increments of 0.25 µg/d over a period of weeks to months until the serum calcium is normalized; the patient is maintained on this dose, which is usually in the range of 0.5 to 2.0 µg/d (33).

Patients with other disorders of vitamin-D metabolism have also benefited from this therapy. Patients with hypo- and pseudoparathyroidism with low or low-normal serum 1,25-$(OH)_2$-D levels normalize their serum calcium with 1,25-$(OH)_2$-D_3 therapy (28, 33). Children with vitamin-D-dependent rickets Type I have dramatic healing of their rachitic lesions within months after treatment with as little as 0.25 µg/d of 1,25-$(OH)_2$-D_3 (33). Many of the other vitamin-D metabolites have been investigated in rats and chicks to see whether they possess any special biologic effects. To date, only 24,25-$(OH)_2$-D_3 has been carefully scrutinized in man and the results are still preliminary. Extensive long-term studies need to be done to determine whether this metabolite or any other vitamin-D metabolite has a therapeutic action that is distinct from that of 1,25-$(OH)_2$-D_3 (55).

References

1. Foote, J.A.: Evidence of rickets prior to 1650. Am. J. Dis. Child 34, 443-452 (1927).
2. Griffenhagen, G.: A brief history of nutritional diseases. II. Rickets. Bull. natn. Inst. Nutr. 2, No.9 (1952).
3. Guthrie, D.: A History of Medicine. Nelson, London, p. 69 (1945).
4. Park. E.A.: The etiology of rickets. Physiol. Rev. iii, 106-159 (1923).
5. Sniadecki, J. (1840).: Cited by W. Mozolowski (1939): Jedrzej Sniadecki (1768-1838) on the cure of rickets. Nature 143, 121 (1939).
6. Palm, T.A.: The geographic distribution and etiology of rickets. Practitioner 45, 270-279, 321-342 (1890).

7. Huldchinsky, K.: Heilung von Rachitis durch künstliche Höhensonne. Dt. med. Wschr. xiv, 712-713 (1919).

8. Hess, A.F., Unger, L.G.: Cure of infantile rickets by sunlight. J. Am. med. Ass. 77, 39 (1921).

9. Mellanby, E.: The part played by an "accessory factor" in the production of experimental rickets. J. Physiol. 52, 11-14 (1918).

10. Mellanby, E.: An experimental investigation on rickets. Lancet 1, 407-412 (1919).

11. McCollum, E.V., Simmonds, N., Becker, J.E., Shipley, P.G.: Studies on experimental rickets. An experimental demonstration of the existence of a vitamin which promoted calcium deposition. J. biol. Chem. 53, 293-312 (1922).

12. Powers, G.F., Park, E.A., Shipley, P.G., McCollum, E.V., Simmonds, N.: The prevention of rickets in the rat by means of radiation with the mercury vapor quartz lamp. Proc. Soc. exp. Biol. Med. 19, 120-121 (1921).

13. Steenbock, H., Black, A.: The reduction of growth-promoting and calcifying properties in a ration by exposure to ultraviolet light. J. biol. Chem. 61, 408-422 (1924).

14. Hess, A.F., Weinstock, M.: Antirachitic properties imparted to inert fluids and green vegetables by ultraviolet irradiation. J. biol. Chem. 62, 301-313 (1924).

15. Havinga, E.: Vitamin D, example and challenge. Experientia 29, 1181-1193 (1973).

16. Okano, T., Yasumura, M., Mizuno, K., Kobayashi, T.: Photochemical conversion of 7-dehydrocholesterol into vitamin D_3 in rat skins. J. Nutr. Sci. Vitaminol. 23, 165-168 (1977).

17. Esvelt, R.P., Schnoes, H.K., DeLuca, H.F.: Vitamin D_3 from rat skins irradiated in vitro with ultraviolet light. Arch Biochem. Biophys. 188, 282-286 (1978).

18. Rauschkolb, E.W., Winston, D., Fenimore, D.C., Black, H.S., Fabre, L.F.: Identification of vitamin D_3 in human skin. J. invest. Dermatol. 53, 289-293 (1969).

19. Holick, M.F., Frommer, J.E., McNeill, S.C., Richtand, N.M., Henley, J.F., Potts, J.T.: Photometabolism of 7-dehydrocholesterol to previtamin D_3 in skin. Biochem. biophys. Res. Commun. 76, 107-114 (1977).

20. Holick, N.F., Richtand, N.M., McNeill, S.C., Holick, S.A., Frommer, J.E., Henley, J.W., Potts, J.T.: Isolation and identification of previtamin D_3 from the skin of rats exposed to ultraviolet irradiation. Biochemistry 18, 1003-1008 (1979).

21. Holick, M.F., McNeill, S.C., MacLaughlin, J.A., Holick, S.A., Clark, M.B., Potts, J.T.: The physiologic implications of the formation of previtamin D_3 in skin. Trans. Ass. Am. Physns. 92, 54-63 (1979).

22. Holick, M.F., Holick, S.A., McNeill, S.C., Richtand, N., Clark, M.B., Potts, J.T.: The Photo-biochemistry of Vitamin D_3 in vivo in the skin. In: "Proceedings of the Fourth Workshop on Vitamin D, Berlin, February 18-22", Eds. Norman, A.W., Schaefer, K., von Herrath, D., Coburn, J.W., Grigoleit, H.G., Mawer, E.B., Suda, T., Walter de Gruyter, Berlin, New York, pp. 173-176 (1979).

23. Elias, P.M., Fritsch, P., Epstein, E.H.: Staphyloccocal scalded skin syndrome. Clinical features, pathogenesis, and recent microbiological and biochemical developments. Arch. Dermatol. 113, 207-211 (1977).

24. Scheuplein, R.J.: Mechanism of percutaneous adsorption. Routes of penetration and the influence of solubility. J. invest. Dermatol. 45, 334-346 (1965).

25. Holick, M.F., McNeill, S.C., MacLaughlin, J., Clark, M.B., Holick, S.A., Potts, J.T.: The Epidermis : A Unique Organ Responsible for the Photo-biosynthesis of Vitamin D_3 . In: "Endocrinology '79" - Proceedings of the 7th International Congress, London 1979., Ed. MacIntyre, I., Elsevier/North-Holland Biomedical Press, Amsterdam, pp. 301-308 (1979).

26. Holick, M.F., Clark, M.B.: The photobiogenesis and metabolism of vitamin D. Fed. Proc. 37, 2567-2574 (1978).

27. DeLuca, J.F.: The vitamin D system in the regulation of calcium and phosphorus metabolism. Nutrition Rev. 37, 161-193 (1979).

28. Haussler, M.R., McCain, T.A.: Basic and clinical concepts related to vitamin D metabolism and action. New Engl. J. Med. 297, 974-983, 1041-1050 (1977).

29. Neer, R., Clark, M., Friedman, V., Belsey, R., Sweeney, M., Buonchristiani, J., Potts, J.T.: Environmental and nutritional influences on plasma 25-hydroxyvitamin D concentration and calcium metabolism in man. In: "Proceedings of the Third Workshop on Vitamin D", Eds. Norman, A.W., Schaefer, K., Coburn, J.W., DeLuca, H.S., Fraser, D., Grigoleit, H.G., von Herrath, D., Walter de Gruyter, Berlin, New York, pp. 595-606 (1977).

30. Holick, M.F., de Blanco, M.C., Clark, M.B., Henley, J.W., Neer, R.M., DeLuca, H.F., Potts, J.T.: The metabolism of $[6\text{-}^3H]1\alpha$,hydroxycholecalciferol to $[6\text{-}^3H]1\alpha$,25-dihydroxycholecalciferol in a patient with renal insufficiency. J. clin. Endocrinol. Metab. 44, 595-598 (1977).

31. Long, R.G., Wills, M.R., Skinner, R.K.: Serum-25-hydroxyvitamin-D in untreated parenchymal and cholestatic liver-disease. Lancet 2, 650-652 (1976).

32. Pietrek, J., Kokot, F.: Serum 25-hydroxyvitamin D in patients with chronic renal disease. Europ. J. Clin. Invest. 7, 283-287 (1977).

33. Frame, B., Parfitt, M.A.: Osteomalacia: Current concepts. Ann. intern. Med. 89, 966-982 (1978).

34. Hahn, J.J., Birge, S.J., Scharp, C.R.: Phenobarbital-induced alterations in vitamin D metabolism. J. clin. Invest. 51, 741-748 (1972).

35. Gascon-Barre, M., Glorieux, F.H.: The effect of phenobarbital treatment on the biliary excretion of cholecalciferol and 25-hydroxycholecalciferol in the D-repleted rat. In: "Proceedings of the Third Workshop on Vitamin D", Eds. Norman, A.W., Schaefer, K., Coburn, J.W., DeLuca, H.S., Fraser, D., Grigoleit, H.G., von Herrath, D., Walter de Gruyter, Berlin, New York, pp. 781-783 (1977).

36. Delvin, E.E., Bourbonnais, F., Glorieux, F.H.: Effect of phenobarbital on hepatic vitamin D-25-hydroxylase activities in vitro. In: "Proceedings of the Third Workshop on Vitamin D", Eds. Norman, A.W., Schaefer, K., Coburn, J.W., DeLuca, H.S., Fraser, D., Grigoleit, H.G., von Herrath, D., Walter de Gruyter, Berlin, New York, pp. 767-769 (1977).

37. Corradino, R.A.: Diphenylhydantoin: direct inhibition of the vitamin D_3 mediated calcium absorptive mechanism in organ-cultured duodenum. Biochem. Pharmacol. 25, 863-864 (1976).

38. Harrison, H.C., Harrison, H.E.:Inhibition of vitamin D-stimulated active transport of calcium of rat intestine by diphenylhydantoin-phenobarbital treatment (39514). Proc. Soc. exp. Biol. Med. 153, 220-224 (1976).

39. Villareale, M., Gould, L.V., Wasserman, R.H.: Diphenylhydantoin: effects on calcium metabolism in the chick. Science 183, 671-674 (1974).

40. Jenkins, M.V., Harris, M., Wills, M.R.: The effect of phenytoin on parathyroid extract and 25-hydroxycholecalciferol-induced bone resorption adenosine 3',5' cyclic monophosphate production. Calcif. Tissue Res. 16, 163-166 (1974).

41. Wark, J.D., Larkins, R.G., Perry-Keene, D., Peter, C.T., Ross, D.L., Sloman, J.G.: Chronic diphenylhydantoin therapy does not reduce plasma 25-hydroxyvitamin D. Clin. Endocr. 11, 267-274 (1979).

42. Avioli, L.V., Birge, S.J., Lee, S.W.: Effects of prednisone on vitamin D metabolism in man. J. clin. Endocrinol. Metab. 28, 1341-1346 (1968).

43. Jowsey, J., Riggs, B.L.: Bone formation in hypercortisolism. Acta Endocrinol. 63, 21-28 (1970).

44. Peck, W.A., Brant, J., Miller, I.: Hydrocortisone-induced inhibition of protein synthesis and uridine incorporation in isolated bone cells in vitro. Proc. natn. Acad. Sci. U.S.A. 57, 1599-1606 (1967).

45. Manolagas, S.C., Anderson, D.C., Lumb, G.A.: Glucocorticoids regulate the concentration of 1,25-dihydroxycholecalciferol receptors in bone. Nature 277, 314-315 (1979).

46. Chesney, R.W., Mazess, R.B., Hamstra, A.J., O'Regan, S., DeLuca, H.F.: Subnormal serum 1,25-dihydroxyvitamin D_3 levels in children with glomerular disease receiving corticosteroids. In: "Proceedings of the Fourth Workshop on Vitamin D", Eds. Norman, A.W., Schaefer, K., von Herrath, D., Coburn, J.W., Grigoleit, H.G., Mawer, E.B., Suda, T., Walter de Gruyter, Berlin, New York, pp. 935-938 (1979).

47. Norman, A.W.: A synopsis of vitamin D, its endocrine system and human disease states. Aust. N.Z. J. Med. 9, 9-16 (1979).

48. Bilezikian, J.P., Canfield, R.E., Jacobs, T.P., Polay, J.S., D'Adamo, A.P., Eisman, J.A., DeLuca, H.F.: Response of 1α,25-dihydroxyvitamin D_3 to hypocalcemia in human subjects. New Engl. J. Med. 299, 437-441 (1978).

49. Kenny, A.D.: Vitamin D metabolism: physiological regulation in egg-laying Japanese quail. Am. J. Physiol. 230, 1609-1615 (1976).

50. Horiuchi, N., Takahashi, H., Matsumoto, T., Takahashi, N., Shimazawa, E., Suda, T., Ogata, E.: Salmon calcitonin-induced stimulation of 1α,25-dihydroxycholecalciferol synthesis in rats involving a mechanism independent of adenosine 3', 5' cyclic monophosphate. Biochem. J. 184, 269-275 (1979).

51. Garabedian, M., Bailly du Bois, M., Corvol, M.T., Pezant, E., Balsan, S.: Vitamin D and cartilage. I. *In vitro* metabolism of 25-hydroxycholecalciferol by cartilage. Endocrinology 102, 1262-1268 (1978).

52. Ornoy, A., Goodwin, D., Noff, D., Edelstein, S.: 24,25-dihydroxyvitamin D essential for bone formation. Nature 276, 517-519 (1978).

53. Norman, A.W., Henry, H.L.: Both 24R,25-dihydroxyvitamin D_3 and 1α,25-dihydroxyvitamin D_3 are indispensable for normal calcium and phosphorus homeostasis. In: "Proceedings of the Fourth Workshop on Vitamin D", Eds. Norman, A.W., Schaefer, K., von Herrath, D., Coburn, J.W., Grigoleit, H. G., Mawer, E.B., Suda, T., Walter de Gruyter, Berlin, New York, pp. 571-578 (1979).

54. Bordier, O., Rasmussen, H., Marie, P., Miravet, L., Gueris, J., Rychwaert, A.: Vitamin D metabolites and bone mineralization in man. J. clin. Endocrinol. Metab. 46, 284-294 (1978).

55. Kanis, J.A., Heynen, G., Russell, R.G.G., Smith, R., Walton, R.J., Warner, G.T.: Biological effects of 24,25-dihydroxycholecalciferol in man. In: "Proceedings of the Third Workshop on Vitamin D", Eds. Norman, A.W., Schaefer, K., Coburn, J.W., DeLuca, H.S., Fraser, D., Grigoleit, H.G., von Herrath, D., Walter de Gruyter, Berlin, New York, pp. 793-795 (1977).

56. Corvol, M.T., Dumontier, M.F., Garabedian, M., Rappaport, R.: Vitamin D and cartilage. II. Biological activity of 25-hydroxycholecalciferol and 24,25- and 1,25-dihydroxy-cholecalciferols on cultured growth plate chondrocytes. Endocrinology 102, 1269-1274 (1978).

57. Gray, T.K., Lester, G., Lorenc, R.: Evidence for extra-renal 1α-hydroxylation of 25-hydroxyvitamin D_3 in pregnancy. Science 204, 1311-1313 (1979).

58. Halloran, B.P., DeLuca, H.F.: Vitamin D deficiency and reproduction in rats. Science 204, 73-74 (1979).

59. Lester, G., Lorenc, R.S., Gray, T.K.: Evidence of maternal and fetal differences in vitamin D metabolism. Proc. Soc. exp. Biol. Med. 159, 303-307 (1978).

60. Weisman, Y., Vargas, A., Duckett, G., Reiter, E., Root, A.W.: Synthesis of 1,25-dihydroxyvitamin D in the nephrectomized pregnant rat. Endocrinology 103, 1992-1996 (1978).

61. Weisman, Y., Harell, A., Edelstein, S., David, M., Spirer, Z., Golander, A.: 1α,25-dihydroxyvitamin D_3 and 24,25-dihydroxyvitamin D_3 *in vitro* synthesis by human decidua and placenta. Nature 281, 317-319 (1979).

62. Tanaka, Y., Halloran, B., Schnoes, H.K., DeLuca, H.F.: *In vitro* production of 1,25-dihydroxyvitamin D_3 by rat placental tissue. Proc. natn. Acad. Sci. U.S.A. 76, 5033-5035 (1979).

63. Frolik, C.A., DeLuca, H.F.: 1,25-dihydroxycholecalciferol: the metabolite of vitamin D responsible for increased intestinal calcium transport. Arch. Biochem. Biophys. 147, 143-147 (1971).

64. Harden, D., Kumar, R., Holick, M.F., DeLuca, H.F.: Side chain metabolism of 25-hydroxy-[26,27-^{14}C] vitamin D_3 and 1,25-dihydroxy-[26,27-^{14}C] vitamin D_3 *in vivo*. Science 193, 493-494 (1976).

65. DeLuca, H.F., Schnoes, H.K.: Recent developments in the metabolism of vitamin D. In: "Proceedings of the Fourth Workshop on Vitamin D", Eds. Norman, A.W., Schaefer, K., von Herrath, D., Coburn, J.W., Grigoleit, H.G., Mawer, E.B., Suda, T., Walter de Gruyter, Berlin, New York, pp. 445-458 (1979).

66. Jones, G.: Assay of vitamin D_2 and D_3 and 25-hydroxyvitamins D_2 and D_3 in human plasma by high-performance liquid chromatography. Clin. Chem. 24, 287-298 (1978).

67. Belsey, R., Clark, M.B., Bernat, M., Glowacki, J., Holick, M.F., DeLuca, H.F., Potts, J.T.: The physiologic significance of plasma transport of vitamin D and metabolites. Am. J. Med. 57, 50-56 (1974).

68. Haddad, J.G., Chyu, K.J.: Competitive protein binding radioassay for 25-hydroxycholecalciferol. J. clin. Endocrinol. Metab. 33, 992-996 (1971).

69. Clemens, T.L., Hendy, G.N., Papapoulos, S.E., Fraher, L.J., Care, A.D., O'Riordan, J.L.H.: Measurement of 1,25-dihydroxycholecalciferol in man by radioimmunoassay. Clin. Endocr. 11, 225-234 (1979).

70. Holick, M.F., Potts, J.T.: Vitamin D (Chapter 351). In: "Harrison's Principles of Internal Medicine", Eds. Isselbacher, K.J., Adams, R.D., Braunwald, E., Petersdorf, R.G., Wilson, J.D., McGraw Hill Book Company, New York (in press).

71. Papapoulos, S.E., Fraher, L.J., Sandler, L.M., Clemens, T.L., Lewin, I.G., O'Riordan, J.L.H.: 1,25-dihydroxycholecalciferol in the pathogenesis of the hypercalcemia of sarcoidosis. Lancet i, 627-630 (1979).

72. Holick, M.F., DeLuca, H.F.: Chemistry and biological activity of vitamin D, its metabolites and analogs. In: "Steroid biochemistry and pharmacology", vol. 4, Eds. Briggs, M.H., Christie, G.A., Academic Press, New York, pp. 111-155 (1974).

RECEPTORS AND MECHANISM OF ACTION OF STEROID HORMONES IN THE FOETAL COMPARTMENT

J. R. Pasqualini and C. Sumida
CNRS Steroid Hormone Research Unit, Foundation for Hormone Research, 26 Boulevard Brune, 75014 Paris, France

I. Introduction

Steroid hormones play an important role not only in basal physiology but also during the crucial periods of gestation; conception, nidation, embryonic development and foetal maturation. During the course of normal pregnancy, the production rates and plasma concentrations of these steroid hormones can vary significantly, sometimes increasing 100-300 times at the end of gestation as in the case of oestrogens and progesterone in pregnant women. The production rates of some steroid hormones during human pregnancy are indicated in Table 1 and plasma concentrations in various animal species are given in Table 2.

Hormones in Normal and Abnormal Human Tissues, Vol. II

TABLE 2

PLASMA CONCENTRATION OF VARIOUS STEROIDS DURING PREGNANCY IN DIFFERENT ANIMAL SPECIES

ANIMAL SPECIES	STEROID	PREGNANCY (EARLY)	(MID)	(END)	REF
GUINEA PIG	CORTISOL	20	120	180	8
RAT	PROGESTERONE (ng/ml)	87	118	5	9
	OESTROGENS (ng/ml)	600	500	3000	10
GOLDEN HAMSTER	PROGESTERONE (ng/ml)	12	-	26	11
SHEEP	PROGESTERONE (ng/ml)	3	20	5	12
GOAT	OESTROGENS (pg/ml)	5	271	622	13

While the production rates of some steroid hormones increase during human pregnancy, the production rates of cortisol at the end of gestation remain similar to those in non-pregnant women. However, the plasma concentration of cortisol increases 4 to 5 times in pregnant women from 100 µg/l in non-pregnant women to 400-600 µg/l at the end of gestation. Despite this increase in circulating cortisol, there is no manifestation of hypercorticism during pregnancy. This is due to an increase in the production of transcortin which is stimulated by oestrogens, indicating the importance of the interaction between hormones in the control of pregnancy.

Polypeptide hormones also increase very significantly during pregnancy. For example, at term, human chorionic somatomammotrophin (HCS) secreted by the placenta reaches a value of 1 g/24 h which represents a 1000-fold rise throughout pregnancy.

The endocrine control of the beginning of pregnancy is the result of the biological synchronization of hormones from the pituitary, the ovary and the placenta and in late pregnancy hormones produced by the foetus itself also become involved. Progesterone and the oestrogens are two of these steroid hormones which play a basic role in pregnancy. Progesterone has been recognized for many decades as being the principal hormone which maintains pregnancy. The action of progesterone starts at the implantation of the blastocyst and a very attractive hypothetical mechanism suggests that progesterone, at this step, can induce the synthesis of new proteins involved in the process of implantation. The complementary action between progesterone and oestrogens in pregnancy is recognized in most animal species, but it is interesting to note the intriguing exception of the elephant which produces very little progesterone before and throughout gestation (14). Very probably, the gestational effect in this animal species is carried out by an unknown hormone.

Before describing various aspects of receptors and the mechanism of action of steroid hormones in the foetal compartment, it is of interest to review the general outline of the interrelation of steroid hormones between the foetal, placental and maternal compartments.

II. Steroids in the Foetal-Placental-Maternal Unit

The production rates of various steroids indicated in Table 1 are the contribution of the secretion of three compartments : maternal, placental and foetal. The production of the different steroid hormones, by these three compartments, is different both qualitatively and quantitatively and also depends on the period of pregnancy as well as the species considered. The present summary is mainly concerned with human pregnancy which has been studied the most extensively and where the concepts of the origin of these hormones, their transformation and the interrelation between these three compartments are the best understood (15, 16).

The foetus, at least from mid-gestation, has all the enzymatic systems necessary for biosynthesis of steroid hormones such as testosterone, corticosterone, cortisol, aldosterone, but "placental progesterone" is required for this biosynthesis. The placenta makes most of the progesterone and oestrogens produced during pregnancy. However, to make progesterone, it uses cholesterol which is of both foetal and maternal origin and pregnenolone and pregnenolone sulfate which are produced mainly in the foetus. For the synthesis of oestrogens, it uses precursors (e.g. dehydroepiandrosterone, dehydroepiandrosterone sulfate, 16α-hydroxy-dehydroepiandrosterone, 16α-hydroxy-dehydroepiandrosterone sulfate) which are produced mainly in the foetal compartment.

The foetus has a very intense sulfokinase activity and most of the steroids circulate in this compartment as sulfates; on the other hand, the placenta contains a very high concentration of sulfatase and most of the steroid sulfates are hydrolyzed in this compartment. This hydrolysis of steroid sulfates by the placenta is selective : the sulfatase is very active for oestrogen sulfates (arylsulfatase) and for sulfates of steroids with a 3β-hydroxy-5-ene function (17) but very little, if any, sulfatase activity is found in the placenta for the 21-sulfates (e.g. cortisol sulfate, corticosterone sulfate) (18), for the 3α-hydroxy sulfate (e.g. androsterone sulfate) (18) or for testosterone sulfate (19).

The foetal compartment until mid-gestation converts cortisol into cortisone, but the reverse reaction is limited (20). The conversion of cortisone to cortisol becomes active in the third trimester of pregnancy in the human (21) or at the end of gestation in guinea pig (22). It is suggested that this increase in the production of the active corticosteroid at the end of gestation could be related to the action of this hormone in lung maturation (23) (See Section V of this Chapter).

III. Steroid Hormone Receptors in the Foetal Compartment

The classical studies of Jensen and Jacobsen (24) and of Glascock and Hoekstra (25) demonstrated for the first time that steroid hormones were selectively retained in their target organs and not in other body tissues. This experiment opened a new era in the studies of the molecular events of hormonal action. In 1963, Edelman et al. (26), using an autoradiographic technique, established that the radioactive hormone (^{3}H-aldosterone) was localized in target tissues. Talwar et al. (27) suggested that oestradiol was bound to a macromolecule in the cytosol of the uterus and in 1966, Toft and Gorski (28) separated the hormone-receptor complexes from other large molecules by ultracentrifugation in a sucrose density gradient. Another step further in the knowledge of hormonal action was the demonstration by autoradiography that the hormones are accumulated in the nuclei of target tissues and that this transfer of the hormone to the nuclei is very rapid (29). Subsequently, the existence of receptors for other steroid hormones was demonstrated : for glucocorticoids in the thymus (30), for mineralocorticoids in the kidney (31), for progesterone in the chick oviduct (32) and for androgens in the prostate (33). Most of these studies on receptors and the mechanism of action of steroid hormones were carried out in immature or adult animals, but very little information is available concerning the presence of steroid hormone receptors during intra-uterine life. In 1971, in this laboratory, we found that binding of steroids can be detected in the foetal compartment of guinea pig for different steroids : for aldosterone in the foetal kidney (34) and for oestradiol in the foetal brain (35).

Steroid hormones circulate in the foetus as a complex bound to plasma proteins which may sometimes have a high binding affinity (e.g. α-foeto-protein, PBG : progesterone binding globulin). This must be taken into consideration when carrying out steroid-receptor binding assays since it is essential to differentiate between receptor-binding and possible contamination or interference from plasma steroid binding proteins.

A. Binding of steroid hormones to plasma proteins during pregnancy

As a consequence of the significant increase in the production of steroid hormones during pregnancy, a mechanism of protection should normally be present to protect foetal tissues from the biological activities of these hormones. The binding of steroid hormones to plasma proteins is one of these protective mechanisms. These proteins also increase during pregnancy and, consequently, some hormones circulate in the foetal or maternal compartment in a very high concentration but in bound form.

The limited length of this chapter allows us to give just some examples of the interaction of hormones with plasma proteins which could be related to or even interfere with putative receptors in the target tissues of the foetus.

Transcortin, which binds principally corticosteroids and to a lesser extent progesterone, increases during pregnancy in the human (36) and in other animal species (37). In the baboon, the interesting observation was made that at mid-pregnancy the capacity for cortisol binding was similar in maternal and foetal plasma, but at the end of gestation the values were twice as high on the maternal side (38). The higher quantity of unbound cortisol circulating in the foetal compartment could be related to some aspects of foetal lung maturation or to the onset of parturition. Another interesting plasma protein is PBG (progesterone binding globulin) which is found in the maternal compartment of the guinea pig (39) and which reaches very high concentrations at 45-55 days of gestation (1 g/l) (8). Recently, a protein with the same physico-chemical characteristics as PBG has been found in foetal plasma of the same animal species (40) but its concentration is 300-500 times less than in the maternal compartment. Androgens can also circulate bound to foetal and maternal proteins and the capacity of this binding could be involved in the control of sex differentiation. It is interesting that testosterone in pregnant guinea pigs, for example, circulates to a great extent in bound form in maternal plasma but very little or no binding is found in foetal plasma proteins or in the amniotic fluid (41, 42). Finally, one should mention α-foetoprotein, an important protein present in the foetal plasma of many animal species. This protein binds oestradiol with very high affinity ($K_D = 10^{-10}$M) in some species (e.g. rat, mouse) (43, 44) but not in others (e.g. human, guinea pig). Since this chapter will describe various aspects of steroid receptors in the foetal compartment of guinea pig, Table 3 indicates the relative percentage of binding of some steroids to foetal plasma proteins of this species. Progesterone and cortisol can be seen to be bound to a great extent but, in contrast,

TABLE 3

RELATIVE PERCENTAGE BINDING OF DIFFERENT STEROIDS TO FOETAL AND MATERNAL PLASMA PROTEIN AND IN THE AMNIOTIC FLUID OF GUINEA PIG (55-65 DAYS OF GESTATION)

STEROID	FOETAL PLASMA (DILUTED 1/10)	MATERNAL PLASMA (DILUTED 1/10)	AMNIOTIC FLUID (NOT DILUTED)
	%	%	%
^{3}H-OESTRADIOL	1 - 3	1 - 2	3 - 4
^{3}H-OESTRONE	0.5 - 2	1 - 2	-
^{3}H-OESTRADIOL SULFATE	3 - 5	-	-
^{3}H-OESTRONE SULFATE	3 - 4	1 - 3	1 - 3
^{3}H-PROGESTERONE	16 - 24	75 - 86	27 - 30
^{3}H-CORTISOL	10 - 18	15 - 18	-
^{3}H-TESTOSTERONE	N.D.	24 - 33	3 - 4
^{3}H-ALDOSTERONE	N.D.	-	N.D.

The plasmas or amniotic fluid were incubated with the radioactive steroid (4×10^{-9}M) for 4h at 4ºC. The total binding was calculated after separation of the unbound steroid using the columns of Sephadex G-15 or adsorption by charcoal-dextran.

only a small proportion of oestrogens circulate in a bound form in the foetal or maternal compartments.

B. Oestrogen receptors in the foetal compartment

Since 1971, when the first observations were made in this laboratory on the binding of oestradiol to macromolecular components in the cytosol of foetal guinea pig brain (35), oestrogen binding has subsequently been found in varying quantities in a whole range of foetal tissues : uterus (45-48), lung (46, 47, 49, 50), kidney (46, 47, 49-51), testis (46) and brain (52, 53). In this section, the physico-chemical properties of oestrogen receptors in several tissues of the guinea pig foetus will be compared, including information on the changes in receptor values as foetal development progresses and the relationship between receptor concentrations in foetal uterus and plasma and tissue concentrations of oestrogens in the intact, developing foetus.

1. <u>Physico-chemical properties of oestrogen receptors in various foetal tissues of the guinea pig</u>. Both the cytosol and nuclear binding of oestradiol in various foetal tissues were studied by incubating whole cell suspensions of the foetal tissues with 5×10^{-8}M ^{3}H-oestradiol (with and without a 100 to 300-fold molar excess of unlabelled oestradiol to be able to calculate

saturable, specific binding) in Krebs-Henseleit buffer at 37°C for 15 min. The values of specific oestradiol binding in uterus, lung, kidney and brain of foetuses of approximately the same gestational age are indicated in Table 4. In the foetus, as in the adult, a typical target organ like the uterus contains 30 to 100 times greater concentration of oestradiol binding sites in the cytosol fraction and 100 to 850 times in the nuclear extract than in other tissues. Nevertheless, specific binding can be measured in lesser but significant quantities in other foetal tissues. Binding can be found not only in the cytosol but also in the nucleus where one would hope to find binding if this receptor-like binding is to have further biological and physiological implications. The values of total oestrogen binding in the uterus measured under conditions which permit translocation of cytosol receptor into the nucleus have been found to be less than those measured in the cytosol of uterus never exposed to oestradiol before the binding determination (48).

By competition studies to test the specificity of the sites to which ^{3}H-oestradiol was binding in these foetal tissues, it was found that in all tissues, including the uterus, other oestrogens such as oestrone and oestriol were able to compete effectively for ^{3}H-oestradiol binding sites. Other steroids had no significant effect (54).

TABLE 4

COMPARATIVE BINDING OF ^{3}H-OESTRADIOL IN CYTOSOL AND NUCLEUS OF FOETAL GUINEA PIG UTERUS, LUNG, KIDNEY AND BRAIN (54)

	CYTOSOL fmole/mg DNA	NUCLEUS fmole/mg DNA
UTERUS	6920	5940
LUNG	210	60
KIDNEY	53	44
BRAIN	110	7

100-150 mg of foetal uterus, 1g of foetal kidney and lung or 2g of foetal brain were incubated with 5×10^{-8}M ^{3}H-oestradiol with and without a 100 or 300-fold excess of unlabelled oestradiol in 4-5 ml of Krebs-Henseleit buffer at 37°C for 15 min. The values represent the average of 2 to 3 experiments at ~ 50 days of gestation.

TABLE 5

PHYSICO-CHEMICAL CHARACTERISTICS OF ^{3}H-OESTRADIOL SPECIFIC BINDING IN THE DIFFERENT FOETAL TISSUES OF GUINEA PIG (50-55 DAYS OF GESTATION)

	Kd M x 10^{-10}	n (fmoles/mg protein)	S	pI
UTERUS	2 - 5	70 - 88	8	6.1 - 6.2
KIDNEY	2.5 - 8.9	1.1 - 4.5	8	6.1 - 6.2
BRAIN	5 - 8	1.5 - 5.0	7 - 8	6.1 - 6.2
LUNG	4 - 8	2.0 - 3.7	8	6.1 - 6.2

Kd : Dissociation constant   n : Number of specific sites

S : Sedimentation coefficient   pI : Isoelectric point

The binding affinity of ^{3}H-oestradiol to these oestrogen-specific binding sites was also compared in the four foetal tissues studied and with values published in the literature for binding affinities in adult uterine cytosol. The dissociation constants of specific ^{3}H-oestradiol binding at 4°C in the cytosols of foetal uterus, kidney, brain and lung (Table 5) show similar binding of high affinity in all tissues, although the foetal uterus has a much higher binding capacity for the same high affinity binding. Similar values have been found in cytosol of immature and adult rat uterus (55, 56).

The sedimentation coefficients of the ^{3}H-oestradiol macromolecule-complexes in all four foetal tissues determined by ultracentrifugation in sucrose density gradients is 8S in low salt gradients which is like that of the oestradiol receptor in calf uterus (57, 58). There has been a report, however, that 8-9S binding of oestradiol in foetal guinea pig brain has been found only in the hypothalamus-preoptic area-amygdala and not in the cerebral cortex and that this macromolecular component represents a lower affinity, higher capacity binder (53). Autoradiographic studies of foetal mouse brain have shown the localization of ^{3}H-oestradiol in the nuclei of cells of certain hypothalamic and extra-hypothalamic regions and in the anterior pituitary (59).

Therefore, in terms of binding specificity, affinity and molecular size, oestradiol binding sites are similar in the four foetal tissues studied and in immature or adult tissues of other animal species.

2. Ontogeny of oestrogen receptor concentrations in foetal uterus, lung, kidney and brain. In the preceding section we have seen that specific, high affinity oestradiol binding sites are present in differing concentrations in four foetal tissues at one time point during gestation. Since the foetus is a developing organism, it was also of interest to study changes in oestradiol binding during the course of foetal development. Table 6 shows that there is a marked increase in oestradiol binding from mid-gestation (34-35 days) to the end (60-65 days) in all four foetal tissues studied. After birth, there is a sharp decline except in foetal lung cytosol which continues to increase. The physiological significance of this increase remains to be elucidated since the relationship between levels of oestradiol and oestradiol receptors and the biological action of oestradiol in the foetus is not yet known. However, the developmental biology of hormone receptors in the foetus could prove to be a useful model in studying the mechanisms of action of hormones in physiological conditions.

TABLE 6

ONTOGENY OF OESTRADIOL BINDING SITES IN FOETAL UTERUS, LUNG, KIDNEY AND BRAIN

	SPECIFIC ^{3}H-OESTRADIOL BINDING (fmole/g TISSUE)							
	UTERUS		LUNG		KIDNEY		BRAIN	
AGE	CYTOSOL	NUCLEUS	CYTOSOL	NUCLEUS	CYTOSOL	NUCLEUS	CYTOSOL	NUCLEUS
DAYS OF GESTATION								
34 - 35	1100	-	170	84	6	45	43	24
37 - 38	2100	-	158	164	297	40	140	12
44 - 45	9500	-	380	430	263	245	117	8
49 - 50	12000	3700	1500	282	289	160	180	7
60 - 65	23000	6400	2500	330	610	460	280	11
AFTER BIRTH								
24 h	13500	3200	8000	145	329	130	113	3
4 WEEKS	10120	520	13800	54	170	150	52	2

Cell suspensions of foetal tissue were incubated with 8×10^{-9}M or 5×10^{-8}M ^{3}H-oestradiol in the presence or absence of a 100 or 300-fold excess of unlabelled oestradiol. Incubations were carried out in Krebs-Henseleit buffer at 37°C for 15 min. The values represent the average of 3 experiments with 36 foetuses at 34 to 35 days, 42 at 37 to 38 days, 10 at 45 days, 6 at 50 days, 2 at 60 to 65 days and 2 newborns and 1 immature female.

3. Subcellular distribution of ^{3}H-oestradiol binding sites in foetal uterus. In these studies using foetuses, one must remember that the foetuses are constantly in the presence of a certain endogenous concentration of hormones which are subsequently being used to measure binding. It is therefore important to take into account the possible effect of endogenous oestradiol on the actual binding assay or on the subcellular distribution of the oestradiol binding sites. Recent technical improvements have made it feasible to differentiate between oestradiol binding sites which are available for binding *in vitro* and those which were previously occupied by endogenous hormone. These determinations were carried out in the foetal uterus since previous studies had shown such high concentrations of oestradiol binding sites in this organ.

Cytosol fractions and 0.6M KCl nuclear extracts of uterus of guinea pig foetuses were prepared and protamine sulfate precipitates of these fractions were incubated with ^{3}H-oestradiol under conditions enabling exchange of ^{3}H-oestradiol with previously bound endogenous hormone (48, 60, 61). Unoccupied cytosol ^{3}H-oestradiol binding sites represent 80.7% of all the oestradiol binding sites in the foetal uterus (Table 7); 12.7% are occupied cytosol binding sites and only 6.7% are in the nucleus (both occupied and unoccupied) (48). This subcellular distribution of available and occupied binding sites correlates well with the low circulating oestrogen concentrations in foetal plasma (54), and with the hypothesis of a hormone-mediated translocation of cytosol receptor into the nucleus to bind to nuclear acceptor sites. The concentration of occupied sites in the cytosol and nuclear fractions (9pmoles/g tissue) also corresponds to the concentration of endogenous oestradiol plus oestrone (7pmoles/g tissue) measured in foetal uterine tissue (54). The occupied oestradiol binding sites thus represent only a fraction of the total in the foetal uterus but are still in the range of values of total oestradiol receptor concentrations in immature or adult rat uterus (62), receptor values which have been found to agree well with what is required to elicit a biological response to oestradiol (63, 64).

TABLE 7

SUBCELLULAR DISTRIBUTION OF ^{3}H-OESTRADIOL BINDING IN FOETAL GUINEA PIG UTERUS

	pmole/mg DNA	pmole/g TISSUE	pmole/UTERUS
CYTOSOL			
UNOCCUPIED	15.43	66.0	2.92
OCCUPIED	2.42	9.0	0.40
NUCLEUS			
UNOCCUPIED	1.27	4.9	0.21
OCCUPIED	0.02	0.07	0.003
TOTAL	19.14	80.4	3.56

Protamine sulfate precipitates of cytosol fractions and nuclear extracts of foetal uterus were incubated with 1 x 10^{-8}M ^{3}H-oestradiol with and without a 100-fold excess of unlabelled oestradiol. Incubations were carried out at 4°C to measure unoccupied binding sites and at 30°C or 37°C to measure total binding sites. The values are the average of 7 determinations.

In conclusion, the apparent ubiquity of oestrogen binding now awaits further study on the physiological action of oestrogens in the foetus, especially in organs previously considered "non-target" organs. However, the similarity of this binding among all of these tissues and their apparent similarity to oestrogen receptor binding described in adult target organs has been shown. Finally, the most recent work in our laboratory has demonstrated that at least two biological actions of oestradiol which have been well established in the uterus of adult animals can now also be evoked in foetal guinea pig uterus whose receptor binding has been studied extensively and which will be discussed in Section V.

C. Androgen receptors

It is well known that androgens, particularly testosterone, play an important role in sex differentiation. The androgens secreted by the foetal testis direct the transformation of the Wolffian ducts into epididymis, seminal vesicles and vas deferens (65). Foetal androgens could contribute also by inducing the regression of the Müllerian ducts (66). The mechanism of this process is not well known at present but this action could be by a series of molecular events which start with the uptake and binding of androgens to specific receptors in the foetal reproductive tracts. It was demonstrated in foetal rats of 14-21 days of gestation that the different tissues of the male genital tract (genital ducts, mesonephric tubules, urogenital sinus and tubercule) have specific high affinity testosterone binding macromolecules in the cytosol fractions and this specific binding increases five times from 14 to 20 days of gestation (67). At the same comparative period no increase was observed in the specific binding of testosterone in the female genital tract. It is noteworthy that in these tissues the binding capacity was limited to 15 fmole/mg protein, which corresponds to 4 pg testosterone and represents only 0.1% of the concentration of the hormone in the tissues. The increase of specific binding for androgens coincides with the increase of testosterone biosynthesis by the foetal testis from day 15 of gestation (68).

Interesting information has also been obtained in foetal rabbits whose maximal uptake of ^{3}H-testosterone in foetal reproductive tracts occurs just before sex differentiation (17-21 days of gestation in this species) (69). A close correlation has also been observed between the appearance of LH-HCG receptors and testosterone biosynthesis at the moment of the formation of Leydig cells in the foetal rabbit (17-19 days of gestation) suggesting that these receptors and the secretion of testosterone are important biochemical factors in sex differentiation (70).

Specific ^{3}H-testosterone binding has also been found in the foetal testis of guinea pig between 36 and 50 days of gestation (46), but these studies need complementary information to be correlated with sex differentiation, particularly the data on the androgen concentration in the foetal reproductive tract. It is concluded that androgens and androgen receptors could play an important role in sex differentiation and maturation of the sexual organs during embryonic life.

D. Progesterone receptors

The uterus of the guinea pig foetus has served as a good model for the study of progesterone receptors in the foetal compartment especially since very large concentrations of oestrogen receptor have been found in this tissue and since a positive relationship between oestrogen and progesterone receptors was studied in postnatal life in the guinea pig and other animal species (71-76).

Specific, high affinity binding for progesterone and the synthetic progestin R-5020 (17α,21-dimethyl-19-norpregnane-4,9-diene-3,20-dione) was found in the uterus of foetal guinea pig (42, 78, 79). This binding showed competition for ^{3}H-progesterone and ^{3}H-R-5020 binding sites by progesterone, R-5020 and 5α-dihydroprogesterone but not by other steroids such as 20α-dihydroprogesterone, oestrone, oestradiol, oestriol, testosterone and cortisol. The lack of competition by cortisol indicates that this binding in the foetal uterus is not due to a contamination by transcortin, which is known to circulate in high concentration in foetal blood of guinea pigs (8). The specific progesterone binding sites in foetal uterus have a high affinity for progesterone ($K_D = 3.3 \pm 1.7(S.D.) \times 10^{-9}$M) and slightly higher for R-5020 ($K_D = 0.7 \pm 0.3 \times 10^{-9}$M) (42). This high affinity binding could possibly have resulted from binding to a foetal progesterone binding globulin (PBG) which also binds progesterone (but not R-5020) with high affinity in foetal guinea pig plasma (40) but 90-97% of the foetal uterine binding protein is destroyed by heating while plasma PBG is heat stable (42). The quantities of progesterone binding sites present in foetal uterine cytosol at the end of gestation are in the order of 60 fmoles/mg protein which is substantially less than the concentration of oestrogen binding sites (77).

As for the oestrogen receptor in foetal uterus, a developmental study of progesterone receptors during gestation was carried out which has yielded very interesting results with reference to the oestrogen receptor (Table 8). Specific binding

TABLE 8

CYTOSOL SPECIFIC ^{3}H-OESTRADIOL AND ^{3}H-PROGESTERONE BINDING IN THE UTERUS OF GUINEA PIG DURING DEVELOPMENT (42)

	fMOLES/MG PROTEIN	
DAYS OF GESTATION	$R\text{-}E_2$	R-P
34 - 35	85 - 95	N.D.
36 - 37	140 - 200	N.D.
44 - 45	300 - 490	N.D.
50 - 54	550 - 680	30 - 45
55 - 65	580 - 880	70 - 140
NEW BORNS		
1 DAY	380 - 460	160 - 220
2 - 3 DAYS	340 - 420	200 - 250
7 - 8 DAYS	300 - 400	200 - 230

N.D. = NOT DETECTABLE
$R\text{-}E_2$ = OESTROGEN RECEPTOR
R-P = PROGESTERONE RECEPTOR

Cytosol was incubated with 4×10^{-9}M of ^{3}H-oestradiol or ^{3}H-progesterone with or without a 100-fold excess of unlabelled oestradiol or progesterone for 4h at 4°C. Specific binding was calculated from the differences between the two determinations after adsorption of the unbound radioactive steroid using the charcoal-dextran method. Values are ranges of 4-5 determinations.

of progesterone in foetal uterine cytosol can only be detected from ~50 days of gestation, unlike the oestrogen receptor which already appears at 34-35 days of gestation (just after mid-gestation in the guinea pig) (42, 77, 78). This temporal relationship is suggestive of the causal relationship between oestradiol treatment and the stimulation of progesterone receptors (71-76), a subject which will be treated in Section V.

Therefore, the observation that foetal uterus not only contains oestrogen receptors but also progesterone receptors has important biological implications, especially in light of the different developmental curves of the two receptors. The foetal guinea pig uterus could thus serve as a good model for the demonstration of a biological action of a steroid hormone in the foetus and for a study of the regulation of two receptors.

E. Glucocorticoid receptors

Glucocorticoids play an important role during foetal development, one of which is their selective action on the maturation of the lung. Specific binding sites for cortisol (79, 80) and dexamethasone in rabbit foetal lung have been demonstrated (81). At 28-30 days of gestation, binding in the foetal lung was found to be higher than in the other foetal tissues studied (82). The number of glucocorticoid receptors in the rabbit foetal lung increased during foetal development as has been shown for estradiol receptors in foetal guinea pig uterus (46).

Quantitative evaluation of glucocorticoid receptors in the foetal lung of different species (rabbit, rat, human) showed an increase in the concentration of binding sites with foetal evolution (Table 9) (83). Similarly, in foetal small intestine of rabbits, the maximum concentration of specific binding sites (1.75 pmol/mg DNA) for dexamethasone occurs on day 26; decreasing to 0.2 pmol/mg DNA at birth (84). This evolution of glucocorticoid receptors could be related to the increase in the conversion of cortisone to cortisol at the end of gestation (20, 21, 22).

Studies on the ontogenesis of glucocorticoid receptors in the rat liver showed that during foetal development maximum values were obtained at 18 days of gestation, were undetectable just before and after parturition and increased at 2-5 days. It was suggested that the undetectable binding sites close to the

TABLE 9

CYTOPLASMIC GLUCOCORTICOID RECEPTORS IN FOETAL LUNG DURING DEVELOPMENT (83)

Species	Developmental Stage	Dexamethasone specific binding sites (pmols/mg DNA)
Rabbit	Foetus 21 days	0.45
	Foetus 29 days	0.52
	Adult	0.27
Rat	Foetus 20 days	0.22
	Newborns	0.05
Human	Foetus 10 weeks	0.07
	Foetus 17 weeks	0.18

time of birth were due to the increase of endogenous corticoids which may occupy the binding sites (85). It is interesting that the rat foetal liver has a higher affinity for corticosterone than for cortisol, while in the adult liver the reverse is true (85); this fact could be related to the maturation of this tissue.

F. Mineralocorticoid receptors

The previous section on oestradiol receptors in various tissues of the guinea pig foetus indicated that besides the uterus, other tissues, such as the kidney, contain small but reproducibly detectable quantities of oestradiol binding sites. The kidney, being a mineralocorticoid target organ, has mineralocorticoid receptors in significant amounts. It is, thus, interesting to note that specific receptors of more than one steroid hormone may be present simultaneously in the same tissue.

The specific binding of ^{3}H-aldosterone has been determined in the kidney of foetal guinea pigs and found to be relatively specific and of high affinity (86). Competition studies have shown that unlabelled aldosterone and to some extent, cortisol, both compete for the ^{3}H-aldosterone binding sites. The weak mineralocorticoid activity of cortisol explains this apparent binding of a glucocorticoid to a mineralocorticoid binding site. Moreover, adult rat kidney has both mineralocorticoid (Type I) and glucocorticoid (Type II) binding sites, the latter being of lower affinity (87). The dissociation constant of the binding of ^{3}H-aldosterone in the cytosol fraction of foetal kidney is 4×10^{-9}M at 4°C which is similar to the affinity of the aldosterone receptor in the kidney of adult adrenalectomized rats (88). The concentration of specific aldosterone binding sites in the cytosol of foetal kidney is about 160 fmoles/mg DNA and the nucleus binds about 23 fmoles/mg DNA when whole kidney cell suspensions are incubated with ^{3}H-aldosterone (47). This is about twice as much as the binding of oestradiol in foetal kidney under the same experimental conditions.

Whether mineralocorticoid binding sites observed in the foetal kidney have a physiological meaning is not yet clear. It has, however, been shown in the kidney of foetal rats that aldosterone can stimulate the activity of Na^{+}-K^{+} dependent ATPase which is involved in sodium transport (89).

IV. Steroid Hormone Receptor in the Plancenta

Early studies have suggested the presence of specific binding sites for oestrogens in the "maternal placenta" of rats, and it was also observed that these receptors decrease in the rat with the advance of pregnancy (90). More recently it has been established that oestrogen receptors are also present in the basal zone of the trophoblast (91). At day 10 of gestation in the rat there are 14,000 sites/cell in the cytosol of the whole placenta (90) and in the basal zone; at day 11 the values were 12,000 sites/cell in the cytosol and 21,000 in the nucleus (91). This oestradiol-macromolecule complex was found to be a 4S component with an affinity (K_d) of $1\text{-}1.8 \times 10^{-10}$M. Studies throughout pregnancy show that in the cytosol the number of sites per cell is 30,000 at day 9, which falls to 600 at the 15th day of gestation; in the nuclei the values are 3400 and 200 respectively (92). This drastic decrease in the number of oestrogen receptors could be explained by the increase of progesterone in trophoblast giant cells at that period. This hypothetical action of progesterone on the oestradiol receptor could be similar to that found in uterine tissue (93).

Glucocorticoid receptors have also been found in the placenta of rabbit, the concentration of sites is 0.26 pmol/mg protein in the foetal side of the placenta (16-26 days of gestation), but was not detectable in the maternal side (81). At present there is no clear explanation for the presence of steroid receptors in the placental compartment and their relationship to receptors in the foetal compartment is to be explored.

V. Steroid Receptors and Biological Activity in the Foetus

A. Glucorticoid receptors and lung maturation

In 1968, Liggins observed that the administration of cortisol to pregnant sheep expanded the foetal lung (23) which is correlated with the maturation of pulmonary surfactant. Glucocorticoids have been found to increase the synthesis of lecithin (phosphatidyl choline) (94) which is the major component of pulmonary surfactant. This action of glucocorticoids has been applied to the treatment of respiratory distress syndrome (RDS) in premature infants. The incidence of RDS is substantially reduced by administration of glucocorticoids to women in premature labor (95). The action of cortisol on the incorporation of ^{3}H-choline into lecithin of foetal lung cells of rabbit was largely confirmed by tissue culture studies (96). Brehier et al. (97) suggested that glucocorticoids stimulate phosphatidic acid phosphatase (PAPase) activity in the foetal lung, which is the regulatory enzyme in surfactant synthesis during lung maturation.

Consequently, the hypothetical mechanism of glucocorticoid action could be as follows : in the early stage of foetal development, the biological action of cortisol, permissive at that embryonic stage, is neutralized by its conversion to inactive cortisone (20, 21). At the end of gestation, the circulating cortisone can be converted to cortisol in the different foetal tissues including the lung (21, 22). This cortisol is bound to specific cytosol receptors in this tissue, translocates to the nuclei to initiate the different steps of transcription and stimulates the synthesis of proteins involved in lecithin synthesis for surfactant.

Despite the fact that these studies are very stimulating for the knowledge of corticoid action in the foetal compartment, some contradictions have been observed concerning the biological effect of glucocorticoids in the foetus, e.g. corticoids injected to the mother diminish immune responses (98), reduce foetal body weight (99) and decrease the content of cerebral DNA (100).

B. Oestradiol-induced responses in foetal guinea pig uterus and ovary

The appearance of measurable receptor levels earlier in gestation than detectable concentrations of progesterone receptor, suggested that the foetal uterus could respond to oestrogen treatment by an increase in progesterone receptor concentration, as has been well established in adult guinea pig uterus (75), in chick oviduct (71) and in mouse and rat uterus (72). Guinea pig foetuses were treated for three consecutive days with oestradiol by administration to the mother and a significant increase in progesterone receptor levels could be observed, even at 37-42 days of gestation when progesterone receptor levels are barely detectable normally (Table 10) (78). This same effect of oestradiol on progesterone receptor levels could also be provoked by a single injection of oestradiol after 24h showing the rapid response of foetal uterus to oestradiol.

Foetal uterus also responds to oestradiol treatment by a 70 to 90% increase in uterine wet weight after three consecutive days of treatment. However, this uterotrophic response was not observed in animals treated for only 24h, indicating a slower uterotrophic response. Thus, two parameters of oestrogenic response in the foetal uterus can be separated temporally.

TABLE 10

SPECIFIC BINDING OF ^{3}H-PROGESTERONE IN THE CYTOSOL FRACTION OF FOETAL UTERUS IN CONTROL AND OESTRADIOL-TREATED(E_2) ANIMALS (78)

Gestational age	Control fmole/mg protein	E_2-Treated fmole/mg protein
37-42 days	2.9 ± 2	30.8 ± 6.8
50-52 days	35.4 ± 6.3	307.7 ± 103.5
55-65 days	85.6 ± 15.7	549 ± 87.9

Pregnant guinea pigs were injected with 1 mg/kg/day of oestradiol in 40% ethanol-saline (controls received vehicle alone) for 3 days. On day 4, foetuses were separated and a cytosol fraction of foetal uterus was prepared in 0.01M Tris-HCl buffer pH 7.4. Aliquots of cytosol were incubated in 4×10^{-9}M ^{3}H-progesterone for 4h at 4°C with or without a 100-fold excess of unlabelled progesterone. Values are mean ± S.D. of 5-7 determinations.

Progesterone receptors are also present in foetal ovaries; the concentration of specific progesterone binding sites at the end of gestation is 20-30 fmol/mg protein, 2-3 times less than the concentration of progesterone receptors in foetal uterus. In oestradiol-primed animals, there is a 3-5 fold increase in progesterone receptors in the ovaries.

Studies in the uterus of newborn animals (2-7 days old) show that, in contrast to oestradiol receptors, progesterone receptor concentrations remain high. However, the oestrogenic response is limited and doses of 1 to 100 µg of oestradiol only stimulate the progesterone receptor 1.5 to 2 times.

At the moment the physiological significance of the oestradiol-induced responses in the foetal female reproductive organs has not been definitely established, but the present data suggest that, during foetal life, oestrogens can be involved in biological effects related to sexual maturity. The action of oestradiol on progesterone receptors in the foetal compartment could be one of the first events in this biological response.

VI. Conclusions

At the present time, it is well established that receptors for different steroid hormones are present in the foetus of various animal species. Two model systems have been well developed from studies of these receptors and their biological implications : the foetal lung as a target tissue for glucocorticoids, mainly studied in the rabbit, and the foetal uterus of guinea pig as a target tissue for oestrogens as shown by the presence of oestrogen receptors and the effect of oestrogens on uterotrophic responses and the stimulation of progesterone receptors.

The complexity of the inter-relationship between maternal, placental and foetal compartments requires more knowledge of the metabolic transformations of steroid hormones and circulating hormone concentrations in these compartments and their correlations with receptor concentrations and ultimately the biological activities of steroid hormones in the target tissues of the foetus. Further investigations on the control of the biosynthesis of receptors in the foetus, the transformations and ultimate fate of these receptors and their interaction with the genome and effect on transcription and translation are necessary in order to elucidate the mechanism, as well as the role, of steroid hormones in foetal tissues. A better understanding will thus be acquired on such important aspects of embryonic life as the mechanism of implantation, foetal sexual differentiation and organ growth and maturation during the normal and pathological development of the foetus.

Acknowledgements

This work was supported in part by a grant from the "Centre National de la Recherche Scientifique, Equipe de Recherche No. 187", France.

References

1. Cope, C.L., Black, E.: Hydrocortisone production in late pregnancy. J. Obstet. Gynacc. Br. Commonw. 66, 404-408 (1959).

2. Migeon, C.J., Kenny, F.M., Taylor, F.H.: Cortisol production rate. VIII. Pregnancy. J. clin. Endocr. Metab. 28, 661-666 (1968).

3. Watanabe, M., Meeker, C.I., Gray, M.G., Sims, E.A.H., Solomon, S.: Aldosterone secretion rates in abnormal pregnancy. J. clin. Endocr. Metab. 25, 1665-1670 (1965).

4. Brown, R.D., Strott, C.A., Liddle, G.W.: Plasma deoxycorticosterone in normal and abnormal human pregnancy. J. clin. Endocr. Metab. 35, 736-742 (1972).

5. Vande Wiele, R.L., Gurpide, E., Kelly, W.G., Laragh, J.H., Lieberman, S.: The secretion rate of progesterone and aldosterone in normal and abnormal late pregnancy. Ist Int. Congr. Endocr., Ed. Fuchs, F., Periodica, Copenhagen, p. 159 (1960).

6. Gurpide, E., Angers, M., Vande Wiele, R.L., Lieberman, S.: Determination of secretory rates of estrogens in pregnant and non-pregnant women from the specific activities of urinary metabolites. J. clin. Endocr. Metab. 22, 934-945 (1962).

7. Simmer, H.H., Easterling, W.E., Pion, R.J., Dignam, W.J.: Neutral C_{19} steroids and steroid sulfates in human pregnancy. I. Identification of dehydroepiandrosterone sulfate in fetal blood and quantification of this hormone in cord arterial, cord venous and maternal peripheral blood in normal pregnancies at term. Steroids 4, 125-135 (1964).

8. Westphal, U.: Steroid protein interaction. In: "Monographs on Endocrinology", vol. 4, Springer Verlag, Heidelberg/ New York, pp. 298-299 (1971).

9. Pepe, G., Rothchild, I.: The effect of hypophysectomy on day 12 of pregnancy on the serum progesterone level and time of parturition in the rat. Endocrinology 91, 1380-1385 (1972).

10. Yoshinaga, K., Hawkins, R.A., Stocker, J.F.: Estrogen secretion by the rat ovary in vivo during the estrous cycle and pregnancy. Endocrinology 85, 103-112 (1969).

11. Leavitt, W.W., Blaha, G.C.: Circulating progesterone levels in the golden hamster during the oestrous cycle, pregnancy and lactation. Biol. reprod. 3, 353-361 (1970).

12. Fylling, P.: The effect of pregnancy, ovariectomy and parturition on plasma progesterone levels in sheep. Acta endocr. 65, 273-283 (1970).

13. Challis, J.R.G., Lindzell, J.L.: The concentration of total unconjugated oestrogens in the plasma of pregnant goats. J. Reprod. Fert. 26, 401-404 (1971).

14. Smith, J.G., Hanks, J., Short, R.V.: Biochemical observations on the corpora lutea of the African elephant. J. Reprod. Fert. 20, 111-117 (1969).

15. Diczfalusy, E.: Steroid metabolism in the foeto-placental unit. Excerpta Medica Int. Congr. Ser. 183, 65-109 (1968).

16. Pasqualini, J.R.: Metabolic conjugation and hydrolysis of steroid hormones in the fetoplacental unit. In: "Metabolic Conjugation and Metabolic Hydrolysis", vol. 2, Ed. Fishman, W.H., Academic Press, New York, pp. 153-259 (1970).

17. Schwers, J., Govaerts-Videtzky, M.: Métabolisme des oestrogènes par le placenta humain.I. Hydrolyse de l'oestriol-3-sulfate du sang foetal par le placenta in vivo. Ann. Endocr. (Paris) 24, 920-924 (1963).

18. Pasqualini, J.R., Cédard, L., Nguyen, B.L., Alssatt, E.: Differences in the activity of human term placenta sulfatases for steroid ester sulphates. Biochim. biophys. Acta 139, 177-179 (1967).

19. French, A.P., Warren, J.C.: Sulfatase activity in the human placenta. Steroids 8, 79-85 (1966).

20. Pasqualini, J.R., Nguyen, B.L., Ulrich, F., Wiqvist, N., Diczfalusy, E.: Cortisol and cortisone metabolism in the human foeto-placental unit at mid-gestation. J. Steroid Biochem. 1, 209-219 (1970).

21. Murphy, B.E.P.: Cortisol and cortisone in human fetal development. J. Steroid Biochem. 11, 509-513 (1979).

22. Pasqualini, J.R., Costa Noves, S., Ito, Y., Nguyen, B.L.: Reciprocal cortisol-cortisone conversion in the total tissue and subcellular fractions of foetal and adult guinea pig liver. J. Steroid Biochem. 1, 341-347 (1970).

23. Liggins, G.C.: Premature parturition after infusion of corticotrophin or cortisol into foetal lambs. J. Endocr. 42, 323-329 (1968).

24. Jensen, E.V., Jacobson, H.I.: Biological activities of steroids in relation to cancer. In: "Fate of Steroid Estrogens in Target Tissues", Eds. Pincus, G., Vollmer, E.P., Academic Press, New York, pp. 161-178 (1960).

25. Glascock, R.F., Hoekstra, W.G.: Selective accumulation of tritium labelled hexestrol by the reproductive organs of immature female goats and sheep. Biochem. J. 72, 673-682 (1959).

26. Edelman, I.S., Bogoroch, R., Porter, G.A.: On the mechanism of action of aldosterone on sodium transport. Proc. natn. Acad. Sci. U.S.A. 50, 1169-1177 (1963).

27. Talwar, G.P., Segal, S.J., Evans, A., Davidson, O.W.: The binding of estradiol in the uterus : a mechanism for derepression of RNA synthesis. Proc. natn. Acad. Sci. U.S.A. 52, 1059-1066 (1964).

28. Toft, D., Gorski, J.: A receptor model for estrogens, isolation from the rat uterus and preliminary characterization. Proc. natn. Acad. Sci. U.S.A. 55, 1574-1581 (1966).

29. Stumpf, W.E.: Subcellular distribution of ^{3}H-estradiol in rat uterus by quantitative autoradiography - a comparison between ^{3}H-estradiol and ^{3}H-nerethynodrel. Endocrinology 83, 777-782 (1968).

30. Munck, A.: Specific metabolic and physico-chemical interactions of glucocorticosteroids in vivo and in vitro with rat adipose tissue and thymus cells. Excerpta Medica Int. Congr. Ser. 132, 472-481 (1966).

31. Fanestil, D.D., Edelman, I.S.: Characteristics of the renal nuclear receptors for aldosterone. Proc. natn. Acad. Sci. U.S.A. 56, 872-879 (1966).

32. O'Malley, B.W., McGuire, W.L., Kohler, P.D., Korenman, S.G.: Studies on the mechanism of steroid hormone regulation of synthesis of specific proteins. Recent Progr. Hormone Res. 25, 105-160 (1969).

33. Fang, S., Anderson, K.M., Liao, S.: Receptor proteins for androgens. On the role of specific proteins in selective retention of 17β-hydroxy-5α-androstan-3-one by rat ventral prostate in vivo and in vitro. J. biol. Chem. 244, 6584-6595 (1969).

34. Pasqualini, J.R., Sumida, C.: Formation de récepteurs spécifiques aldostérone-macromolécules au niveau du cytosol et du noyau du tissu rénal du foetus de cobaye. C.R. Acad. Sci. (Paris) 273, 1061-1063 (1971).

35. Pasqualini, J.R., Palmada, M.: Etude du récepteur de l'oestradiol dans le cerveau du foetus de cobaye. C.R. Acad. Sci. (Paris) 274, 1218-1221 (1972).

36. Slaunwhite, W.R. Jr., Sandberg, A.A.: Transcortin : A corticosteroid binding protein of plasma. J. clin. Invest. 38, 384-391 (1959).

37. Seal, U.S., Doe, R.P.: The role of corticosteroid-binding globulin in mammalian pregnancy. Excerpta Medica Int. Congr. Ser. 132, 697-706 (1967).

38. Oakey, R.E.: Serum cortisol binding capacity and cortisol concentration in the pregnant baboon and its fetus during gestation. Endocrinology 97, 1024-1029 (1975).

39. Diamond, M., Rust, N., Westphal, U.: High affinity binding of progesterone, testosterone and cortisol in normal and androgen treated guinea pig during various reproductive stages : relationship to masculinization. Endocrinology 84, 1143-1151 (1969).

40. Millet, A., Pasqualini, J.R.: Liaison spécifique de la ^{3}H-progestérone à une protéine du plasma du foetus de cobaye. C.R. Acad. Sci. (Paris) 287, 1429-1432 (1978).

41. Pasqualini, J.R., Sumida, C., Gelly, C.: Cytosol and nuclear ^{3}H-oestradiol binding in the foetal tissues of guinea pig. Acta endocr. 83, 811-828 (1976).

42. Pasqualini, J.R., Sumida, C., Nguyen, B.L., Tardy, J., Gelly, C.: Estrogen concentrations and effect of estradiol on progesterone receptors in the fetal and newborn guinea pigs. J. Steroid Biochem. 12, 65-72 (1980).

43. Nunez, E., Engelmann, F., Benassayag, C., Jayle, M.F.: Identification et purification préliminaire de la foeto protéine liant les oestrogènes dans le sérum de rats nouveau-nés. C.R. Acad. Sci. (Paris) Série D 273, 831-834 (1971).

44. Uriel, J., De Nechaud, B., Dupiers, M.: Estrogen binding properties of rat, mouse and man fetospecific serum proteins. Demonstration by immuno-autoradiographic method. Biochem. biophys. Res. Commun. 46, 1175-1180 (1972).

45. Pasqualini, J.R., Nguyen, B.L.: Mise en évidence des récepteurs cytosoliques et nucléaires de l'oestradiol dans l'utérus de foetus de cobaye. C.R. Acad. Sci. (Paris) Série D 283, 413-416 (1976).

46. Pasqualini, J.R., Sumida, C., Gelly, C., Nguyen, B.L.: Specific ^{3}H-estradiol binding in the fetal uterus and testis of guinea pig. J. Steroid Biochem. 7, 1031-1038 (1976).

47. Pasqualini, J.R., Sumida, C., Gelly, C., Nguyen, B.L.: A general view of the quantitative evaluation of cytosol and nuclear steroid hormone receptors in the fetal compartment of guinea pig. J. Steroid Biochem. 8, 445-451 (1977).

48. Sumida, C., Pasqualini, J.R.: Determination of cytosol and nuclear estradiol-binding sites in fetal guinea pig uterus by ^{3}H-estradiol exchange. Endocrinology 105, 406-413 (1979).

49. Pasqualini, J.R., Sumida, C., Gelly, C., Nguyen, B.L., Tardy, J.: Specific binding of estrogens in different fetal tissues of guinea pig during fetal development. Cancer Res. 38, 4246-4250 (1978).

50. Sumida, C., Gelly, C., Pasqualini, J.R.: DNA, protein and specific ^{3}H-oestradiol binding in the nuclear fractions of fetal guinea pig kidney and lung during development. Biol. of Reprod. 19, 338-345 (1978).

51. Pasqualini, J.R., Sumida, C., Gelly, C.: Steroid receptors in fetal guinea pig kidney. J. Steroid Biochem. 5, 977-985 (1974).

52. Pasqualini, J.R., Sumida, C., Nguyen, B.L., Gelly, C.: Quantitative evaluation of cytosol and nuclear ^{3}H-estradiol specific binding in the fetal brain of guinea pig during fetal ontogenesis. J. Steroid Biochem. 9, 443-447 (1978).

53. Plapinger, L., Landau, I.T., McEwen, B.S., Feder, H.H.: Characteristics of estradiol-binding macromolecules in fetal and adult guinea pig brain cytosols. Biol. of Reprod. 16, 586-599 (1977).

54. Sumida, C., Pasqualini, J.R.: Relationship between cytosol and nuclear oestrogen receptors and oestrogen concentrations in the fetal compartment of guinea pig. J. Steroid Biochem. 11, 267-272 (1979).

55. Steggles, A.W., King, R.J.B.: The use of protamine to study [6,7-^{3}H]-oestradiol binding in rat uterus. Biochem. J. 118, 695-701 (1970).

56. Lee, C., Jacobson, H.J.: Uterine estrogen receptors in rats during pubescence and the estrous cycles. Endocrinology 88, 596-601 (1971).

57. Puca, G.A., Nola, E., Sica, V., Bresciani, F.: Studies on isolation and characterization of estrogen binding protein of calf uterus. In: "Advances in the Biosciences", Ed. Raspe, F., Pergamon Press, Oxford, 7, 97-118 (1971).

58. Jensen, E.V., Mohla, S., Gorell, T., Tanaka, S., De Sombre, E.R.: Estrophile to nucleophile in two easy steps. J. Steroid Biochem. 3, 445-458 (1972).

59. Stumpf, W.E., Narbaitz, R., Sar, M.: Estrogen receptors in the fetal mouse. J. Steroid Biochem. 12, 55-64 (1980).

60. Chamness, G.C., Huff, K., McGuire, W.L.: Protamine-precipitated estrogen receptor : a solid phase ligand exchange assay. Steroids 25, 627-635 (1975).

61. Zava, D.T., Harrington, N.Y., McGuire, W.L.: Nuclear estradiol receptor in adult rat uterus : a new exchange assay. Biochemistry 15, 4292-4297 (1976).

62. Anderson, J., Clark, J.H., Peck, E.J.: Oestrogen and nuclear binding sites. Determination of specific sites by ^{3}H-oestradiol exchange. Biochem. J. 126, 561-567 (1972).

63. Anderson, J.N., Peck, E.J., Clark, J.H.: Nuclear receptor oestrogen complex; relationship between concentration and early uterotrophic responses. Endocrinology 92, 1488-1495 (1973).

64. Clark, J.H., Eriksson, H.A., Hardin, J.W.: Uterine receptor-estradiol complexes and their interaction with nuclear binding sites. J. Steroid Biochem. 7, 1039-1044 (1976).

65. Jost, A.: The problems of fetal endocrinology, the gonadal and hypophysial hormones. Recent Prog. Horm. Res. 8, 379 (1953).

66. Wilson, J.D.: Metabolism of testicular androgens. In: "Handbook of Physiology", Section 7 : Endocrinology, vol. V. Eds. Greep, R.O., Astwood, E.B., American Physiological Society, Washington D.C., p. 491 (1975).

67. Gupta, C., Bloch, E.: Testosterone-binding protein in reproductive tracts of fetal rats. Endocrinology 99, 389-399 (1976).

68. Noumura, T., Weisz, J., Lloyd, C.W.: In vitro conversion of 7-^{3}H-progesterone to androgens by the rat testis during the second half of fetal life. Endocrinology 78, 245-253 (1966).

69. Wilson, J.D.: Testosterone uptake by the urogenital tract of the rabbit embryo. Endocrinology 92, 1192-1199 (1973).

70. Catt, K.J., Dufau, M.L., Neaves, W.B., Walsh, P.C., Wilson, J.D.: LH-hCG receptors and testosterone content during differentiation of the testis in the rabbit embryo. Endocrinology 97, 1157-1165 (1975).

71. Sherman, M.R., Corvol, P.L., O'Malley, B.W.: Progesterone binding components of chick oviduct. I. Preliminary characterization of cytoplasmic components. J. biol. Chem. 245, 6085-6096 (1970).

72. Feil, P.D., Glasser, S.R., Toft, D.O., O'Malley, B.W.: Progesterone binding in mouse and rat uterus. Endocrinology 91, 738-746 (1972).

73. Philibert, D., Raynaud, J-P.: Progesterone binding in the immature mouse and rat uterus. Steroids 22, 89-98 (1973).

74. Leavitt, W.W., Toft, D.O., Strott, C.A., O'Malley, B.W.: A specific progesterone receptor in the hamster uterus : physiological properties and regulation during the estrous cycle. Endocrinology 94, 1041-1053 (1974).

75. Corvol, P., Falk, R., Freifeld, M., Bardin, C.W.: In vitro studies of progesterone binding proteins in guinea pig uterus. Endocrinology 90, 1464-1469 (1972).

76. Vu Hai, M.T., Logeat, F., Warenbourg, M., Milgrom, E.: Hormonal control of progesterone receptors. Ann. N.Y. Acad. Sci. 286, 199-209 (1977).

77. Pasqualini, J.R., Nguyen, B.L.: Uterine progesterone receptors in the guinea pig foetus : changes in gestational age and induction by oestrogens. J. Endocr. 81, 144P-145P (1979).

78. Pasqualini, J.R., Nguyen, B.L.: Progesterone receptors in the foetal uterus of guinea pig : its stimulation after oestradiol treatment. Experientia 35, 1116-1117 (1979).

79. Giannopoulus, G., Mulay, S., Solomon, S.: Cortisol receptors in rabbit fetal lung. Biochem. biophys. Res. Commun. 47, 411-418 (1972).

80. Giannopoulus, G.: Glucocorticoid receptors in lung. Mechanism of specific glucocorticoid uptake by fetal lung nuclei. J. biol. Chem. 250, 2896-2903 (1975).

81. Ballard, P.L., Ballard, R.A.: Glucocorticosteroid receptors and the role of glucocorticosteroids in fetal development. Proc. natn. Acad. Sci. U.S.A. 69, 2668-2672 (1972).

82. Giannopoulus, G., Hassan, Z., Solomon, S.: Glucocorticosteroid receptors in fetal and adult rabbit tissues. J. biol. Chem. 249, 2424-2427 (1974).

83. Giannopoulus, G.: Early events in the action of glucocorticoids in developing tissues. J. Steroid Biochem. 6, 623-631 (1975).

84. Lee, D.K.H., Solomon, S.: Characteristics and ontogeny of nuclear receptor for glucocorticoids in the rabbit fetal small intestine. Endocrinology 102, 312-320 (1978).

85. Giannopoulus, G.: Ontogeny of glucocorticoid receptors in rat liver. J. biol. Chem. 250, 5847-5851 (1975).

86. Pasqualini, J.R., Sumida, C.: Mineralocorticoid Receptors in Target Tissues. In: "Receptors and Mechanism of Action of Steroid Hormones", Ed. Pasqualini, J.R., Marcel Dekker, Inc., New York, pp. 399-511 (1977).

87. Funder, J.W., Feldman, D., Edelman, I.S.: The roles of plasma binding and receptor specificity in the mineralocorticoid action of aldosterone. Endocrinology 92, 994-1004 (1973).

88. Rousseau, G., Baxter, J.D., Funder, J.W., Edelman, I.S., Tomkins, G.M.: Glucocorticoid and mineralocorticoid receptors for aldosterone. J. Steroid Biochem. 3, 219-227 (1972).

89. Geloso, J-P., Bassett, J-C.: Role of adrenal glands in development of foetal rat kidney Na-K-ATPase. Pflügers Arch. ges. Physiol. 348, 105-113 (1974).

90. Feherty, P., Robertson, D.M., Waynforth, H.B., Kellie, A.E.: Changes in the concentration of high affinity oestradiol receptors in rat uterus supernatant preparations during the oestrous cycle, pseudopregnancy, pregnancy, maturation and after ovariectomy. Biochem. J. 120, 837-844 (1970).

91. McCormack, S.A., Glasser, S.R.: A high-affinity estrogen-binding protein in rat placental trophoblast. Endocrinology 99, 701-712 (1976).

92. McCormack, S.A., Glasser, S.R.: Ontogeny and regulation of a rat placental estrogen receptor. Endocrinology 102, 273-280 (1978).

93. Hsueh, A.J.W., Peck, E.J., Clark, J.H.: Control of uterine estrogen receptor levels by progesterone. Endocrinology 98, 438-450 (1976).

94. Farrell, P.M., Zachman, R.D.: Induction of choline phosphotransferase and lecithin synthesis in the fetal lung by corticosteroids. Science 179, 297-298 (1973).

95. Liggins, G.C., Howie, R.N.: A controlled trial of antepartum glucocorticosteroid treatment for prevention of the respiratory distress syndrome in premature infants. Pediatrics 50, 515-525 (1972).

96. Torday, J.S., Smith, B.T., Giroud, C.J.P.: The rabbit fetal lung as a glucocorticoid target tissue. Endocrinology 96, 1462-1467 (1975).

97. Brehier, A., Benson, B.J., Williams, M.C., Mason, R.J., Ballard, P.L.: Corticosteroid induction of phosphatidic acid phosphatase in fetal rabbit lung. Biochem. biophys. Res. Commun. 77, 883-890 (1977).

98. Clarman, H.N.: Corticosteroids and lymphoid cells. New Engl. J. Med. 287, 388-397 (1972).

99. Carson, S.H., Taeush, H.W., Avery, M.E.: Inhibition of lung cell division after hydrocortisone injection into fetal rabbits. J. appl. Physiol. 34, 660-663 (1973).

100. Cotterell, M., Balazs, R., Johnson, A.L.: Effects of corticosteroids on the biochemical maturation of rat brain : Postnatal cell formation. J. Neurochem. 19, 2151-2167 (1972).

CIRCULATING AND TISSUE THYROID HORMONES IN RELATION TO HORMONE ACTION : PATHOPHYSIOLOGIC SIGNIFICANCE

B. N. Premachandra, I. B. Perlstein, Kelley Williams
Veterans Administration Hospital, St. Louis, Missouri 63125, U.S.A.

Introduction

Tissue cells may be considered to be in equilibrium with interstitial fluid (ISF) which in turn is in equilibrium with the circulating blood. Hence, it is customary to think of changes in plasma as faithfully reflecting changes in the corresponding constituents of the ISF compartment which may allow an evaluation of cellular changes of these constituents. With regard to hormones, however, it is becoming increasingly apparent that circulating hormone concentrations alone, often fail to adequately reflect hormone action at the cellular level. This is particularly true in the case of thyroid hormones, thyroxine (T_4) and triiodothyronine (T_3), whose measurements in plasma or serum in various diseases and in patients during thyroid therapy often fail to mirror clinical thyroid status accurately. Thus, it is possible to delineate a number of disease states where euthyroidism, as diagnosed clinically, is accompanied by low circulating T_3 levels ("low T_3 syndrome", 1). Similarly, one often encounters low circulating T_4 levels in so-called euthyroid, sick subjects (2). Conversely, in patients maintained euthyroid on 1-thyroxine treatment, Kahn (3) noted several subjects whose plasma T_4 concentration was in the frank hyperthyroid range (> 15µg/100 ml) in the absence of any evidence of abnormalities in peripheral T_4 to T_3 conversion. Numerous other investigators have also reported the increased tolerance of obese individuals for thyroid medication, i.e. clinically diagnosed as euthyroid

Hormones in Normal and Abnormal Human Tissues, Vol. II

despite elevated plasma thyroid hormone concentrations, and indeed Cornman and Alexander (4) treated obese subjects with 300 µg T_3/day, about 3 times the replacement dosage in athyreotic patients and found no thyrotoxic effects.

Some of these inconsistencies between clinical and laboratory thyroid function assessments can be explained by the relatively recent recognition that the active form of the thyroid hormone (TH) is the unbound moiety, i.e. the non-protein bound thyroxine and triiodothyronine (free T_4-FT_4; free T_3-FT_3). In the case of thyroxine for example, the reason for considering circulating FT_4 concentration as the single most accurate index of the true thyro-metabolic status (5) is (a) it is only in the free form that T_4 diffuses into the tissue cells to exert its action, (b) the FT_4 concentration is more closely correlated to thyroxine turnover rates than is T_4 itself and (c) anomalies in T_4 binding protein do not normally affect free hormone concentration. The free T_4 hypothesis has not been without challenge however (6, 7, 8) and there are situations where even the circulating free T_4 concentration fails to correlate with clinical status and with tissue hormone action (5, 9). Thus, one often finds high serum FT_4 concentration, accompanied by low total T_4, in sick people who are nevertheless clinically euthyroid and without apparent thyroid disease (9). Similarly, we have recently described a euthyroid patient who had low thyroxine binding globulin (TBG) and free T_4 levels in the frank hyperthyroid range (10). It seems that some of these discrepancies may be partly reconciled by recent advances made in the understanding of metabolic pathways of thyroid hormones in tissues. First, there is evidence that T_4 must be mono-deiodinated by the cell to T_3 for full expression of its biologic activity. Second, there are probably separate tissue deiodinating enzymes for the inner (tyrosyl) and outer (phenolic) ring mono-deiodination of T_4, thereby allowing the generation of either the active form of the hormone T_3 (5'-T_4 mono-deiodination) or the calorigenically inactive hormone rT_3 (5-mono-deiodination of T_4). Nutritional and environmental factors, as well as some drugs, can differentially affect T_4 mono-deiodination pathways. Finally, the provocative possibility has been suggested that calorigenically inactive iodothyronines may influence the biologically significant cellular T_4 to T_3 mono-deiodinating pathways (19).

The purpose of this chapter is to review briefly the relevant clinical and experimental studies bearing on the above statements and to elaborate on the relative significance of circulating and tissue TH levels in the overt expression of biologic activity. While the binding of thyroid hormones to putative cellular receptors and their significance in the expression of cellular hormone action in various pathophysiologic states are discussed, it is not our goal to provide a detailed survey of TH action at the cellular level. This topic has been reviewed recently (11, 12, 13, 177).

Source of Thyroid Hormones in Extrathyroidal Tissues

Thyroidal secretion

The only hormone known to be secreted from the thyroid gland was T_4 until the discovery of a second hormone, T_3 (14), which was shown to be 3-4 times more potent than T_4 (15). Recent investigations in man and animals have conclusively shown that T_3 in tissue is not derived primarily from thyroidal secretion; rather T_3 is largely a product of peripheral mono-deiodination of T_4 in extrathyroidal tissues.

Thyroglobulin (TG) hydrolysis yields T_4 and T_3 in the thyroid gland and since recent studies have established that TG is normally released into the circulation via the thyroid lymphatics (16), one might wonder whether TG hydrolysis could result in circulating T_4, T_3 and other TH analogs. Based on a serum concentration of about 10 ng/ml TG as noted in radioimmunoassays (RIAs) (17), and considering 2 to 3 residues of T_4/mole TG, the T_4 formed from TG, even assuming its complete hydrolysis at the periphery, is very small compared to the total plasma T_4 concentration.

Extrathyroidal generation

Braverman et al. (18) obtained evidence for the presence of both stable and radioactively labeled T_3 in athyreotic humans administered highly purified mixtures of stable and radioactive T_4. The amounts of T_3 detected were far beyond the levels that could be ascribed to ^{125}I-T_3 contamination in the tracer radioactivity or to the impurities in the stable T_4 used in their studies. More recent studies have established that 35% of daily secreted T_4 is mono-deiodinated peripherally to T_3 and accounts for approximately 80% of the total daily T_3 production (19). Deiodination of T_4 has been shown to occur in various tissues such as liver, kidney and leucocytes. As studied in homogenates, T_4 to T_3 converting activity on a per gram basis was highest in liver and kidney (20).

Thyroid Hormone Analogs in Tissues

The recognized paths of T_4 metabolism are deiodination, decarboxylation, deamination and conjugation (Fig. 1). Of these metabolic pathways, deiodination is by far the most important. Recent studies suggest that as much as 85% of T_4 undergoes sequential mono-deiodination (19). The various analogs resulting from T_4 metabolism that have been measured in circulation by RIA are noted in Table 1. Although most of the TH derivatives are generated in peripheral tissues as a result of T_4 metabolism, some of them may result from thyroidal secretion as well, although the contribution from this source is very small (19).

Iodothyronine deiodination reactions are enzymatically catalyzed. This has been shown by Chopra (19) and Cavalieri et al. (21) who measured T_3 generation from T_4 incubated with subcellular fractions derived from rat liver homogenates. T_3 generation (a) had a pH optimum, (b) was proportional to cellular protein concentration in the medium, (c) was thiol dependent and (d) was reduced markedly at 56-60°C. In addition, Cavalieri et al. (21) found different pH optima for T_4 conversion to T_3 and rT_3, respectively, suggesting that separate deiodinases are involved in the inner and outer ring T_4 mono-deiodination. However, the deiodinating enzymes have not been isolated.

The study of the various deiodinated iodothyronines is important for understanding the pathways of deiodination and for assessing the quantitative importance of each pathway, for determining conditions which alter the kinetics of these pathways and for examining how deiodinated thyronines may control cellular hormone metabolism. Iodothyronines have been shown to modulate T_4 to T_3 conversion _in vitro_. Of the various substances tested using liver homogenates and appropriately controlled assay conditions, 3', 5'T_2 and rT_3 have been shown to be potent inhibitors of the T_4 to T_3 conversion while 3, 3'T_2 has been shown to be a weak inhibitor (20). In these _in vitro_ systems rT_3 has been found to be very unstable and this might cast doubt on its speculated role as a regulator of T_4 to T_3 conversion in peripheral tissues. However, it has been suggested that the transiency of cellular rT_3 would provide a means for rapid modulation of T_4 deiodination within the cell (22). Stimuli regulating T_4 to T_3 conversion include diet, drugs, pathophysiology and other factors. In general, one of the two pathways, T_4 to T_3 or T_4 to rT_3, is activated while the other is inhibited. These observations suggest that there may be extra-thyroidal mechanisms capable of modulating TH influence at the periphery by controlling the amounts of T_3 and rT_3 formed from T_4. As TH effects are ultimately perceived in peripheral tissues, the peripheral regulation of T_4 to T_3 conversion might be deemed more important for hormonal action than the rate of thyroidal secretion modulated by the hypothalamo-pituitary-thyroid axis. A major drawback in the hypothesis of peripheral iodothyronine regulation of T_4 to T_3 conversion is the relatively large dose of the analogs required _in vitro_ to demonstrate inhibition of

TABLE 1 CONCENTRATIONS OF IODOTHYRONINES IN NORMAL AND PATHOLOGIC STATES IN MAN

Iodothyronine/ Analog	EUTHYROID Iodothyronine/analog conc. in Thyroid	EUTHYROID Serum/Plasma	HYPOTHYROID Iodothyronine/analog conc. in Thyroid	HYPOTHYROID Serum/Plasma	HYPERTHYROID Iodothyronine/analog conc. in Thyroid	HYPERTHYROID Serum/Plasma	References
3:3':5:5' Tetraiodo-thyronine (T_4) µg/gm - thyroid µg/100 ml - serum	172.0 ± 22.1 232 137.5±15.8 146 ± 15	8.0 ± 1.6 (5.5 - 12.4)	1.7 ± 1.5† 20, 45††	2.5 ± 1.3 (N.D. - 5.5)	18.6 ± 1.99†††	18.7 ± 4.8 (12.7 - 28.4)	51, 125 50, 51 126 52
3:3':5:5' Tetraiodo-thyroacetic acid (Tetrac) ng/100 ml		121 ± 62 8.6 ± 2.0		73 ± 54		122 ± 62	127 128
3:3':5 Triiodothyro-nine (T_3) ng/100 ml	11.0 ± 1.97 21.3 15.1 ± 1.4 11.7 ± 0.6	142 ± 29.8 (82 - 217)	0.021 ± .017† 1.68, 2.19††	55 ± 32.1 (8 - 128)	7.71 ± 2.27	411 ± 188 (222 - 970)	51, 129 50, 51 126 52
3:3':5' Triiodothyro-nine (rT_3) ng/100 ml	6.5 ± 1.5 1.9* ± 0.45	26 ± 4 (21-37) 40.5 ± 10.4 (27-62) 20 (8-26)		8 ± 4 (<3-16)		77 ± 33 (41-160)	126, 130 131, 132 133
3:3':5 Triiodothyro-acetic acid (Triac) ng/100 ml		8.7 (<5.5-15.2)		7.4 (< 5.5-9.0)		9.7 (<5.5-15.2)	134
3:3':5 Triiodothyro-propionic acid ng/100 ml		<8.8 (1.8) **		< 8.8		< 8.8 (≤ 2.7)**	134
3:3' Diiodothyro-nine (3:3' T_2) ng/100 ml	0.16 0.40 ± .03	6.0 ± 1.0 (4.5-7.8) 7.2 (3-11) 7.6 ± 2.4 17.0 ± 4 (9-28) 4.3 ± 2		2.7 ± 1.1 (<2.0-6.0) <3 6 ± 2.2 9 ± 1 (<6-22) 1.7 - 2.3		9.0 ± 4.6 (3.0-21.0) 11 - 64 20.2 ± 7.5 29 ± 2 11.8 ± 2.7	135, 130 136 137 138 139
3':5' Diiodothyro-nine (3':5' T_2) ng/100 ml	0.22	6.4 ± 2.4 (2.7-13.0) 5.0 ± 0.3 (<2-12.2)		4.2 ± 3.5 (2.3-10.0) N.D.		14.9 ± 7.7 (3.6-32.0) 10.8 ± 0.8 (7.8-14.8)	135, 140 141
3:5 Diiodothyro-nine (3:5 T_2) ng/100 ml	0.32	≤5.2				20.0	142
3' Monoiodothyro-nine (3' T_1) ng/100 ml		< 2.5 < 10					143 140

* Autonomous adenoma
** Concentrated extracts

† Hashimoto's thyroiditis
†† Colloid goiter
††† Graves' disease

Serum T_3 and T_4 concentrations from our laboratory are provided for comparison with other serum iodothyronine values.

N.D. Nondetectable

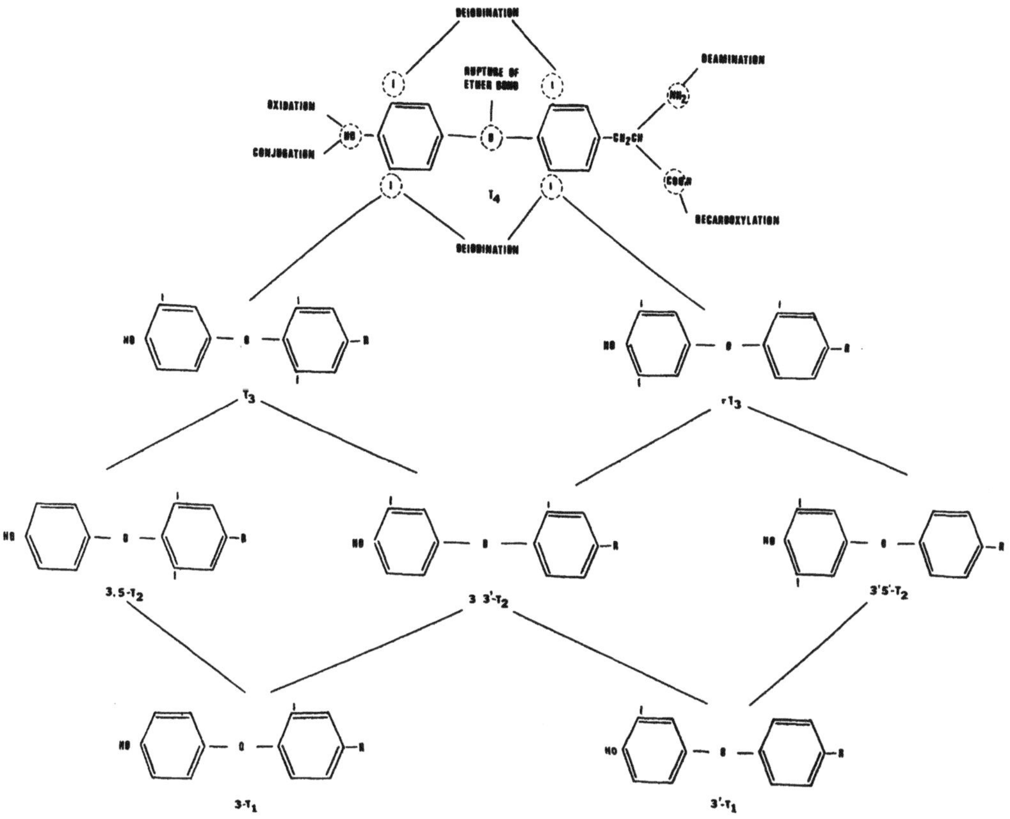

Fig. 1. Pathways of T_4 Metabolism

T_4 to T_3 conversion (17). Injection of relatively large doses of rT_3 in vivo (320 µg/day for 4 days) in man has been shown to have no effect on circulating T_3 levels (23). However, infusion of a pharmacological dose (100 µg rT_3/100 g body weight for 4 h) but not a physiological concentration of rT_3 (3 µg/100 g body weight for 4 h) in the rat did inhibit T_4 to T_3 monodeiodination (180). Perhaps the intracellular generation of iodothyronine intermediates in vivo differs sharply from what is produced by injection or infusion of the compounds in the blood stream.

Although the metabolic degradation products of T_4 are, with some exceptions, calorigenically inactive, some of these metabolites (rT_3, $3,3'T_2$, $3',5'T_2$, tetrac (tetraiodo thyroacetic acid) and triac (triiodo thyroacetic acid)) have been shown to augment or inhibit one or more specific biological responses in vitro, e.g. rT_3 stimulates the activity of L-T_3 amino transferase as effectively as T_3 (24) and stimulates thymocyte uptake of amino acids (25); as noted above, $3',5'T_2$ has been shown to be an effective inhibitor of T_4 to T_3 conversion (20). Obviously, much further study is required to definitively assess the significance of the deiodinated iodothyronines/analogs both in the control of T_4 mono-deiodination and peripheral cellular metabolism.

Measurement of Circulating and Tissue Thyroid Hormones

RIA techniques for measuring circulating hormones and analogs have largely supplanted other techniques because of their simplicity, sensitivity and specificity. Thyroid hormones can be easily measured without extraction of serum in the absence of abnormal TH binding proteins in plasma (vide infra).

Procedures for assay of hormones in tissues have not been reviewed previously. The techniques utilized by various workers can be classified into 3 categories:

Isotopic equilibrium method. Van Middlesworth (26) described a method for achieving radioiodine equilibration in the rat. Radioiodine is incorporated in the diet or injected and when the specific activity of radioiodine in plasma and in tissues approximates that in the diet, isotopic equilibration is considered attained. T_3 and T_4 in tissues of animals injected with radioiodine are separated by chromatographic procedures and radioiodine in the T_3 and T_4 areas is quantitated. From this information and the known specific activity in the diet, one can quantitatively relate T_3 and T_4 concentration in tissues in terms of their T_3 iodine ($T_3$1) or T_4 iodine ($T_4$1) content.

Kinetic assays. Radiolabeled TH is administered and a time period is determined experimentally when plasma and tissue labeled hormone are in equilibrium. Gordon and Spira (27) found that 2-1/2 h after labeled T_3 administration to rats, the disappearance rates of radioactivity from plasma and tissues had become exponential and parallel. Exponential disappearance rates were extrapolated to zero time and the ratio of percent dose in plasma and tissues was multiplied by the plasma hormone concentration. Hennemann et al. (28) criticised this method because of the rapid rate of T_3 metabolism. Instead they calculated T_3 distribution space by dividing metabolic clearance rate of T_3 by the exponential fractional clearance rate obtained 1-2 days after labeled T_3 administration. From this space was subtracted long term distribution space of labeled human albumin to obtain intracellular T_3 volume which, when multiplied by plasma T_3 concentration, yielded what was termed exchangeable intracellular T_3. Oppenheimer et al (29) used a kinetic assay to measure total and rapidly exchangeable subcellular hormone concentration. They determined "equilibrium" time point when labeled hormone concentration in a subcellular fraction was maximal after pulse tracer injection. At such time it was assumed that subcellular labeled hormone influx equalled efflux, although these rates were not measured. The ratio of subcellular labeled hormone and plasma hormone radioactivity measured at this time was multiplied by total plasma hormone concentration to obtain total subcellular hormone concentration. In order to determine the concentration of rapidly exchangeable subcellular hormone, a correction was made for non-specifically bound hormone in tissue subcellular fractions by using a combination of a tracer with increasing quantities of unlabeled hormone until a constant, minimum value of the subcellular/plasma ratio was obtained. This value was then subtracted from uncorrected values of the ratio prior to multiplying by plasma hormone concentration to obtain rapidly exchangeable subcellular hormone concentration.

Radioimmunoassay techniques. RIA methods for tissues are similar to those employed for plasma or sera. Unlike plasma hormone assays where extraction is unnecessary, tissue extraction is essential due to unknown hormone binding sites. The two extractants commonly used are ethanol alone or acidified butanol in combination with ammonium hydroxide and chloroform (Flock-Bollman's reagent) (30). The latter reagent has the advantage of separating hormone into a medium containing minimal lipids. PTU (propylthiouracil) 10^{-4}M is usually added to the extracting media to minimize hormone mono-deiodination. The dried residue is assayed for hormone concentration.

Takaishi et al. (31) employed three different RIA procedures to compare the accuracy of T_3 measurements in tissues. In two methods with ethanolic extraction, the results failed to show parallelism between standards and serially diluted tissue extracts. The third procedure showed parallelism but gave a value twice that obtained with a kinetic assay and 2 of 3 RIAs with Flock-Bollman's reagent which also showed parallelism. This suggested the presence of an interfering substance in the assay when ethanol alone was used for extraction. Irvine (109) had previously reported that a plasma substance resembling a phospholipid interfered with the competitive binding T_4 assay, an observation consistent with the findings of Takaishi et al. (31) who used Folch's procedure (33) to separate lipids from non-lipids; they (31) showed that the amount of labeled hormone bound to the antibody was approximately 50% greater in the lipid free fraction. These results show the necessity of using an appropriate combination of extracting agents and RIA for tissue hormone assay.

Correction of total tissue hormone concentration for hormones in ISF and blood trapped in tissues is necessary in order to yield cellular hormone concentration. Prior to hormone measurements in tissues some investigators employed exsanguination to minimize hormone content in trapped plasma. However, Irvine (32) found in sheep that after exsanguination a significant quantity of plasma was trapped in some tissues. Other workers have perfused animals with saline after killing (34). It may be noted that while this procedure may eliminate trapped plasma, saline perfusion may result in a loss of intracellular hormone and thus artifactually lower tissue hormone concentration. Irvine (32) reported methods for measuring total hormone concentration in trapped plasma and ISF separately in sheep whereas Hasen et al. (35) described a procedure to correct for thyroid hormones bound to plasma protein (albumin) in ISF and trapped plasma combined, in a kinetic assay in the rat.

RIA techniques similar to those used for serum or plasma can be used to measure hormone concentration in tissue fluids. As protein concentration in tissue fluids is very low it is imperative to establish that the RIA technique is not affected by low protein concentration.

Thyroid hormone binding affinity and capacity in cells and cellular fractions have been generally determined by Scatchard analysis (36) in conjunction with a kinetic assay.

Thyroid Hormone Concentrations in Tissue Fluids in Man and in Animals

Studies of TH levels in fluids bathing or surrounding cells are of interest as they indicate the concentration of hormones available for direct cellular uptake and metabolism. The free TH concentration in ISF is presumably a major determinant of cellular uptake. TH concentration in interstitial as well as other fluids in various species are listed in Table 2.

Lymph

Daniel and co-workers (16) found thyroglobulin, the prothyroid hormone, to be present in thyroidal lymph of animals. This demonstration shattered the belief that TG was a secluded or sequestered antigen and forced a revision of fundamental concepts regarding TG antibody formation in individuals with thyroid

TABLE 2 THYROID HORMONE CONCENTRATIONS

Species & Source	LYMPH		INTER-STITIAL FLUID	CEREBROSPINAL FLUID				SYNOVIAL (JOINT) FLUID	ASCITIC FLUID
	T_4	T_3	T_4	T_4	FT_4	T_3	FT_3	T_4	T_4
Man									
Thyroidal	219 ± 118	4.3 ± 2.8							
Inguinal	10	0.70							
Thoracic lymph	11*								
Fembral lymph	55*								
Rheumat. arthritis								132*	
Hepatic cirrhosis									100*
Euthyroid with neuro-logical disorder				1.9 ± 0.7	0.051 ± 0.012				
Hyperthyroid				3.0 ± 0.7	0.123 ± 0.035				
Hypothyroid				0.6 ± 0.02	0.011				
During neurological exam				1.9 ± 0.4 3	0.058	0.174 ± 0.015	0.018		
During physical exam									
Post Operative Chylous Hydrothorax and/or Ascites									
Nontoxic goiter Yellow cyst fluid									
Brown cyst fluid									
Dog				2.2 ± 0.8	0.238 ± 0.096	0.266 ± 0.14	0.032 ± 0.017		
Sheep									
Liver	46		0.9						
Kidney	25		1.6						
Intestine	16		3.8						
Testicular	52								
Prescapular	32								
Cervical	49								
Lumbar	25								
Prefemoral	35								
Popliteal	32								
Rumen			3.4						
Abomasum			4.5						
Salivary gland			4.1						
Lung			3.0						
Skeletal muscle			1.4						
Heart			2.1						
Bone			1.4						
Skin			3.8						
Fat			0.3						
Brain			0.1						
Cattle								46 ± 35*	

*Derived from PBI

(ng/ml) IN TISSUE FLUIDS IN MAN AND ANIMALS

CHYLE	THYROID CYST FLUID		PERIPHERAL PLASMA OR SERUM				THYROIDAL VENOUS PLASMA		Reference
	T_4	T_3	T_4	FT_4	T_3	FT_3	T_4	T_3	
			103 ± 45		1.5 ± 0.6				144
							123 ± 54	2.0 ± 0.67	144
									144
									43
									43
									43
									43
			90 ± 15	0.049 ± 0.013					40
			171 ± 19	0.119 ± 0.020					40
			24 ± 11	0.011					40
									39 47
			74.00	0.024	1.68 ± 0.53	0.003			39
55									47
	66	2.11							48
	307	11.0							48
			27.3 ± 8.1	0.0390 ± 0.010	2.58 ± 1.24	0.007 ± 0.0003			41
			49 (37 - 63)						37, 145, 146
									37, 32
									37, 32
									37, 32
									37, 145
									37
									37
									37
									37
									37, 145
									32
									32
									32
									32
									32
									32
									32
									32
									32
									32
			126 ± 52*						45

autoimmune and other diseases. Thyroid hormones also are released into thyroidal lymph and the recorded concentrations (T_4= 219 ng/ml, T_3= 4.3 ng/ml) are greater than in thyroidal venous plasma (T_4= 123 ng/ml; T_3= 1.5 ng/ml) (144). However, it has been estimated that thyroidal lymph flow rate is about 1000 times less than thyroidal venous blood flow (110); thus, the lymphatic contribution of TH to ISF is probably minor. Whether or not hydrolysis of TG occurs in thyroidal lymph is not known. Although the significance of small differences in T_4 concentration in various lymphatic vessels is not clear, it is certain that the lymph after leaving the thyroid is diluted with lymph from peripheral sources; the thoracic lymph duct concentration represents a mean concentration as lymph from various areas drains into the thoracic duct. Although differences in T_4 concentration among lymphatic vessels have been observed, FT_4 concentration in these vessels and plasma was the same in sheep (37).

Interstitial fluid (ISF)

Irvine (32) measured ISF T_4 concentration in various tissues in sheep (Table 2). ISF T_4 concentrations found in various tissues were markedly lower than in lymph but were similar to CSF values. This undoubtedly reflects the low protein concentrations of CSF and ISF.

Cerebrospinal fluid (CSF)

As there is continuous interchange of the CSF with the ISF of brain at the ependymal and subjacent glial interface, studies of thyroid hormones in CSF are of interest in relating hormonal effects on the brain. Bound and free TH concentration in CSF as noted in several studies in man and in animals are recorded in Table 2. In earlier investigations of the CSF, Alpers and Rall (38) reported a PBI concentration of 0.12 µg% in the euthyroid state, 0.005% (mean) in myxedema and 0.083% in Graves disease in relation to corresponding PBI concentrations in serum of

7.5 μg%, 1.3 μg% and 10.4 μg% respectively. In more recent studies in euthyroid patients with neurologic disorders or in patients undergoing neurologic examinations, a CSF T_4 concentration of 1.9 ng/ml, 30-50 times lower than plasma T_4 concentration was observed (39, 40). The low total T_4 concentration was mirrored by reduced thyroxine binding globulin (TBG) and thyroxine binding prealbumin (TBPA) concentrations in CSF. TBPA in CSF was 1/12 and TBG 1/75 of the levels in normal serum but their binding affinity for T_4 was similar in CSF and serum (39). In CSF Hagen and Elliott (39) observed a 2-fold and a 6-fold higher FT_4 and FT_3 concentration respectively in comparison to serum free TH concentration (Table 2). However, Siersbaek-Nielsen and Hansen (40) found no difference between FT_4 in CSF and in serum. Both groups of workers found similar FT_4 concentrations in CSF in euthyroid subjects; their results differed about 2-fold only in serum FT_4 values. Methodological or other variables affecting FT_4 measurements in serum or CSF would naturally influence the interpretation of CSF-serum FT_4 relationships.

Elevated free TH concentration in the CSF (39) has also been shown in the dog by Hagen and Solberg (41). FT_4 and FT_3 values in CSF were 6 and 5 times greater respectively than in serum. FT_4 in dog CSF was 4 times greater than that in man and FT_3 10 times greater which may reflect differences in TH binding proteins in serum and in CSF between the two species.

Siersbaek-Nielsen and Hansen (40) concluded from their finding of equivalent FT_4 concentrations in CSF and in serum that FT_4 in both compartments were in equilibrium. Hagen and Solberg (41) suggested that active transport of free TH from blood to CSF at the blood-CSF and/or blood-brain barrier might occur, given the findings of higher FT_4 and FT_3 concentrations in CSF in man and dog (39, 41). They also calculated that in man total bulk efflux rates of T_3 and T_4 (bound and free) from CSF to blood were greater than influx rates of protein bound hormone from blood to CSF (41). This implied that the influx of free TH at the blood-CSF and/or blood-brain barrier was greater than efflux in order to maintain a steady state total TH level in the CSF. Since infusion of a large dose of unlabeled T_4 with tracer T_4 reduced the rate constant of FT_4 transfer from blood to CSF, a saturable transport mechanism for T_4 was indicated. In a more recent investigation in the rat, Pardridge (42) used tracer T_3 and graded doses of unlabeled T_3 and demonstrated a saturable transport system for T_3 at the blood-brain barrier. Since influx and efflux rates of T_3 were similar, transport was considered carrier mediated but not active. Thus if influx of free T_4 and free T_3 from blood to CSF is greater than efflux, as suggested by Hagen and Solberg, the blood-CSF barrier is a more likely location for active transport of T_3.

Synovial fluid

In rheumatoid arthritis, Freinkel et al. (43) found a PBI value of 8.6 µg% in synovial fluid, a concentration which was approximately twice that noted in serum (PBI = 5 µg%). The relatively high PBI in synovial fluid may be due to an increase in binding sites. Since T_3 increased hyaluronidase activity (44) and this enzyme can reduce fluid viscosity by hydrolysing hyaluronic acid, one might speculate that high T_4 binding in this pathological state reflects control of synovial fluid viscosity. In cattle, Neuhaus and Sogoian (45) measured T_4 in synovial fluid and the value noted (3 µg% PBI) was less than half of that noted in serum (8.2 $\pm$ 3.4 µg%). Although considerable variation in PBI concentration in synovial fluid was noted, mean values when expressed on the basis of total protein (2.6 µg 1/g) was twice that in serum (1.2 µg 1/g protein).

Ascitic fluid

T_4 concentration in ascitic fluid (43) from patients with hepatic cirrhosis were in the range of serum TH concentration in normal subjects. The equivalent plasma and ascitic fluid T_4 concentrations might be due to the normally greater permeability of liver capillaries to T_4 binding proteins. The similarity of plasma and ascitic fluid T_4 concentrations in cirrhosis may also reflect decreased hepatocyte T_4 uptake in this pathological condition.

Chyle

Robbins and Rall (47) reported a mean T_4 concentration of 50 ng/ml in two patients with chylous hydrothorax and/or ascites. The T_4 concentration in chyle was only slightly lower than the mean plasma T_4 concentration implying a slightly reduced level of T_4 binding protein in chyle.

Thyroid cyst fluid

Galvan et al. (48) measured T_4, T_3 and rT_3 concentration in yellow and brown thyroid cyst fluids in patients with nontoxic goiter (Table 2). The high levels of thyroid hormones in brown cyst fluid were believed to be caused by destruction of thyroid follicles and surrounding blood and lymph vessels as well as by direct secretion of hormones from the thyroid tissue in the cyst wall into the tissue fluid. Clark et al. (171) observed T_4, T_3 and rT_3 concentrations of 235 µg/100 ml, 175 ng/ml and 89 ng/ml respectively in thyroid cyst fluid obtained from euthyroid patients. These values were 10-100 fold higher than serum levels. Hence, these authors suggested that thyroid hormones are sequestered within the cyst. However, graded release of thyroid hormones from the cyst wall into the circulation need not produce long-term serum TH elevations given negative hormonal feedback.

Thyroid Hormones in Tissues

Thyroid hormone concentration in human thyroid gland

Thyroidal T_3 and T_4 concentrations and T_3/T_4 ratios are not only of interest in relation to circulating levels and daily hormonal production rates, but also are of significance in understanding abnormal iodothyronine secretion in pathologic states. With the development of competitive binding assays for T_4 and T_3, direct quantitative estimates of TH levels in thyroidal tissues became possible.

Nagataki et al. (50) separated T_3 and T_4 in pronase digests of the human thyroid glands by paper chromatographic techniques and determined T_4 and T_3 in methanol-ammonia eluates by competitive binding assays. They reported T_4 and T_3 concentrations of 232 $\pm$ 29.2 and 21.3 $\pm$ 2.0 µg/g respectively. The T_3/T_4 ratio was 0.092 (Table 1). Chopra et al. (51) measured TH levels by RIA in the thyroid gland from patients dying of nonthyroidal illnesses and from patients undergoing surgery for Graves' or Hashimoto's disease as well as other pathologic states. T_4 and T_3 content in euthyroid gland (µg/g) was 172.2 $\pm$ 22.1 and 11.0 $\pm$ 1.97 respectively. The T_3/T_4 ratio was 0.064 while in Graves' disease the ratio was 0.41 (51). This increase may have been due to the disease process itself and/or antithyroid or other therapy (51). Larsen et al. (52) reported a T_3/T_4 ratio of 0.07-0.08 in normal thyroids and thyroidal T_4 and T_3 concentrations of 3.8 µg/g and 0.66 µg/g respectively in an adenomatous patient who was clinically euthyroid. The T_3/T_4 ratio in thyroglobulin varied from 0.51-0.96 in different laboratories (50, 51, 52), a value higher than that noted for the whole thyroid tissue.

Although in several kinetic studies it has been assumed that the thyroidal release of T_3 and T_4 normally is in the same relative proportion as they are present in the thyroid, and some animal observations support this assumption (53), other animal results suggest that T_3 is preferentially secreted over T_4 (49, 54, 55). These latter observations along with normal blood T_3 levels noted in patients with elevated TSH (56) have suggested that in pathophysiological states the thyroid gland may secrete disproportionately more T_3 than T_4 and preferential T_3 secretion might explain the degree of overlap in circulating T_3 levels between normal and hypothyroid subjects. Apart from T_4 and T_3, other iodothyronines in the thyroid (Table 1) appear to have no significance relative to their circulating levels in pathologic states, a situation almost surely due to the fact that these thyronines are formed virtually exclusively by deiodination in extrathyroidal tissues.

Thyroid hormone concentrations in extrathyroidal tissues in man

Reichlin et al. (57) reported RIA T_3 and T_4 concentrations in liver, kidney, brain and heart. In liver and kidney, T_4 concentration exceeded T_3 whereas in heart T_3 concentration was greater (Table 3). In patients dying after long wasting illness, the marked reduction in T_3 and increase in T_4 in some tissues were noteworthy. Reichlin et al. (57) speculated that these changes are most likely related to a tissue deiodinase deficiency, though a decrease in cellular T_3 binding protein was not excluded. The reduction in T_3 in liver accompanied by a minimal increase in T_4 may also signify diversion of T_4 mono-deiodination to the metabolically inactive T_4-rT_3 pathway in tissues. In patients undergoing surgery for hernia, T_4 and T_3 concentrations measured _in vitro_ in adipose tissue were the same whereas in muscle and leucocyte the T_3 concentrations were higher (58).

Two groups of workers (59, 60) have studied T_3 and T_4 binding affinity and capacity in lymphocyte nuclei from normal and dysthyroidal subjects. Lymphocyte nuclear binding capacity in hypothyroid patients was 2-3 fold greater than normal although nuclear binding affinity was unchanged in both hypo- and hyperthyroid patients. No differences in binding affinity or capacity were noted between intact lymphocytes and isolated nuclei in either hypo- or eu-thyroid subjects (59). The intact lymphocyte binding capacity in hypothyroid subjects approached normal levels after more than 8 months of therapy (59, Table 3).

Thyroid hormone concentration in extrathyroidal animal tissue

Most measurements of thyroid hormones in whole tissues have been carried out in the rat (Table 4). The technique used, together with information on dietary iodine, has been noted in the table to facilitate appropriate comparisons. All investiga-

TABLE 3 TISSUE THYROID HORMONE CONCENTRATION IN HUMAN PATHOLOGY

Subjects	Liver		Kidney		Brain		Heart		Adipose		Muscle		Leucocyte		Lymphocyte				Reference
															T_4		T_3		
	T_4	T_3	T_4	T_3	T_4	T_3	T_4	T_3	T_4	T_3	T_4	T_3	T_4	T_3	Ka(10^n/M)	Binding Cap.	Ka(10^n/M)	Binding Cap.	
Control	48	9.4	15	7.0	-	2.8	0.5	2.4											57
(Patients dying relatively suddenly)																			
Sick Euthyroid	55.5	1.4	41.0	0.09	34	1.6	27	1.0											57
(Patients dying after long wasting illness)																			
Hernia Patients									2.21 ± 0.81	2.16 ± 0.49	2.86 ± 0.78	4.32 ± 0.95	1.12 ± 0.42	2.86 ± 0.91					58
(Tissues obtained preoperatively)																			
Euthyroid															9.8×10^9	0.013	2.28×10^{10}	0.012	59
Hyperthyroid															8.6×10^9	0.013	1.58×10^{10}	0.011	59
Hypothyroid															1.2×10^{10}	-	1.79×10^{10}	0.034	59
Hypothyroid (Treated for > 8 months)															-	-	2.19×10^{10}	0.015	59

All values are concentration measures (ng/g) except Ka (liters/mole) and binding capacity (ng/mg DNA)

TABLE 4 THYROXINE AND TRIIODOTHYRONINE CONCENTRATION IN CIRCULATION (ng/ml) AND IN EXTRATHYROIDAL TISSUES (ng/g) IN ANIMALS

Tissue	Reichlin et al (57) &		Nejad et al (61)	Gordon & Spira (27)		Oppenheimer et al (29)	Obregon et al (64)		Heninger et al (147)			Heninger & Albright (63)		Janssen et al (34)		Albright et al (65)			Takaishi et al (31)			Winder & Heninger (148)		Irvine (32)
	Low iodine diet		High iodine diet				Low iodine diet		High iodine diet	Low iodine diet		10 μg iodine /day	10 μg iodine /day	High iodine diet		Low iodine diet			High iodine diet			Low iodine diet		Low iodine diet
	RIA	RIA	RIA	Kinetic study	RIA	Kinetic study	IE	RIA	IE	IE	IE	RIA	RIA	RIA	RIA	IE	.E	IE	RIA	RIA	RIA	IE	IE	IE
	T_4	T_3	T_3	T_3[a,b]	T_3[a,b]	T_3	T_3[a,c]	T_3[a,c]	T_4	T_4	T_3	T_4	T_3	T_4[a,c]	T_3[a,c]	T_4	T_3	T_3[a]	T_3[a]	T_3[a]	T_3[a]	T_4	T_3	T_4[a,b,d]
Serum or Plasma	50	0.14	0.2 ± 0.02		0.8 ± 0.05		1.0 ± 0.1	0.6 ± 0.1	5*	21.9 ± 4.4	0.7 ± 0.7	39 ± 12	1.0 ± 0.7	22.6 ± 5.2	0.6 ± 0.1	23.5 ± 3.7	0.6 ± 0.5					43.5 ± 7.7	0.8 ± 0.4	44.6
Liver	13.0	1.5 ± 0.1	1.7 ± 0.1			6.45	3.9 ± 0.7	3.9 ± 0.7	11.2 ± 4.4	11.1 ± 1.6	2.0 ± 0.3	25.6 ± 3.9	4.6 ± 1.1			13.4 ± 2.9	2.4 ± 1.3	2.2 ± 0.1	2.1 ± 0.6	2.2 ± 0.2	4.6 ± 0.4	14.3 ± 2.2	3.5 ± 0.7	24.1
Kidney	5.5	1.9 ± 0.3	1.9 ± 0.1			10.15	5.0 ± 0.8	5.2 ± 1.1	6.9 ± 2.0	9.3 ± 2.1	5.1 ± 1.8	22.8 ± 3.9	9.1 ± 2.7			10.7 ± 3.3	3.4 ± 1.0					15.2 ± 1.5	6.5 ± 0.9	23.0
Brain	8.3	1.2 ± 0.1	1.2 ± 0.1		2.2 ± 0.3	1.21	1.2 ± 0.2	1.3 ± 0.3	0.8 ± 0.3	1.2 ± 0.1	1.0 ± 0.2	2.5 ± 0.3	1.5 ± 0.5			1.5 ± 0.2	0.9 ± 0.4							3.9
Heart						2.29	0.8 ± 0.1	0.7 ± 0.1	1.7 ± 0.9	3.6 ± 1.3	1.5 ± 0.4	6.3 ± 2.0	1.6 ± 0.8			4.3 ± 1.0	1.0 ± 0.3					6.2 ± 0.8	1.7 ± 0.3	0.6
Lung							1.3 ± 0.1	1.4 ± 0.2	4.5 ± 1.9	6.5 ± 1.0	1.8 ± 0.9													0.9
Mixed muscle							0.6 ± 0.3	0.9 ± 0.3	0.9 ± 0.4	1.2 ± 0.3	0.6 ± 0.3	2.3 ± 0.8	0.6 ± 0.3			1.3 ± 0.3	0.3 ± 0.1					2.2 ± 0.4	0.7 ± 0.1	0.4
Red muscle														1.9 ± 0.3	2.1 ± 0.3									
White muscle														1.9 ± 0.3	1.7 ± 0.2									
Ant. Pituitary				6.4	6.8 ± 0.1	6.00																		
Post. Pituitary				2.6	2.6 ± 0.7																			
Median eminence				0.9	1.5 ± 0.4																			
Frontal lobe brain				0.4	0.55																			
Small intestine									2.3 ± 1.0	5.5 ± 1.9	3.4 ± 1.9													1.8
Intestine																4.8 ± 1.2	1.9 ± 0.5							
Spleen						1.19			2.3 ± 1.1	3.2 ± 0.1	1.4 ± 0.7					4.0 ± 1.2	1.0 ± 0.2							
Testis									1.4 ± 0.7	2.7 ± 0.4	0.4 ± 0.3					3.5 ± 0.2	0.3 ± 0.1							
Salivary gland									1.6 ± 1.0	3.5 ± 1.1	1.3 ± 0.3					4.1 ± 0.3	1.0 ± 0.4							2.6
Fat										4.5 ± 1.9	0.8 ± 0.2													0.3
Epididymal Fat																3.1 ± 1.5	0.2 ± 0.2							
Bone																								0.03
Skin																								0.5

With the exception of Irvine's results, all values in the table were obtained in the rat.

IE - Isotopic Equilibrium

RIA - Radioimmunoassay

High iodine diet refers to commonly used rat diets containing approximately 1.4-1.7 μg iodine/g diet.

*Authors (147) reported that in animals fed high iodine diet T_4 measurements in plasma and tissues were less accurate due to the interference of radioactive iodide in the chromatographic separation of iodothyronines.

(a) Corrected for extraction efficiency
(b) Corrected for trapped blood
(c) Utilized saline perfusion to eliminate trapped blood.
(d) Corrected for interstitial fluid

tors found high T_3 concentrations in kidney and liver which were more than 10-fold greater than in plasma in one study (61). As judged by limited observations of T_3 concentration in the anterior and posterior pituitary, values reported may equal or even exceed T_3 concentrations in liver and kidney. Janssen et al. (34) observed a higher T_3 concentration in skeletal muscle than in plasma and the concentration in red muscle (2.1 ng/g) was higher than in white muscle (1.7 ng/g). The consistently higher T_3 concentrations in liver and kidney in relation to circulating levels originally suggested that T_3 was largely an intracellular hormone. T_3 concentrations in lung, intestine, pituitary, brain and heart have also been reported to be higher than in plasma, although not all investigators have found higher values in brain and heart (Table 4). Only three groups of workers have measured T_3 concentrations in spleen, a TH non-responsive tissue. Compared to the concentration in spleen, all groups found higher values for kidney, whereas some reported higher concentrations in liver, intestine, and anterior pituitary (Table 4).

It may also be noted that the effect of low or high iodine diets on T_3 concentrations in kidney and liver is not impressive (Table 4). These observations are consistent with those of Heninger and Albright (63) who reported that although the total iodine in peripheral tissues increased directly with iodine intake, this increase was largely inorganic. In their studies, tissue TH concentrations increased within a relatively narrow range of iodine intake with the maximum concentrations at an iodine intake level of 3-10 µg/day.

That higher T_3 concentrations in liver and kidney might not be due primarily to active transport was shown by Nejad et al. (61) who administered T_3 and T_4 to groups of rats. Liver and kidney T_3 concentrations were the same in T_3 (10 µg/day) or T_4 (25 µg/day) treated rats though plasma T_3 concentration in T_3 administered rats was 2.4 times higher than in T_4 treated animals. This indicated that intracellular T_4 to T_3 conversion rather than sequestration from plasma may have been a more important determinant of tissue T_3 concentrations. It should also be noted that tissue hormone levels as determined by isotopic techniques correlate well with RIA values (64, Table 4). With respect to RIA, a note of caution is suggested by Takaishi et al. (31, Table 4) as discussed in the section on tissue RIA.

In contrast to T_3, T_4 concentrations in plasma are higher than in any other tissue because of greater binding of T_4 by plasma proteins. Among tissues measured, high T_4 concentrations were found in kidney and liver (Table 4); the latter tissue is the source of TBG. Reichlin et al. (57) reported a brain T_4 concentration (8.3 ng/g) comparable to kidney (5.5 ng/g); however this observation was not confirmed by IE determinants of other workers, e.g. Heninger et al. (147) found T_4 concentration of 1.2 ng/g in brain and of 9.3 ng/g in kidney. Both Irvine and Heninger et al. found intermediate values for T_4 in small intestine (Table 4). In two studies (63, 65) T_4 concentrations were measured in both TH responsive tissues and spleen. Liver, kidney, lung and small intestine tissue T_4 concentrations were higher compared to spleen (3.2-4.0 ng, Table 4); Albright et al. (65) found higher T_4 values for liver and kidney but not intestine.

In many tissue hormone measurements, appropriate corrections have not been made for interstitial fluid and trapped plasma. Failure to account for TH contained in these two fluids may lead to a misleading estimate of cellular T_4 concentration, e.g. Irvine (32) found a T_4 concentration of 2 ng/g in sheep skeletal muscle when correction was made for only trapped plasma and a 6-fold lower value when correction was also made for T_4 in interstitial fluid. When hormone measurements in other sheep tissues were corrected for ISF and trapped plasma, only kidney, liver, fat and brain had higher cellular than ISF T_4 concentrations; it may also be noted that the corrected values are lower than those in several tissues in the rat (Table 4).

In both rats and sheep, the highest TH concentrations were found in liver and kidney. However, given the larger mass of skeletal muscle, it might be thought that this tissue contains a higher quantity of T_4. Irvine's corrected T_4 values for liver and skeletal muscle in sheep showed liver to have a larger total amount of T_4; if corrections of a similar magnitude are made for the results of Heninger and Albright (63) and Albright et al. (65), it may be assumed that in the rat, also, more T_4 is contained in liver. However, given the lower binding of T_3 by plasma proteins, T_3 in total skeletal muscle may be higher than in liver.

Thyroid hormone subcellular concentrations and binding characteristics in extrathyroidal tissues

Cellular TH concentrations represent both unbound hormone and hormone bound to structurally specific and non-specific sites. Of the hormone that is specifically bound, it will be assumed that only the portion bound to subcellular receptors including plasma membranes, exerts direct metabolic effects (179). Studies of subcellular binding of TH are a prerequisite for characterization and identification of putative receptors which in turn are essential for elucidation of mechanisms of hormone action. Criteria for receptor status as modified from Hechter (66) are as follows: (a) Structural and steric specificity:binding affinity correlated with hormone and analog mimetic potency, (b) saturability, (c) cell specificity, (d) high affinity:consistent with physiologic hormone concentration, (e) reversibility: kinetics consistent with the reversal of physiologic effects observed when hormone removed from system and (f) parallelism between hormone binding and an early chemical event associated with hormone action. These criteria are necessary but not sufficient for receptor definition since, to demonstrate causality, one must additionally determine a mechanism relating hormone binding to early hormone action.

All subcellular fractions (see Table 5) have been shown to contain high affinity, saturable binding sites. Given binding sites of similar high affinity in different tissues and that these are receptors, binding capacity (or receptor number) is likely to be proportional to TH responsiveness. However, in general, higher binding capacity is associated with lower binding affinity which indicates a lesser likelihood that such a binding site is a receptor. Mitochondria appear to have satisfied more criteria than other cellular fractions although not all laboratories have found specific saturable binding in mitochondria (67, 68, 161). Only plasma membranes have exhibited marked steric specificity for T_3 (162). Putative, nuclear receptors have not rigorously satisfied the criterion of cell specificity.

Using similar experimental conditions, Tata (70) demonstrated high affinity saturable T_3 binding sites in all subcellular fractions of rat liver and found only a 10-fold difference in binding affinities (8.0×10^7 - 8.2×10^8) among fractions. However, the affinity constants for T_3 in subcellular fractions of rat liver determined in vitro in different studies have varied from a minimum of $2.3 \times 10^6 M^{-1}$ in cytosol to a maximum of $3.5 \times 10^{10} M^{-1}$ in the nucleus and $1.9 \times 10^{11} M^{-1}$ in mitochondria. In each of the subcellular fractions for which more than one laboratory has reported specific saturable binding, affinity values have differed by at least 100-fold which could reflect methodological and tissue variations. One group of workers found a 1000-fold higher Ka for T_3 nuclear binding in vivo (29) than in vitro (71) and suggested less favorable in vitro conditions for nuclear binding of T_3. It is particularly noteworthy that in the former study (29) equilibrium affinity values of T_3 nuclear binding (Ka or Kd) for TH responsive and non-responsive tissues were similar. Although Oppenheimer et al. (29) measured fewer high affinity saturable sites in non-responsive tissues, Eberhardt et al. (72) found a greater number of high affinity saturable T_3 nuclear binding sites in the cerebral hemisphere than in liver. Whether or not the cerebral hemisphere in contradistinction to the whole brain is TH responsive merits further investigations. The affinity constant for TH binding to non-histone protein obtained from rat liver nuclei has been found to be similar to that of the nucleus. When affinity constants of microsomes and mitochondria were measured under the

TABLE 5 SUBCELLULAR BINDING AND

Tissue	NUCLEUS T3 Ka(10^n/M) Kd(10^{-n}M)	NUCLEUS T3 Binding Capacity ng T3/mg DNA	NUCLEUS T3 Binding Capacity ng T3/mg prot.	NUCLEUS T3 Binding Capacity ng T3/gm tissue	NUCLEUS T4 Ka(10^n/M) Kd(10^{-n}M)	NUCLEUS T4 Binding Capacity ng T4/gm DNA	NUCLEUS T4 Binding Capacity ng T4/gm tissue	THYROID HORMONE BINDING NUCLEAR PROTEIN T3 Ka(10^n/M) Kd(10^{-n}M)	THBNP T3 Binding Capacity ng T3/mg prot.	THBNP T3 Binding Capacity ng T3/gm tissue	THBNP T4 Kd(10^{-n}M)	THBNP T4 Binding Cap. ng T4/mg prot.	THBNP rT3 Kd(10^{-n}M)	PLASMA MEMBRANE T3 Ka(10^n/M) Kd(10^{-n}M)	PLASMA MEMBRANE T3 Binding Capacity ng T3/mg prot.
In Vitro															
Rat liver	6.1×10^8			1.11				1.6×10^{-9} – 5×10^{-9}	.65						
Rat kidney															
Rat liver	2.4×10^8		1.13					1.0×10^{-9}			5×10^{-9}		3.0×10^{-8}	8.2×10^8	0.21
Rat liver*	1.3×10^8		1.93					9.3×10^7	0.10						
Rat liver														5.2×10^{-8} (1)	
Rat liver														1.5×10^{-6} (1)	
Rat kidney															
Rat liver*	5.0×10^8				1.9×10^8										
Rat kidney*															
Dog kidney															
Dog kidney															
Porcine ant. pit.															
Porcine post. pit.															
Porcine frontal lobe brain															
GH_1 cells															
Rat liver														3.2×10^{-9}	1.63
Rat liver	1.4×10^9			2.0										2.2×10^{-7}	71.61
Rat liver														3.5×10^{-7} (2)	
Rat liver														5.0×10^{-6} (2)	
IM-9 human cultured lymphocyte														2.0×10^{-7}	
Rat liver															
Rat kidney															
Rat myocardium ventricular															
Rat myocardium atrial															
Rat skeletal musc.															
Rat neonatal brain															
Rat lung															
Rat sm. intestinal wall with mucosa															
Rat sm. intestinal mucosa															
Rat adipose															
Rabbit kidney															
Human liver															
Human kidney															
GH_1 cell	2.9×10^{-11}	0.42			2.6×10^{-10}	0.51									
GH_1 cell	2.9×10^{-11}	0.65													
GH_1 cell	1.7×10^{-10}	0.68													
Rat liver	2.1×10^{-10}	0.65													
Rat liver (3)	2×10^9	0.35		0.51											
Rat liver (4)	7×10^8	0.59		1.2											
Rat liver	5.6×10^8			0.85											
Rat liver*	4.3×10^8			1.14											
Rat liver	1.9×10^{-10}	0.65													
Rat liver*	1.9×10^{-10}	0.65													
Rat liver (5)	3.5×10^{10}	0.02													
Rat liver (6)	2.5×10^8	2.02													
Rat liver (5)	3.3×10^{10}	0.02			2.8×10^8	0.03									
Rat kidney (5)	2.8×10^{10}	0.02													
Rat liver (6)	4.8×10^8	0.80													
Rat kidney (6)	4.8×10^8	0.80													
Rat liver	2.2×10^{-10}	0.13													
Rat cerebral hemisp.	1.5×10^{-10}	0.65													
Rat hypothalamus	2.9×10^{-10}	0.10													
Rat pituitary	1.8×10^{-10}	0.89													
Human lymphocyte	3.1×10^{-11}	0.03													
Human lymphocyte	4×10^9	0.03													
Human lymphocyte	2.2×10^{10}	0.01													
Human lymphocyte*	1.9×10^{10}	0.03													
Human polymorphonuclear leukocyte	1.1×10^{-10}	0.03													
Rat liver (7)								2×10^9	0.32	0.87					
Rat liver (8)								8×10^9	0.30	0.78					
Rat liver*								1.6×10^{-10}	0.19		2.0×10^{-9}	0.19			
GH_1 cell								1.8×10^{-10}	0.29		1.2×10^{-9}	0.46			
Human liver	9.3×10^8	0.68													
Rat liver	1.2×10^9	0.76													
Human kidney	8.4×10^8	0.24													
Rat kidney	8.7×10^8	0.26													
Human lymphocyte	3.3×10^{10}	0.03			1.7×10^{10}	0.04									
Human lymphocyte*	3.5×10^{10}	0.05			1.4×10^{10}	0.06									
Human lymphocyte**	$3.2 \wedge 10^{10}$	0.03			1.8×10^{10}	0.03									
In Vivo															
Rat liver*	1.5×10^{-9}	0.43													
Rat kidney*	1.0×10^{-9}	0.13													
Rat pituitary*	1.4×10^{-9}	0.96													
Rat liver		0.37													
Rat kidney		0.13													
Rat ant. pit.		0.77													
Rat liver*				2.4											
Rat liver	4.7×10^{11}	0.52		1.60											
Rat liver	4.7×10^{11}	0.61		1.77											
Rat brain	3.3×10^{11}	0.27		0.42											
Rat heart	4.7×10^{11}	0.40		0.80											
Rat spleen	5.6×10^{11}	0.018		0.31											
Rat testis		0.002		0.02											
Rat kidney	2.8×10^{11}	0.53		2.61											
Rat ant. pit.	4.7×10^{11}	0.79		6.58											

* Hypothyroid
** Hyperthyroid

1. K_I
2. K_m
3. Incubated with SMT, pH 7.85, + 5mM DTT
4. Incubated with SMCT, pH 7.4
5. Incubated with EDTA
6. Incubated with free Mg^{2+}
7. Incubated with KMP, pH 7.4
8. Incubated with TGKM, pH 8.5

In vitro data include incubation of intact cells with labelled TH prior to subcellular fractionation, or incubation of subcellular fractions with labelled TH.

CONCENTRATION OF THYROID HORMONE

Tissue	CYTOSOL T_3 Ka(10^n/M) Kd(10^{-n}M)	CYTOSOL T_3 Binding Capacity ng T_3/ mg prot.	CYTOSOL T_3 Binding Capacity ng T_3/ ml	CYTOSOL T_4 Ka(10^n/M) Kd(10^{-n} M)	CYTOSOL T_4 Binding Capacity ng T_4/ mg prot.	MICROSOME T_3 Ka(10^n/M)	MICROSOME T_3 ng T_3/ mg prot.	MITOCHONDRIA T_3 Ka(10^n/M)	MITOCHONDRIA T_3 Binding Capacity ng T_3/ mg prot.	MITOCHONDRIA T_3 Binding Capacity ng T_3/ gm tissue	MITOCHONDRIA T_4 Ka(10^n/M)	THYROID HORMONE NUCL. BINDING CONC. AT ENDOGENOUS LEVELS Method	T_3 ng T_3/ mg DNA	T_3 ng T_3/ gm tissue	T_4 ng T_4/ mg DNA	Reference
In Vitro																
Rat liver	4.3×10^7															
Rat kidney	2.5×10^7		0.03	9.8×10^6												149, 150, 1
Rat liver	8.0×10^7		0.19	8.1×10^6								IE	0.18 ± 0.07		0.02 ± 0.01	149, 78
Rat liver*	2.3×10^8	0.44						7.3×10^7	0.18							70, 152
Rat liver		0.45				5.9×10^8	0.05	2.2×10^{11}								70, 153
Rat liver	4.8×10^7	1.6														154, 74
Rat kidney	1.8×10^7	2.8														155, 74
Rat liver*	2.3×10^6	21.6														155
Rat kidney*	3.3×10^6			2.0×10^5				1.9×10^{11}			9.4×10^{10}					156,
Dog kidney	2.3×10^7			8.9×10^5				2.0×10^{11}			6.2×10^{10}					156
Dog kidney		488		2×10^9	12.4											77
Porcine ant. pit.	4×10^8			9.2×10^7	117-155											77
Porcine post. pit.				1.4×10^9	0.09											158
Porcine frontal lobe brain					0.05											158
GH_1 cells	1.1×10^{-9}				0.02											158
Rat liver		0.14		2.9×10^{-10}	0.19											157
Rat liver												RIA		0.6		69, 159
Rat liver												RIA	0.33 + 0.12		0.06 + 0.04	69, 160, 78
Rat liver												IE	0.33 ± 0.09		0.07 ± 0.03	75, 78, 161
IM-9 human cultured lymphocyte												Kinetic	0.34 ± 0.08		0.06 ± 0.02	75, 78
Rat liver																162
Rat kidney								1.9×10^{11}								73
Rat myocardium ventricular								2.0×10^{11}								73
Rat myocardium atrial								2.0×10^{11}								73
Rat skeletal musc.								1.6×10^{11}								73
Rat neonatal brain								3.7×10^{11}								73
Rat lung								2.8×10^{11}								73
Rat sm. intestinal wall with mucosa								1.8×10^{11}								73
Rat sm. intestinal mucosa								2.3×10^{11}								73
Rat adipose								3.6×10^{11}								73
Rabbit kidney								2.4×10^{11}								73
Human liver								1.6×10^{11}								73
Human kidney								2×10^{11}								73
GH_1 cell								2×10^{11}								73
GH_1 cell																163
GH_1 cell																164
Rat liver																164
Rat liver(3)																164
Rat liver(4)																165
Rat liver																165
Rat liver*																71
Rat liver																71
Rat liver*																96
Rat liver(5)																96
Rat liver(6)																155
Rat liver(5)																155
Rat kidney(5)																76
Rat liver(6)																76
Rat kidney(6)																76
Rat liver																76
Rat cerebral hemisp.																72
Rat hypothalamus																72
Rat pituitary																72
Human lymphocyte.																72
Human lymphocyte																166
Human lymphocyte																159
Human lymphocyte*																59
Human polymorphonuclear leukocyte																59
Rat liver(7)																167
Rat liver(8)																168
Rat liver*																168
GH_1 cell																157
Human liver																157
Rat liver																169
Human kidney																169
Rat kidney																169
Human lymphocyte																169
Human lymphocyte‡																60
Human lymphocyte**																60
																60
In Vivo																
Rat liver*																173
Rat kidney*																173
Rat pituitary*																173
Rat liver																62
Rat kidney																62
Rat ant. pit.																62
Rat liver*																170
Rat liver																172
Rat liver												Kinetic	0.29	0.83		29
Rat brain												Kinetic	0.11	0.16		29
Rat heart												Kinetic	0.18	0.35		29
Rat spleen												Kinetic	0.009	0.16		29
Rat testis																29
Rat kidney												Kinetic	0.19	0.91		29
Rat ant. pit.												Kinetic	0.38	3.16		29

same conditions, mitochondrial Ka was lower than that of microsomes (70). However Sterling et al. (73, 156) reported affinity constants for mitochondria in the high range of nuclear values. Although high affinity binding was noted in rat liver cytosol (Table 5), no one has demonstrated a correlation of cytosol binding affinity and thyromimetic potency of analogs. In rat liver some workers (69, 74, 75) have indicated that the plasma membrane has two T_3 specific binding sites with different affinities. Similarly, two different T_3 binding sites have been reported in the nucleus (76, 161). Davis et al. (77) have described two different classes of binding sites for T_4 in dog kidney cytosol (Table 4). The lower affinity class in rat liver nucleus and plasma membrane was shown to have a markedly higher binding capacity for T_3 (69, 76). This might reflect a storage rather than a receptor function.

In the euthyroid state, endogenous T_4 and T_3 concentrations in the nucleus as determined by RIA are identical to that obtained by kinetic methods (Table 5, ref. 78). Endogenous nuclear T_3 in rat liver represents 30-50% of nuclear binding capacity (29, 62, 177). A knowledge of endogenous hormone concentrations together with binding capacities is of significance in relation to cellular metabolic expression. Maximal metabolic effect is believed to result when all binding receptors are occupied (11). However Oppenheimer et al. (68) notes that partial receptor occupancy permits a control mechanism for cellular metabolism. Endogenous/maximum hormone binding ratios may also be of clinical significance, e.g. if the ratios in lymphocytes from euthyroid subjects are known, alteration in this ratio may serve as an index of abnormality. Change in T_3 binding affinities might also indicate endocrine pathology. Bernal et al. (80) found in children with inherited partial T_3 resistance, an affinity constant approximately 70 times lower than that of normal children. They attributed the decrease in T_3 binding affinity to either an abnormality in nuclear T_3 binding protein or an absence of normal T_3 binding protein in the nucleus.

The T_3 capacity in all subcellular fractions varied from 0.002 ng T_3/mg DNA in testis to 488 ng T_3/mg protein in dog kidney cytosol. Under the same experimental conditions Tata (70) found the highest binding capacity in rat liver nucleus and the lowest binding capacity in microsomes. T_3 binding capacities in plasma membranes in rat liver in various studies have ranged from 0.05 to 71.6 mg T_3/ng protein. However, the highest value for plasma membrane binding capacity was associated with a lower affinity site whereas, for the higher affinity binding site, the capacity was only 1.63 ng T_3/mg protein (69). Binding capacities in rat liver nuclei have varied from 0.02 to 0.61 ng T_3/mg DNA and from 0.30 to 0.65 ng T_3/mg protein. With the exception of some studies with cytosol, T_4 binding affinity in all subcellular fractions measured has been less than that of T_3. Correspondingly, binding capacity of T_4 has been generally higher compared to T_3.

In studies listed in Table 5 significant differences in T_3 nuclear binding capacity between normal and hypothyroid rats have not been observed. However, in neonatal rat liver and cerebral hemisphere, but not in adult tissue, Valcana and Timiras (46, 81 results not shown in table) found a higher binding capacity in nuclei from hypothyroid animals. In human lymphocytes two groups obtained a 2-3 fold increase in binding capacity in hypothyroid subjects (59, 60). Higher binding capacity in hypothyroid states may be related to a decreased turnover of high affinity binding sites.

Alteration of Receptor Bound Hormone in Pathophysiological States

The amount of hormone bound to receptor sites is determined by receptor binding affinity and capacity, as well as cellular free hormone concentrations. In recent investigations, hormone receptor capacity variations with no change in binding affinity has been reported in some pathological states.

Starvation

Several investigators have reported a decrease in putative nuclear receptors during fasting. Burman et al. (82) reported a 35% decrease in nuclear binding capacity in 3 day fasted rats. Similar observations were reported independently by De Groot et al. (83) and Schussler and Orlando (84) in 2 and 5 day fasted rats respectively.

Obesity

The enhanced tolerance of obese subjects to TH administration has already been noted. A recent investigation in genetically obese mice has shown a decrease in specific T_3 nuclear binding (85). The similarity of observations of hepatic nuclear T_3 specific binding decrease in both starvation and obesity prompted these authors (85) to speculate that in obesity some cells are misdirecting their metabolism as if they were in a fasting state, when in fact the animal is not fasting, thereby increasing metabolic efficiency for storage as the energy intake exceeds the animal's needs.

Partial hepatectomy

Dillmann et al. (86) found that 12 h after partial hepatectomy there was a 50% decrease in regenerating liver nuclear T_3 specific binding capacity in euthyroid and hypothyroid rats. Since starvation for 17 h produced only a 31% decrease in capacity it was suggested that food deprivation alone did not fully account for the surgically produced change.

In starvation and in partial hepatectomy, the decrease in nuclear T_3 specific binding sites has been accompanied by a decrease in circulating T_3 concentration. However, it should be emphasized that these two events are not causally related. The relation of circulating TH concentration and hormone binding to receptors has been discussed separately (vide infra).

Experimental diabetes and glucagon infusion

Dillman et al. (88) reported a 35% reduction in liver nuclear receptor concentrations after streptozotocin-induced diabetes in rat. Dillmann and Oppenheimer (89) infused rats with glucagon for 16-65 h at a dosage (1 ng/100 g body weight) sufficient to approximate the elevated plasma levels reported for this hormone after partial hepatectomy (90) and starvation (91). Liver nuclear T_3 specific binding capacity was decreased approximately 33% at 17 h and 30% at 65 h after initiation of the infusion. Since plasma glucagon is also elevated in streptozotocin-induced diabetes which decreases liver nuclear capacity (88), it appears that in starvation, partial hepatectomy and streptozotocin-induced diabetes, glucagon elevation might contribute to the observed reductions in liver nuclear T_3 specific binding capacity without altering binding affinity (89). This is of particular relevance since in man, starvation also increases plasma glucagon concentration (178); an increase in this hormone can occur in some patients with diabetes (93) and obesity (94). However, whether glucagon is a direct causal antecedent of nuclear binding capacity reduction in the infusion experiments or merely correlative in the other cases noted is unknown.

Animals bearing neoplasms

Surks et al. (87) reported a decrease in hepatic nuclear T_3 receptors in athyreotic mice transplanted with thyrotropic tumors as well as in intact rats with Walker 256 carcinoma. In mice with TSH secreting tumors, Surks et al. (87) found an approximately 51% decrease of hepatic putative nuclear T_3 receptors. In intact rats with Walker 256 carcinoma, a 34% decrease was found. It was speculated that these reductions might have been due to generalized catabolic effects of the neoplasms.

Hypo- and hyper-thyroidism

Several groups of workers (81, 95, 96, 97) have determined specific nuclear T_3 binding in liver from adult hypothyroid rats.

No change in binding capacity (81, 95, 96, 97) or affinity (81, 95, 96) was observed. However, Valcana and Timiras (81) found an increased binding capacity in liver and cerebral nuclei (46, 81) from thyroidectomized, neonatal rats. In hypothyroidism in man two groups of workers have reported a 2-3 fold increase in lymphocyte nuclear T_3 binding capacity (59, 60). The reasons for apparent differences in T_3 nuclear binding capacity in hypothyroidism are not known. In hyperthyroidism, no change in nuclear T_3 binding capacity or affinity was seen in human lymphocytes (60) and similar observations were made by Oppenheimer et al. (95) in liver from hyperthyroid rats.

Relation of Tissue Hormone Action to Circulating Thyroid Hormone

a. Failure of circulating thyroid hormone concentrations to accurately reflect cellular action as determined by clinical diagnosis

In hypo- and hyper-thyroidism, measurements of circulating total or free thyroid hormones usually correlate with clinical diagnosis and tissue metabolic activity. However, in several pathophysiological states and in some patients receiving thyroid therapy, there are discrepancies between circulating hormone concentrations and clinical assessment of metabolic activity (see also Table 6). Some of the factors that affect total TH concentrations are listed below.

Thyroid hormone alterations due to changes in protein binding

That an increase in T_4 and T_3 binding by proteins may increase the corresponding hormone concentrations to hyperthyroid levels is well known e.g. in pregnancy, familial increase in TBG, etc. In addition, total T_4 levels are increased in conditions with circulating TH binding antibodies (98, 99), abnormal non-antibody T_4 binding protein (100) and alterations in the affinity of normal T_4 binding proteins (101). The increase in T_4 binding

TABLE 6 REPRESENTATIVE DATA SHOWING LACK OF CORRELATION BETWEEN HIGH CIRCULATING TRIIODOTHYRONINE LEVELS AND CLINICAL THYROID STATUS IN OBESE SUBJECTS **

Obese Subjects	Serum T_3 (ng/100 ml)	Pulse	Blood Pressure	Tremor	Sweating	Half-relaxation time (msec.)
PK	250	74	110/70	0	0	250
NR	280	69	120/80	0	0	300
MN	225	66	140/90	+	0	290
BR	246	75	130/90	0	0	325
AC	260	72	135/85	0	0	300
During T_3 Therapy*						
BD	350	76	145/90	0	+	280
LN	280	72	135/95	0	0	360
EA	295	69	125/75	0	0	325
NK	325	70	140/85	+	0	335
ST	450	74	120/90	0	0	290

* 75-150 µg/day ** Premachandra and Perlstein (unpublished observations)

Normal T_3 range (80-200) ng/100 ml

Half-relaxation times (photomotographic times) were all in the normal range

0 Absence
+ Presence

proportionately decreases the percentage of free hormone with the result that the free hormone concentrations remain unchanged; this is consistent with the observed clinical euthyroid status. Similarly, there are other pathologic states (e.g. euthyroid illness) wherein opposite changes are found, viz. protein binding of TH is decreased resulting in decreased total hormone levels, the percentage of free hormone is increased and the net amount of free T_4 in circulation remains within the normal range. There are many drugs available that can contribute to an increase or decrease in TH binding (102) but in all these cases, free TH concentrations remain normal.

Methodological factors influencing circulating thyroid hormones

In addition to endogenous or drug induced variations in circulating TH levels, recent studies have also disclosed methodological factors contributing to an artifactual change in hormone levels, e.g. the presence of T_3/T_4 antibodies has been shown to contribute to an over- or under-estimation of RIA TH levels depending on the technique used to separate free and bound hormone thus confounding diagnosis (103, 104). In sera containing T_3/T_4 antibodies, RIA of protein free extracts has yielded values consistent with clinical diagnosis. Tamagna et al. (105) have shown that high plasma protein concentrations in macroglobulinemia can cause interference in RIA TH estimations resulting in artifactually high values. These observations underline the necessity for appropriate assay controls to avoid misinterpretation of laboratory results.

Alterations in circulating hormone levels due to factors other than protein binding

Alterations in metabolic clearance of thyroid hormones in pathophysiologic states are well known (79, 106). The metabolic clearance of T_4, T_3, rT_3, may be altered producing changes in circulating hormone levels which often do not correlate with tissue hormone mediated action. Recent investigations in a number of laboratories have shown that T_4 conversion to T_3 or rT_3 is influenced by a variety of pathophysiological states (106). The changes in peripheral conversion of T_4 to T_3 and rT_3 would be reflected in circulating levels of corresponding hormones. In these cases measurements of circulating total T_4 or T_3 alone give no precise information of cellular hormone mediated metabolism. If T_4 to T_3 conversion is inhibited in a pathophysiological state, even high T_4 concentrations may not be accompanied by clinical thyrotoxicity. The lack of thyrotoxic effect of elevated T_4 levels in the presence of reduced or normal T_3 levels bears an interesting comparison to the experiments of Chopra et al. (19) which suggest that T_3, and not T_4, is catabolic. In their experiments (Fig. 2) groups of rats were injected with saline, T_4 alone, or T_4 and ipodate (oragrafin). Oragrafin was used to prevent T_4 to T_3 conversion. In rats treated with T_4 alone there was a significant reduction in growth and an increase in urinary urea nitrogen compared to control rats. In rats treated with T_4 and oragrafin the circulating T_3 levels were similar to that in control animals and much lower than that noted in animals treated with T_4 alone, but the serum T_4 levels were six times greater than in control animals. Despite this hyperthyroxinemia, body growth was not impaired and no increase in urinary urea nitrogen was observed suggesting a lack of direct catabolic effect of T_4. In similar experiments injection of T_3 alone caused a marked reduction in body growth and an increase in urinary urea nitrogen. These experiments, therefore, suggest that the catabolic activity of T_4 is brought about only by its conversion to T_3. Drugs, contrast media, etc, in addition to inducing alterations in TH protein binding, also inhibit deiodination of thyroid hormones (19).

It should be stressed that in all of the above cases of discordance between total TH levels and clinical signs, free TH concentrations were generally in the normal range; thus the cells are exposed to normal concentrations of free TH which probably accounts for the clinical euthyroid state. However even free TH concentration is not always a valid indicator of clinical thyroid status as has been observed in various pathophysiological states (vide infra).

b. Failure of circulating free thyroid hormone to accurately reflect cellular action as determined by clinical diagnosis

Free thyroid hormones in plasma may be assumed to be in equilibrium with interstitial and intracellular free TH, provided that they cross the plasma membrane by passive or facilitated diffusion. That the situation may not be as simple has been shown in the investigations of Obregon et al. (107) who demonstrated that intracellular T_3 formed from T_4 is not readily and completely exchangeable with extracellular T_3. These investigations are at variance with the conclusions of Oppenheimer et al.(108) who have reported rapid exchange of plasma and intracellular T_3. In hyperthyroidism the high free T_4 and free T_3 in ISF and cytoplasm enables greater, relative saturation of the cellular receptors thus increasing cellular response. The converse situation would prevail in hypothyroidism where decreased free TH levels would result in relative undesaturation of cellular sites mediating hormone action. As already noted in several clinical conditions there is apparently a dissociation between free hormone concentration and metabolic activity. This suggests a discordance between plasma free hormone levels and relative saturation of cellular receptors and the reasons for such a discrepancy are not known. However, various factors which may act singly or in combination to explain these discordances are; receptor binding affinity and capacity, post receptor events, tissue sensitivity, reduced receptor binding capacity followed by amplification, nonthyroid hormonal modulation of receptors, drug effects on receptor, cellular deiodination, availability of hormone to receptors and nonreceptor binding.

In the syndrome of partial TH resistance where elevated free thyroid hormones are accompanied by either clinical hypo- or eu-thyroidism, Bernal et al. (80) described alterations in lymphocyte nuclear specific T_3 binding characteristics and suggested that the putative nuclear receptor is either abnormal or absent in some cases of this syndrome. Although alterations in receptor affinity have been shown (e.g. insulin, 173) which might regulate target cell sensitivity to hormonal stimulation, the majority of studies of TH binding by putative receptors in pathophysiological states have revealed no changes in binding affinity.

Schwartz et al. (111) studied hepatic mitochondrial malic and alpha GPD enzyme responses to T_3 administration in one to six month old rats. They found an age related decrease in basal enzyme activities but no change in hepatic nuclear T_3 receptor binding capacity and affinity or in the concentration of T_3

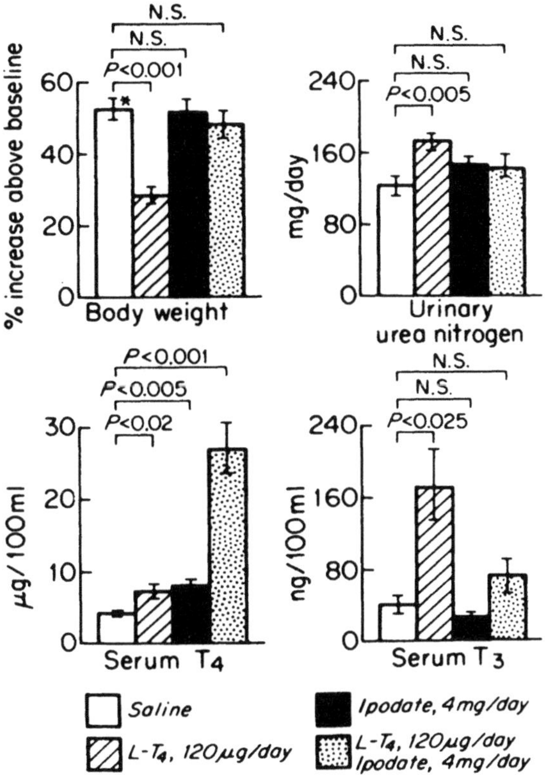

Fig. 2. Metabolic effects of thyroxine (from Chopra et al. (19).
(Reproduced with the permission of the authors and publishers).

bound to the putative nuclear receptors. The increase of the enzymes 24 h after a single large T_3 dose (200 µg T_3/100 g body weight) was 60 to 80% less in six months old compared to one month old rats. Since the decrease in enzymatic activity was not accompanied by changes in nuclear occupancy or number of receptor sites, these authors suggested that modulation of TH action may occur at a postreceptor level. Denckla (112) also showed that the responsiveness to TH decreased with increasing age in the rat as measured by minimal oxygen consumption.

Whether this reflects a decrease in tissue sensitivity to TH or alterations in other metabolic pathways controlling oxidation is not clear. Starvation can affect oxygen consumption independently of TH (113). However, the observations of Wimpheimer et al. (174) indicate a reduced tissue sensitivity to T_3 in starvation. Relative increases in oxygen consumption were measured in fed and starved thyroidectomized rats administered a single dose of 1.825 or 9.125 μg T_3/100 g body weight. An additional increase in oxygen consumption was not observed at the higher dosage in fed animals. However in starved rats the relative increase was less than that of fed animals at the lower dosage of T_3 but equivalent at the higher level.

On the other hand, Oppenheimer et al. (114) have shown that rat liver T_3 responses, as measured by cytosolic malic enzyme and mitochondrial GPD increased 16-fold when receptor saturation was increased from euthyroid levels (~50%) to maximal saturation; i.e. significant amplification of hormone response appears to occur with receptor saturation above 50%. Similar observations have been made by Mariash et al. (175) in the case of four lipogenic hepatic enzymes. Oppenheimer (115) has suggested that amplification of yet undetermined enzymes might explain the multiplicity of effects of thyroid hormones. Such enzymes would necessarily be rate limiting in thyrotoxic catabolism. In partial hepatectomy and starvation (86) an increased sensitivity to T_3 administration has also been shown for alpha-GPD response in rat liver. Oppenheimer (11) has suggested that analogously, an increased sensitivity to T_3 might occur in the low T_3 syndrome to explain normal TSH and TRH responsiveness. One might further speculate that increased sensitivity to TH generally might occur in low T_3 syndrome due to a relative increase in receptor saturation corresponding to a decrease in number of receptors. Thus tissue response commensurate with circulating free TH may not obtain if there is alteration in tissue sensitivity.

That the expression of TH activity at the cellular level may be modulated by other hormones is known from the investigations of Samuels et al. (116) and Martial et al. (117), who demonstrated a synergistic action of T_3 and cortisol in the production of mRNA for growth hormone in GH_1 cells. Dillmann and Oppenheimer (89) reported that glucagon infusion reduced the malic enzyme response to T_3 with the alpha GPD enzyme response either unchanged or increased, both at dosage levels which did and did not decrease rat liver nuclear T_3 specific binding capacity. Since glucagon reduced malic enzyme response to T_3 without changing nuclear T_3 specific binding capacity, the authors suggested that glucagon might modify the effect of T_3 at a postreceptor level. These results bear interesting similarities to the differential malic and GPD enzyme alterations noted in experimental diabetes, where glucagon elevation is also possible (118). Such observations are of particular interest regarding the expression of TH action in various pathological states, i.e. its action at the cellular level may be mediated in a highly differential manner leading to selective inhibition or preservation of responsiveness to T_3 of specific metabolic pathways (89).

It was previously noted that various drugs affect total TH levels in the circulation by influencing the binding of the hormone to plasma proteins. Similarly, some drugs can also compete with hormones for specific binding sites in rat liver nuclei (119). Certain roentogenographic contrast agents competed with T_3 for binding to putative nuclear receptor sites _in vitro_ although apparently not _in vivo_. It is possible, therefore, that some drugs by interfering with T_3 receptor binding may contribute to disparate expressions of cellular activity in relation to free hormone levels.

Alterations in T_4 deiodination in pathophysiological states may also explain the lack of correlation between an abnormally high free T_4 concentration and euthyroid metabolic activity; in this condition, the lack of thyrotoxic effects may in part be due to reduced T_4 mono-deiodination to T_3 (176); correspondingly, in cases with low circulating FT_4, T_4 mono-deiodination may be increased sufficiently to produce normal intracellular T_3

concentrations. Similarly changes in T_3 deiodination might explain euthyroidism accompanied by low circulating T_3.

Alteration in the access of FTH to receptors due to permeability and/or carrier-mediated transport change might occur at the capillary or cellular membrane levels. Additionally, altered metabolic factors in pathophysiology may change the number of high capacity cellular sites. Docter et al. (120) stated that in vivo, cytosol binding proteins and nuclear binding sites are in equilibrium with the same free hormone pool outside the cell; therefore, they have assumed that a change in the number of binding sites outside the nucleus probably would have no effect on the degree of T_3 saturation of nuclear sites. However, in cases where circulating TH antibodies are present in high titres, hormone binding to TBG, which has an affinity comparable to putative receptors, is reduced in the presence of unaltered free T_4 concentration (121). Thus, it seems in principle that a large increase in low affinity binding sites might also decrease hormone bound to TBG; analogously an increase in cellular, nonreceptor binding might decrease hormone bound to receptors in the presence of a constant free TH concentration. Such an increase in nonreceptor binding may assume particular importance in regard to relative saturation of receptors by hormones in cases where the number of receptors is altered (Fig. 3).

Schwartz et al. (122) demonstrated increased T_4 binding by liver microsomes in rats treated with phenobarbital. The increased microsomal binding was associated with increased metabolic clearance of T_4 (8, 123), and an increase in the rate of deiodination of T_4 and T_3 (8). However, no change was observed in oxygen consumption in the intact rat or in mitochondrial GPD activity in rat liver, kidney and heart (124).

c. Is total cellular hormone concentration a better indicator of metabolic activity than circulating free hormone levels?

Our assumption has been that only the concentration of hormones bound to the receptors is of direct metabolic significance.

However, the receptor hormone concentration probably is only a small fraction of the total cellular hormone with the possible exception of the anterior pituitary (29). Furthermore, any change in non-receptor binding could alter the percentage of total cellular hormone bound to receptors thus reducing the relation between total cellular hormone concentration and hormone action (Fig. 3). If plasma free hormone is assumed to be in equilibrium with the cellular free hormone, which is in equilibrium with the receptor bound hormone (Fig. 4), one would expect plasma free hormone to be a valid indicator of hormone mediated metabolic activity. That this is not always the case has been noted above. In view of this, a knowledge of putative receptor affinity, capacity and relative saturation should yield the highest correlation with hormonal metabolic activity. That even this knowledge may not be adequate has been shown by experiments using glucagon (89) described previously; a reduction of the malic enzyme response to T_3 administration was not accompanied by a change in putative nuclear receptor binding affinity or capacity. In conclusion, though measurements of total cellular hormone concentration might yield useful information related to pathology, it is likely that it is less indicative of hormone mediated action than circulating free TH.

Concluding Remarks

Although the dissociation between circulating thyroid hormones and clinical status or tissue metabolic activity has been known for some time, only recent studies of subcellular and plasma membrane binding of TH have suggested possible paths for the understanding of this dichotomy at the molecular level. Fundamental to this understanding is the current belief that only hormone bound to cellular receptors is of direct metabolic significance. Recent studies of TH in pathophysiologic states have provided a basis for this hypothesis, e.g. increased levels of free thyroid hormones in the syndrome of partial TH resistance

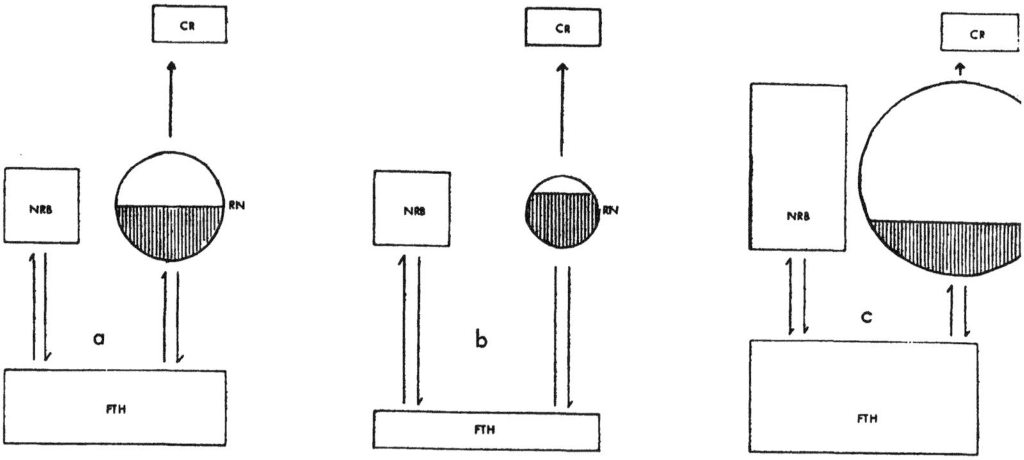

FTH-Free Thyroid Hormone
NRB-Non-Receptor Binding
RN-Receptor Number
CR-Cellular Response

Fig. 3. Euthyroid metabolic response with hypo- and hyperthyroid circulating levels of FTH.
This speculative scheme illustrates how alterations in TH receptor number and/or TH non-receptor binding might yield a normal metabolic response with abnormal circulating FTH levels. It is assumed that ISF and cellular FTH are in equilibrium. (a) Normal FTH with approximately 50% saturation of receptors. (b) Low circulating FTH. Non-receptor binding is unchanged, but a reduced receptor population has allowed increased relative saturation producing sufficient amplification of response to maintain a euthyroid metabolic status. (c) High circulating FTH. The non-receptor population, specific binding sites (deiodinases and cytosol protein) and/or non-specific sites, has increased reducing the amount of TH that otherwise would be bound to receptors. Additionally, the receptor population has increased sufficiently to prevent amplification of response. This combination has allowed maintenance of a euthyroid state. Direct and indirect evidence for these speculations is outlined in the text.

along with putative nuclear receptor abnormality by clinical euthyroidism. Experimental and clinical studies have suggested that TH receptors lend themselves to modulation by hormonal and pathophysiological factors which presumably alter hormone concentration at these sites. The studies reviewed suggest that a

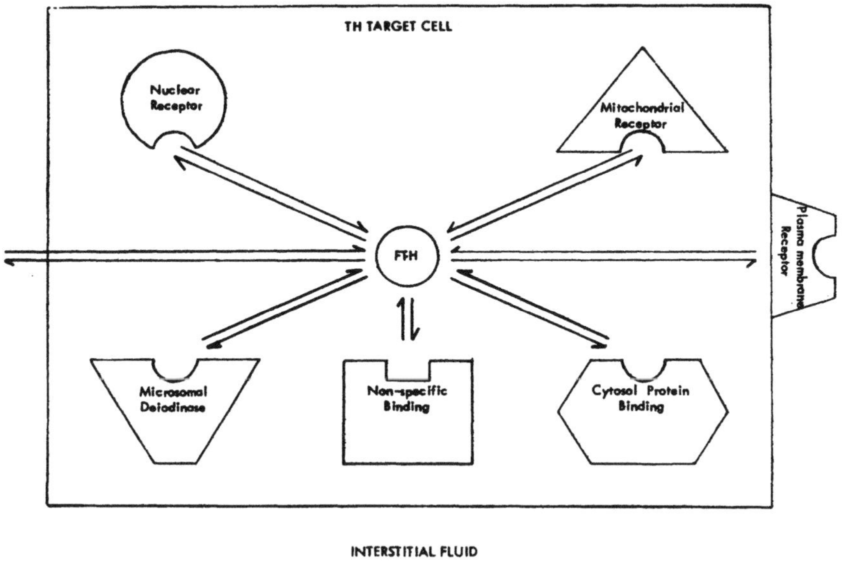

Fig. 4. Multiple equilibria between FTH and cellular receptor and non-receptor binding sites.
Intracellular FTH is shown in equilibrium with putative receptors in the nucleus, mitochondria, and plasma membrane; with non-receptor, specific binding sites of cytosol protein and microsomal deiodinase, with non-specific binding sites and with interstitial FTH.

receptor bound hormone assay would be highly correlated with clinical assessment and tissue metabolic activity. Another aspect of tissue iodothyronines that has stimulated current interest is the possibility that some of the calorigenically inactive products of T_4 metabolism may regulate the generation of calorigenically active T_3. The evidence from in vivo studies is still rudimentary and has been negative. Nevertheless, the provocative suggestion of peripheral control of TH metabolism has stimulated much research which has brought new insights into the physiology of thyroid hormones and their analogs. Should evidence for peripheral T_3 regulation by calorigenically inactive iodothyronines be established, the peripheral means of regulation of cellular TH metabolism may prove to be more crucial than the regulation of thyroidal secretion of hormones by the hypothalamo-pituitary-thyroid axis.

Acknowledgements

Part of the authors' investigations were supported by the Narveen Medical Research Foundation, St. Louis, Missouri. The authors thank Dr. S. Lang, Department of Physiology, Washington University School of Medicine, St. Louis, Missouri and Dr. P. G. Walfish, Department of Medicine, University of Toronto, Canada for a critical reading of the manuscript and for constructive comments and suggestions.

References

1. Bermudez, F., Surks, M.I., Oppenheimer, J.H.: High incidence of decreased serum triiodothyronine concentration in patients with nonthyroidal disease. J. clin. Endocr. Metab. 41, 27-40 (1975).

2. Chopra, I.J., Solomon, D.H., Hepner, G.W., Morgenstein, A.A.: Misleadingly low free thyroxine index and usefulness of reverse triiodothyronine measurement in nonthyroidal illnesses. Ann. intern. Med. 90, 905-912 (1979).

3. Kahn, A.: Serum thyroxine levels in patients receiving L-thyroxine suppression or replacement therapy. Canad. med. Ass. J. 109, 279-281 (1973).

4. Cornman, H.D., Alexander, F.: Effects of L-triiodothyronine alone in the treatment of obesity. Fed. Proc. 24, 189 (1965).

5. Premachandra, B.N., Gossain, V.V., Perlstein, I.B.: Free thyroxine index vs. free thyroxine concentration in inherited partial thyroxine binding globulin deficiency. Clin. Chem. 22, 1408 (1976).

6. Harland, W.A., Orr, J.S.: The role of thyroxine binding in the establishment of thyroid status. Scot. med. J. 14, 375-380 (1969).

7. Lewis, M.: Measurements of free thyroid hormones in health and disease. In: "Free Thyroid Hormones", Proceedings of the International Symposium, Venice, Eds. Ekins, R., Foglia, G., Pennisi, F., Pinchera, A., Excerpta Medica, Amsterdam, pp. 167-180 (1979).

8. Oppenheimer, J.H., Surks, M.I., Schwartz, H.L.: The metabolic significance of exchangeable cellular thyroxine. Recent Prog. Horm. Res. 25, 381-422 (1969).

9. Chopra, I.J., Solomon, D.H., Chopra, U., Young, R.T., Teco, G.N.C.: Alterations in circulating thyroid hormones and thyrotropin in hepatic cirrhosis: Evidence for euthyroidism despite subnormal serum triiodothyronine. J. clin. Endocr. Metab. 39, 501-511 (1974).

10. Premachandra, B.N., Gossain, V.V., Perlstein, I.B.: Increased free thyroxine in a euthyroid patient with thyroxine-binding globulin deficiency. J. clin. Endocr. Metab. 42, 309-318 (1976).

11. Oppenheimer, J.H.: Thyroid hormone action at the cellular level. Science 203, 971-979 (1979).

12. Sterling, K.: Thyroid hormone action at the cell level. New Engl. J. Med. 300, 117-123; 173-177 (1979).

13. De Groot, L.J.: Thyroid hormone action. In: "Endocrinology" vol.1, Eds. De Groot, L.J., Cahill, G.F., Martini, L., Nelson, D.H., Odell, W.D., Potts, J.T., Steinberger, E., Winegrad, A.I., Grune and Stratton, N.Y., pp. 357-363 (1979).

14. Gross, J., Pitt-Rivers, R.: The identification of 3:5:3'-L-triiodothyronine in human plasma. Lancet 1, 439-441 (1952).

15. Gross, J., Pitt-Rivers, R.: Physiological activity of 3:5:3'-L-triiodothyronine. Lancet 1, 593-594 (1952).

16. Daniel, P.M., Pratt, O.E., Roitt, I.M., Torrigiani, G.: Thyroglobulin in the lymph draining from the thyroid gland and in the peripheral blood of rats. Quart. J. exp. Physiol. 52, 184-199 (1967).

17. Premachandra, B.N.: Significance of reverse triiodothyronine (RT_3) in the physiologic and metabolic actions of thyroid hormones. In: "Proceedings 6th Asia and Oceania Congress of Endocrinology", Singapore, Eds. Seng, C.J., Pin, L., Tambyah, J.A., Shanmugaratnam, S., Boon, P.Y.P., Ark, C.N.S., Foo, K.N.K., Stamford College Press (Pte) Ltd., Singapore, pp. 533-541 (1978).

18. Braverman, L.E., Ingbar, S.H., Sterling, K.: Conversion of thyroxine to triiodothyronine in athyreotic human subjects. J. clin. Invest. 49, 855-864 (1970).

19. Chopra, I.J., Solomon, D.H., Chopra, U., Wu, S.Y., Fisher, D.A., Nakamura, Y.: Pathways of metabolism of thyroid hormones. Recent Prog. Horm. Res. 34, 521-567 (1978).

20. Chopra, I.J.: A study of extrathyroidal conversion of thyroxine to 3,3',5-triiodothyronine in vitro. Endocrinology 101, 453-463 (1977).

21. Cavalieri, R.R., Gavin, L.A., Bui, F., McMahon, F., Hammond, M.: Conversion of thyroxine to 3,3',5'-triiodothyronine by a soluble enzyme system of rat liver. Biochem. biophys. Res. Commun. 79, 897-902 (1977).

22. Ramsden, D.B.: "Peripheral Metabolism and Action of Thyroid Hormones", vol. 2, Eden Press, Montreal (1977).

23. Nicod, P., Burger, A., Strauch, G., Vagenakis, A.G., Braverman, L.E.: The failure of physiologic doses of reverse T_3 to effect thyroid-pituitary function in man. J. clin. Endocr. Metab. 43, 478-481 (1976).

24. Fishman, N., Huang, Y.P., Tergis, D.C., Rivlin, R.S.: Relation of triiodothyronine and reverse triiodothyronine administration in rats to hepatic L-triiodothyronine aminotransferase activity. Endocrinology 100, 1055-1059 (1977).

25. Goldfine, I.D., Smith, G.J., Simons, C.G., Ingbar, S.H., Jorgensen, E.C.: Activities of thyroid hormones and related compounds in an in vitro thymocyte assay. J. biol. Chem. 251, 4233-4238 (1976).

26. Van Middlesworth, L.: A method for iodide balance studies in animals on low iodide diets. Endocrinology 58, 235-242 (1956).

27. Gordon, A., Spira, O.: Triiodothyronine binding in rat anterior pituitary, posterior pituitary, median eminence and brain. Endocrinology 96, 1357-1365 (1975).

28. Hennemann, G., Smeulers, J., van der Does, I., Docter, R., Visser, T.J.: Measurement of intracellular T_3 and T_3 disposal in normal subjects. Acta endocr. 82, 92-97 (1976).

29. Oppenheimer, J.H., Schwartz, H.L., Surks, M.I.: Tissue differences in the concentration of triiodothyronine nuclear binding sites in the rat. Endocrinology 95, 897-903 (1974).

30. Flock, E.V., Bollman, J.L.: The metabolism of thyroxine and triiodothyronine in the eviserated rat. J. biol. Chem. 214, 709-721 (1955).

31. Takaishi, M., Miyachi, Y., Aoki, M., Shishiba, Y.: Comparison of the methods for tissue triiodothyronine extraction and subsequent radioimmunoassay. Acta endocr. 87, 125-132 (1978).

32. Irvine, C.H.G.: Concentration of thyroxine in cellular and extracellular tissues of the sheep and the rate of equilibration of labeled thyroxine. Endocrinology 94, 1060-1071 (1974).

33. Folch, J., Lees, M., Stanley, G.H.S.: A simple method for the isolation and purification of total lipids from animal tissues. J. biol. Chem. 226, 497-509 (1957).

34. Janssen, J.W., van Hardeveld, C., Kassenaar, A.A.H.: A methodological study in measuring T_3 and T_4 concentration in red and white skeletal muscle and plasma of euthyroid rats. Acta endocr. 90, 81-89 (1979).

35. Hasen, J., Bernstein, G., Volpert, E., Oppenheimer, J.H.: Analysis of the rapid interchange of thyroxine between plasma and liver and plasma and kidney in the intact rat. Endocrinology 82, 37-46 (1968).

36. Scatchard, G.: The attraction of proteins for small molecules and ions. Ann. N.Y. Acad. Sci. 51, 660-672 (1949).

37. Simpson-Morgan, M.W., Sutherland, R.L.: The transcapillary exchange of thyroid hormones and thyroxine binding proteins between blood and tissue fluids. J. Physiol. 257, 123-136 (1976).

38. Alpers, J.B., Rall, J.E.: The metabolism of iodine in cerebrospinal fluid. J. clin. Endocr. Metab. 15, 1482-1498 (1955).

39. Hagen, G.A., Elliott, W.J.: Transport of thyroid hormones in serum and cerebrospinal fluid. J. clin. Endocr. Metab. 37, 415-422 (1973).

40. Siersbaek-Nielsen, K., Hansen, J.M.: The binding capacity of thyroxine-binding globulin in cerebrospinal fluid. Acta endocr. 67, 616-624 (1971).

41. Hagen, G.A., Solberg,Jr. L.A.: Brain and cerebrospinal fluid permeability to intravenous thyroid hormones. Endocrinology 95, 1398-1410 (1974).

42. Pardridge, W.M.: Carrier-mediated transport of thyroid hormones through the rat blood-brain barrier; primary role of albumin bound hormone. Endocrinology 105, 605-612 (1979).

43. Freinkel, N., Ingbar, S.H., Dowling, J.T.: The influence of extracellular thyroxine-binding protein upon the accumulation of thyroxine by tissue slices. J. clin. Invest. 36, 25-37 (1957).

44. Baxter, J.D., Eberhardt, N.L., Apriletti, J.W., Johnson, L.K., Ivarie, R.D., Schachter, B.S., Morris, J.A., Seeburg, P.H., Goodman, H.M., Latham, K.R., Polansky, J.R., Martial, J.A.: Thyroid hormone receptors and responses. Recent Prog. Horm. Res. 35, 97-153 (1979).

45. Neuhaus, O.W., Sogoian, V.: The thyroxine-binding protein of bovine synovial fluid. J. biol. Chem. 234, 821-823 (1959).

46. Valcana, T., Timiras, P.S.: Nuclear triiodothyronine receptors in the developing rat brain. Molecular and Cellular Endocr. 11, 31-41 (1978).

47. Robbins, J., Rall, J.E.: The interaction of thyroid hormones and protein in biological fluids. Recent Prog. Horm. Res. 13, 161-208 (1957).

48. Galvan, G., Balcke, Ch., Fritz, H., Maier, F.: Triiodothyronine, reverse-triiodothyronine, thyroxine, resin-triiodothyronine-uptake and protein bound iodide in the fluid of thyroid cysts. Klin. Wschr. 56, 617-621 (1978).

49. Studer, H., Greer, M.A.: "The Regulation of Thyroid Function in Iodine Deficiency", Hans Huber Publishers, Bern (1968).

50. Nagataki, S., Uchimura, H., Masuyama, Y., Nakao, K., Ito, K.: Triiodothyronine and thyroxine in thyroid gland of euthyroid Japanese subjects. J. clin. Endocr. Metab. 35, 18-23 (1972).

51. Chopra, I.J., Fisher, D.A., Solomon, D.H., Beall, G.N.: Thyroxine and triiodothyronine in the human thyroid. J. clin. Endocr. Metab. 36, 311-316 (1973).

52. Larsen, P.R., Yamashita, K., Dekker, A., Field, J.B.: Biochemical observations in functioning human thyroid adenomas. J. clin. Endocr. Metab. 36, 1009-1018 (1973).

53. Abrams, G.M., Larsen, P.R.: Triiodothyronine and thyroxine in the serum and thyroid glands of iodine-deficient rats. J. clin. Invest. 52, 2522-2531 (1973).

54. Haibach, H.: Free iodothyronines in the rat thyroid gland. Endocrinology 88, 149-154 (1971).

55. Taurog, A., Chaikoff, I.L.: The nature of the circulating thyroid hormone. J. biol. Chem. 176, 639-656 (1948).

56. Larsen, P.R.: Triiodothyronine: Review of recent studies of its physiology and pathophysiology in man. Metabolism 21, 1073-1092 (1972).

57. Reichlin, S., Bollinger, J., Nejad, I., Sullivan, P.: Tissue thyroid hormone concentration of rat and man determined by radioimmunoassay. Mt. Sinai J. Med. 40, 502-510 (1973).

58. Felt, V., Husek, P.: The different uptake of triiodothyronine and thyroxine by adipose tissue as compared with muscle or leucocytes in man. Physiol. bohemoslov. 22, 51-53 (1973).

59. Lemarchand-Béraud, Th., Holm, A.-Ch., Scazziga, B.R.: Triiodothyronine and thyroxine nuclear receptors in lymphocytes from normal, hyper- and hypothyroid subjects. Acta endocr. 85, 44-54 (1977).

60. Liewendahl, K., Rosengard, S., Lamberg, B.A.: Nuclear binding of triiodothyronine and thyroxine in lymphocytes from subjects with hyperthyroidism, hypothyroidism and resistance to thyroid hormones. Clin. chim. Acta 83, 41-48 (1978).

61. Nejad, I.F., Bollinger, J.A., Mitnick, M., Reichlin, S.: Importance of T_3 secretion in altered states of thyroid function in the rat: Cold exposure, subtotal thyroidectomy and hypophysectomy. Trans. Assoc. Am. Physicians 85, 295-308 (1972).

62. Silva, J.E., Dick, T.E., Larsen, P.R.: The contribution of local tissue thyroxine monodeiodination to the nuclear 3, 5,3'-triiodothyronine in pituitary, liver and kidney of euthyroid rats. Endocrinology 103, 1196-1207 (1978).

63. Heninger, R.W., Albright, E.C.: Alteration in tissue and serum concentrations of TSH, iodide, T_4 , and T_3 induced by various dietary iodide levels. Proc. Soc. exp. Biol Med. 150, 137-141 (1975).

64. Obregon, M.J., de Escobar, M., Escobar del Rey, F.: Concentrations of triiodo-L-thyronine in the plasma and tissues of normal rats, as determined by radioimmunoassay: Comparison with results obtained by an isotopic equilibrium technique. Endocrinology 103, 2145-2153 (1978).

65. Albright, E.C., Heninger, R.W., Larson, F.C.: Effect of cold-induced hyperthyroidism on iodine-containing compounds of extrathyroid tissues. In: "Current Topics in Thyroid Research", Eds. Cassano, C., Andreoli, M., Academic Press, N.Y., pp. 346-355 (1965).

66. Hechter, O.M.: The receptor concent: Prejudice, prediction, and paradox. In: "Hormone Receptors", Advances in Experimental Med. and Biol. vol. 96, Eds. Klachko, D.M., Forte, L.R., Franz, J.M., Plenum Press, N.Y., pp. 1-43 (1978).

67. Grief, R.L., Sloane, D.: Mitochondrial binding sites for triiodothyronine. Endocrinology 103, 1899-1902 (1978).

68. Oppenheimer, J.H., Schwartz, H.L., Surks, M.I., Koerner, D., Dillmann, W.H.: Nuclear receptors and the initiation of thyroid hormone action. Recent Prog. Horm. Res. 32, 529-565 (1976).

69. Pliam, N.B., Goldfine, I.D.: High affinity thyroid hormone binding sites on purified rat liver plasma membranes. Biochem. biophys. Res. Commun. 79, 166-172 (1977).

70. Tata, J.R.: How specific are nuclear "receptors" for thyroid hormones ? Nature 257, 18-23 (1975).

71. Surks, M.I., Koerner, D., Oppenheimer, J.H.: In vitro binding of L-triiodothyronine to receptors in rat nuclei. J. clin. Invest. 55, 50-60 (1975).

72. Eberhardt, N.L., Valcana, T., Timiras, P.S.: Hormone-receptor interactions in brain. Psychoneuroendocrinol. 1, 399-409 (1976).

73. Sterling, K., Lazarus, J.H., Milch, P.O., Sakurada, T., Brenner, M.A.: Mitochondrial thyroid hormone receptor: Localization and physiological significance. Science 201, 1126-1129 (1978).

74. Rao, G.S., Eckel, J., Rao, M.L., Breuer, H.: Uptake of thyroid hormone by isolated rat liver cells. Biochem. biophys. Res. Commun. 73, 98-104 (1976).

75. Docter, R., Krenning, E.P., Bernard, H.F., Visser, T.J., Hennemann, G.: Uptake of triiodothyronine by isolated rat liver cells. Ann Endocrinol. 38, 59A (1977).

76. Docter, R., Visser, T.J., Stinis, J.T., van den Hont-Goemaat, N.L., Hennemann, G.: Binding of L-triiodothyronine to isolated rat liver nuclei under various circumstances. Acta endocr. 81, 82-95 (1976).

77. Davis, P.J., Handwerger, B.S., Glaser, F.: Physical properties of a dog liver and kidney cytosol protein that binds thyroid hormone. J. biol. Chem. 249, 6208-6217 (1974).

78. Surks, M.I., Oppenheimer, J.H.: Concentration of L-thyroxine and L-triiodothyronine specifically bound to nuclear receptors in rat liver and kidney. J. clin. Invest. 60, 555-562 (1977).

79. Bianchi, R., Zucchelli, G.C., Giannessi, D., Pilo, A., Mariani, G., Carpi, A., Toni, M.G.: Evaluation of triiodothyronine kinetics in normal subjects, in hypothyroid, and hyperthyroid patients using specific antiserum for the determination of labeled T_3 in plasma. J. clin. Endocr. Metab. 46, 203-214 (1978).

80. Bernal, J., De Groot, L.J., Refetoff, S., Fang, V.S., Barsano, C.: Absent nuclear thyroid hormone receptors and failure of T_3 -induced TRH suppression in the syndrome of peripheral resistance to thyroid hormone. Abstracts of the 7th International Thyroid Conference, Excerpta Medica, Amsterdam, 361, 66 (1975).

81. Valcana, T., Timiras, P.S.: Triiodothyronine receptors in liver nuclei from developing and aging rats. Abstracts of the V International Congress of Endocrinology, Hamburg, Bruhlsche Universitätsdruckerei, Giessen, pp.237-238 (1976).

82. Burman, K.D., Lukes, Y., Wright, F.D., Wartofsky, L.: Reduction in hepatic triiodothyronine binding capacity induced by fasting. Endocrinology 101, 1331-1334 (1977).

83. De Groot, L.J., Coleoni, A.H., Rue, P.A., Seo, H., Martino, E., Refetoff, S.: Reduced nuclear triiodothyronine receptors in starvation-induced hypothyroidism. Biochem. biophys. Res. Commun. 79, 173-178 (1977).

84. Schussler, G.C., Orlando, J.: Fasting decreases triiodothyronine receptor capacity. Science 199, 686-688 (1978).

85. Guernsey, D.L., Morishige, W.K.: Na^+ pump activity and nuclear T_3 receptors in tissues of genetically obese mice. Metabolism 28, 629-632 (1979).

86. Dillmann, W.H., Schwartz, H.L., Oppenheimer, J.H.: Selective alterations in hepatic enzyme response after reduction of nuclear triiodothyronine receptor sites by partial hepatectomy and starvation. Biochem. biophys. Res. Commun. 80, 259-266 (1978).

87. Surks, M.I., Grajower, M.M., Tai, M., DeFesi, C.R.: Decreased hepatic nuclear L-triiodothyronine receptors in rats and mice bearing transplantable neoplasms. Endocrinology 103, 2234-2239 (1978).

88. Dillmann, W.H., Schwartz, H.L., Bonner, R.A., Oppenheimer, J.H.: Glucagon reduces hepatic nuclear T_3 receptors: Possible role of glucagon in mediating the decreased nuclear T_3 binding capacity in hepatectomized, starved and diabetic animals. Clin. Res. 26, 490A (1978).

89. Dillmann, W.H., Oppenheimer, J.H.: Glucagon influences the expression of thyroid hormone action: Discrepancy between nuclear triiodothyronine receptor number and enzyme responses. Endocrinology 105, 74-79 (1979).

90. Morley, C.G.D., Kuku, S., Rubenstein, A.H., Boyer, J.L.: Serum hormone levels following partial hepatectomy in the rat. Biochem. biophys. Res. Commun. 67, 653-661 (1975).

91. Grey, N., McGuigan, J.E., Kipnis, D.M.: Neutralization of endogenous glucagon by high titer glucagon antiserum. Endocrinology 86, 1383-1388 (1970).

92. Unger, R.H., Aguilar-Parada, E., Muller, W.A., Eisentraut, A.M.: Studies of pancreatic alpha cell function in normal and diabetic subjects. J. clin. Invest. 49, 837-848 (1970).

93. Gossain, V.V., Matute, M.L., Kalkhoff, R.K.: Relative influence of obesity and diabetes on plasma alpha-cell glucagon. J. clin. Endocr. Metab. 38, 238-243 (1974).

94. Goldfine, I.D., Kirsteins, L., Lawrence, A.M.: Excessive glucagon response to arginine and active acromegaly. Horm. Metab. Res. 4, 97-100 (1972).

95. Oppenheimer, J.H., Schwartz, H.L., Surks, M.I.: Nuclear binding capacity appears to limit the hepatic response to L-triiodothyronine. Endocrine Res. Commun. 2, 309-325 (1975).

96. Spindler, B.J., MacLeod, K.M., Ring, J., Baxter, J.D.: Thyroid hormone receptors. Binding characteristics and lack of hormonal dependency for nuclear localization. J. biol. Chem. 250, 4113-4119 (1975).

97. Bernal, J., Coleoni. A.H., De Groot, L.J.: Thyroid hormone receptors from liver nuclei: Characteristics of receptor from normal, thyroidectomized, and triiodothyronine-treated rats; Measurement of occupied and unoccupied receptors, and chromatin binding of receptors. Endocrinology 103, 403-413 (1978).

98. Premachandra, B.N., Blumenthal, H.T.: Abnormal binding of thyroid hormone in sera from patients with Hashimoto's disease. J. clin. Endocr. Metab. 27, 931-936 (1967).

99. Ochi, Y., Shiomi, K., Hachiya, T., Yoshimura, M., Miyazaki, T.: Immunological analysis of abnormal binding of thyroid hormone in the gamma globulin. J. clin. Endocr. Metab. 35, 743-752 (1972).

100. Lee, W.N.P., Golden, M.P., Van Herle, A.J., Lippe, B.M., Kaplan, S.A.: Inherited abnormal thyroid hormone-binding protein causing selective increase of total serum thyroxine. J. clin. Endocr. Metab. 49, 292-299 (1979).

101. Hennemann, G., Docter, R., Krenning, E.P., Bos, G., Otten, M., Visser, T.J.: Raised total thyroxine and free thyroxine index but normal free thyroxine. Lancet 1, 639-642 (1979).

102. Sunderman, Jr. F.W.: Drug interference in clinical biochemistry. Crit. Rev. Clin. Lab. Sci. 1, 427-449 (1970).

103. Hermann, J., Rudorff, K.H., Kroner, H., Premachandra, B.N.: Antibody binding of thyroid hormone in juvenile goitrous hypothyroidism. Horm. Metab. Res. 9, 394-400 (1977).

104. Ginsberg, J., Segal, D., Ehrlich, R.M., Walfish, P.G.: Inappropriate triiodothyronine and thyroxine radioimmunoassay levels secondary to circulating thyroid hormone autoantibodies. Clin. Endocr. 8, 133-139 (1978).

105. Tamagna, E., Hershman, J., Premachandra, B.N.: Circulating thyroid hormones in a patient with hyperviscosity syndrome. Clin. chim. Acta 93, 263-268 (1979).

106. Suda, A.K., Pittman, C.S., Shimizu, T., Chambers, Jr.J.B.: The production and metabolism of 3,5,3'-triiodothyronine and 3,3',5'-triiodothyronine in normal and fasting subjects. J. clin. Endocr. Metab. 47, 1311-1319 (1978).

107. Obregon, M.J., Roelfsema, F., de Escobar, G.M., Escobar del Rey, F., Querido, A.: Exchange of triiodothyronine derived from thyroxine with circulating triiodothyronine as studied in the rat. Clin. Endocr. 10, 305-315 (1979).

108. Oppenheimer, J.H., Schwartz, H.L., Koerner, D., Surks, M.I.: Limiting binding capacity sites for L-triiodothyronine in rat liver nuclei. J. clin. Invest. 53, 768-777 (1974).

109. Irvine, C.H.G.: The effect of an ethanol-extractable thyroxine binding substance in plasma on the measurement of thyroxine by competitive binding. J. clin. Endocr. Metab. 38, 468-475 (1974).

110. Daniel, P.M., Plaskett, L.G., Pratt, O.E.: The lymphatic and venous pathways for the outflow of thyroxine, iodoprotein, and inorganic iodide from the thyroid gland. J. Physiol. 188, 25-44 (1967).

111. Schwartz, H.L., Forciea, M.A., Mariash, C.N., Oppenheimer, J.H.: Age-related reduction in response of hepatic enzymes to 3-5-3'-triiodothyronine administration. Endocrinology 41-46 (1979).

112. Denckla, W.D.: Role of the pituitary and thyroid glands in the decline of minimal O_2 consumption with age. J. clin. Invest. 53, 572-581 (1974).

113. Sisson, R.G., Lang, S.: Oxygen consumption in the rat during prolonged, acute starvation. Proc. Soc. exp. Biol Med. 93, 173-174 (1956).

114. Oppenheimer, J.H., Coulombe, P., Schwartz, H.L., Gutfeld, N.W.: Nonlinear (amplified) relationship between nuclear occupancy by triiodothyronine and the appearance rate of hepatic alpha-glycerophosphate dehydrogenase and malic enzyme in the rat. J. clin. Invest. 61, 987-997 (1978).

115. Oppenheimer, J.H.: Initiation of thyroid-hormone action. New Engl. J. Med. 292, 1063-1068 (1975).

116. Samuels, H.H., Horwitz, Z.D., Stanley, F., Casanova, J., Shapiro, L.E.: Thyroid hormone controls glucocorticoid action in cultured GH_1 cells. Nature 268, 254-257 (1977).

117. Martial, J.A., Seeburg, P.H., Guenzi, D., Goodman, H.M., Baxter, J.D.: Regulation of growth hormone gene expression: Synergistic effects of thyroid and glucocorticoid hormones. Proc. natn. Acad. Sci. U.S.A. 74, 4293-4295 (1977).

118. Ruegamer, W.R., Newman, G.H., Richert, D.A., Westerfeld, W.W.: Specificity of the alpha-glycerophosphate dehydrogenase and malic enzyme response to thyroxine. Endocrinology 77, 707-715 (1965).

119. De Groot, L.J., Rue, P.A.: Roentgenographic contrast agents inhibit triiodothyronine binding to nuclear receptors in vitro. J. clin. Endocr. Metab. 49, 538-542 (1979).

120. Docter, R., Visser, T.J., Henneman, G.: How specific are nuclear "receptors" for thyroid hormones ? Nature 259, 345-346 (1976).

121. Premachandra, B.N., Ginsberg, J., Walfish, P.G.: Binding of reverse triiodothyronine to serum immunoglobulins in man and the rabbit. J. clin. Endocr. Metab. (in press).

122. Schwartz, H.L., Bernstein, G., Oppenheimer, J.H.: Effect of phenobarbital administration on the subcellular distribution of ^{125}I-thyroxine in rat liver: Importance of microsomal binding. Endocrinology 84, 270-276 (1969).

123. Oppenheimer, J.H., Bernstein, G., Surks, M.I.: Increased thyroxine turnover and thyroidal function after stimulation of hepatocellular binding of thyroxine by phenobarbital. J. clin. Invest. 47, 1399-1406 (1968).

124. Oppenheimer, J.H., Shapiro, H.C., Schwartz, H.L., Surks, M.I.: Dissociation between thyroxine metabolism and hormonal action in phenobarbital-treated rats. Endocrinology 88, 115-119 (1971).

125. Premachandra, B.N., Ibrahim, I.I.: A simple and rapid thyroxine radioimmunoassay in unextracted human serum. Clin. chim. Acta 70, 43-60 (1976).

126. Burman, K.D., Dimond, R.C., Wright, F.D., Earll, J.M., Bruton, J., Wartofsky, L.: A radioimmunoassay for 3,3', 5'-triiodothyronine: Assessment of thyroid gland content and serum measurements in conditions of normal and altered thyroidal economy and following administration of thyrotropin releasing hormone and thyrotropin. J. clin. Endocr. Metab. 44, 660-672 (1977).

127. Burger, A.: The pathophysiological significance of tetraiodothyroacetic acid. Abstracts of the V International Congress of Endocrinology, Hamburg, Bruhlsche Universitätsdruckerei, Giessen, p. 52 (1976).

128. Crossley, D.N., Ramsden, D.B.: Serum tetraiodothyroacetate levels in normal healthy euthyroid individuals determined by gas chromatography-mass fragmentography. Clin. chim. Acta 94, 267-272 (1979).

129. Premachandra, B.N.: A simple and rapid radioimmunoassay of triiodothyronine in unextracted serum. J. Nucl. Med. 17, 411-416 (1976).

130. Gavin, L.A., Hammond, M.E., Castle, J.N., Cavalieri, R.R.: 3,3'-Diiodothyronine production, a major pathway of peripheral iodothyronine metabolism in man. J. clin. Invest. 61, 1276-1285 (1978).

131. Reinwein, D., Durrer, H., Emrich, D., Meinhold, H., Wenzel, K.W.: The thyroidal production of reverse triiodothyronine in autonomous adenoma. Clin. Endocr. 7, 171-173 (1977).

132. Chopra, I.J.: A radioimmunoassay for measurement of 3,3', 5'-triiodothyronine. J. clin. Invest. 54, 583-592 (1974).

133. Premachandra, B.N.: Radioimmunoassay of reverse triiodothyronine. J. clin. Endocr. Metab. 47, 746-750 (1978).

134. Nakamura, Y., Chopra, I.J., Solomon, D.H.: An assessment of the concentration of acetic acid and propionic acid derivatives of 3,5,3'-triiodothyronine in human serum. J. clin. Endocr. Metab. 46, 91-97 (1978).

135. Geola, F., Chopra, I.J., Solomon, D.H., Maciel, R.M.B.: Metabolic clearance and production rates of 3',5'-diiodothyronine and 3,3'-diiodothyronine in man. J. clin. Endocr. Metab. 48, 297-301 (1979).

136. Grussendorf, M., Hufner, M.: Radioimmunoassay for 3,3'-diiodothyronine in human serum. Clin. chim. Acta 88, 81-88 (1978).

137. Wu, S.Y., Chopra, I.J., Nakamura, Y., Solomon, D.H., Bennett, L.R.: A radioimmunoassay for measurement of 3,3'-L-diiodothyronine. J. clin. Endocr. Metab. 43, 682-685 (1976).

138. Burman, K.D., Strum, D., Dimond, R.C., Djuh, Y.Y., Wright, F.D., Earll, J.M., Wartofsky, L.: A radioimmunoassay for 3,3'-L-diiodothyronine. J. clin. Endocr. Metab. 45, 339-352 (1977).

139. Burger, A., Sakoloff, C.: Serum 3,3'-L-diiodothyronine, a direct radioimmunoassay in human serum: Method and clinical results. J. clin. Endocr. Metab. 45, 384-391 (1977).

140. Chopra, I.J., Geola, F., Solomon, D.H., Maciel, R.M.B.: 3',5'-Diiodothyronine in health and disease: Studies by a radioimmunoassay. J. clin. Endocr. Metab. 47, 1198-1207 (1978).

141. Burman, K.D., Wright, F.D., Smallridge, R.C., Green, B.J., Georges, L.P., Wartofsky, L.: A radioimmunoassay for 3', 5'-diiodothyronine. J. clin. Endocr. Metab. 47, 1059-1064 (1978).

142. Meinhold, H., Schurnbrand, P.: A radioimmunoassay for 3, 5-diiodothyronine. Clin. Endocr. 8, 493-497 (1978).

143. Smallridge, R.C., Wartofsky, L., Dimond, R.C., Burman, K.D.: 3',5'-Diiodothyronine and 3'-monoiodothyronine: development of radioimmunoassays and demonstration of in vivo peripheral conversion. Abstracts of the 60th Meeting of the Endocrine Society, Miami, p. 125 (1978).

144. Ljunggren, J.G., Persson, B., Granberg, P.O.: Thyroxine, triiodothyronine, and thyroglobulin in the human thyroid lymph. In: "Thyroid Research", Proceedings of the 7th International Thyroid Conference, Boston, Mass., Eds. Robbins, J., Braverman, L.E., Excerpta Medica, Amsterdam, pp. 211-212 (1976).

145. Sutherland, R.L., Irvine, C.H.G,: Total plasma thyroxine concentrations in horses, pigs, cattle, sheep: Anion-exchange resin chromatography and ceric-arsenite colorimetry. Amer. J. vet. Res. 34, 1261-1265 (1973).

146. Sutherland, R.L., Simpson-Morgan, M.W.: The thyroxine-binding properties of serum proteins. A competitive binding technique employing Sephadex G-25. J. Endocr. 65, 319-332 (1975).

147. Heninger, R.W., Larson, F.C., Albright, E.C.: Iodine-containing compounds of extrathyroidal tissues. J. clin. Invest. 42, 1761-1768 (1963).

148. Winder, W.W., Heninger, R.W.: Effect of exercise on tissue levels of thyroid hormones in the rat. Amer. J. Physiol. 221, 1139-1143 (1971).

149. Dillmann, W., Surks, M.I., Oppenheimer, J.H.: Quantitative aspects of iodothyronine binding by cytosol proteins of rat liver and kidney. Endocrinology 95, 492-498 (1974).

150. Koerner, D., Surks, M.I., Oppenheimer, J.H.: In vitro demonstration of specific triiodothyronine binding sites in rat liver nuclei. J. clin. Endocr. Metab. 38, 706-709 (1974).

151. Thomopoulos, P., Dastugue, B., Defer, N.: In vitro triiodothyronine binding to non-histone proteins from rat liver. Biochem. biophys. Res. Commun. 58, 499-506 (1974).

152. Latham, K.R., Ring, J.C., Baxter, J.D.: Solubilized nuclear "receptors" for thyroid hormones. J. biol. Chem. 251, 7388-7397 (1976).

153. Sterling, K., Milch, P.O.: Thyroid hormone binding by a component of mitochondrial membrane. Proc. natn. Acad. Sci. U.S.A. 72, 3225-3229 (1975).

154. Defer, N., Dastugue, B., Sabatier, M.M., Thomopoulos, P., Kruh, J.: Triiodothyronine binding proteins in rat liver cytosol. Biochem. biophys. Res. Commun. 67, 995-1004 (1975).

155. Visser, T.J., Docter, R., Stinis, J.T., Bernard, B., Hennemann, G.: Binding of L-triiodothyronine to rat liver cytosol and nuclei. In: "Thyroid Hormone Metabolism", Eds. Harland, W.A., Orr, J.S., Academic Press, N.Y. pp. 35-45 (1975).

156. Sterling, K., Milch, P.O., Brenner, M.A., Lazarus, J.H.: Thyroid hormone action: The mitochondrial pathway. Science 197, 996-999 (1977).

157. Samuels, H.H., Tsai, J.S., Casanova, J., Stanley, F.: Thyroid hormone action. In vitro characterization of solubilized nuclear receptors from rat liver and cultured GH_1 cells. J. clin. Invest. 54, 853-865 (1974).

158. Sufi, S.B., Toccafondi, R.S., Malan, P.G., Ekins, R.P.: Binding of thyroid hormones to a soluble fraction from porcine anterior pituitary. J. Endocr. 58, 41-52 (1973).

159. De Groot, L.J., Bernal, J., Refetoff, S.: Liver nuclear binding proteins; basic and clinical aspects. In: "Biochemical Basis of Thyroid Stimulation and Thyroid Hormone Action", Eds. von zur Muhlen, A., Schleusener, H., Georg Thieme Publishers, Stuttgart, pp. 143-156 (1976).

160. Bernal, J., De Groot, L.J.: Thyroid hormone receptors: Release of receptors to the medium during in vitro incubation of isolated rat liver nuclei. Endocrinology 100, 648-655 (1977).

161. Nauman, J., Nauman, A., Kubica, A., Witkowska, E., Wasiak, U., Posepna, K., Konador, A.: The binding of T_3 in liver nuclei and other intracellular organelles. In: "Biochemical Basis of Thyroid Stimulation and Thyroid Hormone Action", Eds. von zur Muhlen, A., Schleusener, H., Georg Thieme Publishers, Stuttgart, pp. 169-179 (1976).

162. Holm, A., Jorgenson, E.C., Pliam, N.B., Goldfine, I.D.: Membrane transport and the cellular effects of thyroid hormone. Annls Endocr. 38, 59A (1977).

163. Samuels, H.H., Tsai, J.S.: Thyroid hormone action in cell culture: Demonstration of nuclear receptors in intact cells and isolated nuclei. Proc. natn. Acad. Sci. U.S.A. 70, 3488-3492 (1973).

164. Samuels, H.H., Tsai, J.S.: Demonstration of similar receptors in isolated nuclei of rat liver and cultured GH_1cells. J. clin. Invest. 53, 656-659 (1974).

165. De Groot, L.J., Torresani, J.: Triiodothyronine binding to isolated liver cell nuclei. Endocrinology 96, 357-369 (1975).

166. Tsai, J.S., Samuels, H.H.: Thyroid hormone action: Demonstration of putative nuclear receptors in human lymphocytes. J. clin. Endocr. Metab. 38, 919-922 (1974).

167. Woeber, K.A., Maddux, B.A.: Observations concerning the binding of L-triiodothyronine in the human polymorphonuclear leukocyte. J. clin. Endocr. Metab. 44, 62-68 (1977).

168. Torresani, J., De Groot, L.J.: Triiodothyronine binding to nuclear solubilized proteins in vitro. Endocrinology 96, 1201-1209 (1975).

169. Schuster, L.D., Schwartz, H.L., Oppenheimer, J.H.: Nuclear receptors for 3,5,3'-triiodothyronine in human liver and kidney: Characterization, quantitation and similarities to rat receptors. J. clin. Endocr. Metab. 48, 627-632 (1979).

170. De Groot, L.J., Strausser, J.L.: Binding of T_3 in rat liver nuclei. Endocrinology 95, 74-83 (1974).

171. Clark, O.H., Okerlund, M.D., Cavalieri, R.R., Greenspan, F.S.: Diagnosis and treatment of thyroid, parathyroid, and thyroglossal duct cysts. J. clin. Endocr. Metab. 48, 983-988 (1979).

172. Silva, J.E., Larsen, P.R.: Contribution of plasma triiodothyronine and local thyroxine monodeiodination to triiodothyronine to nuclear triiodothyronine receptor saturation in pituitary, liver, and kidney of hypothyroid rats. J. clin. Invest. 61, 1247-1259 (1978).

173. Jarett, L.: Pathophysiology of the insulin receptor. Human Pathology 10, 301-311 (1979).

174. Wimpfheimer, C., Saville, E., Voirol, M.J., Danforth,Jr., E., Burger, A.G.: Starvation-induced decreased sensitivity of resting metabolic rate to triiodothyronine. Science 205, 1272-1273 (1979).

175. Mariash, C.N., Kaiser, F.E., Oppenheimer, J.H.: Comparison of the response characteristics of four lipogenic enzymes to 3,5,3'-triiodothyronine administration. Endocrinology 106, 22-27 (1980).

176. Maxon, H.R., Burman, K.D., Premachandra, B.N., Chen, I.W., Levy, P., Georges, L.P.: Euthyroid, familial hyperthyroxinemia. New Engl. J. Med. (submitted for publication).

177. De Groot, L.J.: Mechanism of action of thyroid hormone. In: "Free Thyroid Hormones", Proceedings of the International Symposium, Venice, Eds. Ekins, R., Foglia, G., Pennisi, F., Pinchera, A., Excerpta Medica, Amsterdam, pp. 28-44 (1979).

178. Aguilar-Parada, E., Eisentraut, A.M., Unger, R.H.: Effects of starvation on plasma pancreatic glucagon in normal man. Diabetes 18, 717-723 (1969).

179. Roth, J., Lesniak, M.A., Bar, R.S., Muggeo, M., Megyesi, K., Harrison, L.C., Flier, J.S., Wachslicht-Rodbard, H., Gorden, P.: An introduction to receptors and receptor disorders. Proc. Soc. exp. Biol Med. 162, 3-12 (1979).

180. Coiro, V., Harris, A., Goodman, H.M., Vagenakis, A., Braverman, L.: Effect of pharmacological quantities of infused 3,3',5'-triiodothyronine on thyroxine monodeiodination to 3,5,3'-triiodothyronine. Endocrinology 106, 68-75 (1980).

ALDOSTERONE SECRETION UNDER PHYSIOLOGICAL AND PATHOLOGICAL CONDITIONS

T. J. McKenna
Department of Endocrinology, St. Vincent's Hospital, Elm Park, Dublin 4, Ireland.

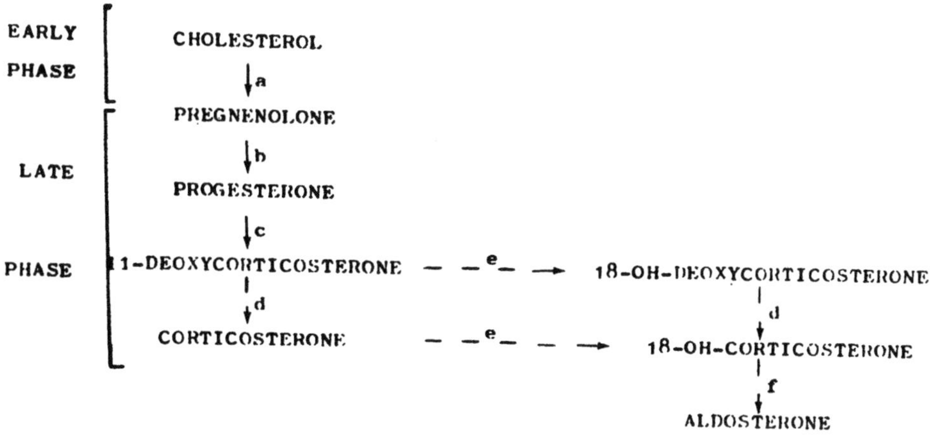

Fig. 1. Biosynthetic Pathways of Aldosterone. Letters a-f represent various enzymes controlling biosynthetic steps: a, 20-22 desmolase (side-chain cleavage); b, 3β-ol-dehydrogenase, $\Delta 4$-5 isomerase; c, 21-hydroxylase; d, 11-hydroxylase; e, 18-hydroxylase (or methyl oxidase type I); f, 18-dehydrogenase (or methyl oxidase, type II). Relative biological significance of steps indicated by broken lines has yet to be established.

Hormones in Normal and Abnormal Human Tissues, Vol. II

Introduction

Physiological Considerations

Aldosterone, the most potent naturally occurring mineralocorticoid is synthesized in the zona glomerulosa of the adrenal cortex. The biosynthetic steps to aldosterone are depicted in Figure 1. Aldosterone biosynthesis has been arbitrarily subdivided into an early phase and a late phase. The early phase of aldosterone biosynthesis is confined to the conversion of cholesterol to pregnenolone; the late phase consists of all the steps in aldosterone biosynthesis subsequent to pregnenolone production (Fig. 1). The sequence of intermediate precursors and the enzymes responsible for the biosynthetic steps from cholesterol up to and including 11-deoxycorticosterone is generally accepted (1-4) but some uncertainty surrounds the biosynthetic events subsequent to 11-deoxycorticosterone production. 11-Deoxycorticosterone may be hydroxylated to form corticosterone which is then hydroxylated at C-18. While 18-hydroxycorticosterone is secreted by the adrenal cortex its role as an obligatory precursor of aldosterone has not been established. Alternative hypotheses include a two-step mixed function oxidation of corticosterone to aldosterone (5) or conversion of 11-deoxycorticosterone to 18-hydroxy-11-deoxycorticosterone and then to 18-hydroxycorticosterone and aldosterone (6, 7). It is possible that more than one biosynthetic pathway to aldosterone may operate under physiological conditions.

Aldosterone stimulates sodium re-absorption in exchange for potassium and hydrogen ions in the distal tubule of the kidney. Aldosterone biosynthesis and secretion are predominantly influenced by the renin-angiotensin cascade. Renin is secreted by the juxtaglomerular apparatus of renal afferent arterioles and the associated macula densa (8). The stimuli may be conveyed to the afferent arterioles by changes in barometric pressure and by changes in intracellular electrolyte concentrations

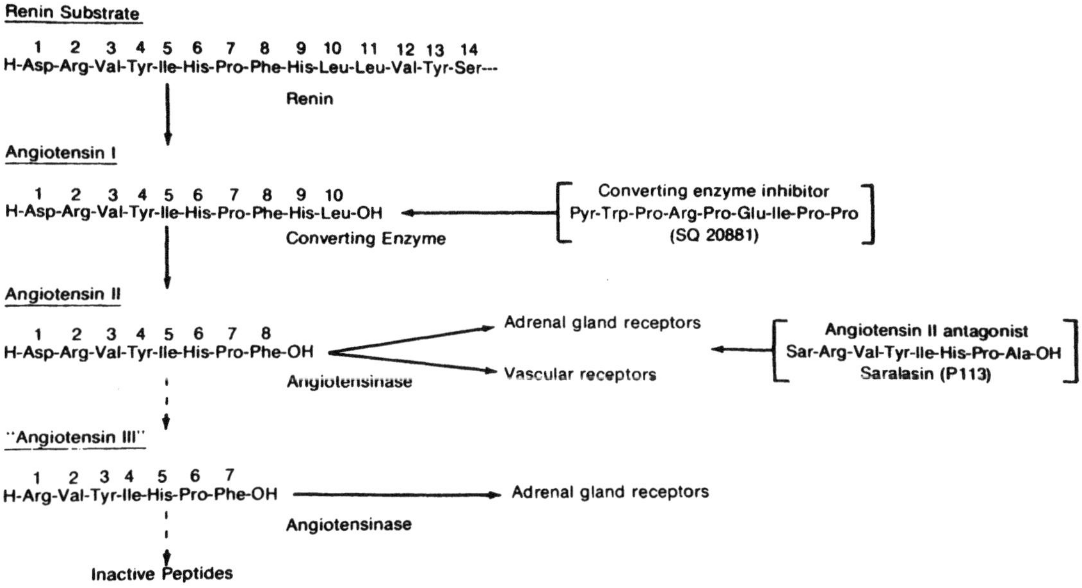

Fig. 2. The renin-angiotensin system and its effector peptides and sites of blockade. Reprinted with permission from Biglieri, 1978 (8a).

resulting in renin secretion. Renin release by the kidney is in part dependent on the integrity of the renal sympathetic nerves (8). Renin stimulates the conversion of circulating renin-substrate (angiotensinogen) to angiotensin I (Fig. 2). Angiotensin I is a decapeptide from which two amino acids are cleaved during its passage through the pulmonary circulation under the influence of the converting enzyme (Fig. 2) to produce angiotensin II. Angiotensin II has a variety of biological functions including the stimulation of intense arteriolar constriction and the stimulation of aldosterone biosynthesis (Fig. 3). The loss of another amino acid from angiotensin II yields the heptapeptide angiotensin III (Fig. 2). Angiotensin III

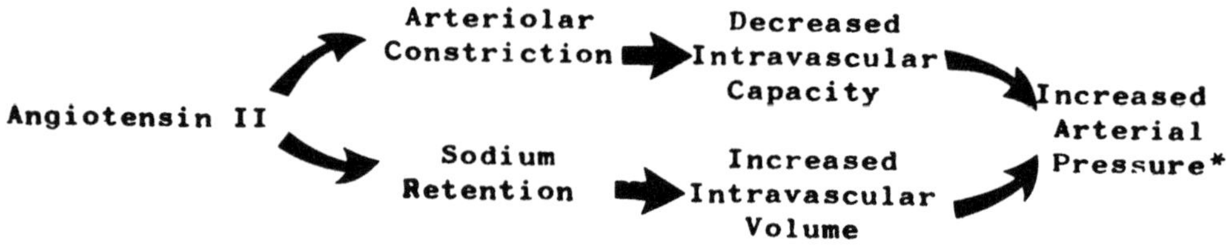

Fig. 3. The vascular and salt and water responses to angiotensin which lead to alterations in blood pressure. * Normotensin will be maintained when adequate physiological (appropriate) mechanisms operate. Hypertension may develop when non-physiological (inappropriate) mechanisms are operative.

while retaining the ability to stimulate aldosterone biosynthesis is not a potent vasoconstrictor (9).

Salt and water depletion leads to generation of angiotensins II and III which stimulate contraction of the arteriolar tree and increase conservation of sodium via the action of aldosterone, responses which maintain arterial pressure (Fig. 3). In addition to angiotensin, aldosterone biosynthesis is responsive to changes in circulating levels of potassium and ACTH. Dopamine, serotonin and catecholamines may also be involved in modulating aldosterone biosynthesis.

Angiotensin

The precise intracellular events initiated by angiotensin in glomerulosa cells is unsettled. _In vitro_ studies using glomerulosa cells have provided conflicting results suggesting that angiotensin-stimulated aldosterone biosynthesis is cyclic AMP dependent (10) or independent of nucleotide generation (11). However, extensive in vivo and in vitro evidence exists to suggest that angiotensin stimulates independently both the early and late phases of aldosterone biosynthesis. These actions of angiotensin have recently been definitively demonstrated in vitro. Chemical inhibitors of some of the enzymatic steps in aldosterone biosynthesis facilitated these studies. Trilostane, a cyanoketone derivative, inhibits the conversion of pregnenolone to progesterone. Aldosterone and pregnenolone were measured in bovine glomerulosa cells with and without the addition of angiotensin II and/or trilostane. The addition of angiotensin stimulated aldosterone biosynthesis; when angiotensin was added to trilostane-treated cells the aldosterone response was abolished while pregnenolone accumulated (12). Thus angiotensin stimulates steroidogenesis at a point prior to pregnenolone production i.e. the early phase of aldosterone biosynthesis (Table 1). However, these findings do not exclude an additional effect of angiotensin on the late phase. The late phase of aldosterone biosynthesis was examined using aminoglutethimide which inhibits the conversion of cholesterol to pregnenolone. Although aldosterone production did not increase in vitro in response to angiotensin, aldosterone was produced when precursors subsequent to cholesterol were added to aminoglutethimide-treated glomerulosa cells. Measurement of the amount of aldosterone derived from various precursors with and without the addition of angiotensin provided an index of activity in the isolated late phase of steroidogenesis. More aldosterone was derived from 11-deoxycorticosterone when angiotensin was added to the cell suspension than when it was omitted (12). These studies demonstrate that angiotensin can exert a direct stimulatory effect on the late phase of aldosterone biosynthesis (Table 1).

Sodium depletion

Sodium depletion and the associated dehydration provide intense stimuli to renin secretion and to the generation of angiotensin II. However, plasma renin activity and angiotensin levels do not

Table 1. Site of Action of Various Modulators on Aldosterone Biosynthetic Pathway

Modulators	Net Aldosterone Production	Aldosterone Biosynthesis: Early Phase	Aldosterone Biosynthesis: Late Phase
Angiotensin	*↑	↑	↑
Potassium			
0-6 mEq/l	↑	↑	↑
6-12 mEq/l	—	↑	↓
Dopamine			
Basal	—	—	—
Stimulated	↓	—	↓

*↑ Stimulated, ↓ Inhibited, — Unaffected.

correlate well with aldosterone secretion (8, 13). In addition, infusion of angiotensin into salt-depleted animals or man is associated with greater aldosterone secretion than is seen in the sodium replete state (14). These findings have stimulated a search for factors other than angiotensin which may be involved in priming aldosterone secretion in sodium deficiency. Patients with hypopituitarism and hypophysectomized animals were reported to have a blunted *in vivo* aldosterone response to salt depletion. Replacement of all known pituitary factors failed to return the aldosterone response to normal (15). However, other investigators have been unable to confirm these findings (16). Failure of angiotensin levels to correlate with aldosterone production might reflect changing sensitivity of the adrenal to angiotensin under various conditions. Angiotensin receptors have been examined in adrenal tissue obtained from salt replete and from salt deplete animals. Angiotensin receptor number and affinity were significantly influenced by the sodium content of the diet of the animals from which the adrenals were obtained (17). Increasing angiotensin receptor numbers and increased affinity of the angiotensin receptor greatly amplified the effects of angiotensin in the salt depleted state.

The renin-angiotensin system plays the dominant role in stimulating aldosterone biosynthesis in the salt depleted state. Speculation on the possible existence of unidentified aldosterone stimulators, perhaps of pituitary origin, is less justified since the recognition of the increased sensitivity of glomerulosa cells to angiotensin as a result of sodium depletion-induced changes in angiotensin receptors. Changes in serum sodium concentrations are unpredictable during salt depletion and depend upon the relative degree of associated dehydration. However hyponatraemia may stimulate aldosterone secretion directly (18).

Potassium

Increasing concentrations of potassium within the physiological range stimulate aldosterone biosynthesis (8, 13). This can be demonstrated in normal subjects *in vivo* and also *in vitro*. Indeed potassium deficiency occurring as a consequence of aldosterone excess may modify aldosterone biosynthesis. The action of potassium on aldosterone biosynthesis is probably not mediated by cyclic AMP (11) and may be mediated by changes in cell charge dependent upon transmembrane potassium flux. Similar experiments to those previously described to identify the site of action of angiotensin have been employed to examine the enzymatic steps in aldosterone biosynthesis which are influenced by increasing concentrations of potassium. When the potassium concentration in the buffer bathing glomerulosa cells *in vitro* is increased from 0 to 6 meq/l, aldosterone production increases. Treatment of glomerulosa cells with trilostane abolishes the aldosterone response to increasing concentrations of potassium but is associated with accumulation of pregnenolone (19). Therefore, increasing potassium concentrations from 0 to 6 meq/l is associated with stimulation of the early phase of aldosterone biosynthesis (Table 1). The effect of potassium on the late phase of aldosterone biosynthesis was examined by measuring the effect of increasing concentrations of potassium on the conversion of corticosterone to aldosterone in aminoglutethimide-treated cell suspensions. The amount of aldosterone derived from corticosterone increased as the potassium concentration in the cell suspension rose from 0 to 6 meq/l. In contrast, when the potassium concentration was increased from 6 to 12 meq/l net aldosterone production was not significantly altered, but pregnenolone production was markedly stimulated. Therefore, although the early phase of aldosterone biosynthesis was stimulated, aldosterone production did not increase. To explain this apparent discrepancy events in the late phase of aldosterone biosynthesis were examined. As the potassium concentration was increased from 6 to 12 meq/l, significantly less corticosterone was converted to aldosterone (Table 1).

ACTH

ACTH exerts a transient stimulatory effect on aldosterone biosynthesis that is probably mediated by cyclic AMP production (8, 13). After the initial response aldosterone production returns to basal levels although ACTH administration is continued. 17-Hydroxylase deficiency, in which cortisol biosynthesis is impaired while the biosynthetic pathway to aldosterone is intact, is associated with chronically elevated ACTH values and normal or suppressed aldosterone levels (20). In this condition

11-deoxycorticosterone accumulates. This compound has weak mineralocorticoid properties and when produced in excess, promotes salt retention with expansion of the blood volume and potassium loss. As a consequence of sodium and water retention plasma renin activity and angiotensin generation is suppressed. When glucocorticoids are used to treat the cortisol deficiency occurring in 17-hydroxylase deficiency, ACTH secretion is suppressed, deoxycorticosterone levels fall, salt and water retention are corrected and plasma renin activity and aldosterone levels increase. These findings are compatible with the hypothesis that impaired aldosterone biosynthesis in normal subjects chronically treated with ACTH, is due to suppression of angiotensin levels occurring as a consequence of salt retention. It is possible therefore that ACTH may stimulate early steps in aldosterone biosynthesis with a consequent accumulation of deoxycorticosterone since the subsequent conversion of late precursors to aldosterone is dependent on a permissive concentration of angiotensin. During chronic stimulation with ACTH the plasma volume may expand and as a consequence angiotensin levels may fall below the critical concentration required for stimulation of the late steps in aldosterone biosynthesis. However, the alternative possibility exists that the high concentrations of deoxycorticosterone observed in patients chronically stimulated with ACTH, may be derived from fasciculata cells. Since deoxycorticosterone does not provide a specific marker of the activity of the aldosterone biosynthetic pathway it is possible that neither early nor late phases of aldosterone biosynthesis are stimulated chronically by ACTH.

An alternative explanation for the transient nature of the aldosterone response to ACTH is the emergence of enzymatic defects in the final steps of aldosterone biosynthesis (21). Although deoxycorticosterone levels remain markedly elevated after 30 hours of stimulation with ACTH, corticosterone and 18-hydroxy-11-deoxycorticosterone levels fall from peak values to plateau at levels clearly above basal while aldosterone and 18-hydroxycorticosterone levels return to basal values. These findings suggest a decreased activity of 11- and 18-hydroxylations in the aldosterone biosynthetic pathway. However the origin of 11-deoxycorticosterone and 18-hydroxy-11-deoxycorticosterone has not been established and these steroids may be derived from zona fasciculata. Therefore, while the foregoing observations are compatible with suppression of enzymatic activity in the final portion of the late phase of aldosterone biosynthesis, this explanation awaits definitive proof.

Another possible explanation has been suggested by a recent morphological study of adrenal architecture before and after stimulation of sheep with ACTH (22). The width of the zona glomerulosa decreases during stimulation with ACTH while an increase in the number of cells with characteristics intermediate between glomerulosa and fasciculata cells occurs. These cells may be transitional. It is possible therefore, that ACTH stimulates conversion of the aldosterone-producing glomerulosa cell into another type of cell which loses the capacity to secrete aldosterone and perhaps acquires 17-hydroxylase activity which will facilitate cortisol biosynthesis. Thus, the number of cells capable of secreting cortisol may increase and aldosterone-secreting cells may decrease in number during sustained adrenal stimulation with ACTH and this may account for the transient nature of the aldosterone response.

Dopamine and other neurogenic amines

The observation that patients treated with bromocryptine, a dopaminergic agonist, developed symptomatology suggestive of mineralocorticoid deficiency lead to examination of the effect of the drug on aldosterone levels in normal subjects. The aldosterone response to diuresis was blunted during bromocryptine administration (23). Aldosterone levels are elevated during administration of the dopamine antagonist, metoclopromide (24) and this effect could be inhibited by simultaneous administration of dopamine (25). Administration of bromocryptine to patients with primary aldosteronism proved to be beneficial particularly for patients with bilateral adrenal hyperplasia (26). In addition, Kuchel et al. (27) made the intriguing observation that two patients with fluctuating primary aldosteronism demonstrated inverse relationships between plasma dopamine and aldosterone levels. The effect of dopamine might be to interfere with the renin-angiotensin cascade or with the action of potassium or ACTH on aldosterone biosynthesis, and dopamine might directly affect one or more of the enzymes involved in aldosterone biosynthesis. It is also possible that dopamine influences aldosterone biosynthesis only indirectly; prolactin was suggested as a possible mediator of the dopamine effect. Alternatively, non-dopamine related properties of bromocryptine and metaclopromide may have been responsible for the effects of the drugs on aldosterone secretion. To examine some of these possibilities, aldosterone production was measured in glomerulosa cells *in vitro* under basal conditions and during stimulation with angiotensin, with and without the addition of dopamine (28). Basal aldosterone biosynthesis was not affected by dopamine but the aldosterone response to angiotensin was markedly blunted. Dopamine did not affect the early phase of aldosterone biosynthesis nor the conversion of deoxycorticosterone to aldosterone under basal conditions. However, the stimulatory effect of angiotensin on the conversion of deoxycorticosterone to aldosterone was almost entirely blocked by dopamine (Table 1). These findings suggest that dopamine *in vitro* has a highly specific effect on aldosterone biosynthesis. Although these observations provide a basis for speculation, the role of dopamine *in vivo* in the physiological or pathological modulation of aldosterone biosynthesis remains to be established. However, changes in aldosterone levels in man treated with dopaminergic agonists and antagonists support the concept that dopamine exerts an inhibitory influence on aldosterone biosynthesis in normal subjects.

Preliminary *in vitro* studies have examined the possibility that neurogenic amines other than dopamine might be involved in the control of aldosterone secretion (29). These studies showed stimulatory effects of both epinephrine and norepinephrine on aldosterone biosynthesis in bovine glomerulosa cells. Other *in vivo* observations have been attributed to the effect of catecholamines on renin release (30-32). Specific α- and β- sympathetic receptor agonists also proved stimulatory; although α- and β- sympathetic antagonists blocked these effects, the actions were not entirely specific. The possible physiological implications for the role of catecholamines in aldosterone biosynthesis remain speculative.

Serotonin

Serotonin will stimulate aldosterone biosynthesis (2, 33). Serotonin agonists and antagonists have predictable effects on aldosterone production *in vitro* and *in vivo* (34, 35). It has been suggested that the inhibitory effect of bromocryptine on aldosterone biosynthesis is dependent upon anti-serotonin properties of the agent (33). While not entirely excluding the possibility, the observation that dopamine inhibits the effect of bromocryptine suggests that the drug is not acting through a serotonin-dependent mechanism (25). However a role for serotonin in the physiological control of aldosterone secretion in man has not been definitively proven. *In vivo* experiments suggest that histamine may also directly stimulate aldosterone biosynthesis (36).

Pathological Considerations

Hyperaldosteronism

Primary aldosteronism

Primary aldosteronism (37, 38) is characterized by the secretion of aldosterone in excess of physiological requirements in the absence of any identified stimulus. Primary aldosteronism is associated with a unilateral adrenal adenoma in approximately 70% of affected patients while the remaining 30% are almost all accounted for by bilateral adrenal hyperplasia. Adenocarcinoma of the adrenal is a very rare cause of primary aldosteronism. Unilateral adenoma or adenocarcinoma probably arises as a consequence of an isolated event occurring in a glomerulosa cell during mitosis which leads to the assumption of neoplastic characteristics by progeny cells. However, the occurrence of bilateral disease suggests either a congenital abnormality or the presence of a circulating stimulator of glomerulosa cells. The onset of the disorder in adulthood and the absence of a familial pattern in patients with idiopathic bilateral adrenal hyperplasia argues against a congenital disorder. Interesting observations bearing on the possible presence of an adrenal stimulator have been made using sheep with their adrenal glands autotransplanted into their necks. Blood from patients with either tumourous or hyperplastic primary aldosteronism was injected into the artery supplying the adrenal (39). While aldosterone secretion in the sheep was indifferent to serum from patients with tumourous disease, a stimulatory effect was exerted by serum from patients with adrenal hyperplasia. Differences in angiotensin, potassium or ACTH concentrations in the two types of sera could not explain the aldosterone-stimulating properties of sera from patients with hyperplastic disease. These observations suggest the existence of an unidentified stimulator of aldosterone biosynthesis in at least some patients with idiopathic adrenal hyperplasia. The control of aldosterone secretion in patients with tumours and with hyperplastic primary aldosteronism demonstrates a number of characteristic differences. Patients with tumourous disease show a diurnal rhythm in aldosterone levels while this is absent in patients with bilateral disease. After early morning blood sampling in the recumbent position, patients with hyperplastic disease maintained upright will show a further elevation in aldosterone levels during the day while patients with tumourous disease demonstrate a lowering of aldosterone levels (40). In addition, patients with tumourous disease show a transient suppression of aldosterone levels after administration of glucocorticoids (41). Differences in the responsiveness of aldosterone secretion to stimulation also exist in the two disorders. After infusion of angiotensin II, patients with hyperplastic disease showed a marked elevation in blood aldosterone levels while normal subjects showed a lesser response (42) and patients with tumourous primary aldosteronism did not respond (43).

Low renin essential hypertension may be related to idiopathic adrenal hyperplasia. Both disorders are characterized by hypertension and suppressed plasma renin activity (44, 45). They differ however, in that aldosterone production is elevated beyond the range seen in normal subjects and hypokalaemia is present in patients with primary aldosteronism but not in patients with low renin essential hypertension. However, aldosterone production appears to be inappropriately elevated for the simultaneous angiotensin levels in low renin essential hypertension (44, 46). When plasma renin activity is suppressed by salt loading in normal subjects to values seen in patients with low renin essential hypertension, the associated aldosterone levels are lower in the normal subjects. In addition, patients with low renin essential hypertension also demonstrate increased sensitivity to stimulation with angiotensin or ACTH (47). These observations suggest that inappropriate aldosterone production may be of pathogenetic significance in low renin essential hypertension.

The meaning of these various observations is as yet unclear. Hyperplastic primary aldosteronism may be related to the presence of a stimulator of aldosterone biosynthesis so that the adrenals are abnormally primed to respond excessively to some or all stimuli. Since aldosterone secretion in hyperplastic primary aldosteronism appears to be enhanced by upright stance, the putative unidentified stimulator may respond in a manner that would be predicted for angiotensin in normal subjects. The possibility exists that increased sensitivity to minor changes in angiotensin levels may account for the hyperplastic disorder. Such changes might be brought about by alteration in the number and affinity of angiotensin receptors as probably occurs normally in salt depletion (17) or by decreased dopaminergic activity in the adrenal (24, 25). Similar but less fully developed abnormalities may explain the pathogenesis of low renin essential hypertension. A possible role for ACTH in tumourous adrenal hyperplasia is suggested by the presence of a diurnal rhythm of aldosterone similar to that of cortisol and by the suppressive effect of dexamethasone on aldosterone secretion. However, the inhibitory effect of glucocorticoids is only transitory and aldosterone secretion returns to pretreatment levels while ACTH levels are suppressed. These observations suggest that while ACTH may modify aldosterone secretion from adrenal tumours acutely, ACTH is not essential for secretion of the mineralocorticoid.

In summary, while intriguing similarities and differences in aldosterone secretion exist in patients with primary aldosteronism of tumourous and hyperplastic origin and in patients with low renin essential hypertension, a full understanding of the regulatory mechanisms underlying these disorders has not yet been elucidated.

Secondary aldosteronism

Secondary aldosteronism is characterized by hypersecretion of aldosterone in response to a definable stimulus, usually angiotensin (48). Secondary aldosteronism may be appropriate e.g. in patients with salt and water deficiency or with a contracted intravascular volume, or inappropriate e.g. in patients with renal artery stenosis or a renin secreting tumour. The physiological importance of the renin-angiotensin-aldosterone system lies in its ability to protect the organism from salt and water depletion. Renin release is stimulated during sodium deprivation and consequently aldosterone secretion increases (Fig. 4). Aldosterone then stimulates sodium reabsorption by the distal tubule in the kidney. Therefore, elevations of plasma renin activity, angiotensin levels and aldosterone secretion i.e. secondary aldosteronism, function as an effective regulator of

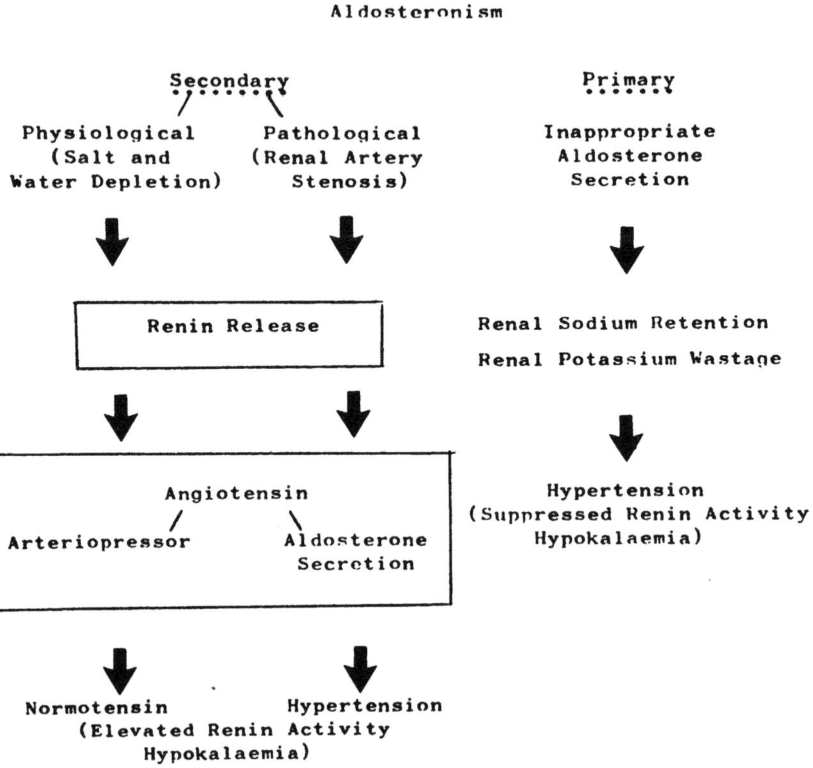

Fig. 4. Schematic comparisons of mechanisms and results in aldosteronism, primary (always pathological) and secondary (physiological and pathological).

salt and water metabolism. However, in oedematous states the organism may not be deficient in salt and water but in these circumstances there is an intense stimulus to the renin-angiotensin-aldosterone system. While this response is appropriate, the attempt to correct for a contracted effective blood volume is frustrated by leakage of retained salt and water from the vascular tree; the intra-arterial blood volume is virtually unchanged but oedema formation increases.

In patients with stenosis affecting a renal artery or one of its branches, that part of the renal parenchyma distal to the arterial blockage perceives the reduced local perfusion as a signal of a generalized reduction in tissue perfusion. In an attempt to correct for this, renin is released from the hypoperfused renal tissue which then stimulates aldosterone biosynthesis via generation of angiotensin. Salt and water are retained, causing an expansion in the intravascular volume. As well as stimulating aldosterone biosynthesis angiotensin exerts a profound arterioconstrictor effect (Fig. 3). The combination of expanding the intravascular volume and contracting the capacity of the vascular tree may lead to variable degrees of hypertension (49, 50). The recognition of renal artery stenosis as a frequent cause of "curable" hypertension has made a significant contribution to the treatment of this common disorder. A much rarer disorder, renin-secreting renal tumours, also produces hypertension by a similar mechanism. In addition to renal tumours, renin is secreted from paragangliomas which are generally seen in children (51).

Bartter's syndrome is characterized by excessive prostaglandin biosynthesis in the kidney which is intimately related to renal salt loss, hyperreninaemia, aldosteronism and hypokalaemia (51, 53). Disabling muscle weakness occurring as a consequence of potassium deficiency is frequently the clinical feature which brings affected patients to medical attention. The precise interrelationships between prostaglandin biosynthesis, renal sodium loss and hyperreninaemia have not been definitely established. Prostaglandin synthetase inhibitors when administered lead to correction of all the clinical features of the syndrome. The attractive hypothesis that excessive prostaglandin biosynthesis results in salt loss and that hyperreninaemia occurs as a consequence of this is not supported by the observation that saline infusion fails to correct the hyperaldosteronism (53). Prior to the recognition of the role of prostaglandin in this disorder, treatment consisted of potassium supplementation and the administration of spironolactone.

Scattered case reports suggest that administration of agents which block sympathetic β-receptors lead to reduced renin secretion, to decreased secondary aldosteronism and to partial correction of hypokalaemia.

Aldosteronism, primary or secondary, is associated with kaliuresis. This leads to hypokalaemia and a total body deficiency of potassium. Potassium deficiency decreases aldosterone biosynthesis. The full expression of aldosteronism may be modified by potassium deficiency. When potassium deficiency is profound in primary aldosteronism, aldosterone production may fall into the normal range. Only when the deficiency of potassium is corrected will the supraphysiological production of aldosterone become fully re-established (52).

Some inhibitors of angiotensin activity are available. Saralasin, an analogue of angiotensin (Fig. 2), has modest agonist properties and competitively inhibits the effect of angiotensin II on its receptor (54). When saralasin is administered to patients with secondary aldosteronism the action of angiotensin is inhibited and blood pressure levels fall (55). However, when saralasin is administered to patients with suppressed angiotensin levels e.g. primary aldosteronism, the antagonist properties of angiotensin cannot be expressed and only the agonist properties are observed. Therefore, in hypertensive patients with suppressed endogenous angiotensin levels saralasin may cause a further rise in blood pressure (56). These responses not only distinguish between the two types of aldosteronism, but they also predict those patients in whom correction of angiotensin excess will lead to a significant reduction in blood pressure levels (55, 57).

Tumourous primary aldosteronism is best treated by removal of the affected adrenal gland (58). Adrenalectomy probably has no role to play in the treatment of bilateral adrenal hyperplasia; even after total bilateral adrenalectomy hypertension may persist although hypokalaemia is corrected (58). Primary aldosteronism due to idiopathic adrenal hyperplasia or tumourous disease not amenable to surgery, is probably best treated with the mineralocorticoid antagonist spironolactone (58). However this agent is not entirely specific and as well as competing for the aldosterone receptor, spironolactone may impair enzymes involved in steroid biosynthesis. This may lead to feminization with the development of gynaecomastia and to impotence in males or to menstrual disorders in females. Other diuretics may be useful but may lead to the development of profound hypokalaemia. When diuretics are used in the treatment of primary aldosteronism additional potassium supplements should be supplied. An alternative method of medical treatment is the use of drugs which inhibit aldosterone biosynthesis. Aminoglutethimide (59), trilostane (60) (see above) and metyrapone which inhibits 11-hydroxylase activity, have all been used with some success. The problem related to the use of many of these agents is the emergence of unpleasant side-effects and the necessity of using multiple doses during a day in order to achieve an adequate effect. As a consequence of these problems the drugs which inhibit aldosterone biosynthesis are not suitable for the indefinite treatment of primary aldosteronism except in very unusual circumstances.

Secondary hyperaldosteronism is best treated by correcting the underlying disorder e.g. congestive heart failure, renal artery stenosis. However this is not always possible and less definitive treatment may be useful. Inhibitors of the converting enzyme necessary for the conversion of angiotensin I to angiotensin II (Fig. 2) have been developed (61). One of these, captopril, is effective when administered orally and when it is used therapeutically angiotensin II-dependent hypertension can be corrected and aldosterone secretion decreased (62). Early reports on the use of captopril suggest that it or similar agents will play a significant role in the management of hypertension in the future.

Aldosterone Deficiency

Total destruction of the adrenal gland as occurs in patients with idiopathic Addison's disease will not be considered here. This review will be confined to those pathological situations in which aldosterone deficiency occurs as an isolated abnormality (Table 2).

Table 2. Aldosterone Deficiency

1. **Global Adrenal Cortical Failure**

   (Antibody-mediated Addison's Disease, tuberculosis etc.)

2. **Isolated Aldosterone Deficiency**

   i. **Hyporeninaemic Hypoaldosteronism**

   ii. **Congenital aldosterone biosynthetic defects in activity of methyl oxidase reactions Types 1 or 2.**

   iii. **Pseudohypoaldosteronism (tissue insensitivity to aldosterone**

Hyporeninaemic hypoaldosteronism

Under certain conditions the juxtaglomerular apparatus appears to lose its capacity to secrete renin. This is seen mainly in older patients, in patients with moderate degrees of renal impairment, and in patients with diabetes mellitus (63, 64). The disorder is probably most common in older diabetic patients with some limitation of renal function. Changes in the small vasculature of the kidney occurring with increasing years may disturb the functioning of the juxtaglomerular apparatus and the macula densa. Primary parenchymal renal disease may also disrupt the activity of these structures. Normal renin secretion can be stimulated by the sympathetic nervous system. In patients with sympathetic neuropathy this stimulatory effect may be removed. As a consequence of all these changes the physiological renin-angiotensin-aldosterone response to salt and water deprivation is blunted and relative or absolute aldosterone deficiency may become manifest. Postural hypotension associated with hyperkalaemia and hyponatraemia provide the clinical setting of mineralocorticoid deficiency. The diagnosis of this disorder is made by demonstrating suppressed renin and aldosterone levels in patients with a reduced blood volume and/or by failure of an adequate renin-angiotensin-aldosterone response to diuresis. The diagnosis of hyporeninaemic hypoaldosteronism will be confirmed by correction of the clinical disorder by administration of a mineralocorticoid. However, it has been noted that patients with hyporeninaemic hypoaldosteronism may require larger doses of mineralocorticoids than those for patients with other forms of mineralocorticoid deficiency (65). A possible explanation for this finding is damage to the distal renal tubules and to the renin-secreting tissues in the kidney. The kidney therefore may lose the normal capacity to secrete renin and to respond to mineralocorticoid replacement.

The aldosterone response to infusion of angiotensin II is blunted in diabetic patients with hyporeninaemic hypoaldosteronism (66, 67). This intriguing observation has been further characterized by the demonstration of an apparent defect in the late steps of aldosterone biosynthesis in these patients i.e. decreased 18-dehydrogenase activity (methyl oxidase type II reaction). This finding may be explained by slow induction of enzymes involved in the late phase of aldosterone biosynthesis when the pathway is re-stimulated. When angiotensin is infused into normal subjects the aldosterone biosynthetic pathway may be primed by endogenous angiotensin; in contrast, aldosterone biosynthesis will not be primed in this way in patients with hyporeninaemic hypoaldosteronism and therefore a different response to exogenous angiotensin may be seen in the two groups.

It is possible that if stimulation with angiotensin had been maintained for several days the apparent enzymatic defect in aldosterone biosynthesis would not have been detectable. An analogous situation was observed when supraphysiological amounts of ACTH were administered over ten days to a normal subject (68). Cortisol levels increased steadily until a plateau was reached after 8 days but the levels of pregnenolone and 17-hydroxypregnenolone rose early and then fell towards basal values after about 7 days. These observations suggested that the intra-adrenal utilization of pregnenolone and 17-hydroxypregnenolone increased with continuing exposure of the biosynthetic pathway to ACTH and this resulted in more efficient cortisol biosynthesis. Alternatively it is tempting to speculate that sympathetic neuropathy, presumably affecting the renin-secreting tissues in the kidney, may also affect aldosterone secreting cells in the adrenal. Since the inhibitory effect of dopamine is specifically exerted on the late phase of aldosterone biosynthesis (28) one might speculate that catecholamines exert their stimulatory effect (29) at the same point. Since the glomerulosa cells are intimately attached to the adrenal capsule it is possible that the capsular sympathetic neurons may be a source of catecholamines which then modulate aldosterone biosynthesis. Based on these assumptions sympathetic neuropathy would deprive the late phase of aldosterone biosynthesis of the stimulatory effect of catecholamines. Angiotensin-stimulated aldosterone precursors would then accumulate at a point prior to the catecholamine-sensitive enzymatic steps e.g. methyl oxidase type 2. If this hypothesis is correct the acquired "enzymatic" defect in aldosterone biosynthesis and the failure to generate renin are due to a common abnormality in diabetic patients with hyporeninaemic hypoaldosteronism i.e. sympathetic neuropathy.

Some patients may have only limited responsiveness of the renin-angiotensin-aldosterone system. Under normal conditions aldosterone biosynthesis may be adequate to meet physiological requirements but increasing the demands may lead to decompensation. The author has seen a patient who enjoyed good health until symptomatology of thyrotoxicosis became evident. At that time atrial fibrillation was present and treatment with propranolol and carbimazole was initiated. The patient developed mineralocorticoid deficiency with hypotension, hyponatraemia, and hyperkalaemia. Plasma renin activity and aldosterone levels were markedly suppressed and failed to respond to diuresis. Treatment with propranolol was discontinued and fludrocortisone and saline were administered. The patient's clinical condition improved rapidly. These findings suggest that this patient had a modest impairment in renin production which was further diminished by treatment with propranolol. In addition, increased metabolic clearance of aldosterone while thyrotoxic contributed to this patient's mineralocorticoid deficiency (69). When the euthyroid status was re-established, treatment with mineralocorticoid was no longer necessary.

Congenital enzymatic defects in aldosterone biosynthesis

18-Hydroxylation and 18-dehydrogenation or their equivalent, methyl oxidase reactions types I and II respectively, are uniquely involved in aldosterone biosynthesis (5). Although 18-hydroxylase activity is present in fasciculata cells, the importance of any 18-hydroxylated compounds from these cells has not been appreciated. Congenital deficiencies in these enzamatic activities are only very rarely encountered. Impaired methyl oxidase type II activity is characterized by accumulation of corticosterone and 18-hydroxycorticosterone while aldosterone blood levels are low. In patients with type I defects both 18-hydroxycorticosterone and aldosterone are present in very low concentrations but corticosterone accumulates (70, 71). As a result of these defects in aldosterone biosynthesis salt and water deficiency and hyperkalaemia occur while plasma renin activity and angiotensin levels are markedly elevated. The affected child develops a state of vascular collapse soon after birth and administration of saline and mineralocorticoids proves life-saving.

Enzymatic defects of the 21-hydroxylase, 11-hydroxylase and 3β-OL-dehydrogenase, Δ4-5 isomerase systems are more common than the isolated enzymatic defects of aldosterone biosynthesis. However, in the former both cortisol and aldosterone biosynthesis is impaired (72). Contrary to previous practice whereby mineralocorticoid replacement was withheld after the very early years, it is now clearly established that treatment of affected individuals should include both glucocorticoids and mineralocorticoids throughout life (73, 74).

Pseudohypoaldosteronism

This very rare disorder is characterised by congenital insensitivity of the distal renal tubule to aldosterone (75, 76). Although the renin-angiotensin-aldosterone system is normal, aldosterone receptors are absent from, or defective in, the renal tubule. Affected children present the same clinical features as those with enzymatic defects. They differ however in that circulating aldosterone levels are markedly elevated in patients with pseudohypoaldosteronism while aldosterone levels are very low in patients with enzymatic defects. Administration of mineralocorticoids will prove ineffective in patients with pseudohypoaldosteronism whose tissues are insensitive to the steroids but they respond to the administration of a high salt diet.

References

1. Samuels, L.T., Uchikawa, T.: Biosynthesis of adrenal steroids. In: "The Adrenal Cortex", Ed. Eisenstein, A.B., Little Brown and Company, Boston, pp. 61-102 (1967).

2. Muller, J.: Factors directly influencing aldosterone biosynthesis in short-term incubation or perfusion experiments. In: "Regulation of Aldosterone Biosynthesis", Springer Verlag Berlin, pp. 11-47 (1971).

3. Ross, E.J.: Biosynthesis and metabolism. In: "Aldosterone and Aldosteronism", Lloyd-Luke Ltd., London, pp. 10-52 (1975).

4. Simpson, E.R., Mason, J.I.: Molecular aspects of the biosynthesis of adrenal steroids. Pharmac. Therap. B. 2, 339-369 (1976).

5. Ulick, S.: Diagnosis and nomenclature of the disorders of the terminal portion of the aldosterone biosynthetic pathway. J. clin. Endocrinol. Metab. 43, 92-96 (1976).

6. Wettstein, A., Kahnt, F.W., Neher, R.: The biosynthesis of aldosterone (electrocortin) in the adrenal. Ciba Found. Coll. Endocr. 8, 170-188 (1955).

7. Muller, J.: Alternate biosynthetic pathway to aldosterone through 18-OH-DOC: influence of precursor concentration and of sodium and potassium status. In: "Programme, 6th International Congress of Endocrinology" Melbourne, p. 403 (1980).

8. Davis, J.O.: Regulation of aldosterone secretion. In: "Handbook of Physiology", Section 7: Endocrinology, vol. 6, Eds. Blaschko, H., Sayers, G., Smith, A.S., American Physiological Society, Washington, pp. 77-106 (1975).

8a. Biglieri, E.: Aldosterone and the renin-angiotensin system. In: "The Year in Endocrinology 1977", Ed. Ingbar, S.H., Plenum Medical Book Co., New York, pp. 191-204 (1978).

9. Kono, T., Oseko, F., Ikeda, F., Nanno, M., Endo, J.: Biological activity of des-asp ileu^8-angiotensin II (ileu^8-angiotensin III) in man. J. clin. Endocrinol. Metab. 43, 940-943 (1976).

10. Peytremann, A., Nicholson, W.E., Brown, R.D., Liddle, G.W., Hardman, J.G.: Comparative effects of angiotensin and ACTH on cyclic AMP and steroidogenesis in isolated bovine adrenal cells. J. clin. Invest. 52, 835-842 (1973).

11. Fujita, K., Aguilera, C., Catt, K.J.: Role of cyclic AMP in aldosterone production by isolated zona glomerulosa cells. J. biol. Chem. 254, 8567-8574 (1978).

12. McKenna, T.J., Island, D.P., Nicholson, W.E., Liddle, G.W.: Angiotensin stimulates both early and late steps in aldosterone biosynthesis in isolated bovine glomerulosa cells. J. Steroid Biochem. 9, 967-972 (1978).

13. Ross, E.J.: The control of aldosterone secretion. In: "Aldosterone and Aldosteronism", Lloyd-Luke Ltd., London, pp. 144-191 (1975).

14. Frazer, R., Buckingham, J.C., Mason, P.A., Semple, P.F.: The influence of sodium, ACTH and angiotensin II on plasma corticosteroids in man: some applications in the control of corticosteroid biosynthesis. In: "The Endocrine Control of The Human Adrenal Cortex", Eds. James, V.H.T., Serio, M., Giusti, G., Martini, L., Academic Press, London, pp. 359-374 (1978).

15. McCaa, R.E., Montalvo, J.M., McCaa, C.S.: Role of growth hormone in the regulation of aldosterone biosynthesis. J. clin. Endocrinol. Metab. 46, 247-253 (1978).

16. Seifert, C., Oelkers, W.: Aldosterone stimulation by angiotensin II in patients with hypopituitarism before and after sodium depletion. In: "Programme, Sixth International Congress of Endocrinology" Melbourne, p. 408 (1980).

17. Catt, K.J., Aguilera, G., Capponi, A., Fujita, K., Schirar, A., Fakunding, J.: Angiotensin receptors and aldosterone secretion. J. Endocrinol. 81, 37P-48P (1979).

18. Davis, J.O., Urquhart, J., Higgins, J.T.Jr.: The effects of alteration of plasma sodium and potassium concentration on aldosterone secretion. J. clin. Invest. 42, 597-609 (1963).

19. McKenna, T.J., Island, D.P., Nicholson, W.E., Liddle, G.W.: The effects of potassium on early and late steps in aldosterone biosynthesis in cells of the zona glomerulosa. Endocrinology 103, 1411-1416 (1978).

20. Biglieri, E.: A perspective on aldosterone abnormalities. Clin. Endocr. 5, 399-410 (1976).

21. Biglieri, E.G., Schambelan, M., Rost, C.R.: A mechanism for the selective inhibition of corticosterone, 18-hydroxycorticosterone, aldosterone and 18-hydroxydeoxycorticosterone by ACTH. In: "Programme, Sixth International Congress of Endocrinology" Melbourne, p. 538 (1980).

22. McDougall, J.G., Butkus, A., Coghlan, J.P., Denton, D.A., Muller, J., Oddie, C.J., Robinson, P.M., Scoggins, B.A.: Effect of ACTH on the biochemistry and morphology of the sheep adrenal cortex. In: "Programme, Sixth International Congress of Endocrinology" Melbourne, p. 629 (1980).

23. Edwards, C.R.W., Miall, P.A., Hanker, J.P., Thorner, M.O., Al-Dufaili, E.A.S., Besser, G.M.: Inhibition of the plasma-aldosterone response to frusemide by bromocriptine. Lancet 2, 903-904 (1975).

24. Norbiato, G., Becilacqua, M., Raggi, U., Micossi, P., Moroni, C.: Metaclopramide increases plasma aldosterone concentration in man. J. clin. Endocrinol. Metab. 45, 1313-1316 (1977).

25. Noth, R.H., McCallum, R.W., Contino, C., Havelick, J.: Tonic dopaminergic suppression of aldosterone in man. Clin. Res. 27, 574A (1979).

26. Mantero, F., Gion, M., Aramanini, D., Opocher, G.: Effect of bromocriptine on plasma aldosterone in primary aldosteronism. Acta Endocrinol. 85 (Suppl. 212) 94 (1977).

27. Kuchel, O., Burn, N.T., Nowaczynski, W., Genest, J.: Episodic primary aldosteronism: a periodic escape from the dopaminergic inhibition of aldosterone. Clin. Res. 27, 505A (1979).

28. McKenna, T.J., Island, D.P., Nicholson, W.E., Liddle, G.W.: Dopamine inhibits angiotensin-stimulated aldosterone biosynthesis in bovine adrenal cells. J. clin. Invest. 64, 287-291 (1979).

29. McKenna, T.J., Island, D.P., Nicholson, W.E., Liddle, G.W.: Stimulation of aldosterone production by catecholamines _in vitro_. In: "Programme, Sixth International Congress of Endocrinology" Melbourne, p. 407 (1980).

30. Laragh, J.H., Anders, M., Kelly, W.G., Lieberman, S.: Hypotensive agents and suppressor substances. The effect of epinephrine, norepinephrine, angiotensin II and others on the secretory rate of aldosterone in man. J. Amer. med. Ass. 174, 234-240 (1960).

31. Gordon, R.D., Kuchel, O., Liddle, G.W., Island, D.P.: Role of the sympathetic nervous system in regulating renin and aldosterone production in man. J. clin. Invest. 46, 599-605 (1967).

32. Michelakis, A.M., Horton, R.: Relationship between plasma renin and aldosterone in normal man. Circulat. Res. 27, (suppl. 1) 185-194 (1970).

33. Mantero, F., Opocher, G., Armanini, D., Boscaro, M., Edwards, C.W.: Effect of serotonin on plasma aldosterone in man. Acta Endocrinol. 225, 345S (1979).

34. Espiner, E.A., Al-Dufaili, E.A.S., Martin, V.I., Edwards, C.R.W.: Indolamines stimulate steroidogenesis in isolated human adrenal cells. In: "Programme, Sixth International Congress of Endocrinology" Melbourne, p. 506 (1980).

35. Mantero, F., Boscaro, M., Opocher, G., Armanini. D., Edwards, C.R.W.: In vitro and in vivo effect of metergoline on aldosterone secretion. In: "Programme, Sixth Internatio-nal Congress of Endocrinology" Melbourne, p. 405 (1980).

36. Aikawa, T., Hirose, T., Matsumoto, I., Suzuki, T.: Secretion of aldosterone in response to histamine in hypophysectomized-nephrectomized dogs. J. Endocrinol. 81, 325-330 (1979).

37. Ross, E.J.: Syndromes of mineralocorticoid excess. In: "Aldosterone and Aldosteronism", Lloyd-Luke Ltd., London, pp. 208-260 (1975).

38. Edmonds, C.J.: Aldosterone secretion and its clinical disorders. In: "General Comparative and Clinical Endocrinology of The Adrenal Cortex", vol. 2, Eds. Jones, I.C., Henderson, I.W., Academic Press, London, pp. 565-599 (1978).

39. Nicholls, M.G., Espiner, E.A., Hughes, H., Ross, J., Stewart, D.T.: Primary aldosteronism: study and contrasts. Amer. J. Med. 59, 334-343 (1975).

40. Luetscher, J.A., Ganguly, A., Malada, G.A., Dowdy, A.J.: Pre-operative differentiation of adrenal adenoma from idiopathic adrenal hyperplasia in primary aldosteronism. Circulat. Res. (Suppl. 1) 34-35, 1175-1182 (1974).

41. Kem, D.C., Weinberger, M.H., Gomez-Sanchez, C., Kramer, M.J., Larmen, R., Furuyama, S., Nugent, C.A.: Circadian rhythm of plasma aldosterone concentration in patients with primary aldosteronism. J. clin. Invest. 52, 2272-2277 (1973).

42. Wisgerhof, M., Carpenter, P.C., Brown, R.B.: Increased adrenal sensitivity to angiotensin II in idiopathic hyperaldosteronism. J. clin. Endocrinol. Metab. 47, 938-943 (1978).

43. Slaton, P.E., Jr., Schambelan, M., Biglieri, E.G.: Stimulation and suppression of aldosterone secretion in patients with an aldosterone producing adenoma. J. clin. Endocrinol. Metab. 29, 239-250 (1969).

44. Luetscher, J.A., Ganguly, A., Malada, G.A., Dowdy, A.J.: Abnormal regulation of aldosterone in hypertension. Advances in Internal Medicine 20, 183-196 (1975).

45. Gunnells, J.C.Jr., McGuffin, W.L.: Low renin hypertension. Annual Review of Medicine 26, 259-275 (1975).

46. Grim, C., Winnacker, J., Peters, T., Gilbert, G.: Low renin, "normal" aldosterone and hypertension: circadian rhythm of renin, aldosterone, cortisol and growth hormone. J. clin. Endocrinol. Metab. 39, 247-256 (1974).

47. Wisgerhof, M., Brown, R.D.: Increased adrenal sensitivity to angiotensin II in low-renin essential hypertension. J. clin. Invest. 61, 1456-1462 (1978).

48. Ross, E.J.: Secondary aldosteronism. In: "Aldosterone and Aldosteronism", Lloyd-Luke Medical Books Ltd., London, pp. 261-295 (1975).

49. Laragh, J.H.: The renin-aldosterone axis and blood pressure homeostasis. In: "Textbook of Endocrinology", Ed. Williams, R.H., W.B. Saunders Co., Philadelphia, pp. 948-962 (1974).

50. Biglieri, E.G.: Renin-angiotensin-aldosterone. In: "Contemporary Endocrinology" Vol. 1, Ed. Ingbar, S.H., Plenum Medical Book Company, New York, pp. 233-243 (1979).

51. Ehrlich, E.N.: Adrenal cortical regulation of salt and water metabolism. In: "Endocrinology" Vol. 3, Eds. DeGroot, L.J., Cahill, G.F., Martini, L., Nelson, D.H., Odell, W.D., Potts, J.T., Steinberger, E., Winegrad, A.I., Grune and Stratton, New York, pp. 1883-1909 (1979).

52. Biglieri, E.G., Forsham, P.H.: Studies on the expanded extracellular fluid and the responses to various stimuli to primary aldosteronism. Amer. J. Med. 30, 564-576 (1961).

53. Bartter, F.C., Gill, J.R.Jr., Frolich, J.C., Boden, R.E., Hollifield, J.W., Radfar, N., Keiser, H.R., Oates, J.A., Seyberth, H., Taylor, A.A.: Prostaglandins are over produced by the kidneys and mediate hyperreninaemia in Bartter's syndrome. Trans. Ass. Amer. Phycns. 89, 77-91 (1976).

54. Pals, D.T., Masucci, F.D., Sipos, F., Denning, G.S.: A specific competitive antagonist of the vascular action of angiotensin II. Circulat. Res. 29, 664-672 (1971).

55. Wilson, H.M., Wilson, J.P., Slaton, P.E., Foster, J.H., Liddle, G.W., Hollifield, J.W.: Saralasin infusion in the recognition of renovascular hypertension. Ann. intern. Med. 87, 36-42 (1977).

56. Streeten, D.H.P., Anderson, G.H. Jr., Delakos, T.G.: Angiotensin blockade: Its clinical significance. Amer. J. Med. 60, 817-824 (1976).

57. Marks, L.S., Maxwell, M.H., Kaufman, J.J.: Renin, sodium, and vasodepressor response to saralasin in renovascular and essential hypertension. Ann. intern. Med. 87, 176-182 (1977).

58. Ferriss, J.B., Brown, J.J., Fraser, T., Haywood, E., Davis, D.L., Kay, A.W., Lever, A.F., Robertson, J.I.S., Owen, K., Peart, W.S.: Results of adrenal surgery in patients with hypertension, aldosterone excess, and a low plasma renin concentration. Brit. med. J. 1, 135-138 (1975).

59. Liddle, G.W.: Management of aldosteronism. Amer. J. clin. Pathol. 54, 331-332 (1970).

60. Hollifield, J.W., McKenna, T.J., Wolff, J. McD., Chick, W.T., Liddle, G.W.: New adrenal inhibitor effective in the treatment of primary aldosteronism. Clin. Res. 23, 237A (1975).

61. Ondetti, M.A., Williams, M.J., Sabo, E.S., Pluseuc, J., Weaver, E.R., Kocy, O.: Angiotensin-converting enzyme inhibitor from the venom of vothrops fararaca: isolation, elucidation of structure and synthesis. Biochemistry 10, 4033-4039 (1971).

62. Brunner, H.R., Gavras, H., Waber, B., Kershaw, G.R., Turini, G.A., Vukovich, R.A., McKinstry, D.N., Gavras, I.: Oral angiotensin-converting enzyme inhibitor in long-term treatment of hypertensive patients. Ann. intern. Med. 90, 19-23 (1979).

63. Schambelan, M., Sebastian, A.: Hyporeninemic hypoaldosteronism. Adv. intern. Med. 24, 385-405 (1979).

64. Knochel, J.P.: The syndrome of hyporeninemic hypoaldosteronism. Ann. Rev. Med. 30, 145-153 (1979).

65. Sebastian, A., McSherry, E., Schambelan, M., Connor, D., Biglieri, E., Morris, R.C.: Amelioration of metabolic acidosis with fludrocortisone therapy in hyporeninemic hypoaldosteronism. New Engl. J. Med. 297, 576-583 (1977).

66. DeLeiva, A., Christlieb, A.R., Melby, J.C., Graham, C.A., Day, R.P., Luetscher, J.A., Vager, P.G.: Big renin and biosynthetic defect of aldosterone in diabetes mellitus. New Engl. J. Med. 295, 639-693 (1976).

67. Tuck, M.L., Mayes, D.M.: Mineralocorticoid biosythesis in patients with hyporeninemic hypoaldosteronism. J. clin. Endocrinol. Metab. 50, 341-347 (1980).

68. McKenna, T.J., Island, D.P., Nicholson, W.E., Miller, R.B., Lacroix, A., Liddle, W.E.: ACTH stimulates late steps in cortisol biosynthesis. Acta Endocrinol. 90, 122-132 (1979).

69. Visser, H.K.A., Cost, W.S.: A new hereditary defect in the biosynthesis of aldosterone: urinary C_{21}-corticosteroid pattern in 3 related patients with salt-losing syndrome suggesting an 18-oxidation defect. Acta Endocrinol. 47, 589-612 (1964).

70. Luetscher, J.A., Camargo, C.A., Cohn, A.P., Dowdy, A.J., Callaghan, A.: Aldosterone secretion and metabolism in hyperthyroidism and myxoedema. J. clin. Endocrinol. Metab. 23, 873-880 (1963).

71. Rosler, A., Rabinowitz, D., Theodor, R., Ramirez, L.C., Ulick, S.: The nature of the defect in a salt wasting disorder in Jews of Iran. J. clin. Endocrinol. Metab. 44, 279-291 (1977).

72. McKenna, T.J.: The adrenal cortex and the menstrual disorders. In: "Endocrine Causes of Menstrual Disorders", Ed. Givèns, J.R., Year Book Medical Publishers, Chicago, pp. 371-407 (1977).

73. Rosler, A., Levine, L.S., Schneider, B., Movogroder, M., New, M.I.: The interrelation of sodium balance, plasma renin activity and ACTH in congenital adrenal hyperplasia. J. clin. Endocrinol. Metab. 45, 500-512 (1977).

74. Limal, J.M., Rapaport, R., Bayard, F.: Plasma aldosterone, renin activity and 17-hydroxyprogesterone in salt losing congenital adrenal hyperplasia. 1. Response to ACTH in hydrocortisone treated patients and the effects of 9α-fludrocortisol. J. clin. Endocrinol. Metab. 45, 551-559 (1977).

75. Rosler, A., Theodor, R., Boichis, H., Gerty, R., Ulick, S., Alagam, M., Tabachnik, E., Cohen, B., Rabinowitz, D.: Metabolic responses to the administration of angiotensin II, K, and ACTH in two salt-wasting syndromes. J. clin. Endocrinol. Metab. 44, 292-301 (1977).

76. Broesmans, W., Gussens, H., Corbeel, L., Eckels, R.: Pseudohypoaldosteronism. Amer. J. Dis. Child. 126, 510-516 (1973).

SECRETIN AND ITS ROLE IN HEALTH AND DISEASE

J. C. Mason, R. W. Henry*, R. F. Murphy
Departments of Biochemistry and Medicine*, Queen's University, Belfast BT9 7BL, Northern Ireland

Introduction

In 1902 a new branch of science was heralded when Bayliss and Starling (1) reported that an extract of jejunal mucosa stimulated bicarbonate secretion from the pancreas of anaesthetised dogs. The chemical substance thought to be responsible was named secretin and was present only in desquamated epithelial cells from the duodenum and jejunum. It was suggested by Starling (2) that the term hormone be applied to this type of chemical messenger which is produced in one organ and carried in the blood to exert control of the functions of another organ. Numerous preparations of secretin were made available over the years and though they were unstable and had low activity, Chiray and coworkers (3, 4, 5, 6) introduced the secretin test as a diagnostic tool in medicine. Intravenous administration of secretin with measurements of bicarbonate release from the pancreas revealed impaired response to secretin and was an indication of the mass of functioning pancreatic tissue. Later it was shown that cancer of the pancreas (7, 8, 9), gall bladder and bile ducts (7) and some processes involving the liver (10) could be diagnosed with the aid of the secretin test. The history and value of the secretin test for measuring pancreatic function in various diseased states was reviewed by Jorpes and Mutt (11), Zimmerman et al. (12) and Dreiling (13). More recently Noda et al. (14, 15) developed a pancreatic excretion test, using a weak acid of 5,5-dimethyl-2,4-oxazolidinedione (DMO), which may

Hormones in Normal and Abnormal Human Tissues, Vol. II

have advantages over the secretin test for detecting early stages of pancreatic disease including carcinoma and chronic pancreatitis (16). Because of the widespread use of the secretin test there was a need for reliable methods of assay for secretin and for a reference standard to enable some correlation to be made between the various studies on pancreatic function. While the biological assay for secretin is dependent on the measurement of the volume of pancreatic juice released in anaesthetised animals, three different species have been used, dogs (17), cats (17, 18) and rats (19), each with different units of potency. Jorpes and Mutt (20) reviewed the interrelationship between the units and recommended the international acceptance of the clinical unit (CU) defined by Lagerlöf as the quantity of hormone suitable for administration in the routine tests for pancreatic function in man.

The Chemistry of Secretin

Structure

Although secretin was discovered in 1902, early attempts to isolate the hormone in its pure form were unsuccessful because appropriate procedures for polypeptide purification were unavailable. In the early 1960's Jorpes and Mutt (21, 22) took advantage of the newly developed techniques, electrophoresis, ion exchange chromatography and counter current distribution, to isolate porcine secretin in pure form with an activity of 4000 CU/mg peptide. Mutt and Jorpes (23) tentatively proposed the amino acid sequence (Fig. 1) of a strongly basic peptide after studies employing proteolysis and isolation of the resulting fragments by paper chromatography (24). Confirmation of these original findings was obtained with further enzymic hydrolysis when the fragments were purified on ion exchange columns (25).

Synthesis

The importance of synthetic peptide hormones was realised when du Vigneaud et al. (26) synthesised an octapeptide amide with the hormonal activity of oxytocin. It was apparent that this approach could be used to provide proof for proposed amino acid sequences and that studies with synthetic hormone analogues could reveal relationships between hormone structure and function. Two successful attempts at the synthesis of secretin were made by the Squibb group in the 1960's. The first approach (27-29) followed the principle introduced by Bodanszky (30) for the entirely stepwise synthesis of peptides by aminolysis of nitrophenyl esters. This had been used for the synthesis of oxytocin (31) and vasopressin (32). Ondetti et al. (33) synthesised secretin, combining the methods of stepwise synthesis and fragment condensation which had been applied to larger peptides including β-corticotropin (34). Irrespective of the route of synthesis, the synthetic peptides had marked biological activity and the same potency, 4000 CU/mg, as that of the natural hormone. The complete agreement between the physiological, physical and chemical properties of pure natural secretin and synthetic secretin provided conclusive evidence for the structure proposed by Mutt and Jorpes (23). Subsequent preparations of secretin were synthesised by other workers. Wünsch et al. (35) and Jaeger et al. (36) favoured a modification of the fragment condensation approach while Van Zon and Beyerman (37) employed a stepwise procedure in which peptides were coupled by the method of repetitive excess mixed anhydride. Early difficulties with the solid phase synthesis of secretin (38) concerning the removal of the amide form of the peptide from the supports were overcome by Hemmasi and Bayer (39).

Conformation

Bodanszky et al. (40) had sufficient synthetic peptide to carry out optical rotatory dispersion (ORD) and circular dichroism (CD) studies. The spectra were strikingly similar to those of lysozyme (41) for which the three dimensional structures had been established by X-ray crystallography. This led Bodanszky et al. (40) to propose a helical structure for the region between residues 6 and 13 but the exact length of the helix is unknown. They also suggest that the aspartyl residue in position 3 plays no apparent role in stabilizing the conformation since secretin (5-27) exhibits ORD and CD spectra similar to those of the complete sequence. However, the C-terminal end of the molecule is necessary to maintain the helical conformation since the fragment 1-14 showed no helicity in spectral studies. Bodanszky et al. (42) suggest that Glu_9 and Asp_{15} may play an important role in stabilizing the conformation and maintaining the helicity of secretin by forming ion pairs with arginine residues at positions 12 and 18. Substitution of the carboxylic acid residues of secretin (5-27) by the corresponding carboxamides (glutamine and asparagine) or lysine maintains the size, shape and polar character of the side chains but eliminates their ability to form ion pairs (40, 42, 43). These substituted analogues have, therefore, moderately reduced helicity with a single substitution whereas dual substitution reduces helicity substantially. The hydrophobic pocket created by the non-polar side of the helical stretch and by the C-terminal sequence forms the inside of the molecule. The hydrophillic amino acids of the helix and the N-terminal sequence are on the outside and are regarded as suitable for contact with the hormone receptors (40).

Homology

Extensive structural homology exists between secretin and other gastrointestinal hormones; glucagon, vasoactive intestinal peptide (VIP) and gastric inhibitory peptide (GIP) (see Fig. 1). Since secretin, glucagon and VIP have been isolated from both avian and mammalian tissues, with only minor changes in amino acid sequences between species, it was suggested (47-49) that these hormones arose from a common ancestral peptide. The divergence of these peptides was probably much earlier in evolutionary terms since the presence of secretin-like and glucagon-like

Hormone	Amino Acid Sequence
Secretin[25]	[1]His.Ser.Asp.Gly.[5]Thr.Phe.Thr.Ser.Glu.[10]Leu.Ser.Arg.Leu.Arg.[15]Asp.Ser.Ala.Arg. Leu.[20]Gln.Arg.Leu.
VIP[44]	His.Ser.Asp.Ala.Val.Phe.Thr.Asp.Asn.Tyr.Thr.Arg.Leu.Arg.Lys.Gln.Met.Ala. Val.Lys.Lys.Tyr.
Glucagon[45]	His.Ser.Gln.Gly.Thr.Phe.Thr.Ser.Asp.Tyr.Ser.Lys.Tyr.Leu.Asp.Ser.Arg.Arg. Ala.Gln.Asp.Phe.
GIP[46]	Tyr.Ala.Glu.Gly.Thr.Phe.Ile.Ser.Asp.Tyr.Ser.Ile.Ala.Met.Asp.Lys.Ile.Arg. Gln.Gln.Asp.Phe.
Secretin	Leu.Gln.[25]Gly.Leu.ValNH_2
VIP	Leu.Asn.Ser.Ile.Leu.AsnNH_2
Glucagon	Val.Gln.Trp.Leu.Met.Asn.Thr.
GIP	Val.Asn.Trp.Leu.Leu.Ala.Gln.[30]Gln.Lys.Gly.Lys.Lys.[35]Ser.Asp.Trp.Lys.His.[40]Asn. Ile.Thr.Gln.

Figure 1. Amino acid sequences of porcine secretin, VIP, glucagon and GIP.

immunoreactivity has been demonstrated in teleost fish (50, 51).

Analogues of secretin

Studies of pancreatic secretion in cat (52) and dog (53) suggest that the complete amino acid sequence is necessary for biological activity. Secretin (2-27) retained only slight secretory activity and shorter sequences, such as secretin (5-27) and (15-27) had no activity. Recent results, however, suggest that the carboxy-terminal sequences have more biological activity than was first suspected. Makhlouf et al. (54) showed that secretin (5-27) is potent in stimulating pancreatic secretion in rat and guinea pig. They also found that while analogues of secretin with single or dual substitution of the carboxylic residues (55) with the corresponding carboxamides or lysine have reduced helical conformation, biological activity is not reduced. Bodanszky et al. (43) report that secretin (5-27) retains significant activity in gastric circular smooth muscle of rat.

The N-terminal region of secretin appears to be important for the lipolytic effect of secretin on fat cells; Rudman and Del Rio (56) have shown that secretin (1-14) possesses lipolytic activity and stimulates adenylate cyclase in rat adipocytes *in vitro*. On a molar basis, however, the activity is only 1/200 that of the intact molecule.

Stability

Secretin retains biological activity for at least one year when stored dry in sealed glass vials in the presence of cystine HCl at -20°C (57). In sterile neutral saline solutions at 4°C potency is maintained for several hours but is rapidly lost at room temperature (58). Recently, Jaeger et al. (59) showed that in acid solution the Asp_3-Gly_4 of secretin underwent a slow rearrangement to form a cyclic succinimide derivative which retained only 1 to 2% of the biological activity. This was subsequently converted to the β-Asp_3 derivative at pH 7 to 8 and this had

10 to 20% of the original biological activity. Both derivatives had markedly reduced ability to bind to target cells and activate adenylate cyclase indicating that the α-Asp_3 is essential for biological activity.

Radioimmunoassay

The absence of a tyrosyl residue which could be readily iodinated delayed the development of a radioimmunoassay for secretin. Early attempts (60, 61) using chloramine-T to incorporate ^{125}I into the N-terminal histidyl residue were only partly successful because of the more extreme levels of the oxidant and the high pH required with imidazole compared with phenolic groups (62, 63). Holohan et al. (63) used lactoperoxidase to catalyse the iodination of the histidyl residue under mild conditions and this facilitated the first satisfactory radioimmunoassay for secretin. Subsequently, modified methods, in which the pH and levels of chloramine T were reduced, were used to catalyse iodination without undue oxidative damage to the hormone (64-68) but the efficiency of ^{125}I incorporation was still lower than with the enzyme (63, 69). When ion exchange chromatography on SP-Sephadex C-25 (70) was used to separate ^{125}I-labelled secretin from the reactants of either method, however, products with identical specific radioactivity and immunoreactivity were obtained (71).

As an alternative to iodinating the histidyl residue of secretin Schwarz-Mann (Orangeburg, N.Y.) marketed 6-Tyr secretin and Urbach et al. prepared secretin extended at the N-terminus by a des-Tyr-βAla peptide (DATA secretin). Both are readily iodinated with chloramine T (66, 72-74). Iodinated DATA secretin appears to retain immunoreactivity (74) but iodinated 6-Tyr secretin is less immunoreactive than all other iodinated derivatives (66, 72, 74, 75).

Results obtained by radioimmunoassay have limitations mainly because the assay antibodies bind only to a small region rather than to the entire structure of secretin. As discussed previously for glucagon and other polypeptide hormones (76-78), a single antibody may not distinguish between intact secretin, fragments of the hormone, hormone precursors in which the immunogenic site is exposed and related hormones including GIP, VIP and glucagon in which the immunogenic site may be part of homologous sequences. Consequently, while it is desirable to determine the regional specificity of antibodies using selected fragments of secretin, it is essential to exclude the possibility of cross-reactivity of antibodies with other hormones. All antibodies raised against intact secretin appear to bind a structure in the C-terminal sequence (14-27) of the hormone. As in the case with glucagon (78), attempts are being made to raise antibodies against selected overlapping sequences of secretin so that these could be used simultaneously in radioimmunoassay of the intact hormone.

Interfering factors in tissue extracts or biological fluids which prevent the binding of antibody and radiolabelled secretin are a major source of error. Plasma constituents which depress binding include protein, enzymes, salts and urea (76, 79). In these laboratories, plasma samples are either treated with ethanol (1.5 vol) to extract the polypeptide hormone, or immunoactive substances are first purified by affinity chromatography before quantification by radioimmunoassay (70).

Molecular species

It is now well established that large precursors of polypeptide hormones are synthesised in endocrine cells and the biologically active hormones, when required, are released by proteolysis (80, 81). Multiple molecular forms of gastrointestinal hormones including glucagon (77, 78), VIP (82), gastrin (83) and CCK (84) have been detected in tissue extracts and in the circulation. There is controversy, however, as to whether multiple molecular forms of secretin can be isolated. Straus and Yalow (85) could not find immunoreactivity in fractions larger than secretin when extracts of intestinal mucosa from pig, dog, rat, monkey, rabbit and guinea pig were subjected to gel-filtration. Conversely Boden et al. (86) found that only 30-50% of the immunoreactivity in extracts of duodenal mucosa from dog had an apparent molecular weight about 3000. Most of the immunoreactivity was detected in fractions much larger than secretin with molecular weight between 6000 and 21000. Also, a minor fraction (<10% of the total immunoreactivity) was eluted at the void volume of columns of Sephadex G-50 (exclusion limit >30000). The lyophylised fractions retained their relative elution volumes when reapplied to gel-filtration columns. Inter-laboratory discrepancies in results concerning multiple molecular forms of polypeptide hormones, however, may often be attributable to the failure to eliminate the possibility of self-polymerisation or aggregation of hormones with other proteins by using dissociating agents (78).

In these laboratories, secretin and related peptides in plasma (70) and tissue extracts (87) were first purified by immunoaffinity chromatography to avoid possible interference with other proteins during gel-filtration and radioimmunoassays. Furthermore, 2M guanidine hydrochloride and 0.1% sodium dodecyl sulphate were used to confirm that molecular species larger than secretin could not be attributable to non-covalent aggregations. Four discrete fractions of immunoreactivity were detected in extracts of pig duodenum and jejunum. The predominant fraction (70%) had a molecular weight about 6000 while the remainder was present in fractions with molecular weights <2000 (5%), 3000 (20%) and 12000 (5%). Most (>80%) of the immunoreactivity in plasma of fasted human subjects was detected in fractions smaller than secretin (70), presumably C-terminal fragments of the hormone. The remainder was detected in fractions with molecular weight 12000 and 30000. The absence of intact secretin is probably due to its short half-life in the circulation but the significance of the larger forms of immunoreactivity remains unclear. The lack of agreement between workers studying the molecular species of secretin may be due to variations in the specificities of antibodies used in various laboratories. This highlights the need for assay antibodies with a range of specificities to establish the full extent of the multiple forms of secretin in tissues and in the circulation.

The Physiology of Secretin

Distribution in tissues

Prior to the discovery of secretin, Dolinski (88) had shown that acid in the duodenum stimulated release of bicarbonate from the pancreas. Bayliss and Starling (1) confirmed this finding and related the increase of bicarbonate from the pancreas to the stimulation of secretin due to acid infusion of the duodenum. Secretin is released when the duodenal contents have an acidity greater than pH 5 (89) and the rate of release is related to the length of gut acidified (90). Bloom (91) reported that the amount of secretin extractable from the small gut mucosa diminished in tissues distal to the duodenum. Straus and Yalow (85) found that secretin concentrations in rat, monkey and guinea pig tended to be higher in the distal rather than the proximal duodenum and are in agreement with Curtis et al. (92) who reported that the major portion of total mucosa secretin in the dog was found in the jejunum. Both groups emphasise that since acidification of the mucosa is the only stimulus of secretin release and takes place physiologically in only 10-12 cm of duodenum, the majority of secretin remains dormant. Straus and Yalow speculate that the secretin not under physiological stimulus may act as a reserve against the event of acidic abuse (85).

Krawitt et al. (93) sectioned frozen duodenal mucosa from dogs into histologically distinct layers and subjected extracts to bioassay. They suggest that the hormone originates in the stroma of the villi or in the villous epithelial cells. Subsequently the individual secretin cells were clearly identified, first in the dog mucosa (94, 95) and later in human mucosa (96) and were found to be present chiefly in the transitional zone between the crypts and villi. The tissue was treated with fixatives to insolubilize cellular contents and the granules containing secretin were visualised by immunohistochemistry. Identification of the secretin cell was later confirmed (97, 98) and is classified internationally as an S cell (99). The cells with small round or irregular granules, about 200 nm, are found scattered in the duodeno-jejunal mucosa being more abundant in dog and pig than in man (100).

Secretin receptors

Glucagon, secretin and VIP activate adenylate cyclase in hepatocyte or fat plasma membranes. Binding of ^{125}I-labelled glucagon can be inhibited by glucagon but not by secretin or VIP and conversely binding of ^{125}I-labelled VIP can be inhibited by secretin or VIP but not by glucagon (101-103). The binding of ^{125}I-labelled VIP to liver or fat plasma membranes is 100 times greater than that of labelled secretin. It has been concluded therefore that liver and fat plasma membranes possess two distinct classes of receptors, one interacting with glucagon and the other with secretin and VIP. The studies also revealed that there was close correlation between the binding of the hormone to the receptor and the stimulation of adenylate cyclase. Gardner (104, 105) however emphasises that the above results were not obtained under identical incubation conditions.

Plasma membranes from the pancreas also possess a receptor that interacts with secretin and VIP but unlike the receptors in liver and fat cells, it has a 100 times greater affinity for secretin than for VIP (106). There was close correlation between secretin binding and secretin-stimulated adenylate cyclase in pancreatic membranes (106) but as with liver and fat cells (101-103) results were not obtained under identical conditions.

Studies with isolated pancreatic acinar cells (107-108) have revealed two classes of receptors, one with high affinity for VIP and low affinity for secretin, the other with reversed affinities. Results obtained with fragments and analogues of secretin (109-112) have led to the conclusion that the C-terminal region contains the information required for recognition by the receptor site. The N-terminal region is essential for adenylate cyclase activation and also contributes to the affinity of the hormone for the receptor (104, 113, 114).

Gardner et al. (115) investigated the possibility that the structural difference at position 15 might account for the variation in affinities for receptors. Secretin has an acidic aspartyl residue at this position while VIP has a basic lysyl residue. The authors employed secretin (5-27) and two analogues of the fragment, 15-Asn-secretin (5-27) and 15-Lys-secretin (5-27). They conclude that the presence of an acidic residue in position 15 of secretin (5-27) reduces the affinity of the peptide for the VIP-specific receptors while the presence of a basic residue reduces the affinity of the peptide for the secretin-specific receptors. Furthermore, they suggest that the observed increase in amylase secretion caused by VIP and secretin (116) is mediated exclusively by the VIP-specific receptors.

Metabolism and pharmacokinetics

The basal plasma concentrations of secretin in man were initially estimated on the basis of bioassays to be 30-70pmol/l (73). More recently, however, levels below 5pmol/l were reported (67, 117, 118).

Secretin is rapidly removed from the human circulation; using a bioassay, Lagerlöf estimated that the half-life was approximately 17 min (119). However, radioimmunoassay measurements suggest that the half-life is 2 to 5 min in the dog (120) and man (68).

Earlier it was suggested that the degradation of secretin in the dog takes place partly in the liver and kidney (121, 122). Chey et al. reported that in plasma of patients with chronic renal failure secretin has a prolonged half-life, 6 min, compared with 2 min in normal subjects (123). These authors also conclude, however, that secretin is actively catabolised in extra-renal sites. A similar situation exists in dogs and rats (124).

Intravenous infusion of secretin has its most noticeable effect on the function of the pancreas. Doses of less than 1 clinical unit of secretin per Kg body weight increase the secretion of water and electrolyte by the pancreas (125-127), stimulate the release of trypsin (128) and enhance the release of insulin during hyperglycaemia (129). However, less than 1 clinical unit may also control the functions of other organs. Secretin acts on the stomach, reducing the rate of gastric emptying (130), inhibiting submaximal acid secretion (130), and releasing pepsin (131). The liver is stimulated to increase the volume and electrolyte output of the bile (132). Secretin decreases the duodenal motility (133) and acts on the oesophagus to reduce resting and gastrin stimulated pressure of the lower sphincter (134). With doses higher than 1 clinical unit, secretin has an additional effect on various organs. It releases insulin from the pancreas (135, 136) and inhibits maximal acid secretin in the stomach (137) whereas contraction of the gall bladder in response to cholecystokinin is enhanced (138). Secretin also possesses a lipolytic activity as shown in adipocytes of rat and mouse (139). The evaluation of the results from the early studies is hampered by the fact that, in many cases, preparations of impure secretin were used and doses were supraphysiological (140, 141). Since 1 clinical unit per Kg of body weight causes maximal bicarbonate secretion from the human pancreas, Hubel (142) suggests that higher doses are pharmacological rather than physiological. However, recent studies using radioimmunoassay to determine levels of circulating secretin-like immunoreactivity (SLI) indicate that values even lower than 1 clinical unit of secretin per Kg are pharmacological. There is no stimulation of insulin secretion when pure natural porcine secretin is infused in doses which are within this range (143).

The physiological actions of secretin may be affected by other hormones, including potentiation by cholecystokinin (143, 144) and inhibition by somatostatin (145). When secretin is infused intravenously in man at a dose of 0.25 clinical units per Kg, it stimulates the pancreas at half the maximal secretory rate but if given together with cholecystokinin, maximal secretory rate is obtained (146). Since cholecystokinin is released by acid (147), it has been suggested (148) that such action may be physiological.

Both vagal and sympathetic innervation influence hormone release from the gastrointestinal tract and pancreas. Neural control is important for the release of gastrin (149, 150) and possibly glucagon (151). Ward and Bloom (152) observed the effect of vagotomy on secretin release in man and concluded that it is not dependent on intact vagal innervation of the small intestine. McLoughlin et al. (153) investigated the role of neural influences on the release of secretin in man using hypoglycaemia which is a potent autonomic nerve stimulus. They found no alteration in plasma secretin levels and concluded that neural influences are relatively unimportant in the release of secretin.

Secretin in health

Fasting plasma concentrations of SLI in our laboratory fall within the range 0-10 pmol/l. Basal concentrations of SLI are not constant and episodic rises in plasma levels have been shown to coincide with changes in duodenal pH (154). SLI in plasma is released in response to intraduodenal acidification (120, 155) and this release is inhibited by somatostatin (145).

There are, however, no consistent results of plasma SLI concentrations in response to a variety of oral stimuli. O'Connor et al. (156) observed suppression of plasma SLI concentrations whereas episodic rises in plasma SLI after a protein-rich meal with a fall in duodenal pH have been reported (154). Chey and Fahrenkrug (157) report a sustained rise in plasma SLI after a meat-containing meal. Ingestion of lemonade, a commonly used acidic soft drink, causes a bi-phasic rise in plasma SLI concentrations (148). The increase was similar to that observed after intraduodenal acid infusion and is indicative of the lemonade having a pH well below 4.5, the threshold level for stimulation of secretin. The results of an early study in which release of plasma SLI was observed after oral glucose (136) have not been confirmed by subsequent studies (120, 158). Alcohol has been reported to cause an increase in the concentrations of circulating SLI (159) but neither Henry et al. (160) nor

Häcki et al. (148) have been able to confirm this finding. The different results between groups may be due to the variety of stimuli used, different rates of gastric emptying in different subjects or variations in individual gastric responses.
Thus it has been difficult, using radioimmunoassay, to confirm the accepted classical role for secretin in human physiology as a determinant of pancreatic bicarbonate secretion.

A report that plasma SLI concentrations are raised by fasting and lowered by refeeding (161) have not been observed in other laboratories (148, 162). Further studies (70, 163) however, confirmed original findings (161) that increased levels of plasma immunoreactivity after prolonged fasting were manifested by material smaller than secretin. This material may be degradation products of secretin which are still able to cross-react with the assay antibody.

Secretin in disease

Investigation of possible roles for secretin in disease is complicated because of the complex inter-relationship between gastro-entero-pancreatic (GEP) hormones and because it is still not clear whether some of the reported biological actions of the hormone are physiological rather than pharmacological. These problems are increased by the possibility that fragments of GEP hormones may possess biological activity (83, 84) but may not be recognised by individual assay antibodies.

It now seems that secretin is unlikely to be the "incretin" of the 'entero-insular axis'. Secretin "priming" however, enhances early insulin output in response to a subsequent glucose stimulus in normal human subjects (164) and in maturity-onset diabetes (165) but the mechanism of this augmentation is not known. The effects of secretin "priming" upon release of hormones which may be insulinogenic is worthy of investigation.
Elevated levels of SLI have been found in untreated patients with maturity onset diabetes; a significant positive correlation was observed between the fasting glucose and fasting SLI levels

at the time of diagnosis (166). Treatment improved glucose tolerance and reduced the concentrations of plasma SLI.

Secretin in pharmacological doses inhibits gastric acid secretion possibly by a direct effect upon parietal cells and by indirect inhibition of antral gastrin release (167-169). The report that secretin release failed to respond to intraduodenal acidification with 0.1M HCl in duodenal ulcer patients (170) was not confirmed in a later study (171) although basal SLI concentrations were higher in the ulcer group than in controls. The release of secretin in response to duodenal acidification is impaired in both children and adults with coeliac disease but improves with treatment (172-174).

The reports of abnormal plasma SLI concentrations in various diseases failed to demonstrate that secretin was an aetiological factor in any pathological condition. Unlike most other gut hormones (175), abnormal circulating levels of secretin have not been found in association with either endocrine or non-endocrine tumours of the gastro-intestinal tract. It has been observed that the largest molecular species of hormone-like immunoreactivity, including those of insulin and gastrin, are secreted by tumours and are presumably due to the lack of the converting enzymes (77). The larger molecular weight species of secretin may be produced by some tumours but remain undetectable with the available assay antibodies. The biological effects, however, of a tumour primarily producing secretin are likely to be clinically inapparent and could evade detection.

References

1. Bayliss, W.M., Starling, E.H.: The mechanism of pancreatic secretion. J. Physiol. 28, 325-353 (1902).

2. Starling, E.H.: The chemical correlation of the functions of the body. The chemical control of the function of the body. Croonian Lecture I. Lancet ii, 338-341 (1905).

3. Pennau, H., Simmonnet, H.: Secretine duodénale et insuline. Bull. Soc. Chim. biol. 7, 17-25 (1925).

4. Chiray, M., Salmon, A.R., Mercier, A.: Action of purified secretin on external secretion of pancreas in man. Bull. Mém. Soc. méd. Hôp. Paris, 50, 1417-1426 (1926).

5. Chiray, M., Jeandel, A., Salmon, A.R.: L'exploration clinique du pancréas et l'injection intraveineuse de secretine purifiée. Presse méd. 38, 977-982 (1930).

6. Chiray, M., Bolgert, M.: Le diagnostic des affections pancréatiques par l'épreuve à la secretine purifiée. Presse méd. 44, 428-431 (1936).

7. Dreiling, D.A., Nieburgs, H.E., Janowitz, H.D.: The combined secretin and cytology test in the diagnosis of pancreatic and biliary tract cancer. Med. Clins N. Am. 44, 801-815 (1960).

8. Raskin, H.F., Wenger, J., Sklar, M., Pleticka, S., Yarema, W.: The diagnosis of cancer of the pancreas, biliary tract and duodenum by combined cytologic and secretory methods. I. Exfoliative duodenal intubation. Gastroenterology 34, 996-1008 (1958).

9. Werner, B., Raskin, H.F.: The diagnosis of cancer of the pancreas, biliary tract and duodenum by combined cytologic and secretory methods. II. The Secretin Test. Gastroenterology 34, 1009-1019 (1958).

10. Henning, N., Witte, S., Bresset, D.: Ueber den Befund von Leberzellen im Duodenalinhalt und seinen diagnostischen Wert. Med. Klin. 55, 692-694 (1960).

11. Jorpes, J.E., Mutt, V.: Gastrointestinal hormones. In: "The Hormones IV", Eds. Pincus, G., Thimann, K.V., Academic Press, New York, pp. 365-383 (1964).

12. Zimmerman, M.J., Dreiling, D.A., Janowitz, H.D.: The secretin test. In: "Handbook of Experimental Pharmacology. XXXIV" Eds. Jorpes, J.E., Mutt, V., Springer Verlag, Berlin, pp. 218-246 (1973).

13. Dreiling, D.A.: The secretin story. Am. J. Gastroenterol. 70, 455-479 (1978).

14. Noda, A., Hayakawa, T., Nakajima, S., Suzuki, T., Toda, Y.: Pancreatic excretion of 5,5-dimethyl-2,4-oxazolidinedione in normal subjects. Am. J. dig. Dis. 20, 1011-1018 (1975).

15. Noda, A., Hayakawa, T., Aoki, I., Horiguchi, Y., Toda, Y.: Pancreatic excretion of 5,5-dimethyl-2,4-oxazolidinedione in patients with chronic pancreatitis. Am. J. dig. Dis. 20, 1019-1026 (1975).

16. Noda, A., Kamiya, N., Takayama, T., Hayakawa, T.: Pancreatolithiasis and pancreatic carcinoma. Evaluation of pancreatic excretion test with 5,5-dimethyl-2, 4-oxazolidinedione. Arch. intern. Med. 137, 754-760 (1977).

17. Ivy, A.C., Janecek, H.M.: Assay of Jorpes-Mutt secretin and cholecystokinin. Acta physiol. scand. 45, 220-230 (1959).

18. Mutt, V., Söderberg, U.: On the assay of secretin. Ark. Kemi 15, 63-68 (1959).

19. Love, J.W.: A method for the assay of secretin, using rats. Q. Jl. exp. Physiol. 42, 279-284 (1957).

20. Jorpes, J.E., Mutt, V.: On the biological assay of secretin. The reference standard. Acta physiol. scand. 66, 316-325 (1966).

21. Mutt, V.: Electrophoretic purification of highly active secretin preparations. Ark. Kemi 15, 275-278 (1959).

22. Jorpes, E., Mutt, V.: On the biological activity and amino acid composition of secretin. Acta chem. scand. 15, 1790-1791 (1961).

23. Mutt, V., Jorpes, J.E.: Lecture, Presented at the 4th International Symposium on the Chemistry of Natural Products, Stockholm, Sweden Section 2C-3 (1966).

24. Mutt, V., Magnusson, S., Jorpes, J.E., Dahl, E.: Structure of porcine secretin. I. Degradation with trypsin and thrombin. Sequence of the tryptic peptides. The C-terminal. Biochemistry 4, 2358-2362 (1965).

25. Mutt, V., Jorpes, J.E., Magnusson, S.: Structure of porcine secretin. The amino acid sequence. Biochemistry 15, 513-519 (1970).

26. Du Vigneaud, V., Ressler, C.H., Swann, J.M., Roberts, C.W., Katsoyannio, P.G., Gordon, S.: The synthesis of an octapeptide amide with the hormonal activity of oxytocin. J. Am. chem. Soc. 75, 4879-4880 (1953).

27. Bodanszky, M., Ondetti, M.A., Levine, S.D., Narayanan, V.L., von Saltza, M., Sheehan, J.T., Williams, N.J., Sabo, E.F.: Synthesis of a heptacosapeptide amide with the hormonal activity of secretin. Chem. Ind. 1757-1758 (1966).

28. Bodanszky, M., Williams, N.J.: Synthesis of secretin. I. The protected tetradecapeptide corresponding to sequence 14-27. J. Am. chem. Soc. 89, 685-689 (1967).

29. Bodanszky, M., Ondetti, M.A., Levine, S.D., Williams, N.J.: Synthesis of secretin. II. The stepwise approach. J. Am. chem. Soc. 89, 6753-6757 (1967).

30. Bodanszky, M.: Synthesis of peptides by aminolysis of nitrophenyl esters. Nature 175, 685 (1955).

31. Bodanszky, M., Du Vigneaud, V.: A method of synthesis of long peptide chains using a synthesis of oxytocin as an example. J. Am. chem. Soc. 81, 5688-5691 (1959).

32. Bodanszky, M., Meienhofer, J., Du Vigneaud, V.: Synthesis of lysine-vasopressin by the nitrophenyl ester method. M. Am. chem. Soc. 82, 3195-3198 (1960).

33. Ondetti, M.A., Narayanan, V.L., von Saltza, M., Sheehan, J.T., Sabo, E.F., Bodanszky, M.: The synthesis of secretin. III. The fragment condensation approach. J. Am. chem. Soc. 90, 4711-4716 (1968).

34. Schwyzer, R., Sieber, P.: Die Totalsynthese des β-Corticotropins. Helv. chim. Acta 42, 2622-2624 (1959).

35. Wünsch, E., Jaeger, E., Deffner, M., Scharf, A., Lehnert, P.: Zur synthese des sekretino, VI reindarstellung des synthelischen sekretins. Chem. Ber. 105, 2515-2522 (1972).

36. Jaeger, G., Konig, W., Wissmann, H., Geiger, R.: Beitrag zur synthese des sekretins. Chem. Ber. 107, 215-231 (1974).

37. Van Zon, A., Beyerman, H.C.: Synthesis of the gastrointestinal peptide hormone secretin by the repetitive excess mixed anhydride (REMA) method. Helv. chim. Acta 59, 1112-1126 (1976).

38. Bodanszky, M.: The synthesis of (porcine) secretin. In: "Handbook of Experimental Pharmacology. XXXIV", Eds. Jorpes, J.E., Mutt, V., Springer-Verlag, Berlin, pp. 180-194 (1973).

39. Hemmasi, B., Bayer, E.: The solid phase synthesis of porcine secretin with full biological activity. Int. J. Pept. Protein Res. 9, 63-70 (1977).

40. Bodanszky, A., Ondetti, M.A., Mutt, V., Bodanszky, M.: Synthesis of secretin. IV. Secondary structure in a miniature protein. J. Am. chem. Soc. 91, 944-949 (1969).

41. Blake, C.F., Koenig, D.F., Mair, G.A., North, A.C.T., Phillips, D.C., Sarma, V.R.: The structure of hen egg white lysozyme. Nature 206, 757-761 (1965).

42. Bodanszky, M., Fink, M.L., Boden, G.: The role of some polar amino acid residues in secretin. Gastroenterology 72, 801-802 (1977).

43. Bodanszky, M., Fink, M.L., Funk, K.W.: A re-examination of the conformation of secretin in water. Clin. Endocr. 5, 195-200 (1976).

44. Bodanszky, M., Klausner, Y.S., Said, S.I.: Biological activities of synthetic peptides corresponding to fragments of and to the entire sequence of vasoactive intestinal peptide. Proc. natn. Acad. Sci. U.S.A. 70, 382-384 (1973).

45. Bromer, W.W., Sinn, L.G., Behrens, O.K.: The amino acid sequence of glucagon. J. Am. chem. Soc. 79, 2807-2810 (1956).

46. Brown, J.C., Dryburgh, R.J.: A gastric inhibitory peptide. The complete amino acid sequence. J. Biochem. 49, 867-872 (1971).

47. Weinstein, B.: On the relationship between glucagon and secretin. Experientia 24, 406-408 (1968).

48. Dockray, G.J.: Evolution of secretin-like hormones. In: "Gut Hormones", Ed. Bloom, S.R., Churchill Livingstone, Edinburgh, pp. 64-67 (1978).

49. Dockray, G.J.: Evolutionary relationships of the gut hormones. Fed. Proc. 38, 2295-2301 (1979).

50. Barrington, E.J.W., Dockray, G.J.: Gastrointestinal hormones. J. Endocrinol. 69, 299-325 (1976).

51. Dockray, G.J.: Molecular evolution of gut hormones : Application of comparative studies on the regulation of digestion. Gastroenterology 72, 344-358 (1977).

52. Ondetti, M., Sheehan, J.T., Bodanszky, M.: Synthesis of gastrointestinal hormones. In: "Pharmacology of Hormonal Polypeptides and Proteins", Eds. Black, N., Martini, L., Paoletti, R., Plenum Press, New York, pp. 18-31 (1968).

53. Grossman, M.I.: Regulation of glucagon action at its receptor. In: "Structure-Activity Relationships of Protein and Polypeptide Hormones", Eds. Margoulies, M., Greenwood, F.C., Excerpta Medica, Amsterdam, p. 479 (1972).

54. Makhlouf, G.M., Bodanszky, M., Fink, M.L., Schebalin, M.: Pancreatic secretory activity of secretin$_{5-27}$ and substituted analogues. Gastroenterology 75, 244-248 (1978).

55. Fink, M.L., Bodanszky, M.: Secretin VI. Simultaneous "in situ" syntheses of three analogues of the C-terminal tricosapeptide and a study of their conformation. J. Am. chem. Soc. 98, 974-977 (1976).

56. Rudman, D., Del Rio, A.E.: Lipolytic activity of a peptide fragment of porcine secretin. Endocrinology 85, 610-611 (1969).

57. Grossman, M.I.: Stability of secretin. Gastroenterology 57, 767 (1969).

58. Spignola, L.J., Grossman, M.I.: Secretin-measurement. Bioassay. In: "Peptide Hormones", Eds. Berson, S.A., Yalow, R.S., North-Holland Publishing Co., Amsterdam-London, pp. 1066-1068 (1973).

59. Jaeger, E., Knof, S., Scharf, R., Lehnert, P., Schulz, I., Wünsch, E.: Chemical evidence for the mechanism of inactivation of secretin. Scand. J. Gastroenterol. 13, 93 (1978).

60. Young, J.D., Lazarus, L., Chisholm, D.J., Atkinson, F.F.V.: Radioimmunoassay of secretin in human sera. J. Nucl. Med. 9, 641-642 (1968).

61. Berson, S.A., Yalow, R.S.: Progress in gastroenterology. Gastroenterology 62, 1061-1084 (1972).

62. Li, C.H.: Kinetics of reactions between iodine and histidine. J. Am. chem. Soc. 66, 225 (1944).

63. Holohan, K.N., Murphy, R.F., Flanagan, R.W.J., Buchanan, K.D., Elmore, D.T.: Enzymic iodination of the histidyl residue of secretin: A radioimmunoassay of the hormone. Biochim. biophys. Acta 322, 178-180 (1973).

64. Boden, G., Chey, W.Y.: Preparation and specificity of antiserum to synthetic secretin and its use in a radioimmunoassay (RIA). Endocrinology 92, 1617-1624 (1973).

65. Teale, J.D., Buchanan, K.D., Harper, G.: A radioimmunoassay for secretin using antibodies raised to pure natural and synthetic hormone. Gut 13, 849-850 (1972).

66. Schaffalitzky De Muckadell, O.B., Fahrenkrug, J.: Preparation of ^{125}I-labelled synthetic porcine secretin for radioimmunoassay. Scand. J. clin. Lab. Invest. 36, 661-668 (1976).

67. Hanssen, L.E., Torjesen, P.: Radioimmunoassay of secretin in human plasma. Scand. J. Gastroenterol. 12, 481-488 (1977).

68. Kolts, E.B., McGuigan, J.E.: Radioimmunoassay measurement of secretin half-life in man. Gastroenterology 72, 55-60 (1977).

69. Boden, G.: Secretin radioimmunoassay. In: "Gastrointestinal Hormones", Ed. Thompson, J.C., University of Texas Press, Austin and London, pp. 283-294 (1975).

70. Mason, J.C., Murphy, R.F., Henry, R.W., Buchanan, K.D.: Starvation-induced changes in secretin-like immunoreactivity of human plasma. Biochim. biophys. Acta 582, 322-331 (1979).

71. Mason, J.C.: unpublished results.

72. Raptis, S., Leitze, M., Schlegel, W., Pfeiffer, E.F.: Secretin radioimmunoassay using ^{125}I-6-tyrosyl-secretin (6TS). Horm. Metab. Res. 7, 447 (1975).

73. Rayford, P.L., Curtis, P.J., Fender, H.R., Thompson, J.C.: Plasma levels of secretin in man and dogs : Validation of a secretin radioimmunoassay. Surgery 79, 658-665 (1976).

74. Urbach, H.J., Domschke, W., Reiss, M., Domschke, S., Rosselin, G., Wünsch, E., Jaeger, E., Moroder, L., Demling, L.: Superior immunoreactivity of ^{125}I-(des-tyr-βala)-secretin with rabbit anti-secretin sera compared to ^{125}I-secretin and ^{125}I-6-tyrosyl secretin. Horm. Metab. Res. 8, 459-461 (1976).

75. Straus, E., Urbach, H.J., Yalow, R.S.: Comparative reactivities of ^{125}I-secretin and ^{125}I-6-tyrosyl secretin with guinea pig and rabbit antisecretin sera. Biochem. biophys. Res. Commun. 64, 1036-1040 (1975).

76. Rehfeld, J.F.: Problems in the technology of radioimmunoassays for gut hormones. In: "Gut Hormones", Ed. Bloom, S.R., Churchill-Livingstone, Edinburgh, pp. 112-119 (1978).

77. Murphy, R.F.: The chemical characterization of GI hormones. In: "Clinics In Endocrinology And Metabolism", Ed. Buchanan, K.D., W.B. Saunders Co. Ltd., London, pp. 281-298 (1979).

78. Murphy, R.F., Buchanan, K.D., Flanagan, R.W.J.: Glucagon and related peptides. This issue pp. 187-221 (1980).

79. Bryant, M.G.: Plasma artefacts in radioimmunoassay. In: "Gut Hormones", Ed. Bloom, S.R., Churchill-Livingstone, Edinburgh, pp. 120-125 (1978).

80. Geisow, M.J.: Polypeptide secondary structure may direct specificity of prohormone conversion. Febs Lett. 87, 111-114 (1978).

81. Hales, C.N.: Proteolysis and the evolutionary origin of polypeptide hormones. Febs Lett. 94, 10-16 (1978).

82. Dimaline, R., Dockray, G.J.: Multiple immunoreactive forms of vasoactive intestinal peptide in human colonic mucosa. Gastroenterology 73, 387-392 (1978).

83. Dockray, G.J.: Gastrin overview. In: "Gut Hormones", Ed. Bloom, S.R., Churchill-Livingstone, Edinburgh, pp. 129-139 (1978).

84. Rehfeld, J.F.: Multiple molecular forms of cholecystokinin. In: "Gut Hormones", Ed. Bloom, S.R., Churchill-Livingstone, Edinburgh, pp. 213-218 (1978).

85. Straus, E., Yalow, R.S.: Immunoreactive secretin in gastrointestinal mucosa of several mammalian species. Gastroenterology 75, 401-404 (1978).

86. Boden, G., Murthy, N.S., Silver, E.: "Big" secretin. Clin. Res. 23, 245 (1975).

87. Mason, J.C., Murphy, R.F., Buchanan, K.D.: The characterisation of secretin-like peptides from tissue and plasma extracts. Ir. J. med. Sci. 147, 218 (1978).

88. Dolinski, I.L.: Influence of acids on the secretion of the pancreatic gland. Arch. de Soc. Biol. St. Petersburg 3, 399-427 (1894).

89. Thomas, J.E., Crider, J.O.: A qualitative study of acid in the intestine as a stimulus for the pancreas. Am. J. Physiol. 131, 349-356 (1940).

90. Meyer, J.H., Way, L.W., Grossman, M.I.: Pancreatic bicarbonate response to various acids in duodenum of the dog. Am. J. Physiol. 219, 946-970 (1970).

91. Bloom, S.R.: Hormones of the gastrointestinal tract. Br. med. Bull. 30, 62-67 (1974).

92. Curtis, P.J., Rayford, P.L., Thompson, J.C.: Determination of secretin levels in mucosa by radioimmunoassay. Surg. Forum 27, 428-429 (1976).

93. Krawitt, E.L., Zimmerman, G.R., Clifton, J.A.: Location of secretin in dog duodenal mucosa. Am. J. Physiol. 211, 935-938 (1966).

94. Polak, J.M., Bloom, S.R., Coulling, I., Pearse, A.G.E.: Immunofluorescent localisation of secretin in the canine duodenum. Gut 12, 605-610 (1971).

95. Bussolati, G., Capella, C., Solcia, E., Vasallo, G., Vezzadini, P.: Ultrastructural and immunofluorescent investigation on the secretin cell in the dog intestinal mucosa. Histochemie 26, 218-227 (1971).

96. Polak, J.M., Coulling, I., Bloom, S.R., Pearse, A.G.E.: Immunofluorescent localisation of secretin and enteroglucagon in human intestinal mucosa. Scand. J. Gastroenterol. 6, 739-744 (1971).

97. Chey, W.Y., Escoffery, R.: Secretin cells in the gastrointestinal tract. Endocrinology 98, 1390-1395 (1976).

98. Larsson, L.-I., Sundler, F., Alumets, G., Håkanson, R., Schaffalitzky de Muckadell, O., Fahrenkrug, J.: Distribution, ontogeny and ultrastructure of the mammalian secretin cell. Cell Tissue Res. 181, 361-368 (1977).

99. Solica, E., Polak, J.M., Pearse, A.G.E., Forssmann, W.G., Larsson, L.-I., Sundler, F., Lechago, J., Grimelius, L., Fujita, T., Creutzfeldt, W., Gepts, W., Falkmer, S., Lefranc, G., Heitz, Ph., Hage, E., Buchan, A.M.J., Bloom, S.R., Grossman, M.I.: Lausanne 1977 classification of gastroenteropancreatic endocrine cells. In: "Gut Hormones", Ed. Bloom, S.R., Churchill Livingstone, Edinburgh, pp. 40-48 (1978).

100. Capella, C., Solica, E., Frigerio, B., Buffa, R.: Endocrine cells of the human intestine. An ultrastructural study. In: "Endocrine Gut and Pancreas", Ed. Fujita, T., Elsevier Scientific Publishing Co., Amsterdam, pp. 42-59 (1976).

101. Desbuquois, B., Laudat, H.M., Laudat, P.H.: Vasoactive intestinal polypeptide and glucagon: Stimulation of adenylate cyclase activity via distinct receptors in liver and fat cell membranes. Biochem. biophys. Res. Commun. 53, 1187-1194 (1973).

102. Desbuquois, B.: The interaction of vasoactive intestinal polypeptide and secretin with liver cell membranes. Europ. J. Biochem. 46, 439-450 (1974).

103. Bataille, D., Freychet, P., Rosselin, G.: Interaction of glucagon, gut glucagon, vasoactive intestinal polypeptide and secretin with liver and fat cell plasma membranes : Binding to specific sites and stimulation of adenylate cyclase. Endocrinology 95, 713-721 (1974).

104. Gardner, J.D., Long, B.W., Uhlemann, E.R., Peikin, S.R.: Membrane receptors for VIP and secretin. In: "Gut Hormones", Ed. Bloom, S.R., Churchill Livingstone, Edinburgh, pp. 92-96 (1978).

105. Gardner, J.D.: Receptors for Gastrointestinal Hormones. Gastroenterology 76, 202-214 (1979).

106. Milutinovic, S., Schulz, I., Rosselin, G.: The interactions of secretin with pancreatic membranes. Biochim. biophys. Acta 432, 113-127 (1976).

107. Gardner, J.D., Conlon, T.P., Fink, M.L., Bodanszky, M.: Interactions of peptides related to secretin with hormone receptors on pancreatic acinar cells. Gastroenterology 71, 965-970 (1976).

108. Christophe, J.P., Conlon, T.P., Gardner, J.D.: Interaction of porcine vasoactive intestinal peptide with dispersed pancreatic acimar cells from the guinea pig : Binding of radioiodinated peptide. J. biol. Chem. 251, 4629-4634 (1976).

109. Robberecht, P., Conlon, T.P., Gardner, J.D.: Interaction of porcine vasoactive intestinal peptide with dispersed pancreatic acimar cells from the guinea pig : Structural requirements for effects of vasoactive intestinal peptide and secretin on cellular adenosine 3':5'-monophosphate. J. biol. Chem. 251, 4635-4639 (1976).

110. Gardner, J.D., Conlon, T.P., Beyerman, H.C., van Zon, A.: Interaction of synthetic 10-tyrosol analogs of secretin with hormone receptors on pancreatic acinar cells. Gastroenterology 73, 52-56 (1977).

111. Wünsch, E., Jaeger, E., Moroder, L., Schulz, I.: Progress in the problem of structure activity relations of gastro-intestinal hormones. In: "Hormonal Receptors in Digestive Tract Physiology", Eds. Bonfils, S., Fromageot, P., Rosselin, G., North Holland Publishing Co., Amsterdam, pp. 19-27 (1977).

112. Robberecht, P., Deschodt-Lanckman, M., Camus, J., Christophe, J.: Specific binding and mode of action of caerulein on plasma membranes of rat pancreas. In: "Hormonal Receptors in Digestive Tract Physiology", Inserm Symposium No.3, Eds. Bonfils, S., Fromageot, P., Rosselin, G., North Holland Publishing Co., Amsterdam, pp. 261-274 (1977).

113. Robberecht, P., Deschodt-Lanckman, M., Dehaye, J.P., Christophe, J.: Secretin-VIP receptor interactions. In: "Gut Hormones", Ed. Bloom, S.R., Churchill Livingstone, Edinburgh, pp. 97-103 (1978).

114. Christophe, J., Calderon, P., Svoboa, M., Deschodt-Lanckman, M., Robberecht, P.: A working model of stimulus-secretion coupling in pancreatic acimar cells. In: "Gut Hormones", Ed. Bloom, S.R., Churchill Livingstone, Edinburgh, pp. 104-111 (1978).

115. Gardner, J.D., Rothman, A.J., Naṭarajan, S., Bodanszky, M.: Interaction of secretin $_{5-27}$ and its analogues with hormone receptors on pancreatic acini. Biochim. biophys. Acta. 583, 491-503 (1979).

116. Gardner, J.D., Jackson, M.J.: Regulation of amylase release from dispersed pancreatic acinar cells. J. Physiol. 270, 439-454 (1977).

117. Schaffalitzky de Muckadell, O.B., Fahrenkrug, J.: Radio-immunoassay of secretin in plasma. Scand. J. clin. Lab. Invest. 37, 155-162 (1977).

118. Häcki, W.H., Bloom, S.R., Mitznegg, P., Domschke, W., Domschke, S., Belohlavek, D., Demling, L., Wünsch, E.: Plasma secretin and pancreatic bicarbonate response to exogenous secretin in man. Gut 18, 191-195 (1977).

119. Lagerlöf, H., Ek, S.Y., Nyberg, A.: The duodenal secretion in man as a function of secretin dose and secretin inactivation. Gastroenterology 43, 174-180 (1962).

120. Boden, G., Essa, N., Ouwen, O.E., Reichle, F.A.: Effects of intraduodenal administration of HCl and glucose on circulating immunoreactive secretin and insulin concentrations. J. clin. Invest. 53, 1185-1193 (1974).

121. Lehnert, P., Stahlheber, H., Forell, M.M., Fuellner, R., Fruehauf, S., Fritz, H., Hutzel, M., Werle, E.: Studies on the elimination of secretin and cholecystokinin with regard to the kinetics of exocrine pancreatic secretin. Digestion 11, 51-63 (1974).

122. Curtis, P.J., Miller, T.A., Rayford, P.L., Thompson, J.C.: The effect of nephrectomy on the catabolism of secretin. Am. J. Surg. 133, 52-54 (1977).

123. Chey, W.Y., Rhodes, R.A., Tai, H.H.: Role of secretin in man II. In: "Gut Hormones", Ed. Bloom, S.R., Churchill Livingstone, Edinburgh, pp. 193-196 (1978).

124. Thompson, J.C., Llanos, O.L., Schafmayer, A., Teichmann, R.K., Rayford, P.L.: Mechanisms of release and catabolism of secretin. In: "Gut Hormones", Ed. Bloom, S.R., Churchill Livingstone, Edinburgh, pp. 176-181 (1978).

125. Wormsley, K.G.: Response to secretin in man. Gastroenterology 54, 197-209 (1968).

126. Konturek, S.J.: Pancreatic dose-response curves to intravenous secretin in man. Gastroenterology 58, 828-832 (1970).

127. Petersen, H.: The effect of pure natural secretin on the bicarbonate secretion into the duodenum in man. Scand. J. Gastroenterol. 5, 105-111 (1970).

128. Wormsley, K.G.: The action of secretin on the secretion of enzymes by the human pancreas. Scand. J. Gastroenterol. 3, 183-188 (1968).

129. Kraegen, E.W., Chisholm, D.J., Young, J.D., Lazarus, L.: The gastrointestinal stimulus to insulin release II. A dual action of secretin. J. clin. Invest. 49, 524-529 (1970).

130. Chey, W.Y., Hitanant, S., Hendricks, J., Lorber, S.H.: Effect of secretin and cholecystokinin on gastric emptying and gastric secretion in man. Gastroenterology 58, 820-827 (1970).

131. Brooks, A.M., Isenberg, J., Grossman, M.I.: The effect of secretin, glucagon and duodenal acidification on pepsin secretion in man. Gastroenterology 57, 159-162 (1969).

132. Waitman, A.M., Dyck, W.P., Janowitz, H.D.: Effect of secretin and acetazolamide on the volume and electrolyte composition of hepatic bile in man. Gastroenterology 56, 286-294 (1969).

133. Chey, W.Y., Lorber, S.H., Kusakcioglu, O., Hendricks, J.: Effect of secretin and pancreozymin-cholecystokinin on motor function of stomach and duodenum. Fed. Proc. 26, 383 (1967).

134. Cohen, S., Lipshutz, W.: Hormonal regulation of human lower esophageal sphincter competence : Interaction of gastrin and secretin. J. clin. Invest. 50, 449-454 (1971).

135. Dupre, J., Rojas, L., White, J.J., Unger, R.H., Beck, J.C.: Effects of secretin on insulin and glucagon in portal and peripheral blood in man. Lancet ii, 26-27 (1966).

136. Chisholm, D.J., Young, J.D., Lazarus, L.: The gastrointestinal stimulus to insulin release. I. Secretin. J. clin. Invest. 48, 1453-1460 (1969).

137. Brooks, A.M., Grossman, M.I.: Effect of secretin and cholecystokinin on pentagastrin-stimulated gastric secretion in man. Gastroenterology 59, 114-119 (1970).

138. Stening, G.F., Grossman, M.I.: Potentiation of cholecystokinetic action of cholecystokinin (CCK) by secretin. Clin. Res. 17, 528 (1969).

139. Butcher, R.W., Carlson, L.A.: Effects of secretin on fat mobilizing lipolysis and cyclic AMP levels in rat adipose tissue. Acta physiol scand. 79, 559-563 (1970).

140. Botterman, P., Souvatzoglou, A., Schwartz, K.: Stimulirung der beta-cytotropin wirkung von tolbutamide durch secretin beim menschen. Klin. Wochenschr. 45, 549 (1967).

141. Boyns, D.R., Jarrett, R.J., Kun, H.: Intestinal hormones and plasma insulin; an insulinotropic action of secretin. Br. med. J. ii, 676-678 (1967).

142. Hubel, K.A.: Secretin : a long progress note. Gastroenterology 62, 318-341 (1972).

143. Schaffalitzky de Muckadell, O.B., Fahrenkrug, J., Kuhl, C.: Plasma insulin concentration during physiological variations in immunoreactive plasma secretin. Horm. Metab. Res. 8, 253-256 (1976).

144. Brown, J.C., Harper, A.A., Scratcherd, T.: Potentiation of secretin stimulation of the pancreas. J. Physiol. 190, 519-530 (1967).

145. Hanssen, L.E., Hanssen, K.F., Myren, J.: Inhibition of secretin release and pancreatic bicarbonate secretion by somatostatin infusion in man. Scand. J. Gastroenterol. 12, 391-394 (1977).

146. Wormsley, K.G.: A comparison of the response to secretin pancreozymin and a combination of these hormones in man. Scand. J. Gastroenterol. 4, 413-417 (1969).

147. Barbezat, G.O., Grossman, M.I.: Release of cholecystokinin by acid. Proc. Soc. exp. Biol Med. 148, 463-467 (1975).

148. Häcki, W.H., Greenberg, G.R., Bloom, S.R.: Role of secretin in man I. In: "Gut Hormones", Ed. Bloom, S.R., Churchill Livingstone, Edinburgh, pp. 182-192 (1978).

149. Grossman, M.I.: Neural and hormonal stimulation of gastric secretion of acid. In: "Handbook of Physiology : Section 6 vol. 2", Eds. Code, C.F., Heidel, W., American Physiological Society, Washington D.C., pp. 835-863 (1967).

150. Uvnäs-Wallensten, K.: Vagal release of antral hormones. In: "Gut Hormones", Ed. Bloom, S.R., Churchill Livingstone, Edinburgh, pp. 389-393 (1978).

151. Edwards, A.V., Bloom, S.R.: Nervous control of pancreatic hormones. In: "Gut Hormones", Ed. Bloom, S.R., Churchill Livingstone, Edinburgh, pp. 394-405 (1978).

152. Ward, A.S., Bloom, S.R.: Effect of vagotomy on secretin release in man. Gut 16, 951-956 (1975).

153. McLoughlin, J.C., Hayes, J.R., Buchanan, K.D., Kelly, J.G.: Role of neural influences in the release of gastrin, glucagon, and secretin during hypoglycaemia in man. Gut 19, 632-639 (1978).

154. Schaffalitzky de Muckadell, O.B., Fahrenkrug, J.: Role of secretin in man III. In: "Gut Hormones", Ed. Bloom, S.R., Churchill Livingstone, Edinburgh, pp. 197-200 (1978).

155. O'Connor, F.A., Buchanan, K.D., Connon, J.J., Shahidullah, M.: Secretin and insulin: Response to intraduodenal acid. Diabetologia 12, 145-148 (1976).

156. O'Connor, F.A., Buchanan, K.D., Henry, W., Calvert, H.: Secretin: lack of response to oral feeding. Gut 18, A415 (1977).

157. Chey, W.Y., Lee, Y.H., Hendricks, J.G., Rhodes, R.A., Tai, H.H.: Plasma secretin concentrations in fasting and postprandial state in man. Am. J. dig. Dis. 23, 981-988 (1978).

158. Buchanan, K.D., Teale, J.D., Harper, G., Hayes, J.R., Trimble, E.R.: Plasma secretin assay in man. Clin. Sci. Mol. Med. 45, 13-14 (1973).

159. Straus, E., Urbach, H.J., Yalow, R.S.: Alcohol-stimulated secretion of immunoreactive secretin. New Engl. J. Med. 293, 1031-1032 (1975).

160. Henry, R.W., Flanagan, R.W.J., Buchanan, K.D.: The effect of alcohol on gastro-enteropancreatic hormones. Ir. J. med. Sci. 146, 33 (1977).

161. Henry, R.W., Flanagan, R.W.J., Buchanan, K.D.: Secretin - a new role for an old hormone. Lancet ii, 202-203 (1975).

162. Greenberg, G.R., Bloom, S.R.: Plasma-secretin during fasting. Lancet i, 273-274 (1978).

163. Henry, R.W., Mason, J.C., Murphy, R.F., Buchanan, K.D.: Plasma secretin during fasting. Lancet i, 510 (1978).

164. Lerner, R.L.: The augmentation effect of secretin on the insulin responses to known stimuli : specificity for glucose. J. clin. Endocrinol. Metab. 45, 1-9 (1977).

165. Lerner, R.L.: Augmented insulin responses to glucose after secretin priming in diabetic subjects. J. clin. Endocrinol. Metab. 48, 462-466 (1979).

166. Trimble, E.R., Buchanan, K.D., Hadden, D.R., Montgomery, D.A.D.: Secretin : High plasma levels in diabetes mellitus. Acta Endocrinol. 85, 799-805 (1977).

167. Berstad, A., Petersen, H.: Dose response relationship of the effect of secretin on acid and pepsin secretion in man. Scand. J. Gastroenterol. 5, 647-654 (1970).

168. Hansky, J., Soveny, J., Korman, M.G.: Effect of secretin on serum gastrin measured by immunoassay. Gastroenterology 61, 62-68 (1971).

169. Thompson, J.C., Reeder, D.D., Bunchman, H.H., Becker, H.D., Brandt, E.N.: Effect of secretin on circulating gastrin. Ann. Surg. 176, 384-393 (1972).

170. Bloom, S.R., Ward, A.S.: Failure of secretin release in patients with duodenal ulcer. Br. med. J. 1, 126-127 (1975).

171. Isenberg, J.I., Cano, R., Bloom, S.R.: Effect of graded amounts of acid instilled into the duodenum on pancreatic bicarbonate secretion and plasma secretin in duodenal ulcer patients and normal subjects. Gastroenterology 72, 6-8 (1977).

172. O'Connor, F.A., McLoughlin, J.C., Buchanan, K.D.: Impaired immunoreactive secretin release in coeliac disease. Br. med. J. 1, 811 (1977).

173. Rhodes, R.A., Tai, H.H., Chey, W.Y.: Impairment of secretin release in celiac sprue. Am. J. dig. Dis. 23, 833-839 (1978).

174. Signer, E., Girard, J., Birnbaumer, A.: Impaired secretin release in coeliac disease. Europ. J. Pediat. 130, 222 (1979).

175. Holst, J.J.: Gut endocrine tumour syndromes. In: "Clinics In Endocrinology and Metabolism", Ed. Buchanan, K.D., W.B. Saunders Co.Ltd., London, pp. 413-432 (1979).

TESTOSTERONE AND HUMAN SKIN

C. Conti, F. Sciarra, G. Concolino
Istituto di Clinica Medica Generale e Terapia Medica V,
Università degli Studi, Rome, Italy

Introduction

The progress made in molecular endocrinology in recent years has led to a better understanding of the role of steroid hormones in different organs and their metabolism and mechanism of action. The increased knowledge has been derived from in vitro and in vivo studies performed in animals and man. Whilst in vivo experiments may be employed in laboratory animals, in vitro experiments are usually preferred for studies in man. It has thus been possible to establish the physiological role of steroids in man, how these steroids are metabolized in a particular organ, their site of action, and, last but not least, how these hormones act on the genomic expression of the cells to evoke a well defined response. In some cases this response is peculiar to a certain type of cell, with induction of synthesis of some particular enzymatic proteins, in other cases the response is more generalized and also found in other cells possessing steroid-receptors.

The action of testosterone on the skin will therefore be briefly discussed, as well as its metabolism and related enzymes, and also the androgen receptors found mainly in sebaceous glands, dermal and genital tissue.

Hormones in Normal and Abnormal Human Tissues, Vol. II

Testosterone and Skin

Acne-like skin eruptions in women and hypogonadal males treated with androgens is a well known phenomenon. Testosterone acts on the skin through an effect on epidermic and dermal compartments: the sebaceous glands and hair follicles, sudorific glands being unaffected.

A. Epidermis

Testosterone seems to be responsible for increased proliferation of epidermal cells and increased synthesis of keratin. The metabolic effects of testosterone include enhancement of melanin deposits, which is particularly evident in some areas of the body e.g. genitalia and perineal zone where this steroid action is more pronounced and is responsible for sex differentiation commencing before birth. Improved blood flow with a direct action on dermal fibroblasts is also relevant in this respect.(1).

B. Dermis

Testosterone interferes with the mucopolysaccharide composition by interfering with hyaluronidase activity which leads to depolymerization of the mucopolysaccharides. Fibroblast activity and proliferation are also regulated by testosterone or its direct metabolites. Thickening of the skin, related primarily to an increase in the number and strength of reticular and elastic fibres, is a typical feature of men with normal gonadal function.

C. Skin apparatus

Androgens have hardly any effect upon nails and sudorific glands, whereas sebaceous glands and hair follicles are markedly influenced by the action of testosterone or its metabolites. The effect of testosterone on sebaceous glands is revealed by increased secretion from the glands, often accompanied by the appearance of acne (2).

Acne in the male begins uniformly at, or shortly after, puberty, when hypertrophy of the sebaceous glands and increased secretion from them occur. Prepubertal boys and castrated men treated with effective doses of testosterone often develop seborrhea and acne (3), whilst acne improves if estrogens are given to suppress gonadal function and testosterone levels are decreased. Controversy exists regarding the hormones responsible for acne in women. Acne begins at puberty and has exacerbations in the premenstrual phase. As in men, there is no evidence that individuals with acne have a different hormonal status from those without. Factors other than hypertrophy of the sebaceous glands, e.g. abnormal ducts or abnormal secretion of the sebaceous glands, may be involved in its pathogenesis. Studies on the hormonal regulation of sebaceous glands shows that testosterone causes hypertrophy of these glands. In preputial gland, a gland with a similar structure to that of the sebaceous gland, it was demonstrated that testosterone caused enlargement of this gland with increased secretion. It is possible on the basis of certain features to differentiate acne due to androgen excess from that of Cushing's syndrome. The latter is usually due to retention of sebaceous gland secretion, the former to seborrhea, hypertrophy of the sebaceous glands and increased keratin synthesis. The individual genetic composition should also be taken into consideration (4).

The effect of testosterone upon hair growth is still poorly understood, although it is well known that hirsutism usually develops in the presence of excess androgen production by the ovaries or adrenals. Hair growth is predetermined by genetic factors and its expression is related to individual age and the action of androgenic compounds. In some areas of the body, genetic factors are predominant and plasma testosterone levels remain within the normal range e.g. idiopathic hirsutism with hair growth on the legs, anus, sacral area, chest, and shoulders. Testosterone is the most active androgen on hair growth in both sexes (5, 6, 7). The usual type of male baldness seems to require a genetic factor, a hereditary end-organ sensitivity, increased by testosterone administration, but not modified by orchiectomy. Low plasma testosterone levels, in fact, do not interfere with the phenotypic expression of the genetic abnormality (8, 9).

These general morphological changes in skin produced by testosterone action are not as marked as those induced by testosterone on the skin of the genital tract. In this area, testosterone action begins in the fetus and interferes not only with the skin and related structures, but particularly with the conformational changes of the external genitalia, as well as with the Müllerian and Wolffian ducts, leading to the morphological changes which characterize the two sexes.

Metabolism of testosterone and the related products as well as the involved enzymes, will then represent the key point of hormonal action on the skin, whilst the identification of androgen-receptors in the skin will lead to a better understanding of some clinical patterns in patients with end-organ insensitivity due to an abnormal or defective steroid-receptor mechanism that mediates androgen action.

Testosterone Metabolism

In vitro experiments on human skin biopsies in fibroblast cultures over the last 20 years have demonstrated that one of the functions of this tissue is to metabolize androgens and that this metabolism may be altered in some pathological conditions.

A. Testosterone metabolism in normal skin specimens

Skin biopsies, homogenized or cut into 0.5 mm slices, were incubated at 37°C in phosphate buffer containing ^{14}C or ^{3}H labelled steroid precursors with or without co-factors such as ATP, $NADP^{+}$, NADPH, NAD^{+}, NADH. The radiochemical purity of the compounds isolated after chromatography was confirmed by adding appropriate carriers and recrytallizing these materials to constant specific activity.

Normal human skin transformed dehydroepiandrosterone and androstenedione into testosterone. The most important transformations, however, concern testosterone itself, which is converted either to less active or inert metabolites such as 5α-androstane-3α-ol-17-one, 5α-androstane-3,17-dione, androstenedione, etiocholanolone, androsterone and epiandrosterone, or to more active compounds such as dihydrotestosterone (10, 11, 12, 13, 14).

This metabolism is not uniform in all the tissue areas, being more efficient in genital skin, i.e. of the foreskin, labia majora, clitoris and scrotum, than in the non-genital areas, i.e. abdomen, feet, legs, etc.

In scrotal skin testosterone is actively transformed into dihydrotestosterone (32%) and to a lesser extent into 5α-androstanedione (7.9%), androstenedione (6.1%), androsterone (5.3%), and 5α-androstane-3α-17β-diol (5.1%) (14). DHT is also formed from testosterone in the prepuce (383 μμmoles/100 mg per h, compared to 534 μμmoles in the scrotum), clitoris (350 μμmoles) and labia majora (283 μμmoles) (15). In labia majora, testosterone is converted into androstenedione (16%) and in lesser amounts to androsterone (5.1%), 5α-androstanedione (5%) DHT (4.9%) and 5α-androstane-3α,17β-diol (2.9%) (14).

Testosterone metabolism displays a sex difference and appears to be greater in male than in female perineal skin, particularly as far as DHT is concerned. No significant differences in the transformation of testosterone were found, on the contrary, in the corresponding genital areas of skin from male and female fetuses, where this steroid is transformed into androstenedione (29%) and 5α-androstanedione and to DHT (8.7%) (14).

With regard to non-genital skin zones, no significant sex differences were found, testosterone being transformed first into androstenedione (22%) and to a much lesser extent into other compounds with conversions ranging between 1.5-3.7% (14, 16).

It has been observed, moreover, that formation of the metabolites, in these *in vitro* experiments is time dependent. In suprapubic skin, for example, the conversion of testosterone to DHT is optimal after incubation for 1 h at 37°C, thereafter it decreases progressively whilst that of 3α- and 3β-androstanediols, the metabolic derivatives of DHT rises (17). Results and conclusions may therefore vary depending upon the various methodological procedures employed.

Testosterone metabolism in pathological skin specimens

1. Testicular feminization syndrome. This is an inherited disease due to a defect in the metabolism or in the mechanism of action of testosterone at target tissue level. Some of these patients present impaired transformation of testosterone into DHT and show a phenotypic aspect of male pseudohermaphroditism. *In vitro* experiments carried out on suprapubic skin specimens revealed that in testicular feminization syndrome the DHT/T ratio is 1/10 that found in normal subjects (18) due to the inability of this tissue to convert testosterone into DHT and into 3α- and 3β-androstanediol (19, 20, 21). The same finding is observed when testosterone is applied percutaneously (17). Other investigators found normal T→DHT conversion in these patients (16) thus demonstrating that the defect in DHT formation is not a constant finding in patients with male pseudohermaphroditism.

2. Male hypogonadism. *In vitro* experiments on pubic skin obtained from a patient affected by hypogonadotropic hypogonadism showed that the conversion of testosterone to DHT was also deficient, 2% compared to values of 15% in normal men (22). Similar results were obtained in prepubertal children conversion of 0.6 to 3.4% (17). After HCG treatment for three weeks, however, DHT synthesis in pubic skin increased significantly in the hypogonadal male reaching values of 30% conversion (22). In this pathological condition, therefore, the sexual skin areas are still able to synthesize DHT when sufficient amounts of precursors reach the target tissue, contrary to observations in the testicular feminization syndrome.

3. Hirsutism. *In vitro* experiments on the metabolism of testosterone have also been carried out in skin specimens from women presenting idiopathic hirsutism with normal testosterone levels, in order to determine whether the transformation of testosterone into DHT is increased at target tissue level. Results so far obtained are controversial. In a small group of hirsute females (23), testosterone metabolism in skin fragments from linea alba was comparable to that in corresponding zones of normal menstruating women; the same tissue, however, transformed dehydroepiandrosterone into testosterone in amounts comparable to those found in non-genital skin of normal male subjects (23). In virilized women with congenital adrenal hyperplasia, adrenal adenoma or Stein-Leventhal syndrome, dehydroepiandrosterone metabolism by abdominal skin was comparable to that in normal women (24).

An increased conversion rate of androstenedione to testosterone and of testosterone to DHT and androstanediols on the contrary has been reported in pubic skin of patients affected by idiopathic hirsutism (17, 25).

These controversial results may be due either to differences in *in vitro* techniques employed or to the heterogeneity of the cases studied. It cannot be excluded that in some hirsute females, excessive hair growth is due to an altered interaction of normal circulating androgens with cellular receptors of hair follicles.

B. Testosterone metabolism in fibroblast cultures

The metabolism of steroid hormones in human skin has also been studied in monolayer cultures of skin fibroblasts taken from different parts of the body, since all extracellular influences are thus removed and the differences in steroid metabolism occurring in the various cell populations may reflect inheritable differences intrinsic to cell types. Fibroblasts used for these experiments were obtained from explants of genital and non-genital skin of normal and abnormal subjects and maintained in Eagle's minimum essential medium supplemented with non-essential aminoacids, pyruvate and fetal and newborn calf serum. The cells were kept at 37°C in the presence of 5% CO_2 and then dissociated with trypsin. The medium was changed every 2-3 days and when a confluent monolayer appeared, fresh medium containing the radioactive steroid was added. After extraction and purification of each metabolite by multiple chromatography, carrier steroids were added for crystallization to constant specific activity.

1. Testosterone metabolism in cultured fibroblasts from normal subjects. This more sophisticated technique confirmed that subcultured human fibroblasts from genital skin such as labia majora and foreskin metabolised testosterone more actively than those from skin of the abdominal and deltoid region, thus demonstrating that the rate of steroid metabolism by cultured cells is a function of the anatomical site of the primary explant (26).

In vitro incubation of fibroblast monolayers grown from skin biopsies of foreskin and scrotum (27) indicated that DHT was the main product of conversion from testosterone reaching values of 54 pmol/mg protein/h and that its formation was linear for 36 h. Androstenedione, androstanedione and androstanediols were produced in smaller amounts. In contrast with in vitro incubation studies (15), no change in the transformation of testosterone into DHT was observed in fibroblast cultures from genital skin of normal male subjects ranging in age from newborn to 25 y (28).

Other investigators found that the major metabolite (49-57%) with genital skin fibroblasts, was androstenedione which is transformed after 12-24 h into androstanedione and then to androsterone. Other metabolites formed e.g. androstanediols and dihydrotestosterone, represented minor conversion products (about 5%) (26). For fibroblast cultures from non-genital skin, the conversion T$\rightarrow$DHT appears to be significantly lower (about 1 pmole/mg protein/h) than that observed in genital skin (28).

2. Testosterone metabolism in cultured fibroblasts from testicular feminization syndrome. Testosterone has been studied in cultured fibroblasts from foreskin of males with pseudohermaphroditism, the autosomal recessive disorder of phenotypic sexual differentiation, which includes the complete and incomplete forms.

The incomplete form is divided into type I, in which scrotal fibroblast formation of DHT is comparable to that of normal scrotal fibroblasts, and type 2 in which foreskin fibroblast formation of DHT is significantly lower (about 0.8 pmole/mg protein/h) than that observed with normal foreskin fibroblasts.

In the complete form T⟶DHT transformation in fibroblasts from labia majora may be intermediate (0.5-2.4 pmole/mg protein/h) between type I and 2 incomplete male pseudohermaphroditism. Normal formation of DHT however (16) or a deficient synthesis of this androgen (18, 19) have been reported in in vitro experiments. These controversial results are probably due to the different methods employed.

C. Enzymes involved in skin androgen metabolism

In vitro experiments have shown that human skin possesses various enzymes involved in androgen metabolism; in particular 3β-ol-dehydrogenase which plays a fundamental role in the conversion of dehydroepiandrosterone to androstenedione, 17β-ol-dehydrogenase transforming androstenedione to testosterone and 5α-reductase converting testosterone to DHT; these enzymatic sequences are therefore able to transform weak androgens to strong ones.

The skin, however, possesses enzymes which transform active compounds to inactive ones: 5α- and 5β-Δ^4-reductase forming androsterone and etiocholanolone and the 3α- and 3β-hydroxysteroid-dehydrogenases reducing DHT to 3α- and 3β-androstanediols respectively. These enzymes are more active in genital skin areas of both sexes than in non-genital zones and are even more active in male than in female perineal skin.

Enzymatic activity may be altered in some pathological conditions: in incomplete male pseudohermaphroditism type 2 and in some cases of the complete form, for instance, a deficiency in 5α-reductase is observed, whilst in the incomplete form type I, an apparently X-linked disorder of phenotypic sexual differentiation, 5α-reductase is normal and the defect seems to be due to the absence of the cytoplasmic receptor which conveys DHT to the nucleus of target cells.

Finally in secondary male hypogonadism 5α-reductase is low but may increase after HCG stimulation, whilst in some hirsute women this enzyme may be more active than in normal females.

Steroid-Receptors in Human Skin

It was reported above that sebaceous glands, hair follicles and skin of the genital area must be considered androgen-dependent. It was recently found that hormone-dependency of tissues and organs can be monitored by the study of hormone-receptors, which mediate hormone action. Studies on androgen receptors in the skin and skin structures will be briefly reviewed, in order to define the effect that hormones such as testosterone and dihydrotestosterone may have on the skin.

A. Androgen receptors in skin biopsy

The main difficulty, encountered in the measurement of androgen binding sites in the human skin, is the restriction placed upon the location of the biopsy and the number of replicates by the considerable amount of tissues (1/2 cm^2) required for a single assay. Furthermore, the exchange assay must be used (29) to detect the total number of androgen binding sites, since there are no free receptors in the human skin.

Cytosol androgen receptors have been detected in the sebaceous glands of animals (30, 31, 32) and of men (29). Sebaceous glands in both species are, in fact, target organs for androgens (33, 34, 35). Investigations on skin biopsies from the interscapular region in 16 men and 2 women, using tritiated metribolone (RI88I) as radioligand and the exchange assay, revealed no specific binding sites in the skin of subjects without seborrhea, whereas the concentration of binding sites in skin biopsies in 8 of the 11 patients with marked seborrhea ranged between 14 and 230 fmol/mg protein. No quantitative correlation was found between the severity of sebum secretion and the number of binding sites (29).

Unfortunately the exchange assay for the measurement of total receptors was not used in further studies on human genital skin, using RI88I as radioligand (36, 37).

In a comparison made between the androgen binding of prostate, seminal vesicles, epididymis and scrotal skin, and between cytosol and nuclear binding, the binding specificity of RI88I in the cytosol was distinctly different from that in scrotal skin where DHT was more potent than progestins in competition experiments. Androgen receptor binding was detected in 3 out of 4 biopsies of genital skin and the concentration of the binding sites ranged between 9 and 13 fmol/mg protein. In sharp contrast to cytosol, steroid specificity of RI88I binding in the nuclei of male sex accessory tissues and scrotal skin demonstrated that DHT was more potent than progestational agents in competition experiments and was strictly bound to the androgen receptor. In these studies, however, high affinity binding was found only in genital skin specimens (36).

Tritiated RI88I was used in preference to labelled T and DHT in experiments on androgen receptor binding in genital skin because the two latter compounds have a high degree of conversion during the incubation period (respectively, 28 and 68%). The mean androgen receptor values in the cytosol of preputial skin from 11 boys with different types of hypospadias were lower than those from 16 healthy controls (4.0 ± 2.84 vs 6.46 ± 2.79 fmol/mg protein) (37).

It can therefore be concluded that androgen receptors are usually undetectable in biopsies of normal human non-genital skin, even if total receptors are measured, whereas they are present in normal human genital skin. Androgen receptors are found, on the contrary, in non-genital skin of patients with high sebum secretion as well as in the genital skin of male patients with defective organogenesis of the external genitalia, although in these patients androgen receptor concentration is low and could account for the androgen-insensitivity of the cells of the genital area. Further investigations are necessary in order to detect androgen receptors in other pathological conditions of the human skin from the various areas known to be affected by androgens.

It is well known that testosterone has a stimulatory effect on dermal fibroblasts. It was therefore reasonable to seek an androgen receptor in these cells using monolayer dermal fibroblast cultures.

B. Androgen receptor in cultured human fibroblasts

1. Cell strains from normal subjects. The fibroblasts used were cultured from skin explants obtained either at circumcision or in the operating room under sterile conditions. Confluent monolayer cultures in disposable Petri dishes were used for incubation with tritiated steroid in the presence and absence of equivalent unlabelled steroid and at the end of the incubation period bound steroids were separated on Sephadex G-100 columns. One half of the measured binding was nuclear and the rest cytoplasmic. Androgen binding activity was measured in all normal cells including cells from foreskin, inguinal area, wrist, neck and buttocks (0.17-2.58 fmol/μg DNA which corresponded to 1,249-18,616 molecules per whole cell) (38).

Androgen binding on monolayer culture of fibroblasts was further examined in non-genital and genital skin from 14 normal subjects. The Petri dishes were incubated with various concentrations of tritiated DHT (with high specific activity) in the presence and absence of 200-fold excess of unlabelled steroid. The mean androgen-receptor values were lower in non-genital skin fibroblasts than in those from the genital area in all cases (14 vs 37 fmol/mg protein) (39).

The range in the non-genital cell strains from 16 controls varied nine-fold (4-23.3 fmol/mg protein with no sex differences) and threefold in the genital cell strains (15-53 fmol/mg protein) (40).

Androgen binding in fibroblast strains from 21 normal subjects was examined with saturation analysis, sucrose gradient centrifugation and separation on Sephadex G-100 column, or with a single saturating dose using 1mM tritiated steroid with or without 500-fold excess equivalent unlabelled steroid (41).

The values of the dissociation constants for T and DHT were comparable (0.13 and 0.11 x 10^{-9}M respectively for T and DHT) as were the number of binding sites (63.2 and 54.3 fmol/mg protein, respectively). Androgen binding on sucrose gradient centrifugation appeared as an 8S complex in a low ionic strength buffer and as a 4S complex in 0.5M KCl buffer. In five human cell lines it was possible to demonstrate a different number of specific binding sites for T, DHT, and RI88I used as radioligand, whereas no saturable binding was observed with estradiol and 17-epitestosterone. DHT binding (and 5α-reductase activity) was higher in fibroblast lines established from explants of genital skin than in similar lines derived from the non-genital skin (65 vs 4 fmol/mg protein, respectively). No correlation was found between DHT binding and 5α-reductase activity, whilst a correlation was established between T binding and the activity of this enzyme. T binding was also higher in fibroblasts derived from genital skin than in those derived from the non-genital region (59 vs 3 fmol/mg protein).

Although it was demonstrated that T itself was bound to androgen receptors, data on the metabolism of T during the binding assay indicates that DHT accounts for the major part of the intracellular androgen in nearly all cell lines displaying a high binding capacity. Furthermore, androgen-binding was constant in aging cell cultures. The finding that in some fibroblasts strains with high 5α-reductase activity the estimated receptor concentrations are higher when T is used as ligand suggests that the 5α-reductase activity and its subcellular localization are physiologically significant. In many tissues, this enzyme seems to be localized in or near the cell nucleus (42) and may protect intracellular DHT from degradation by the 3α-hydroxydehydrogenase and from low affinity binding in the cytosol (41).

2. Cell strains from androgen-insensitive patients. The types of receptor analysis previously described were employed to investigate different forms of androgen-insensitivity possibly due to a lack of androgen-receptor. Indeed, no specific androgen binding was detectable in fibroblasts from genital and non-genital areas in two siblings with androgen insensitivity (38).

A specific DHT binding to skin fibroblasts from wrist and pubis in the mother of three male pseudohermaphrodites was found to be within the normal range, indicating that androgen-insensitivity is X-linked in man and therefore homologous to the Tfm locus in the mouse. A significant population of clones from the subjects investigated had deficient receptor activity, and this finding is compatible with inactivation of one X-linked allele at this locus (43).

Two subgroups of androgen-insensitive patients have been identified on the basis of specific DHT binding by skin fibroblasts: one with undetectable DHT-receptor and one with normal DHT-receptor, revealing two distinct genetic variants (44). Similar results were found by others. High affinity androgen binding was demonstrated in fibroblasts from patients with incomplete male pseudohermaphroditism type 2 (with a 5α-reductase defect) and from patients with male pseudohermaphroditism (with a 17β-hydroxydehydrogenase defect): mean values ranged between 61 and 17 fmol/mg protein, respectively, for the genital and non-genital areas. Binding was low in fibroblasts from patients with complete testicular feminization and with incomplete male pseudohermaphroditism type I (X-linked recessive disorders) (39). In a study of 11 patients with testicular feminization DHT binding was reported in fibroblasts from 8 patients with mean values of 10-15 and 2 fmol/mg protein respectively, for the genital and non-genital areas (40). Furthermore, DHT binding in the cultured fibroblasts from patients with incomplete testicular feminization and with Reifenstein's syndrome (familial incomplete male pseudohermaphroditism type I) had values between that of normal subjects and most patients with complete testicular feminization. There is no significant change in the affinity constant and the turnover of the binding protein is within the normal range. In these two disorders, therefore, a defective regulation exists in the formation of the active DHT binding complex, i.e. the mutations in the two disorders affect the synthesis of the DHT binding proteins (45).

It would appear that receptor studies in skin biopsies and in cultured human fibroblasts can help to understand the pathogenesis of some familiar disorders related to the genetic information within the cells. These studies may therefore be useful in explaining other disorders with abnormal androgen end-organ sensitivity.

References

1. Edwards, E.A., Hamilton, J.B., Duntley, S.Q., Hubert, G.: Cutaneous vascular and pigmentary changes in castrate and eunuchoid men. Endocrinology 28, 119-125 (1940).
2. Strauss, J.S., Kligman, A.M., Pochi, P.E.: The effect of androgens and estrogens on the human sebaceous gland. J. invest. Derm. 39, 139-155 (1962).
3. Hamilton, J.B.: Male hormone substance; a prime factor in acne. J. clin. Endocrinol. Metab. 1, 570-579 (1941).
4. Voorhees, J.J., Hayes, E., Wilkins, J., Harreli, E.R.: The XYY chromosomal complement and nodulocystic acne. Ann. intern. Med. 73, 271-276 (1970).
5. Ferriman, D., Gallway, J.D.: Clinical assessment of body hair growth in women. J. clin. Endocrinol. Metab. 21, 1440-1447 (1961).
6. Rook, A.: Endocrine influences on hair growth. Br. med. J. 1, 609-614 (1965).
7. Bercovici, J.P., Mauvais-Jarvis, P.: Physiologie et pathologie du récepteur pilo-sébacé. Presse Méd. 78, 2229-2332 (1970).

8. Hamilton, J.B.: Effect of castration in adolescent and young adult males upon further changes in the proportions of bare and hairy scalp. J. clin. Endocrinol. Metab. 20, 1309-1318 (1960).

9. Konigsmark, B.W.: Hereditary deafness in man. New Engl. J. Med. 281, 827-832 (1969).

10. Gallegos, A.J., Berliner, D.L.: Transformation and conjugation of dehydroepiandrosterone by human skin. J. clin. Endocrinol. Metab. 27, 1214-1218 (1967).

11. Sciarra, F., Piro, C., Concolino, G., Conti, C.: Il metabolismo del deidroepiandrosterone a livello cutaneo: esperimenti in vitro. Folia Endocrinol. 21, 423-430 (1968).

12. Gomez, E.C., Hsia, S.L.: In vitro metabolism of testosterone-4-^{14}C and androstenedione-4-^{14}C in human skin. Biochemistry 7, 24-32 (1968).

13. Rongone, E.L.: Testosterone metabolism by human male mammary skin. Steroids 7, 489-504 (1966).

14. Flamigni, C., Collins, W.P., Koullapis, E.N., Craft, I., Dewhurst, C.J., Sommerville, I.F.: Androgen metabolism in human skin. J. clin. Endocrinol. Metab. 32, 737-743 (1971).

15. Wilson, J.D., Walker, J.D.: The conversion of testosterone to dihydrotestosterone by skin slices of man. J. clin. Invest. 48, 371-379 (1969).

16. Jenkins, J.S., Ash, S.: The metabolism of testosterone by skin in normal subjects and in testicular feminization. J. Endocrinol. 49, 515-520 (1971).

17. Mauvais-Jarvis, P., Kuttenn, F., Gauthier-Wright, F.: Testosterone 5α-reduction in human skin as an index of androgenicity. In: "Endocrine function of the human ovary", Eds. James, V.H.T., Serio, M., Giusti, G., Academic Press, London-New York-San Francisco, pp. 481-493 (1976).

18. Northcutt, R.C., Island, D.P., Liddle, G.W.: An explanation for the target organ unresponsiveness to testosterone in the testicular feminization syndrome. J. clin. Endocrinol. Metab. 29, 422-425 (1969).

19. Mauvais-Jarvis, P., Bercovici, J.P., Crepy, O., Gauthier, F.: Studies on testosterone metabolism in subjects with testicular feminization syndrome. J. clin. Invest. 49, 31-40 (1970).

20. Walsh, P.C., Madden, J.D., Harrod, M.J., Goldstein, J.L., MacDonald, P.C., Wilson, J.D.: Familial incomplete male pseudohermaphroditism, type 2. Decreased dihydrotestosterone formation in pseudovaginal perineoscrotal hypospadias. New Engl. J. Med. 291, 944-949 (1974).

21. Wilson, J.D., Harrod, M.J., Goldstein, J.L., Hemsell, D.L., MacDonald, P.C.: Familial incomplete male pseudohermaphroditism. New Engl. J. Med. 290, 1097-1103 (1974).

22. Kutten, F., Mauvais-Jarvis, J.: Testosterone 5α-reduction in the skin of normal subjects and of patients with abnormal sex development. Acta Endocrinol. 79, 164-176 (1975).

23. Oake, R.J., Thomas, J.P.: Androgen metabolism in the skin of hirsute women. In: "Endocrine function of the human ovary", Eds. James, V.H.T., Serio, M., Giusti, G., Academic Press, London-New York-San Francisco, pp. 495-507 (1976).

24. Piro, C., Sciarra, F., Conti, C.: The in vitro metabolism of 4-^{14}C-dehydroepiandrosterone by abdominal skin in hirsute females of adrenal and ovarian origin. Folia Endocrinol. 25, 38-44 (1972).

25. Jenkins, J.S., Ash, S.: The metabolism of testosterone by human skin in disorders of hair growth. J. Endocrinol. 59, 345-351 (1973).

26. Mulay, S., Finkelberg, R., Pinsky, L., Solomon, S.: Metabolism of 4-^{14}C-testosterone by serially subcultured human skin fibroblasts. J. clin. Endocrinol. Metab. 34, 133-143 (1972).

27. Voigt, W., Fernandez, E.P., Hsia, S.L.: Transformation of testosterone into 17β-hydroxy-5α-androstan-3-one by microsomal preparations of human skin. J. biol. Chem. 245, 5594-5599 (1970).

28. Wilson, J.D.: Dihydrotestosterone formation in cultured human fibroblasts. J. biol. Chem. 250, 3498-3504 (1975).

29. Bonne, C., Saurat, J.H., Chivot, M., Lehuchet, D., Raynaud, J.P.: Androgen receptor in human skin. Br. J. Derm. 97, 501-503 (1977).

30. Adachi, K., Kano. M.: The role of receptor proteins in controlling androgen action in the sebaceous glands of hamster. Steroids 19, 567-574 (1972).

31. King, R.J.B., Mainwaring, W.I.P.: Steroid-cell interaction. Eds. King, R.J.B., Mainwaring, W.I.P., Butterworths, London pp. 403-404 (1974).

32. Bonne, C., Raynaud, J.P.: Characterization and hormonal control of the androgen receptor in the hamster sebaceous gland. J. invest. Derm. 68, 215-220 (1976b).

33. Hamilton, J.B., Montagna, W.: The sebaceous glands of the hamster. I. Morphological effects of androgens on integumentary structures. Am. J. Anat. (Amer.) 86, 191-199 (1950).

34. Ebling, F.J.: Hormonal control of the sebaceous gland in experimental animals. Advances in biology of the skin. In: "The Sebaceous Glands", Eds. Montagna, W., Ellis, R.A., Silver, A.F., Pergamon Press, Oxford, vol. IV, pp. 200-211 (1963).

35. Strauss, J.S., Pochi, P.E.: The human sebaceous gland: its regulation by steroidal hormones and its use as end organ for assaying androgenicity in vivo. Recent Prog. Horm. Res. 19, 355-368 (1963).

36. Menon, M., Tananis, C.E., Hicks, L.L., Hawkins, E.L., McLoughlin, M.G., Walsh, P.C.: Characterization of the binding of a potent synthetic androgen, methyltrienolone, to human tissues. J. clin. Invest. 61, 150-162 (1978).

37. Svensson, J., Snochowski, M.: Androgen receptor levels in preputial skin from boys with hypospadias. J. clin. Endocrinol. Metab. 49, 340-345 (1979).

38. Keenan, B.S., Meyer, W.J., Hadjian, A.J., Jones, H.W., Migeon, C.J.: Syndrome of androgen-insensitivity in man: absence of 5α-dihydrotestosterone binding protein in skin fibroblasts. J. clin. Endocrinol. Metab. 38, 1143-1146 (1974).

39. Griffin, J.E., Punyashthiti, K., Wilson, J.D.: Dihydrotestosterone binding by cultured human fibroblasts. Comparison of cells from control subjects and from patients with hereditary male pseudohermaphroditism due to androgen resistance. J. clin. Invest. 57, 1342-1351 (1976).

40. Kaufman, M., Straisfeld, C., Pinsky, L.: Male pseudohermaphroditism presumably due to target organ responsiveness to androgens. Deficient 5α-dihydrotestosterone binding in cultured skin fibroblasts. J. clin. Invest. 58, 345-350 (1976).

41. Lamberigts, G., Dierickx, P., De Moor, P., Verhoeven, G.: Comparison of the metabolism and receptor binding of testosterone and 17β-hydroxy-5α-androstan-3-one in normal skin fibroblast cultures. J. clin. Endocrinol. Metab. 48, 924-930 (1979).

42. Verhoeven, G., Lamberigts, G., De Moor, P.: Nucleus associated steroid 5α-reductase activity and androgen responsiveness. J. Steroid Biochem. 5, 93-100 (1974).

43. Meyer, J.W., Migeon, B.R., Migeon, C.J.: Locus on human X chromosome for dihydrotestosterone receptor and androgen insensitivity. Proc. natn. Acad. Sci. U.S.A. 72, 1469-1472 (1975).

44. Amrhein, J.A., Meyer, W.J., Jones, H.W., Migeon, C.J.: Androgen insensitivity in man; evidence for genetic heterogeneity. Proc. natn. Acad. Sci. U.S.A. 73, 891-894 (1976).

45. Griffin, J.E., Wilson, J.D.: Studies on the pathogenesis of the incomplete forms of androgen resistance in man. J. clin. Endocrinol. Metab. 45, 1137-1143 (1977).

ECTOPIC PRODUCTION OF A GROWTH HORMONE-RELEASING FACTOR BY TUMORS

Marta Szabo and L. A. Frohman
Division of Endocrinology and Metabolism, Department of Medicine, Michael Reese Hospital and Medical Center and the University of Chicago, Chicago, Illinois 60616, U.S.A.

Hypothalamic Growth Hormone Releasing Factor

The existence of a growth hormone (GH)-releasing factor (GHRF) of hypothalamic origin was first demonstrated by Deuben and Meites (1) in 1964 and subsequently confirmed in many laboratories. Attempts to isolate hypothalamic GHRF have been made by several groups but to date none have been successful. A decapeptide from porcine hypothalamus isolated by Schally et al. (2) exhibited biologic activity when a nonspecific bioassay was used but failed to stimulate immunoreactive GH release and was eventually identified as the N-terminal portion of porcine β-hemoglobin. A peptide isolated from ovine hypothalamus by Villareal et al. (3) did release immunoreactive GH but was found to be a fragment of myelin basic protein. Other partially purified factors (4-8) have exhibited immunoreactive GH-releasing activity (GHRA) but none has been isolated in a pure form.

Clinical Evidence for Ectopic Growth Hormone Releasing Factor

The rationale of searching for GHRF in tissues other than hypothalamus was suggested by the recent observations that GH hypersecretion, acromegaly, and pituitary tumors can coexist with carcinoid (9-13) and pancreatic islet tumors (14, 15) and that in a few patients, removal of the extra-pituitary tumor has

Hormones in Normal and Abnormal Human Tissues, Vol. II

been followed by a return of plasma GH levels to normal (12, 13). Beck et al. (16) reported that extracts of lung carcinoma stimulated GH release in a perfused rat pituitary system, though similar effects were also observed in response to surrounding normal lung tissue. Dabek et al. (12) examined extracts of a carcinoid tumor removed from a patient with acromegaly but did not demonstrate GHRA. We initially reported the presence of GHRA in a bronchial carcinoid tumor from a patient who had previously undergone surgical removal of a GH-secreting pituitary tumor and in whom the persistently elevated GH levels postoperatively returned to nearly undetectable levels after excision of the carcinoid tumor (17). Biologic activity was demonstrated in a dispersed pituitary cell monolayer culture. A subsequent report (18) suggested the presence of similar biologic activity in a bronchial carcinoid tumor, though the lack of appropriate controls limited the interpretation of the results.

In this report, we review the results of studies on tissue obtained from additional patients with carcinoid, pancreatic islet or adrenal tumors. In addition, we will describe the results in small cell lung carcinoma tissue obtained at surgery and grown in continuous cell culture (19). The latter studies were prompted by the similarity in morphologic appearance between carcinoid tumors and small cell carcinomas and the known production of numerous peptide hormones by such carcinomas.

Partial Purification and Characterization of Ectopic GHRA

Tumor tissue from patients with or without evidence of GH hypersecretion was obtained at surgery or autopsy and stored at -80°C for up to 10 y until extraction with 2N acetic acid (17). GHRA of tumor extracts was assessed in four day primary cultures of enzymatically dispersed adenohypophyseal cells from estrogen-primed, male rats (20, 21). The minimum quantity of tissue required for the extraction of demonstrable GHRA from seven tumors is listed in Table 1. Five of these tumors were obtained from

Table 1. Growth Hormone-Releasing Activity of Tumor Extracts

Tumor	Plasma GH	Tumor GHRA: Least Detectable Dose, Tissue	Tumor GHRA: Least Detectable Dose, Protein	Tumor GHRA: Maximal Stimulation Above Control
	ng/ml	mg	µg	%
1. Bronchial carcinoid	31	0.25	3	82
2. Pancreatic islet adenoma	24	0.025	0.75	141
3. Liver carcinoid (metastatic)	178	0.33	8.5	119
4. Bronchial carcinoid	1	2.5	33	55
5. Small cell carcinoma of lung	1.2	5.0	82	17
6. Liver carcinoid (metastatic)	176	7.5	128	242
7. Adrenal cortical adenoma	140-180	1.5	25	21

patients with elevated plasma GH and clinical manifestations of acromegaly. The extracts of two tumors, one bronchial carcinoid and one pancreatic islet adenoma from patients whose symptoms of acromegaly had subsided upon surgical excision of the tumor were employed for the majority of characterisation studies described. The extracts of seven additional tumors (two bronchial carcinoids, three small cell carcinomas, one carcinoid of unknown origin metastatic to liver and one pancreatic islet adenoma) obtained from patients with normal GH levels were devoid of biologic activity.

Because of the generally recognized embryological and ultrastructural similarities of carcinoid tumors to small cell carcinoma of the lung, a series of hormone-producing human pulmonary small cell carcinoma cells in continuous culture (22) was also screened for the possible presence of GHRA. Medium was harvested from dense cultures, grown for four days, and after repeated washing, replaced with fresh, serum-free medium and incubated at 37°C for one hour. Three out of ten one hour serum free media significantly stimulated GH release by cultured adenohypophyseal cells (Fig. 1), suggesting the ability of some of these small cell carcinoma cell lines to produce ectopic GHRA. GHRA was not detected in any of the four day culture media; all inhibited GH release, presumably because of the accumulation during the four day culture period of inhibitors and/or enzymes capable of degrading GH release by the adenohypophyseal cells.

Stimulation of GH release by an extract of bronchial carcinoid was dose dependent. However, the dose-response curve plateaued at the highest concentration of extract tested (Fig. 2). The secretion of prolactin (PRL) and thyrotropin (TSH) was not increased, indicating specific stimulation of the somatotroph. Crude or partially purified extracts of the pancreatic islet adenoma also elicited linear log-dose stimulation of GH release. All tumor extracts with GHRA caused a slight suppression of PRL release.

The GHRA of the bronchial carcinoid extract (Fig. 3) and pancreatic islet adenoma extract was confirmed in an additional

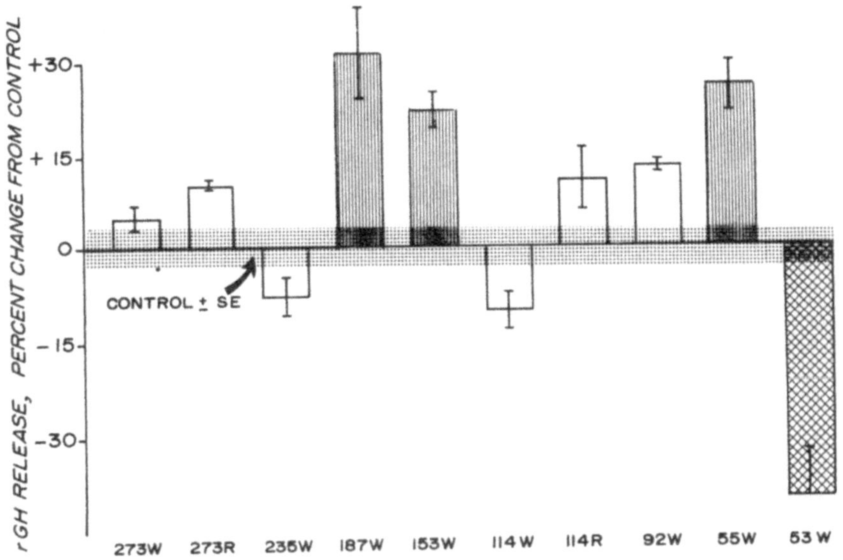

Fig. 1. Effect of media (W=Waymouth MB752/1, R=RPMI 1640) in which pulmonary small cell carcinoma cultures had been incubated for 1 h, on GH release from rat adenohypophyseal cells in 4 day primary culture. Each bar represents the Mean ± SEM of quadruplicate incubations. The shaded area denotes the range of responses to unincubated culture media.

in vitro system which utilized the measurement of immunoprecipitable ^{3}H-GH release from ^{3}H-leu prelabeled, perifused rat pituitary fragments (23). Furthermore, intracarotid administration of a partially purified carcinoid extract to estrogen-primed, urethane anesthetized male rats led to a significantly greater elevation of plasma GH than did the administration of vehicle alone (Fig. 4).

Plateauing of the dose-response curve at the highest concentration of crude bronchial carcinoid extract tested (Fig. 1) suggested the presence of an inhibitor of GH release. The possible presence of somatostatin (SRIF) in this and other extracts was, therefore, examined using a specific radioimmunoassay (24). All extracts contained detectable SRIF-like immunoreactivity

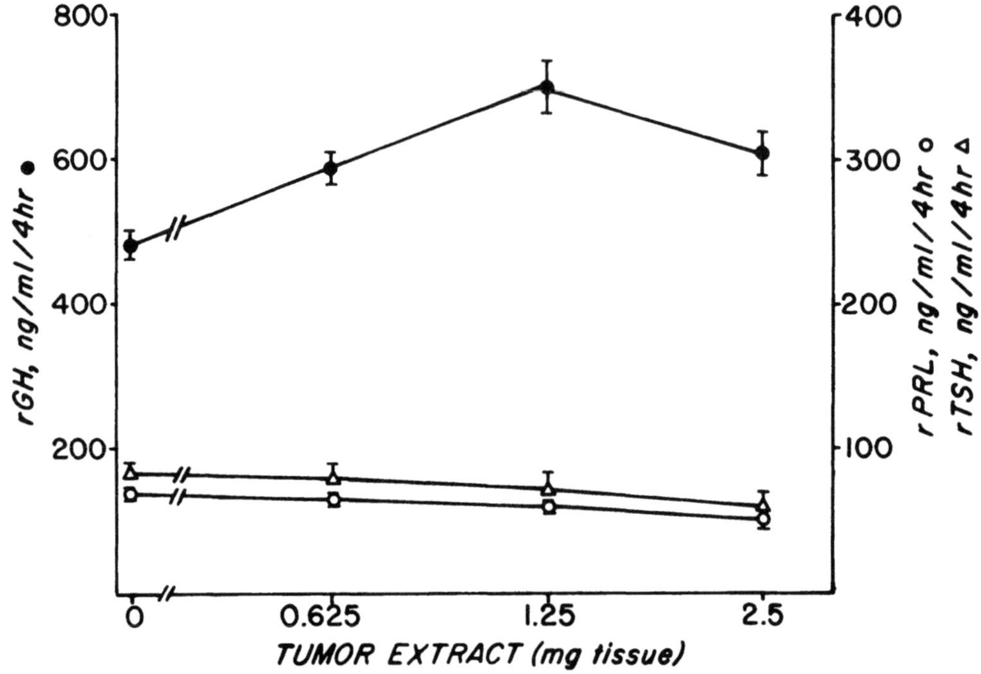

Fig. 2. Dose-related effect of a bronchial carcinoid tumor extract on GH, PRL, and TSH release by rat adenohypophyseal cells in 4 day primary culture. Each point represents the Mean $\pm$ SEM of quadruplicate incubations. Reprinted with permission (17).

(SRIF-LI), several in sufficient quantity to oppose the stimulatory action of the extract at the minimum dose required to demonstrate GHRA (Table 2). The minimum concentration of SRIF required to suppress stimulated GH release by pituitary cell cultures was previously determined as 3×10^{-11}M (21). The stimulation of GH release by all active extracts was completely antagonized by the addition of SRIF, 10^{-9}M. SRIF-LI of the seven additional tumors devoid of GHRA ranged from 1.6 to 96 ng/g.

Compounds known to be produced by carcinoid and pancreatic islet tumors which failed to stimulate GH release by cultured pituitary cells and could thus be excluded as agents responsible for the extracts' releasing activity are listed in Fig. 5. The

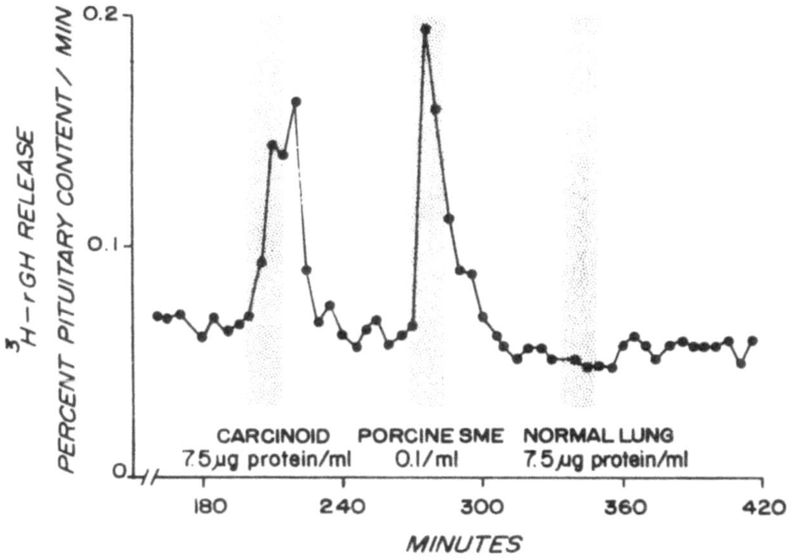

Fig. 3. Effect of extracts of bronchial carcinoid tumor, porcine stalk median eminence, and normal human lung on the release of immunoprecipitable ^{3}H-rGH from perifused rat anterior pituitary fragments prelabeled with ^{3}H-leucine. Pulses of each test agent, indicated by the shaded area, were of 15 min duration. Pituitary fragments were perifused with medium for 3 h to allow a stable basal release rate prior to the introduction of the pulse. Reprinted with permission (21).

peptide nature of the bronchial carcinoid and pancreatic islet tumors' GHRA was indicated by the finding that the broad spectrum peptidase, pronase, completely destroyed the GH stimulatory activity during incubation at 37°C for 30 min. The peptide, bradykinin, also known to be produced by carcinoid tumors, stimulated both GH and PRL release, in contrast to the putative GH-releasing peptide.

The approximate molecular weight of GHRA was determined and partial purification accomplished by gel filtration chromatography. GHRA of the pancreatic islet tumor extract was contained in the void volume of Sephadex G25 equilibrated and eluted with 1 N acetic acid (Fig. 6), indicating an apparent MW >5,000 daltons.

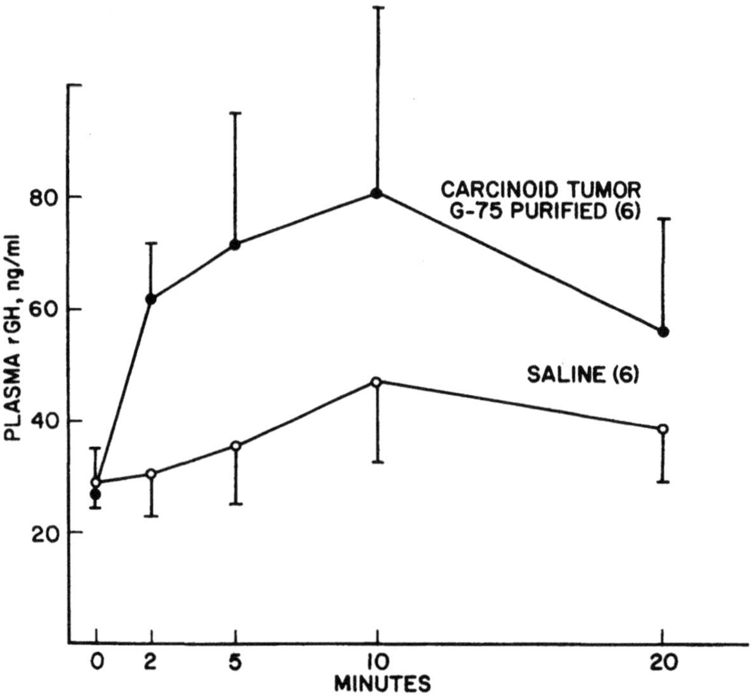

Fig. 4. Effect of intracarotid administration of Sephadex G75-purified extract of a carcinoid tumor on plasma GH levels of estrogen-primed, urethane anesthetized male rats. Control rats received an injection of phosphate buffered saline, used as the vehicle for the tumor extract. The number of rats in each group is indicated in parentheses.

The majority of SRIF-like immunoreactivity, on the other hand, was retarded and, thus, separated from GHRA, leading to a marked rise in specific activity of the void volume peak.

Gel filtration chromatography on Sephadex G75 was carried out in order to achieve more accurate molecular sizing and additional purification (Fig. 7). A major peak of activity was eluted at a Kd of 0.5-0.7 and was separated from two major protein peaks in the void volume resulting in about a 20-fold increase in specific activity. On the basis of its elution position

Table 2. Somatostatin-Like Immunoreactivity of Tumor Extracts with GHRA

Tumor[a]	SRIF-LI ng equiv/g[b]	Tissue Required For Detection of Bioactivity mg
1. Bronchial carcinoid	6.8	8.0
2. Pancreatic islet adenoma	226	0.24
3. Liver carcinoid (metastatic)	20	2.7
4. Bronchial carcinoid	14.4	3.8
5. Small cell carcinoma of lung	14.0	3.9
6. Liver carcinoid (metastatic)	1.6	34
7. Adrenal cortical adenoma	4.1	13.3

[a] The SRIF-LI concentration of normal human lung and pancreas was 2.4 and 880 ng/g, respectively

[b] Least detectable values = 0.1 - 0.2 ng/g at the extract concentration used for assay (100 mg tissue equivalent/ml)

POTENTIAL TUMOR-ASSOCIATED FACTORS WHICH DO NOT STIMULATE GROWTH HORMONE RELEASE

Agent	Concentration
SEROTONIN NOREPINEPHRINE DOPAMINE	10^{-7}-10^{-5}M
5-HYDROXYTRYPTOPHAN	10^{-6}-10^{-4}M
CHOLECYSTOKININ-8 SECRETIN V.I.P. G.I.P. SUBSTANCE P INSULIN GLUCAGON PANCREATIC POLYPEPTIDE CALCITONIN	10^{-8}-10^{-6}M

Fig. 5. Lack of effect of agents, potentially produced by carcinoid and pancreatic islet tumors, on GH release by cultured rat adenohypophyseal cells at the concentrations indicated

the apparent molecular weight of GHRA from this tumor was estimated as 8,000 daltons. GHRA from three other carcinoids eluted from Sephadex G75 with an identical Kd; in addition, a void volume peak of activity was also present in one. Incubation of the pancreatic islet tumor extract with mercaptoethanol did not modify its GHRA or the elution position on Sephadex G75.

Ion exchange chromatography of crude pancreatic islet tumor extract was carried out in order to assess the net charge of the peptide as well as the utility of this procedure for further purification. GHRA was quantitatively retained on DEAE cellulose in 0.001 M NH_4HCO_3, pH 7.6 and could be eluted by

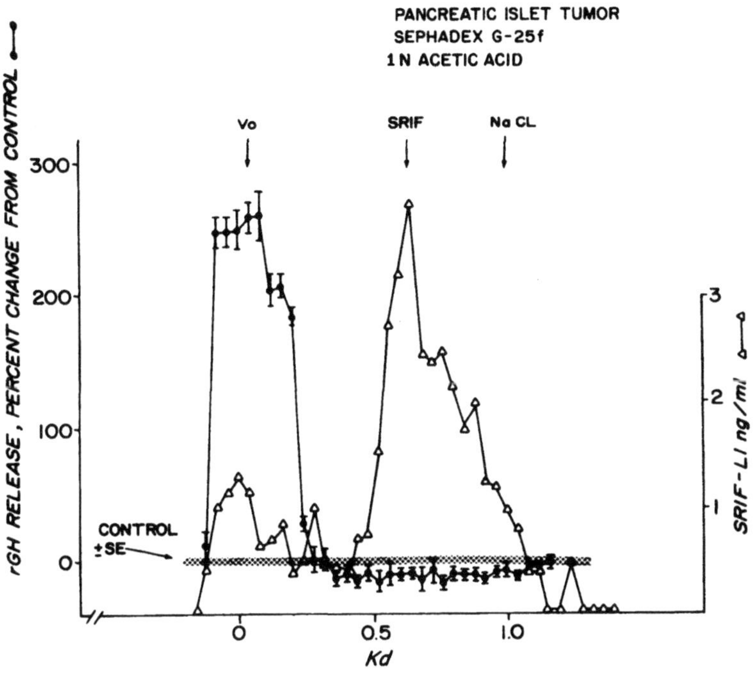

Fig. 6. Gel filtration chromatography of crude pancreatic islet tumor extract on a 2.2 x 90 cm Sephadex G25 column, equilibrated and eluted with 1 N acetic acid. GHRA of 4 ml fractions (solid circles), determined in four replicate rat adenohypophyseal cultures, is shown as the percent change ± SEM compared to control release (shaded area). SRIF-LI is indicated by the open triangles. Reprinted with permission (21).

increasing the buffer concentrations to 0.1 - 1.0 M. No retention of GHRA on CM cellulose was evident at a low ionic strength and slightly acidic pH (0.001M NH_4OAc, pH 6.5). A significant portion of the activity was irreversibly retained on both columns.

Additional purification of the crude pancreatic islet tumor extract was accomplished by reverse phase high performance liquid chromatography (HPLC) on a µ-cyanopropyl column equili-

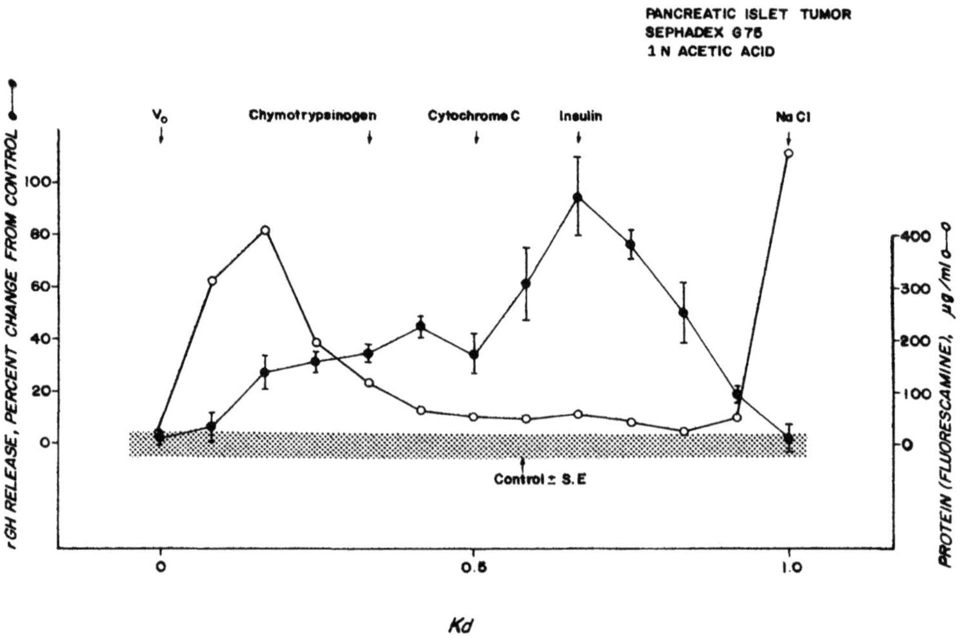

Fig. 7. Gel filtration chromatography of crude pancreatic islet tumor extract on a 0.9 x 55 cm Sephadex G75 column, equilibrated and eluted with 1 N acetic acid. GHRA of 2 ml fractions (solid circles), is expressed as in Figure 6. Protein concentration (open circles) was determined by the fluorescamine assay. Reprinted with permission (21).

brated with 0.25M triethyl-ammonium formate, pH 3.5, 90% - acetonitrile, 10%, and eluted with a 10-50% linear acetonitrile gradient at a flow rate of 2 ml/min (Fig. 8). GHRA, initially determined by bioassay of pooled portions of five successive fractions and subsequently in individual fractions correspon-ding to the active pool, eluted in a single fraction at an ace-tonitrile concentration of 26%. Protein concentration of each fraction was monitored by the highly sensitive fluorescamine assay for primary amines (25). An approximately 50-fold purifi-

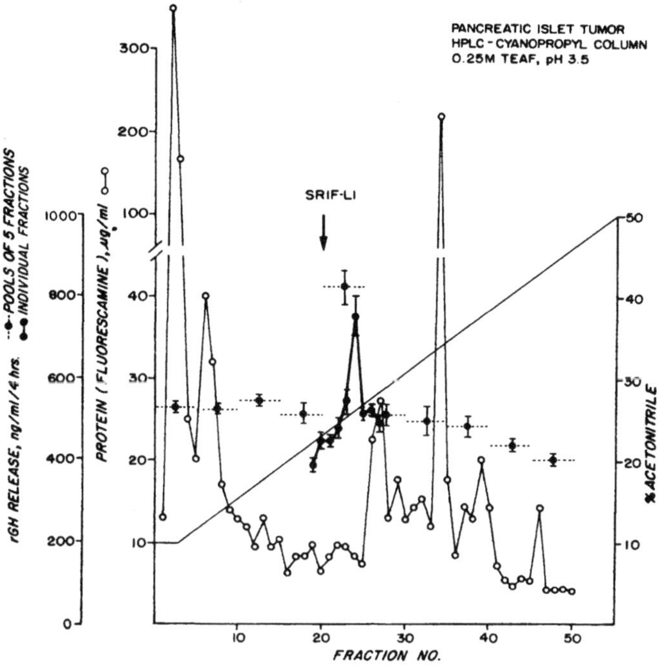

Fig. 8. Purification of pancreatic islet tumor GHRA by HPLC. Two ml fractions were collected at a flow rate of 2 ml/min. Pools of a portion (20%) of 5 successive fractions were assayed initially in 4 replicate cultures of rat adenohypophyseal cells (horizontal broken lines). Individual fractions within and extending slightly beyond the active pool (solid line and circles) were then tested. GH release by control cultures was 519±6 ng/ml/4 h in the assay of pools and 489±10 ng/ml/4 h in the assay of individual fractions. Protein concentration (open circles) was determined by fluorescamine assay. Reprinted with permission (21).

cation was achieved and as little as 40 ng peptide exhibited significant bioactivity in pituitary cell cultures. HPLC is our current method of choice for purification of crude ectopic GHRA on a preparative scale.

Preliminary structural characterization of pancreatic islet tumor extract was obtained by means of treatment with proteolytic enzymes. Incubation of crude pancreatic islet tumor extract with human plasma for 60 min led to a partial loss of activity. Pancreatic islet tumor extract, partially purified on Sephadex G75, was treated with the limited specificity proteolytic enzymes trypsin, chymotrypsin, carboxypeptidases A and B, leucine aminopeptidase and pyroglutamate aminopeptidase. GHRA was completely destroyed by treatment with trypsin and chymotrypsin but was unaffected by incubation with all four exopeptidases (Fig. 9). These findings indicate that internal lysine and/or arginine and aromatic amino acids are required for biologic activity while the COOH and NH_2 terminals are either blocked or non-essential. The failure of pyroglutamate aminopeptidase to alter releasing activity suggests that, in contrast to hypothalamic GHRA (8), an N-terminal pyroglutamate residue is not a part of the active site of the peptide.

Biologic Implications

Peptide hormone secretion by non-endocrine tumors has generally been restricted to those tumors whose cells of origin belong to the amine precursor-uptake-and-decarboxylation (APUD) series of cells as described by Pearse (26), although there exists some uncertainty as to the embryonic origin of the cells, i.e., neural crest or a specialized neuroectoderm. These cells are generally characterized by the presence of specific enzyme systems (i.e. aromatic amino acid decarboxylase, histidine decarboxylase) and the presence of secretory granules. The demonstration of GHRA in the tumors studied is consistent with this hypothesis and adds yet another peptide hormone to the extensive list already recognized (27). The production of GHRA by small cell carcinoma tumors strengthens the link between these tumors and carcinoid tumors, both of which have been proposed to be derived from the Kulchitsky cell in the bronchial epithelium which

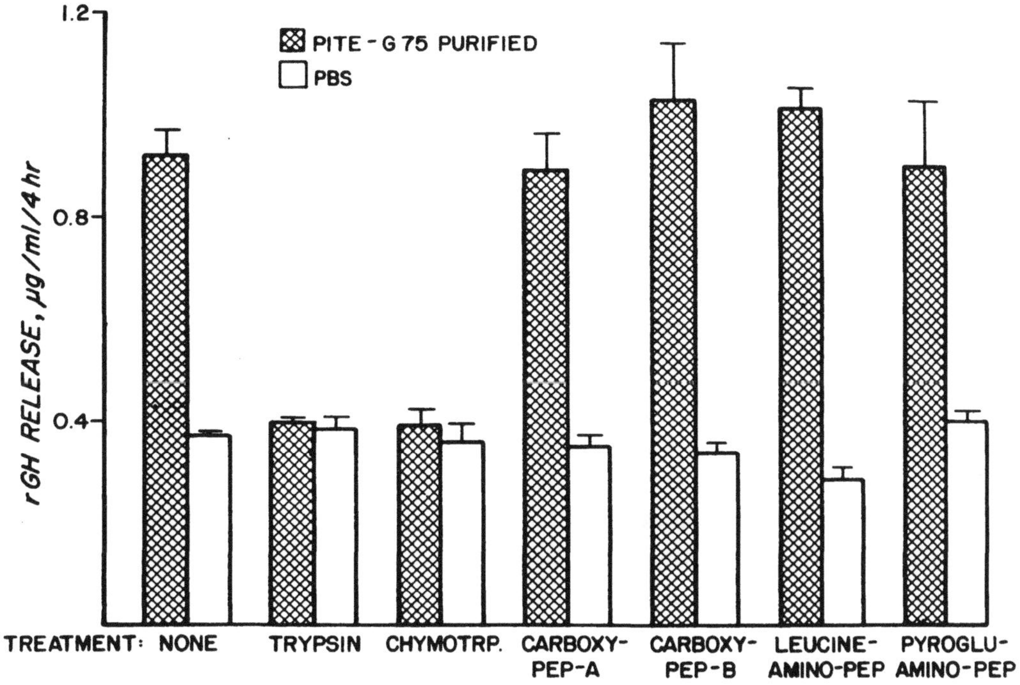

Fig. 9. Effect of enzyme treatment on the GHRA from pancreatic islet tumor. GHRA, partially purified on Sephadex G75, was incubated with enzyme, 50 µg/ml, at 37°C for 60 min, placed into a 100°C water bath for 5 min, and added to quadruplicate cultures of rat adenohypophyseal cells. Control incubations were performed with heat inactivated enzymes.

contains abundant secretory granules (28). The inclusion of an adrenal cortical adenoma in our series appears to represent an exception to the above classification and suggests that others may also be found in the future.

The majority of the studies described were performed in the pituitary culture system because of its technical feasibility for assaying large numbers of samples. It is, of course, a "static" incubation in which the dynamics of GH release cannot be evaluated. We, therefore, used a pituitary perifusion system previously validated with a crude hypothalamic extract possessing GHRA (29). The rapid response of GH release upon exposure to tumor GHRF as well as the demonstration of in vivo GHRA provide for the validation of the results obtained in the cell culture system.

The presence of somatostatin in the islet cell tumor could have been predicted since it is a normal constituent of the pancreatic islet D cells (30), but it was unsuspected in the other tumors. It is of interest that the net expression of biologic activity of each tumor in situ must represent the effects of both GH-releasing and GH-inhibiting activities and that this was reflected better by the concentration of the former than that of the latter. These findings raise the possibility that tumors in which no GHRA was found may contain a GHRF which is obscured by the presence of somatostatin or another inhibitor, the detection of which must await development of a different type of assay system (i.e. radioimmunoassay or receptor binding assay). The presence of the releaser and the inhibitor and, in at least one patient (cf. 21), GH itself in the tumor, raises the intriguing possibility that the genomes which code for a pituitary hormone and its hypothalamic regulatory hormones are closely related to one another and that this arrangement may have been of some evolutionary advantage. It is supported by the occasional association of ACTH and its hypothalamic regulatory factor corticotropin-releasing factor in small cell carcinomas (31).

Although it is premature from the present studies to conclude that the tumor GHRFs are identical to one another or to hypothalamic GHRF, the results are consistent with their being closely related. The tumor GHRFs are all peptides, and where compared, exhibited parallel dose response curves and similar partition coefficients on Sephadex G75. The estimated molecular size ($\pm$ 8,000 daltons) is somewhat larger than expected for a hypothalamic releasing hormone (the maximum size of structurally identified hypophysiotropic hormones is 1,600 daltons). The inability of mercaptoethanol to alter the elution position from

Sephadex is consistent with the tumor GHRF representing a precursor molecule. Plasma from the patient with tumor no.3 has been reported to contain GHRA of a smaller size than that which we have identified in the tumor (32) and suggests further processing of the molecule in association with its release into circulation. The lowest quantity of tumor GHRF required for bioactivity (40 ng protein) is also greater than that of synthetic hypothalamic hormones. This observation could represent decreased bioactivity of a precursor molecule but could also be due to contaminating, biologically inert peptides. Additional evidence in support of the precursor hypothesis is provided by the demonstration that higher molecular weight forms of ACTH (33) and somatostatin (34) are secreted by tumors. This question can, however, be resolved only when the structural identities of both the hypothalamic and tumor GHRFs are known.

The spectrum of biologic activity of the tumor GHRA is also unknown. There is yet no experimental evidence to implicate an action on GH or protein synthesis. However, several of the patients from whom the tissues described in the present report were obtained, as well as others reported in the literature, exhibited pituitary tumor formation as well as GH hypersecretion. The specific mechanism whereby excessive releasing factor stimulation could lead to tumor formation must await further study.

Clinical Considerations

From a clinical standpoint, the present results provide an explanation for the association of GH-secreting pituitary tumors in patients with the Multiple Endocrine Neoplasia Syndrome, Type I and imply that small, otherwise asymptomatic extrapituitary tumors may be the cause of GH hypersecretion in patients with acromegaly. Consideration of the presence of an extrapituitary tumor should, therefore, be given in such patients. Although the nature of the extrapituitary tumor is not necessarily benign, it is unlikely that a rapidly growing malignant lesion which secretes a GHRF will cause acromegaly because of the long duration of time generally required to produce the clinical features of this disease. However, measurement of GH levels in patients with small cell lung carcinomas may provide information as to the frequency of ectopic GHRF secretion.

Finally, the results provide a fresh insight into the question of the role of hypothalamic GHRF in the production of acromegaly. The fact that excessive stimulation by an ectopic GHRF can produce not only GH hypersecretion and acromegaly, but also pituitary tumor formation, suggests that in at least some patients, hypersecretion of hypothalamic GHRF represents the etiologic factor in the development of GH-secreting pituitary tumors.

Acknowledgements

The studies from the authors' laboratory were supported, in part, by United States Public Health Service Grant AM-18722.

References

1. Deuben, R.R., Meites, J.: Stimulation of pituitary growth hormone release by a hypothalamic extract in vitro. Endocrinology 74, 408-414 (1964).
2. Schally, A.V., Baba, Y., Nair, R.M.G.: The amino acid sequence of a peptide with growth hormone-releasing activity isolated from porcine hypothalamus. J. biol. Chem. 246, 6647-6650 (1971).
3. Villareal, J.A., Vale, W., Brown, M., Butcher, M., Brazeau, P., Rivier, C., Burgus, R.: Myelin basic protein: a substance that releases immunoreactive growth hormone in vitro. Biochem. biophys. Res. Commun. 70, 551-558 (1976).
4. Frohman, L.A., Maran, J.W., Dhariwal, A.P.S.: Plasma growth hormone responses to intrapituitary injections of growth hormone-releasing factor in the rat. Endocrinology 88, 1483-1488 (1971).
5. Wilber, J.F., Nagel, T., White, W.F.: Hypothalamic growth hormone-releasing activity:characterization by the in vitro rat pituitary and radioimmunoassay. Endocrinology 89, 1419-1424 (1971).

6. Johansson, K.N-G., Currie, B.L., Folkers, K.: Identification and purification of factor B-GHRH from hypothalami which releases growth hormone. Biochem. biophys. Res. Commun. 60, 610-615 (1974).

7. Takahara, J., Arimura, A., Schally, A.V.: Assessment of GH releasing hormone activity in Sephadex - separated fractions of porcine hypothalamic extracts by hypophyseal portal vessel infusion in the rat. Acta endocr. 78, 428-434 (1975).

8. Nair, R.M.G., DeVillier, C., Barnes, M., Antalis, J., Wilbur, D.L.: A bovine hypothalamic peptide possessing immunoreactive growth hormone-releasing activity. Endocrinology 103, 112-120 (1978).

9. Southern, A.L.: Functioning metastatic bronchial carcinoid with elevated levels of serum and cerebrospinal fluid serotonin and pituitary adenoma. J. clin. Endocrinol. Metab. 20, 298-305 (1960).

10. Weiss, L., Ingram, M.: Adenomatoid bronchial tumors: a consideration of the carcinoid tumors and the salivary tumors of the bronchial tree. Cancer 14, 161-178 (1961).

11. Buse, J., Buse, M.G., Roberts, W.J.: Eosinophilic adenoma of the pituitary and carcinoid tumors of the rectosigmoid area. J. clin. Endocrinol. Metab. 21, 735-738 (1961).

12. Dabek, J.T.: Bronchial carcinoid tumor with acromegaly in two patients. J. clin. Endocrinol. Metab. 38, 329-333 (1974).

13. Sönksen, P.H., Ayres, A.B., Braimbridge, M., Corrin, B., Davies, D.R., Jeremiah, G.M., Oaten, S.W., Lowy, C., West, T.E.T.: Acromegaly caused by bronchial carcinoid tumours. Clin. Endocr. 5, 503-513 (1976).

14. Ballard, H.S., Frame, B., Hartsock, R.J.: Familial multiple endocrine adenoma-peptic ulcer complex. Medicine (Baltimore) 43, 481-516 (1964).

15. Caplan, R.H., Koob, L., Abellera, R.M., Pagliara, A.S., Kovacs, K., Randall, R.V.: Cure of acromegaly by operative removal of an islet cell tumor of the pancreas. Am. J. Med. 64, 874-882 (1978).

16. Beck, C., Larkins, R.G., Martin, T.J., Burger, H.G.: Stimulation of growth hormone release from superfused rat pituitary by extracts of hypothalamus and of human lung tumours. J. Endocrinol. 59, 325-333 (1973).

17. Zafar, M.S., Mellinger, R.C., Fine, G., Szabo, M., Frohman, L.A.: Acromegaly associated with a bronchial carcinoid tumor: evidence for ectopic production of growth hormone-releasing activity. J. clin. Endocrinol. Metab. 44, 66-71 (1979).

18. Shalet, S.M., Beardwell, C.G., MacFarlane, I.A., Ellison, M.L., Norman, C.M., Rees, L.H., Hughes, M.: Acromegaly due to production of a growth hormone-releasing factor by a bronchial carcinoid tumour. Clin. Endocr. 10, 61-67 (1979).

19. Pettengill, O.S., Sorenson, G.D., Wurster-Will, D.H., Curphey, T.J., Noll, W.W., Cate, C.C., Maurer, L.H.: Isolation and growth characteristics of continuous cell lines from small cell carcinoma of the lung. Cancer 45, 906-918 (1980).

20. Rick, J., Szabo, M., Payne, P., Kovathana, N., Cannon, J.G., Frohman, L.A.: Prolactin-suppressive effects of two amino-tetralin analogs of dopamine: their use in characterization of the pituitary dopamine receptor. Endocrinology 104, 1234-1242 (1979).

21. Frohman, L.A., Szabo, M., Berelowitz, M., Stachura, M.E.: Partial purification and characterization of a peptide with growth hormone-releasing activity from extrapituitary tumors in patients with acromegaly. J. clin. Invest. 65, 43-54 (1980).

22. Sorenson, G.D., Pettengill, O.S., Brinck-Johnsen, T., Cate, C.C., Maurer, L.H.: Hormone production by cultures of small cell carcinoma of the lung. Cancer (in press, 1980).

23. Stachura, M.E.: Basal and dibutyryl cyclic AMP-stimulated release of newly synthesized and stored growth hormone from perifused rat pituitaries. Endocrinology 98, 580-589 (1976).

24. Kronheim, S., Berelowitz, M., Pimstone, B.L.: A radioimmunoassay for growth hormone release-inhibiting hormone: method and quantitative tissue distribution. Clin. Endocr. 5, 619-630 (1976).

25. Undenfriend, S., Stein, S., Bohlen, P., Dairman, W., Leimgruber, W., Weigele, M.: Fluorescamine: a reagent for assay of amino acids, peptides, proteins and primary amines in the picomole range. Science 178, 871-872 (1972).

26. Pearse, A.G.E.: The diffuse neuroendocrine system and the APUD concept: Related "endocrine" peptides in brain, intestine, pituitary, placenta, and anuran cutaneous glands. Med. Biol. 55, 115-125 (1977).

27. Sherwood, L.M., Gould, V.E.: Ectopic hormone syndrome and multiple endocrine neoplasia. In: "Endocrinology", Eds. De Groot, L.J., Cahill, G.F., Martini, L., Nelson, D.H., Odell, W.D., Potts, J.T., Steinberger, E., Winegrad, A.I., Grune and Stratton, New York, pp. 1733-1766 (1979).

28. McDowell, E.M., Barrett, L.A., Trump, B.F.: Observations on small granule cells in adult human bronchial epithelium and in carcinoic and oat cell tumors. Lab. Invest. 34, 202-206 (1976).

29. Stachura, M.E., Szabo, M., Frohman, L.A.: Multiphasic effect of porcine stalk-median eminence extract on growth hormone release from perifused rat pituitaries. Endocrinology 102, 1520-1526 (1978).

30. Hökfelt, T., Efendic, S., Hellerström, C., Johansson, O., Luft, R., Arimura, A.: Cellular localization of somatostatin in endocrine-like cells and neurons of the rat with special reference to the A_1-cells of the pancreatic islets and to the hypothalamus. Acta endocr. 80, Suppl.200, 5-41 (1975).

31. Upton, G.V., Amatruda, T.T.Jr.: Evidence for the presence of tumor peptides with corticotropin-releasing-factor-like activity in the ectopic ACTH syndrome. New Engl. J. Med. 285, 419-424 (1971).

32. Leveston, S.A., Lee, Y-C., Jaffe, B.M., Daughaday, W.H.: Massive GH and ACTH hypersecretion associated with a metastatic carcinoid tumor. 60th Annual Meeting of The Endocrine Society, Miami, Fla. p. 371 (1978).

33. Wolfsen, A.R., Odell, W.D.: ProACTH: Use for early detection of lung cancer. Am. J. Med. 66, 765-772 (1979).

34. Szabo, M., Berelowitz, M., Pettengill, O.S., Sorenson, G.D., Frohman, L.A.: Somatostatin secretion by cultured human small cell carcinoma of the lung. 61st Annual Meeting of The Endocrine Society, Anaheim, Calif. p. 144 (1979).

THE USE OF HUMAN CELL CULTURES AS MODEL SYSTEMS FOR STUDYING THE ACTION OF GLUCOCORTICOIDS IN HUMAN LYMPHOBLASTIC LEUKAEMIAS

M. Norman
Department of Chemical Pathology, King's College Hospital Medical School, Denmark Hill, London, SE5 8RX, U.K.

J. Harmon and E. B. Thompson
Biochemistry of Gene Expression Section, Laboratory of Biochemistry, National Cancer Institute, NIH, Bethesda, Maryland 20205, U.S.A.

Early physiological studies on adrenal cortical function provided the first suggestion that steroid hormones might be useful for controlling lympho-proliferative disorders such as leukaemia. In 1937, both Selye (1) and Moon (2) published papers describing the inhibitory effects which adrenal hormones could exert on lymphoid tissue. Later, Dougherty and White (3, 4, 5) made a careful study of these inhibitory responses, and showed that treatment of animals with adrenal steroids caused pyknosis and destruction of lymphocytes, together with involution of the thymus. Since adrenal hormones exerted such a powerful inhibitory effect on some normal lymphoid cells in animals, attempts were made to exploit these effects for the treatment of lymphomas and leukaemias by stimulation of the adrenals with pituitary adrenocorticotrophic hormone (ACTH) or direct injection of adrenal steroids. Early studies on experimental leukaemia were encouraging. For example, administration of adrenal hormones increased survival in rats with transplanted or spontaneous leukaemia (6). Nevertheless, early attempts to treat human patients were disappointing. Dameshek (7) treated two patients with chronic lymphocytic leukaemia (CLL) using crude pituitary extracts without effect. Similarly, Nordenson (8) and Hellman (9)

Hormones in Normal and Abnormal Human Tissues, Vol. II

reported little or no effect when patients with CLL were treated with ACTH. The first encouraging results appear to have been reported by Pearson and coworkers, who noted a dramatic decrease in the size of lymph nodes and spleen in six patients with lymphomatous tumours who were treated with ACTH or cortisone (10). They later described remissions of acute leukaemia in five patients treated with ACTH (11). Subsequent experience showed that response to steroid therapy varied markedly between different types of leukaemias, the best results being obtained with acute lymphocytic leukaemia (ALL). Complete remission was obtained in 40-60% of ALL patients treated with prednisone (12, 13). Unfortunately, remission was never permanent and a second course of steroid treatment after relapse was usually less effective than the first, or even totally ineffective. If steroid administration was continued after remission induction, the risk of undesirable side-effects increased without any obvious decrease in the likelihood of relapse (14). These difficulties were partially overcome by combining steroids with other cytotoxic drugs and with drug regimens currently in use complete remission can be induced in more than 90% of patients with ALL, with the possibility of eventual cure in about 40%.

Paradoxically, the very success of multi-drug treatment now hampers research on the individual components of drug regimens. Direct studies on human patients are now excessively complicated due to the near impossibility of disentangling the metabolic effects and interactions of several drugs being administered simultaneously; yet a logical approach to improving drug therapy must be based on knowledge of the mechanism of action of each drug. Despite a considerable amount of research, the complete sequence of biochemical events leading to the destruction of leukaemic cells exposed to steroid hormones remains obscure. As a result, there is now an urgent need for a reliable model system which resembles the human as nearly as possible, but which can be freely manipulated in order to clarify the factors which might determine the effectiveness of steroids and other drugs.

Before the validity of a model system can be fairly assessed, it is first necessary to determine the characteristics required in order for it to reasonably mimic the pertinent aspects of the disease under consideration. For this purpose, we shall first briefly review the available literature concerning responses of leukaemia cells to steroid therapy.

The Response of Leukaemic Cells to Steroids

It is generally believed that the effective use of glucocorticoids in leukaemia therapy involves a sequence of events which is initiated by direct interaction between steroid and leukaemic cell and which culminates in cell lysis and death. Unfortunately, because of the difficulties involved in studying these processes in human patients on multi-drug therapy, the evidence supporting these assumptions is mainly either indirect or is inferred from effects observed in animal cells.

Inhibition of various metabolic processes occurs when leukaemic cells from patients are incubated *in vitro* with steroids. These inhibitory effects include decreased cellular uptake of glucose, amino acids, and precursors of nucleic acids, as well as decreased exclusion of certain dyes (17, 18, 19). It would seem reasonable to conclude that these responses are precursors of cell death and thus represent the early stages of events which occur *in vivo*. Progression from early inhibitory responses to cell death may not be inevitable, however, since a clear correlation between *in vitro* inhibitory effects and the response of individual patients to steroid therapy has yet to be established. Also, it is well known that glucocorticoids inhibit uptake of various nutrients in cells which may not ultimately die, such as muscle, adipose cells and fibroblasts (20). It is difficult to reproduce steroid-mediated cell death *in vitro* with cells taken from patients, because leukaemic cells do not normally survive long enough in culture for observation of anything but the most rapid responses. Cell death has been observed, however, in several established cell lines derived from leukaemic cells. These include the S49 and W7 mouse lymphoma lines (21, 22) and the human CCRF CEM line, derived from a patient with ALL, which will be discussed later. With the techniques recently devised by Salmon's group (23) it may now be possible to grow in agar gel cells from most leukaemic patients to confirm that cell lysis resulting from direct interaction between steroids and leukaemic cells is a general phenomenon which occurs in all patients who respond to steroid therapy.

When ACTH or glucocorticoids are administered to patients with ALL, the number of leukaemic blast cells in peripheral blood and/or bone marrow usually falls dramatically within five or six days (24, 25). These changes are accompanied by a marked increase in uric acid excretion, presumably reflecting breakdown of nucleic acids from dying leukaemic cells (26). Since direct microscopic observation of cell lysis to our knowledge has not been described in human patients, we have to assume that the process is similar to that which occurs in animal thymus cells exposed to glucocorticoids - i.e. cytoplasmic budding, pyknosis, and karyorrhexis (3, 4, 5).

In addition to these destructive effects, glucocorticoids have also been found to provoke a temporary transfer of animal lymphoid cells from the blood stream to other body compartments, such as bone marrow (27, 28). The transient lymphocytopaenia which occurs about four hours after normal humans are treated with glucocorticoids (29, 30) seems to reflect a similar redistribution phenomenon. It does not seem likely, however, that these short-term sequestration effects play an important role in the gross disappearance of cells which occurs when a patient with leukaemia responds favourably to steroid therapy.

Evidence for the direct interaction between steroids and leukaemic cells is also provided by various studies on intracellular receptors. According to the currently accepted mechanism of steroid hormone action (20, 31, 32, 33), steroid molecules which diffuse into target cells bind tightly to specific receptor proteins. The steroid-receptor complex is then translocated to the cell nucleus where gene activity is modulated to produce the characteristic hormone response. If this mechanism is correct, then responsiveness of cells to steroid should be determined partly by the number and the quality of receptors. At present, we do not know whether steroid action requires a limiting number of receptors in each target cell or whether hormone responsiveness increases with receptor concentration. However, in human breast cancer it has been found that tumours lacking oestrogen receptors rarely respond to endocrine therapy, whereas up to 80% of tumours containing more than 100 f moles oestrogen receptor sites per mg cell protein respond favourably to endocrine therapy (34). In fact, there is now evidence that the probability of breast cancer's responding to endocrine therapy increases in proportion to receptor concentration in the tumour (35, 36, 37). Similar correlations have been found between possession of glucocorticoid receptors by certain types of leukaemic cells and response to multidrug, including steroid, therapy. For example, Lippman et al. (38) found that in ALL, duration of remission correlated well with receptor content. Median duration of complete remission in eleven patients with cellular receptor levels of 0 to 2,500 sites/cell was only 7.6 months, but patients with intermediate receptor levels had a median duration of remission of 21.4 months, and those with high receptor levels (greater than 6,000 sites/cell) had a median duration of remission of 30.4 months.

As with the studies on oestrogen receptors in breast tumours, it is particularly important to note that leukaemic cells lacking receptors are unlikely to respond to drug therapy, but not all cells possessing receptors are responsive. In 1974, mouse and human leukaemic cell lines were found which were resistant to glucocorticoids despite possession of appropriate receptors (39). The presence of large numbers of glucocorticoid receptors has been demonstrated in cells from patients with lympho-proliferative disorders which often do not respond clinically to glucocorticoids, such as acute myelocytic leukaemia and chronic lymphocytic leukaemia (19, 40). A further complication already mentioned, is that in most modern studies cellular receptor content can only be correlated with treatment which includes several drugs other than steroids, so that we cannot be certain that responsiveness correlates with steroids rather than the drugs used. Despite these complications, there is strong evidence that inhibitory effects in thymocytes and killing of cultured rodent cells are mediated by specific receptors, since the potency of various steroids is closely correlated with affinity for receptor binding sites (20, 41). In addition, elegant studies initiated by Tomkins have shown that conversion of S49 mouse lymphoma cells to a resistant phenotype is invariably associated with a measurable abnormality, usually loss, of glucocorticoid receptors (42, 43), and similar results have been obtained with W7 cells (44).

If, as there is good reason to suspect, specific glucocorticoid receptors in target cells are requisite for the effective treatment of leukaemia by steroids, then perhaps the binding characteristics of these receptors can be used to predict some dose-response characteristics of steroid therapy. In making these predictions two ancillary factors must be taken into account. First, although it has been generally observed that fractional occupancy of receptor by steroid correlates well with the extent of observed response, this situation need not always obtain. Thus, assumptions about the extent of response based on measurements of equilibrium binding constants and concentrations of steroid are just that - assumptions. Second, many glucocorticoids bind to serum proteins and specifically to corticosteroid binding globulin (CBG). For example, since only free non-CBG bound steroid will gain entry into target cells and interact with receptor, one must correct total serum levels of steroid for that fraction bound to CBG before attempting to predict the extent of therapeutic response to a given steroid.

If we assume from in vitro studies that occupancy of 95% of all receptors is sufficient for maximal response then, based on measurements of the equilibrium binding constants of glucocorticoid receptors in ALL cells (18, 19), continuous exposure of like cells to about 2×10^{-7} M free prednisolone should ensure lysis of virtually all cells. To achieve this level of free steroid in the presence of CBG, a total circulating level of about 10^{-6} M prednisolone would be required. At lower concentrations, proportionately lower fractions of cells would be affected (Fig. 3). Oral administration of 10 mg prednisone to adults (approximately 0.15 mg/kg) results in a peak total plasma prednisolone concentration of 5.5×10^{-7} M, of which 80% is bound to CBG (45). In early studies, remission of ALL was frequently obtained with doses of 2 mg/kg/day of prednisone, nearly 15 times more each day than the amount needed in a single dose to achieve a peak prednisolone concentration of 5.5×10^{-7} M. Therefore, it appears that effective therapeutic concentrations of steroid approximate those calculated from assumptions based on blood distribution and receptor affinity constants.

Although very high concentrations of steroids (10^{-5} M and above) may exert direct effects on cell membranes and may inhibit glucose uptake by competitive inhibition of glucose transport (46), it is unlikely that these effects play any significant role in the treatment of leukaemia since, as discussed above, the inhibitory response seems to be mediated by specific steroid receptors and to occur at much lower steroid concentrations. In any case, it would be virtually impossible, and probably undesirable, to maintain such high concentrations *in vivo* for prolonged periods.

A further prediction may be made which is based on the assumed requirement for interaction between steroids and their receptors. Because the receptors are highly specific, the glucocorticoid receptor will only bind those steroids with glucocorticoid activity, so that oestrogens and testosterone, for example, should be inactive. There is little direct evidence for this prediction, except that one attempt to treat leukaemic patients with the oestrogen stilboestrol proved unsuccessful (47), and in vitro inhibitory effect on thymocytes and S49 cells are observed only with glucocorticoid hormones and not with steroids such as oestrogen and testosterone, which are devoid of glucocorticoid activity (41, 20). Furthermore, there are no noteworthy sex bias in the incidence or course of major leukaemias.

Of the inhibitory effects which have been observed when leukaemic patients are treated with steroids, one of great interest is the effect on progression of cells through the cell cycle. Two groups independently showed that the fraction of marrow lymphoblasts capable of incorporating ^{3}H-thymidine, i.e. cells in S phase, decreased markedly between 8 and 24 hours after glucocorticoids were administered to patients. At later times, the number of mitotic cells, i.e. cells in M phase, also decreased (48, 49, 50). The most remarkable interpretation of these effects was that steroids either blocked cells in G1 phase or destroyed cells in the later S, G2 and M phases. One important corollary of these observations lies in the implication that steroids could interact with other antileukaemic drugs which act on cells in specific stages of the cell cycle.

One final characteristic of the response of leukaemic cells, a phenomenon of particular importance in clinical practice, is the inevitable emergence within a population of leukaemic cells of variant cell types which are resistant to steroids. This phenomenon is a common complication of drug therapy, but was particularly noticeable in the early days of steroid therapy for leukaemia. Steroids induced complete remission in 40-60% of untreated patients with ALL, but inevitably the patients became refractory to further treatment. This indirect evidence for the emergence of resistant cells is supported by the in vitro resistance of cells to glucocorticoids when leukaemic cells are derived from patients who no longer respond to treatment (18). The mechanism for the emergence of drug resistance is generally assumed to involve the random appearance of variant, possibly mutant, cells in the leukaemic population, followed by selection of drug-resistant clones. Recently it has been possible to observe this process occurring during treatment of leukaemic patients. Using various cell-surface and enzyme markers, two subclones of blast cells could be identified coexisting in one patient with ALL. During chemotherapy, one of these clones was eliminated, while the other, apparently resistant to drugs, became predominant (51).

Requirements of a Model System

From the preceding review, we can briefly summarize the known or surmised responses of sensitive leukaemic cells to steroid therapy:

1. Steroids inhibit various aspects of cellular metabolism, such as uptake of glucose and incorporation of leucine, uridine and thymidine.
2. The inhibitory activity of steroids ultimately results in cellular pyknosis, karyorrhexis and death.
3. The action of glucocorticoids on leukaemic cells requires binding of the hormone to specific cellular receptors, so that dose-response relationships should be determined by the binding affinity and concentration of these receptors.
4. Inhibitory effects are exerted only by steroids with known glucocorticoid activity.
5. The inhibitory effects of glucocorticoids include a specific effect on the cell cycle which could involve either a block in G1 phase or destruction of cells in S, G2 or M phases.

It should be noted that a single model system is probably incapable of representing all forms of leukaemia, since the basic biology as well as the responsiveness of each to steroid therapy is different (52). Even ALL is now known to be a heterogeneous disease, the responsiveness to chemotherapy being different in each form (53). But a single, well-characterized model system may provide rather specific answers for certain leukaemias as well as principles of broad, general relevance to many leukaemias. The strengths and limitations of a given system will only be known fully when the complete mechanism of action of steroids in all leukaemias is known.

Experimental stimulation of human leukaemia could most reasonably be achieved with one of two systems, i.e. animal leukaemia or cultured human leukaemic cells, each of which has various advantages and disadvantages. Animal leukaemia models, such as mouse L1210, have been used extensively for studying drug therapy, but these systems have failed to predict some drug effects in patients (54) and Claman (55) has emphasised the difference in response to steroids between humans and the animals commonly used for experimental purposes.

We chose to concentrate on the development of a suitable human leukaemic cell line because of the potential offered by such a system for exploring the actions of and interactions between various drugs. In addition to more classical techniques, the lethal action of glucocorticoids provides an opportunity for the analysis of steroid hormone action by genetic techniques as pioneered by Tomkins and co-workers with S49 mouse lymphoma cells (43, 44). The use of cultured cells as a model system is inevitably subject to the usual criticisms leveled against all reductionist scientific methods. The relative simplicity of cell cultures greatly facilitates the study of basic molecular processes but this advantage is gained at the expense of one major disadvantage, namely the avoidance of many factors such as drug metabolism and concentration dynamics which can exert a profound influence on drug activity in the whole animal. For this reason, extrapolations from results obtained with cell cultures to the treatment of human patients will always be tentative and require confirmation from animal models and clinical trials.

Cultured human leukaemic cells have not been used extensively for the simulation of leukaemia, partly because leukaemic cells do not usually grow well in culture and partly because most human cell lines which have been established are derived from B cells and consequently are resistant to steroids.

Hirshaut and co-workers (56) measured the ability of 6-mercaptopurine, methotrexate, vincristine and prednisolone to inhibit growth of various cell lines. They found measurable effects at 2.1×10^{-8} M prednisolone with cell lines derived from acute myelogenous leukaemia (RPMI 6410), chronic myelogenous leukaemia (RPMI 8205) and Burkitt's lymphoma (AL-2 and P_3J). These promising results do not appear to have been followed up. Most other studies have found cultured human leukaemic cell lines to be relatively resistant to glucocorticoids. Bird et al. (57) measured ^{3}H-uridine incorporation and nigrosine exclusion in eight human lymphoblastoid cell lines (RUS_1, RUS_2, BLA_1, F89, GS_1, JIJOYE, PEN_2 and YAK_1) but failed to detect inhibition at prednisolone concentrations of less than 10^{-4} M. Gailani et al. (58) observed clear inhibition of ^{3}H-uridine incorporation by HRIK cells derived from a Burkitt lymphoma only when cortisol concentrations greater than 10^{-5} M were used. Rosner et al. (59) used the SK-LN cell line to study interactions between prednisolone and vincristine but 7.8×10^{-6} M prednisolone merely slowed cell growth during the first 24 hours of cell culture and subsequent growth was uninhibited. Drewinko et al. (60) used T_1 cells to assay the effects of various antineoplastic drugs on ability of cells to form colonies but prednisolone at 2.8×10^{-4} M only decreased colony formation to 73%. Our own earlier studies with CCRF CEM cells obtained from the American Type Culture Collection showed that cell growth and ^{3}H-uridine incorporation were not significantly affected by 10^{-6} M dexamethasone (39). As will be discussed more fully later, we suspect that the resistance of many human lymphoid cell lines to glucocorticoids arises either from selection of resistant cells in the donor during chemotherapy or from phenotypic changes occurring in long-term tissue culture.

Most studies of cells freshly isolated from patients have not yielded results capable of discriminating clinical responses in individual patients, probably reflecting the inevitable dependence on short-term tests to predict effects on cell viability. Cline and Rosenbaum (17) attempted to develop a test system to predict responsiveness of individual patients to drug therapy. They found that inhibition by cortisol of ^{3}H-uridine incorporation into bone marrow and peripheral leukocytes correlated reasonably well with _in vivo_ response to steroid therapy though there was a marked variability between individuals. With five patients in whom a reduction of lymphoblastoid cells resulted from prednisone therapy, the mean reduction of ^{3}H-uridine incorporation into RNA was to 29 $\pm$ 11% of controls, whereas the mean reduction in 18 patients who did not respond was only to 97 $\pm$ 42% of controls. However, these results were only seen at extremely high concentrations of cortisol and although there were statistical differences between the groups, individual patients did not always fit the pattern. Our studies in acute lymphoblastic leukaemia of childhood (CALL) were those which first demonstrated a functional relationship between glucocorticoid receptor occupancy by steroids and biological response in human cells (18). In these cells, _in vitro_ inhibition of uridine and thymidine incorporation was seen. Retrospective analysis of the clinical records of the patients studied showed that all the previously untreated patients with CALL responded to multidrug therapy which included glucocorticoids; so did a number of patients after one or more relapses. Lymphoblasts from both groups had receptors and responded to steroids _in vitro_ (18). As yet no other study has attempted to examine systematically the receptor status of CALL patients after treatment and relapse. In our early study on acute myeloblastic leukaemic cells, the majority of such cells lacked cytoplasmic receptors and were unresponsive _in vitro_, while a few contained such receptor sites and were responsive (61). A number of laboratories have now shown that most leukaemic cells do contain receptor sites in varying quantities when assayed in unbroken cells and they do show some _in vitro_ responses to glucocorticoids. Crabtree et al. (19) for example, have examined a variety of leukaemias in this way. There is little correlation between the _quantity_ of receptor sites per cell and the magnitude of _in vitro_ responses in a variety of commonly used tests (19, 62).

There remain general correlations between these various tests and *in vivo* responses to therapy, but the necessary patient-specific prognostic test has not yet been found. It is generally agreed that cells truly lacking receptors are steroid-resistant, at least with doses of steroid now used clinically, but such cells form the minority of those observed by the whole-cell assay method in most leukaemias.

Characterisation of a Cell Line Suitable for Use in Simulation of Leukaemia Therapy

The CCRF CEM cell line was initiated from peripheral blood cells obtained from a 4-year-old patient shortly before death from acute lymphoblastic leukaemia (63). The patient had previously been treated with various drugs, including prednisone, for an unknown dose and duration. The lymphoid cells grew spontaneously in suspension culture and subsequent analysis showed them to have several characteristics associated with T cells, including the ability to form rosettes with sheep erythrocytes (64) and possession of thymic lymphocyte-specific antigens (64, 65). The cells used by us in an earlier study (39) were obtained from the American Type Culture Collection, but the cells discussed in this paper were obtained from Dr. D. Mann, National Cancer Institute. These latter cells express the HLA antigens A1, A10, B8, and BW10 (Dr. Mann, personal communication). The karyotype of CEM cells showed a mode of 47 chromosomes per cell, together with a significant number of tetraploid cells (66).

Although the CEM cells obtained from the American Type Culture Collection proved resistant to dexamethasone, the cells obtained from Dr. Mann were partially sensitive to glucocorticoids (67), as shown by the effect of 10^{-6} M dexamethasone on growth of cells in suspension (Fig. 1a). The transient nature of the response suggested that the observed growth curve could represent the summation of steroid effects on a heterogeneous population of cells, with selective inhibition of sensitive

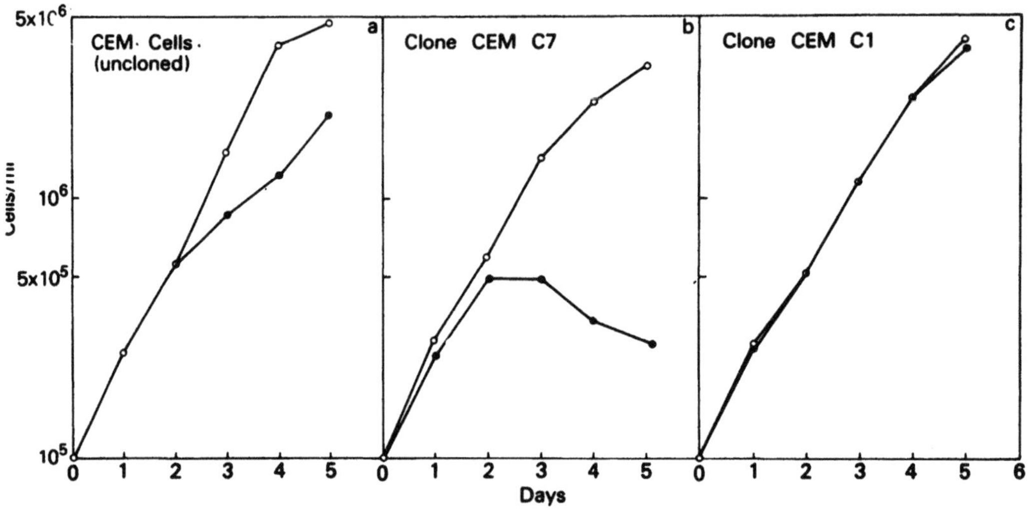

Fig. 1. Effect of dexamethasone on growth of CEM cells in suspension culture.
Each point represents the mean of three replicate cultures. O, growth in the absence of dexamethasone; ●, growth in the presence of 10^{-6}M dexamethasone. [From Norman, M. and Thompson, E.B.: Cancer Res., 37, 3785-3791 (1977)].

cells coupled with continued growth of resistant cells. To test for this possibility, 17 clones were isolated, without selection, in Microtiter dishes. When these clones were examined for sensitivity to steroids, most (Fig. 1b) were markedly more sensitive to dexamethasone than the parental cell line. A few (Fig. 1c) were almost completely resistant to steroid.

The Response of CEM Cells to Steroids

a. Loss of viability

Any investigation into the activity of cytotoxic drugs using cultured cells must depend critically on the availability of an appropriate assay for cell viability. Although various tests are currently in use for this purpose, the only truly satisfactory test is based on the ability of cells to form clones. In addition to being the most sensitive indication of cell viability, cloning efficiency measures the parameter of most interest in chemotherapy, destruction of clonogenic cells. Other tests, such as exclusion of vital dyes, may give misleading results (68). Fortunately, CEM cells form clones in agarose gels with an efficiency of up to 60%, provided a "feeder" layer of human fibroblasts is present (47). They can also be cloned, without "feeder" cells, in multiwell plastic tissue culture dishes.

When a sensitive clone of CEM cells (C7) was exposed to 10^{-6} M dexamethasone, little effect on cloning efficiency was detected for 18-24 h, but cloning efficiency declined logarithmically thereafter. By 60 h, viability was about 1% (Fig. 2). To assess the specificity of this effect, cells were cloned in the presence of various steroids at a concentration of 10^{-6} M. Inhibition of colony formation was closely related to known glucocorticoid activity for dexamethasone, prednisolone and cortisol while testosterone, oestradiol, prednisone, and cortexolone, a known antagonist of glucocorticoids, had no detectable effect (Table 1). CEM C7 cells have no detectable receptor sites for sex steroids (L. Danel and E.B. Thompson, unpublished results).

To determine the effect of steroid dose on cell viability, CEM cells (clone C7) were exposed to dexamethasone for 48 h, then plated in agarose gels after removal of steroid. Loss of cell viability was nearly maximal at a steroid concentration of about 5×10^{-7} M, and half-maximal at a concentration of approximately 2×10^{-8} M. Direct observation by phase microscopy confirmed that cells treated with dexamethasone were ultimately destroyed (Plate 1).

b. Other inhibitory responses

Cellular pyknosis is detectable within 6 h of exposing clone C7 to 10^{-6} M dexamethasone and by 2 days cells have shrunk to

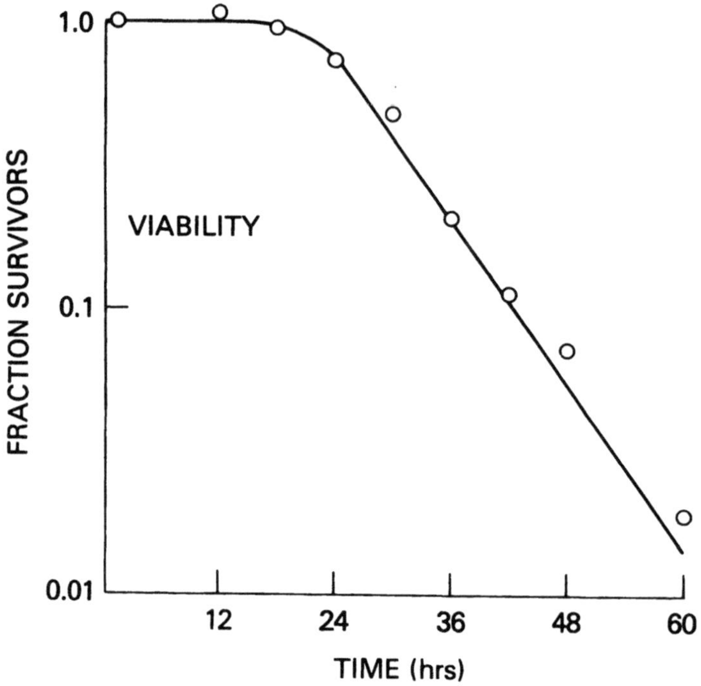

Fig. 2. Effect of dexamethasone on viability of clone C7. Cells were incubated with 10^{-6} M dexamethasone. At various times cells were washed free of steroid and plated in medium containing 0.25% agarose over a layer of human diploid fibroblasts. After two weeks the number of colonies were counted. Viability is expressed as the fraction of colonies formed compared to untreated controls. [From Harmon, J., Norman, M., and Thompson, E.B., In: "Steroid Receptors and the Management of Cancer", Eds. Thompson, E.B., Lippman, M., CRC Press, Boca Raton, FL (1979)]

50% of their normal volume (Fig. 3). Inhibition of radiolabeled thymidine incorporation was also seen after exposure of sensitive clones of CEM cells to glucocorticoid.

Inhibition of protein synthesis, measured by incorporation of radioactive leucine, was usually observed in sensitive leukaemic cells exposed to glucocorticoids. Analysis of polyribosome

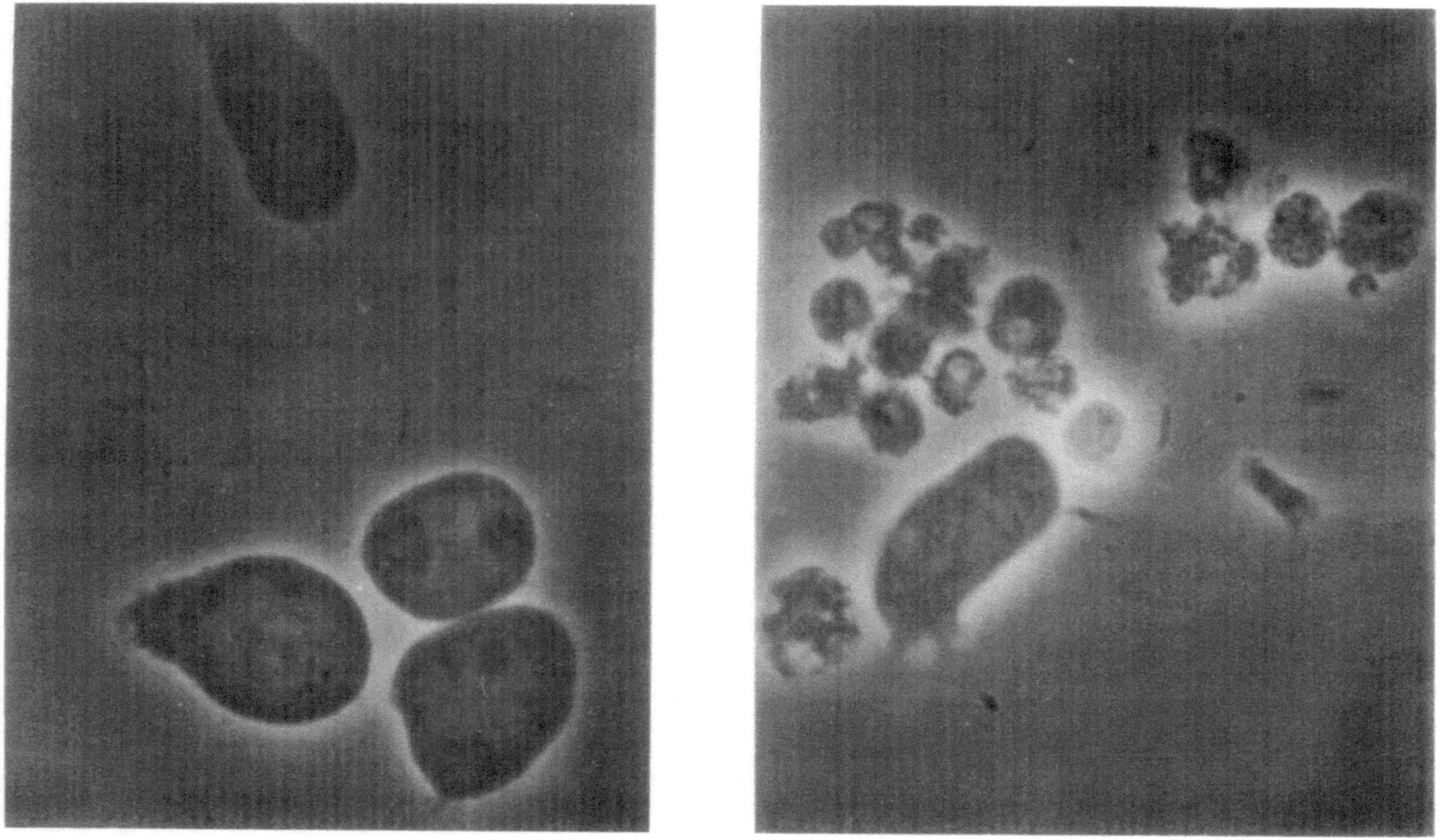

Plate 1. Phase-contrast photomicrographs of CEM cells (clone C13) x 1280. Left panel cells grown in the absence of dexamethasone; right panel cells grown for 4 days in the presence of 10^{-6} M dexamethasone. [From Norman, M. and Thompson, E.B., Cancer Res., 37, 3785-3791 (1977)].

Table 1

Cloning efficiency of CEM cells (clone C7) on agarose gels in the presence of various steroids at 10^{-6} M.
[From Norman, M. and Thompson, E.B., Cancer Res. 37, 3785-3791 (1977)]

Steroid	Relative Cloning Efficiency
Oestradiol	1.086
Dihydrotestosterone	0.975
Cortexolone	0.938
Prednisone	0.926
Cortisol	0.0031
Prednisolone	0.0028
Dexamethasone	0.0008

patterns showed that steroids inhibited protein synthesis in CEM cells since there was a decrease in polyribosomes and a corresponding increase in monomers after 24 h exposure of clone C7 to 10^{-6} M dexamethasone (Fig. 4). The type of polysome pattern observed in inhibited cells was most consistent with either inhibition of initiation of translation or a decreased supply of mRNA. It did not result from increased TNase activity which would increase the number of oligomers, so that activation or release of RNase as a cause of cell death when lymphocytes are exposed to steroids (71) seems unlikely.

c. Glucocorticoid receptors and the response of CEM cells to steroids

Binding of ^{3}H-dexamethasone to the 105,000 x g supernatant of lysed and intact CEM cells (clone C7) revealed the presence of around 20,000 binding sites per cell. The equilibrium dissociation constant (K_D) for these binding sites, determined from the data shown in Fig. 5, was approximately 1.4×10^{-8} M. The binding

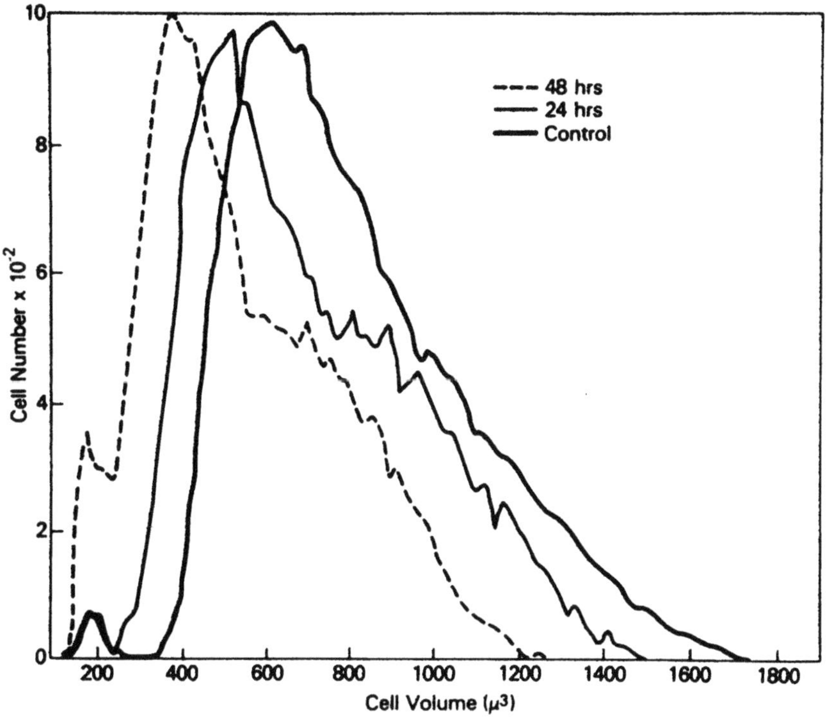

Fig. 3. Effect of dexamethasone on cell volume. Distribution of cell volumes after treatment of clone CEM C13 for various times. [From Norman, M. and Thompson, E.B.: Cancer Res. 37, 3785-3791 (1977)]

measured in these assays was specific, since only steroids with known glucocorticoid or anti-glucocorticoid activity were able to displace ^{3}H-dexamethasone (Fig. 6). Thus CEM cells contain binding sites with the characteristics expected of physiological receptors, namely a small number of binding sites which specifically bind a single type of hormone with high affinity. A further property expected of receptors, transfer to the cell nucleus together with bound steroid, was observed when radioactively labeled dexamethasone was incubated with CEM cells (M. Norman, J. Harmon, and E.B. Thompson, unpublished results).

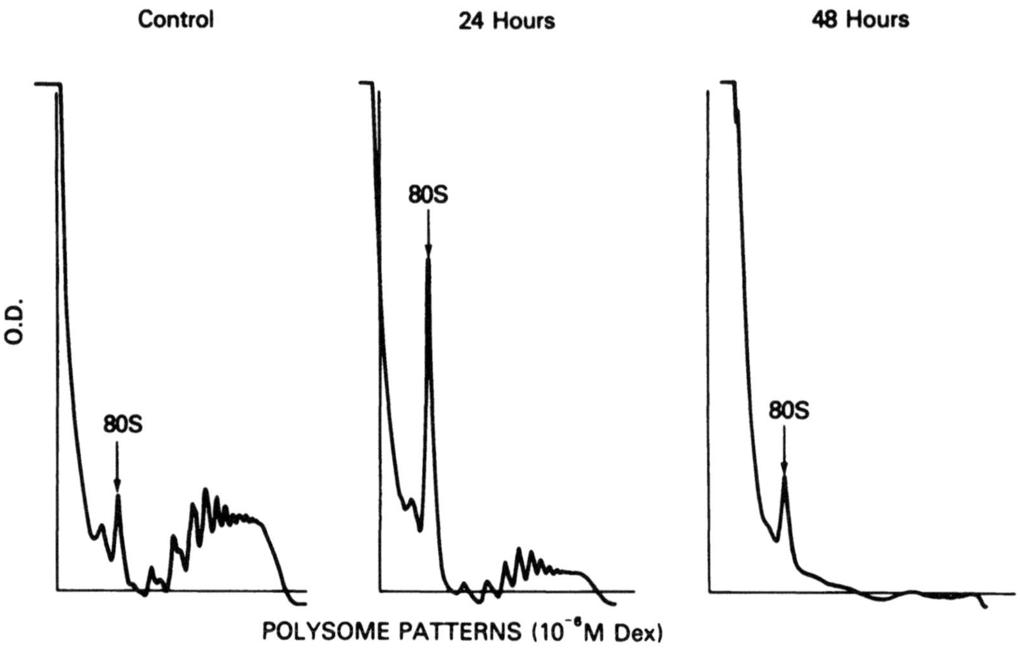

Fig. 4. Effect of dexamethasone (Dex) on polysome profiles obtained from CEM cells (clone C7). 80S, monomeric ribosomes. [From Norman, M. and Thompson, E.B.: Cancer Res. 37, 3785-3791 (1977)]

The mere presence of receptors in sensitive cells does not prove that glucocorticoid action on CEM cells necessarily involves interaction with those receptors. A receptor-mediated mechanism seems likely however, because there was a correlation between the ability of various steroids to bind to the receptor (Fig. 6) and the ability of the same steroids to inhibit cloning of CEM cells (Table 1). Similarly, the dexamethasone concentration required to bind 50% of receptor sites (1.4×10^{-8} M) correlated well with the dexamethasone concentration (about 2×10^{-8} M) required to reduce cloning by 50%.

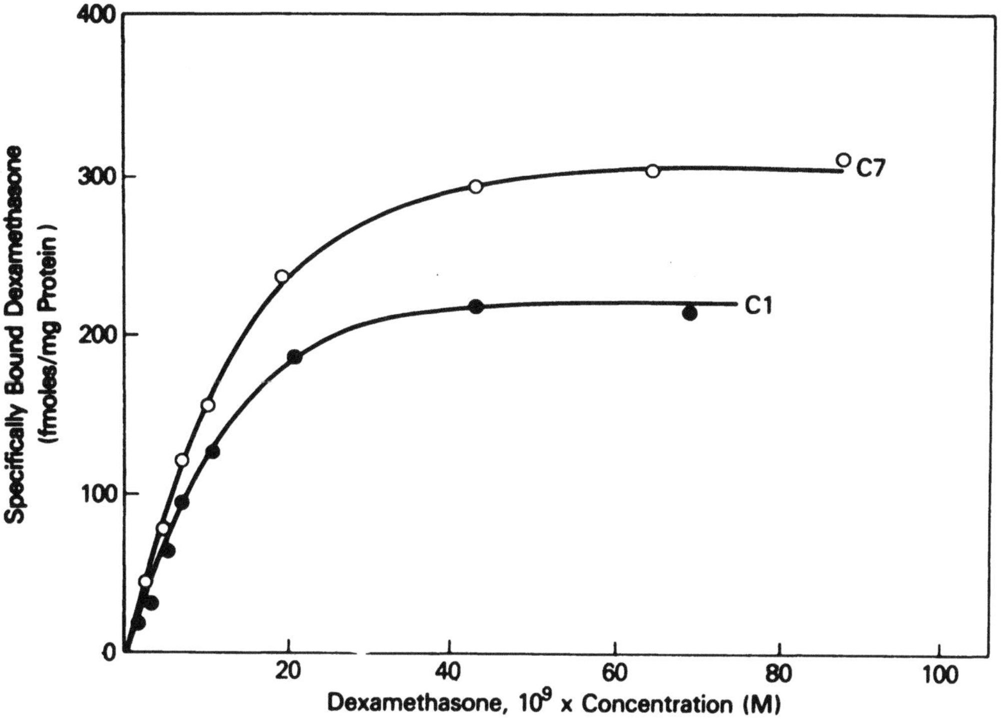

Fig. 5. Specific binding of [^{3}H] dexamethasone to cytoplasmic extracts of CEM cells.
Each point represents the mean of duplicate assays. [From Norman, M. and Thompson, E.B.: Cancer Res. 37, 3785-3791 (1977)]

More direct evidence for the role played by receptors was provided by the characterisation of CEM clones resistant to glucocorticoids, as discussed in the next section

d. The nature of steroid-resistant cells

The lethal activity of glucocorticoids is clearly dependent on the differentiated state of target cells and consequently many established cell lines are not inhibited by steroids simply because they are derived from a cell type which does not respond. Nevertheless, it seems that a cell population which is initially

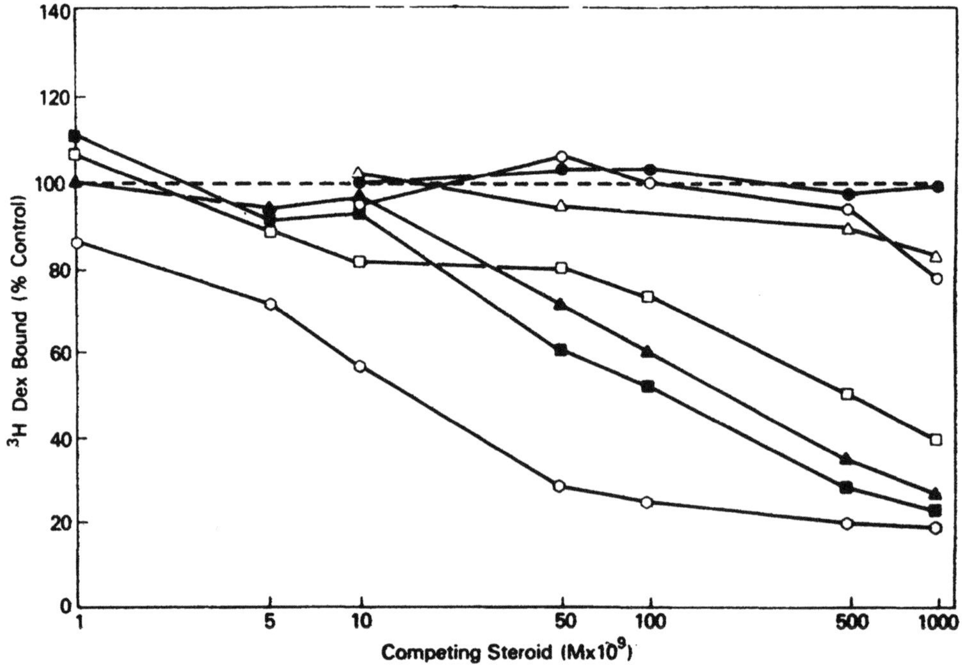

Fig. 6. Displacement of [^{3}H] dexamethasone bound to CEM cells (clone C7) by various steroids.
Each point represents the mean of duplicate determinations.

⧫, dexamethasone; 0, estradiol; ●, dihydrotestosterone; Δ, prednisone; ▲, cortisol; □, cortexolone; ■, prednisolone. [From Norman, M. and Thompson, E.B.: Cancer Res. 37, 3785-3791 (1977)]

sensitive may alter with time and become resistant and this may occur both in leukaemic patients and in tissue culture.

When studying the S49 mouse lymphoma cell line, Sibley and Tomkins (42) found that spontaneous conversion to steroid resistance occurred about once every 3.5 x 10^{6} cell divisions. Statistical analysis of the rate at which resistant cells appeared suggested that conversion was a random event and hence compatible with a mutational origin for resistance. A similar analysis of CEM cells also showed that transition from sensitivity to resistance occurred in a random fashion, the rate of this change being about 1×10^{-5}/cell/generation. Several observations are compatible with the hypothesis that resistance results from mutation: (1) acquisition of the resistant phenotype is random and rare (72); (2) the resistant phenotype is maintained for at least 6 months in continuous culture in the absence of steroid (71) and (3) the frequency of resistance is increased by exposure to known mutagens (J. Harmon and E.B. Thompson, unpublished results). Unequivocal proof of a mutation however, requires biochemical evidence for an abnormal gene, so the possibility remains that steroid resistance results from some mechanism other than mutation, such as a change in state of differentiation.

Whatever the mechanism by which lymphoid cells acquire resistance to steroids, the existence of the phenomenon may provide an explanation both for the resistance of many cultured cell lines and for the frequent failure of a second course of steroid therapy in leukaemia.

It can be shown that if one neglects drift toward mutational equilibrium, the proportion of mutants in a logarithmically growing population increases linearly. If resistant cells arise at a rate of one per 10^{x} cells per division, then when cells have grown for N generations, the number of resistant cells will be N per 10^{x} cells. For CEM cells, with a generation time of about 18 h and a spontaneous rate of appearance of resistance of about 10^{-5}, after culture for one year there should be $\sim\frac{24 \times 365 \times 10^{-5}}{18}$ or about 0.5% resistant cells. This crude estimate assumes, of course, that all cells are actively and constantly doubling. Thus, spontaneous acquisition of resistance is clearly of importance when working with cultured cells and may contribute to the variable characteristics found when the same cell line is obtained from different sources. If spontaneous conversion to resistance were to occur in a patient at a similar rate to that observed in CEM cells, then that patient at diagnosis with a leukaemic cell load of 10^{12} cells (73) might be expected to have about 4×10^{6} cells which are resistant to steroids before treatment begins. A single precursor cell, after 40 doubling times, will produce 1.1 x 10^{12} cells. Then the total number of resistant cells will be N per 10^x cells, or 40 per 10^5, or a total of about 4 x 10^6 resistant cells in a population of 1.1 x 10^{12}. Under selective pressure, of course, conversion of a culture to resistance will be far more rapid. This may have occurred in the individual donor before initiation of a cell line as a result of either endogenous steroids or steroids administered therapeutically, killing sensitive cells.

Recently, Bourgeois and Newby (22) have suggested that the wild-type S49 mouse lymphoma cell line carries a mutation in one allele of the receptor gene so that the cells are effectively haploid at this locus. Another mouse thymoma line, W7, is markedly more sensitive to glucocorticoids than S49 and is presumed to have two functioning receptor genes. Mutation of W7 cells results in resistant cells occurring in two stages, with cells at the intermediate stage resembling S49 cells both in receptor content and sensitivity to steroids.

It is possible that similar events occur in leukaemic patients, and the CEM cell line, which was isolated from a patient who had been treated with steroids, may resemble the partially resistant S49 cell line in this respect. Although showing many similarities, sensitive CEM cells differ from S49 cells in several important respects. The lag of about 24 h before viability of CEM cells is decreased by steroids is much longer than the 3 h lag seen in S49 cells (21). Also, most steroid-resistant clones isolated from S49 cells have a greatly reduced receptor content (23, 43, 44), whereas most spontaneously resistant CEM cells have less dramatic reduction in receptor sites, and are defective in nuclear transfer of steroid/receptor complexes (72).

e. Glucocorticoids and the cell cycle of CEM cells

To determine whether or not glucocorticoids exert a specific effect on the passage of CEM cells through the cell cycle, we analysed cell populations by flow microfluorometry (74). The histogram of cellular DNA content obtained with normal, exponentially growing cells is shown in Figure 7a, where the abscissa is proportional to cellular DNA content and the ordinate represents the number of cells with a given DNA content. The large peak of lower DNA content represents cells in G1 phase and accounts for 55-65% of cells, while the smaller peak corresponds with cells in G2 and M phase which have twice the amount of DNA. The intermediate area represents cells in S phase. Treatment of cells with 10^{-6} M dexamethasone for 48 h alters the distribution of cells between different phases of the cell cycle, so that a greater proportion are in G1 phase and fewer are in S, G2, and M phases (Fig. 7b). To find out whether the altered distribution was the result of a decreased rate of exit from G1 phase, colcemid was used to block cells in mitosis. The result obtained when cells were treated with 10^{-6} M dexamethasone for 48 h followed by colcemid plus dexamethasone for a further 12 h is shown in Figure 7d. When cells were incubated with colcemid alone for 12 h (Fig. 7c) the G1 population was virtually eliminated, the G1 fraction has not been replenished because mitosis was blocked, and cells which were in G1 when colcemid was added have moved into other phases of the cycle. Cells which had been treated with dexamethasone for 48 h before addition of colcemid (Fig. 7d) did not leave G1 phase, confirming that the steroid prevented exit of cells from G1 phase.

Using a range of dexamethasone concentrations, the extent to which cells accumulate in G1 phase was found to be proportional to the fraction of glucocorticoid receptors occupied (74) so that the cell cycle effect, as with the effect of cell viability, is probably dependent on binding of steroid to receptor.

Interference with the cell cycle by steroids raises the question of a possible link between this effect and the lethal response of CEM cells to glucocorticoids, a suspicion which is reinforced by the close temporal relationship between the two effects (74). A change detectable by flow microfluorometry will be delayed by the time normally required for cells to traverse

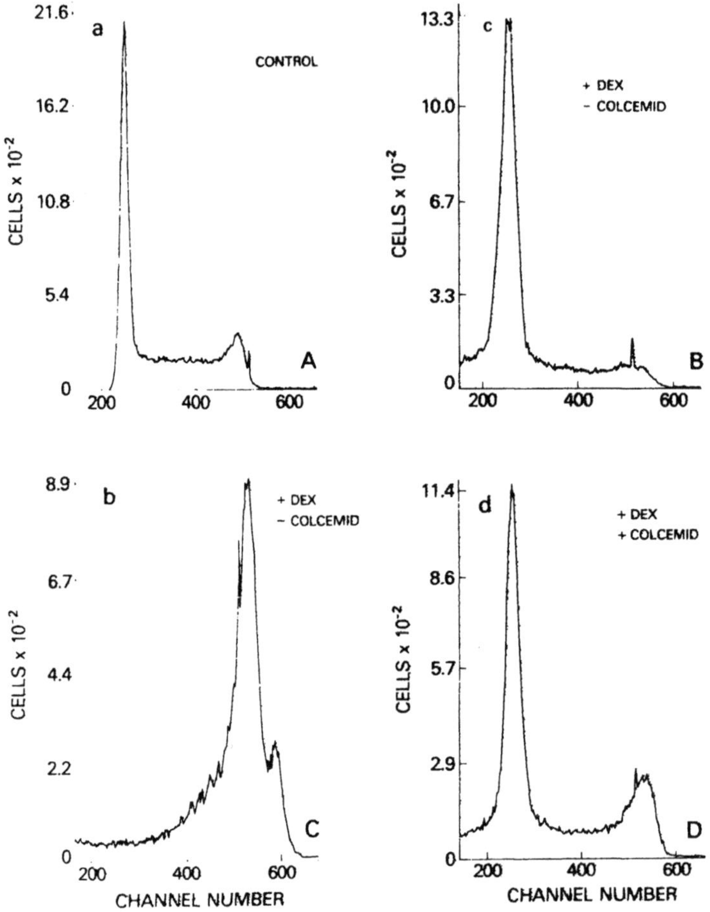

Fig. 7. Cell cycle effect of dexamethasone treatment on CEM-C7.
Cells were grown in the absence (A, C) or presence (B, D) of 10^{-6} M dexamethasone for 48 h. Colcemid was added to cultures C and D for an additional 12 h and all cultures were analysed by FMF.
[From Harmon, J., Norman, M. and Thompson, E.B.: In: "Steroid Receptors and the Management of Cancer" Eds. Thompson, E.B., Lippman, M., CRC Press, Boca Raton, FL (1979)]

each phase of the cell cycle, but direct measurement using colcemid showed that after 24 h treatment with 10^{-6} M dexamethasone, when 24% of cells were no longer capable of forming clones, 20% of cells were arrested in G1 phase. Other experiments which involved measurement of the ability of dexamethasone to protect cells from damage inflicted on cells in the S phase of the cell cycle, showed that arrest in G1 phase results in immediate loss of viability or possibly that loss of viability is a consequence of G1 arrest. For these experiments, 2×10^{-7} bromodeoxyuridine was added to cells for the final 24 h of a 48 h incubation with dexamethasone. The cells were then irradiated with white light, which has a lethal effect on any cells which have incorporated bromodeoxyuridine. (Hoechst 33258 dye was added to amplify this effect). If dexamethasone had arrested cells reversibly in G1 phase, it would by so doing have prevented incorporation of bromodeoxyuridine, which occurs in S phase, and consequently would have protected cells from the effects of irradiation. Since dexamethasone had no protective effect (Fig. 8), we concluded that all cells arrested in G1 phase by dexamethasone were non-viable. This conclusion has important implications for multi-drug chemotherapy of leukaemia, as will be discussed in the next section.

The Use of CEM Cells to Simulate Chemotherapy of Leukaemia

Lampkin et al. (50) suggested that if steroids decreased exit of cells from G1 phase, then the effectiveness of drugs which act on subsequent stages of the cell cycle might be diminished. This prediction depends on the assumption that cell-cycle effects of steroids are reversible, but we have shown that in CEM cultured leukaemic cells, G1 arrest by steroids is an <u>irreversible</u> phenomenon. If our results can be applied to leukaemic patients, then the predicition of Lampkin et al. would be reversed, that is, killing of cells in G1 phase by steroids would present drugs which act in other phases with a greater

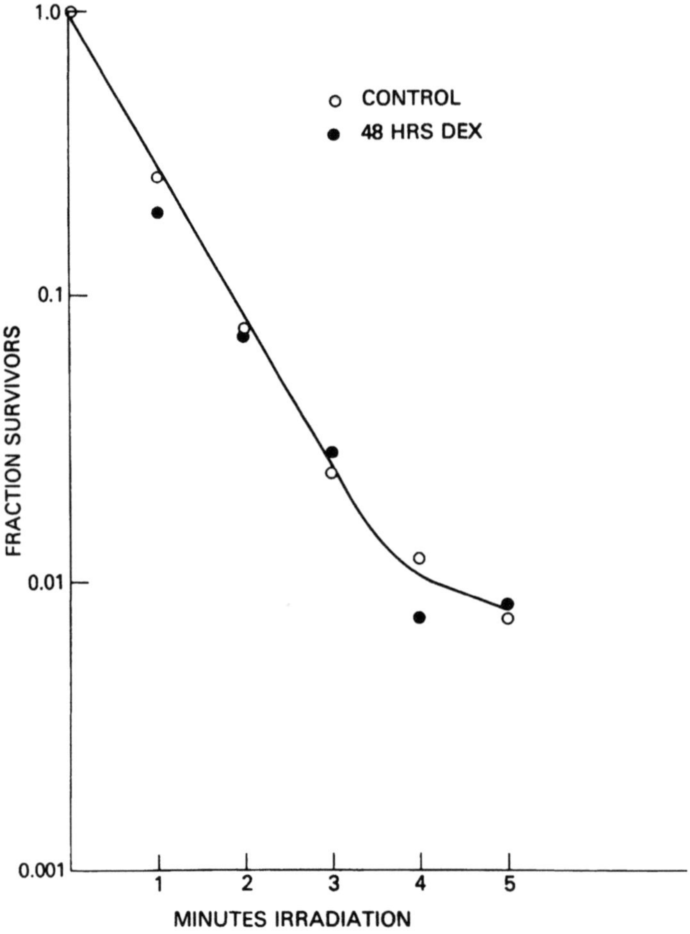

Fig. 8. Effect of dexamethasone on photosensitivity of BrdUrd substituted cells.
Parallel cultures were incubated in the presence (●) or absence (0) of 10^{-6} M dexamethasone for 48 h. BrdUrd (2×10^{-7} M) was added to each culture for the final 24 h followed by 3 h in the presence of 1.5 µg/ml 33258 Hoechst. Survivors are expressed on the basis of unirradiated samples, normalizing for the toxicity of dexamethasone in the dexamethasone Rx'd culture. Survival of the dexamethasone-treated culture was 7.3%. [From Harmon, J., Norman, M., Fowlkes, B.J. and Thompson, E.B.: J. Cell Physiol. 98, 267-278 (1979)]

proportion of viable target cells.

To test these predictions, we measured the effectiveness of prednisolone when combined with vincristine, methotrexate, and 6-mercaptopurine (75), three drugs widely used in the treatment of ALL and which act on phases of the cell cycle other than G1 (76). Using the measured toxicity of individual drugs to CEM cells (S_A, S_B), the predicted combined toxicity ($S_A \times S_B$) was close to the observed combined toxicity (S_{AB}) when prednisolone was used together with vincristine or methotrexate (Table 2). The results obtained when prednisolone was combined with 6-mercaptopurine provide a notable exception, since 15% of cells survived at a drug concentration where predicted survival was only 6% (Table 2). We do not yet know the reason for the observed antagonism between these two drugs, though possible interactions which merit further investigation include inhibition of 6-mercaptopurine transport into cells by steroids, blockage of steroid effects due to interference with RNA synthesis by 6-mercaptopurine and reversible block of cells in S phase by 6-mercaptopurine, with such a block protecting against the steroid effects.

Conclusions

Having reviewed the available information concerning the action of steroids and other cytotoxic drugs on leukaemic cells, it is apparent that there are two main objections to the use of cultured cells as models for leukaemia. Firstly, we cannot exclude the possibility of some antileukaemic properties of drugs resulting from indirect effects which require the participation of cells other than leukaemic cells. If such effects occur, it may be necessary to use linked or co-cultivation tissue culture systems. Secondly, the heterogenicity of the leukaemias might confer limits on the usefulness of a pure cell line. Every patient is different and this may well extend to the leukaemic cells of each individual. The recent introduction of reliable

Table 2

Interactions of prednisolone with other antileukaemic drugs

Definitions

Antagonists	$S_{AB} > S_A \times S_B$
Independent	$S_{AB} = S \times S$
Synergists	$S_{AB} < S_A \times S_B$

Where S = fractional survival in 10^{-6} M prednisolone

Fractional Survivors[a]

	Experimental			Predicted	Interaction
Drug B	S_A	S_B	S_{AB}	$S_A \times S_B$	
VINC (5×10^{-9} M)	0.289	0.161	0.027	0.046	Weak synergists?
MTX (5×10^{-6} M)	0.289	0.183	0.030	0.053	Weak synergists?
6-MP (10^{-4} M)	0.289	0.199	0.155	0.058	Antagonists

[a] Cells were grown in 10^{-6} M prednisolone for 48 h during the last 24 h of which either MTX, VINC, or 6-MP was added. Cells were then assayed for colony forming ability. [From Norman, M., Harmon, J. and Thompson, E.B.: In: "Steroid Receptors and the Management of Cancer", Eds. Thompson, E.B., Lippman, M., CRC Press, Boca Raton, FL (1979)]

methods for growing colonies of leukaemic cells derived from patients (23) provides an opportunity to study this variability under controlled conditions.

Although there is a clear need for the availability of systems which circumvent the known deficiencies of cell lines for the study of leukaemia therapy, we believe that a permanent cultured human cell line offers distinct advantages. Most of the available evidence indicates that chemotherapeutic drugs, including steroids, interact directly with leukaemic cells and although effectiveness may vary between individual patients, the basic mechanism of cell death is probably universal. To our knowledge, CCRF CEM cells provide the only available human cell line which has been fully characterised and found to fulfill the requirements of a model system for studying the use of steroids in the treatment of leukaemia. Sensitive clones of CEM cells exposed to steroids show pyknosis, inhibition of protein synthesis, arrest in G1 phase of the cell cycle and ultimately death. As far as we can tell, similar events occur in sensitive leukaemic cells in patients. There is evidence that in both cases these inhibitory effects result from binding of steroid to specific glucocorticoid receptors and that cells with an altered phenotype which confers resistance to steroids are occasionally produced both by cultured CEM cells and by proliferating leukaemic cells in patients. The parental CCRF CEM cell line is well characterised in other respects since it has been used in many different laboratories for a wide range of investigations, including chromosome banding (66), immunological properties (64, 65, 77), sensitivity to radiation (78), methotrexate (79) and deoxyribonucleosides (80) and interaction with endothelial cells (81).

Our initial studies with CEM cells show that they can be used effectively to study the mechanism by which glucocorticoids inhibit lymphoid cells, to predict interactions between steroids and other drugs which are used to treat leukaemia and to elucidate the mechanism by which leukaemic cells become resistant to steroids and other drugs. Other cell lines from both treated and untreated patients need to be characterised as thoroughly so as to provide a panel of relevant model systems.

References

1. Selye, H.: Studies on adaptation. Endocrinology 21, 169-188 (1937).
2. Moon, H.: Inhibition of somatic growth in castrated rats with pituitary extract. Proc. Soc. exp. Biol. Med. 37, 34-37 (1937).
3. Dougherty, T., White, A.: Effect of pituitary adrenocorticotropic hormone on lymphoid tissue. Proc. Soc. exp. Biol. Med. 53, 132-133 (1943).
4. Dougherty, T., White, A.: Influence of hormones on lymphoid tissue structure and function. Endocrinology 35, 1 (1944).
5. Dougherty, T., White, A.: Functional alterations in lymphoid tissue induced by adrenal cortical secretion. Am. J. Anat. 77, 81-116 (1945).
6. Murphy, J., Sturm, E.: Effect of adrenal cortical and pituitary adrenotropic hormones on transplanted leukemia in rats. Science 99, 303 (1944).
7. Dameshek, 1943 [unpublished observations, quoted in: Rosenthal, M., Saunders, R., Schwartz, L., Zannos, L., Santiago, E., Dameshek, W.: The use of adrenocorticotropic hormone and cortisone in the treatment of leukemia and leukosarcoma. Blood 6, 804-832 (1951)].
8. Nordenson, N.: Clinical experimental observations on the influence of adrenocorticotrophic hormone and desoxycorticosterone on the peripheral blood and bone marrow. Acta med scand. suppl., 196, 419-431 (1947).
9. Hellman, L.: Effect of adrenocorticotropin in human chronic lymphatic leukemia. Fed. Proc. 8, 72 (1949).
10. Pearson, O., Eliel, L., Rawson, R., Dobriner, K., Roads, C.: ACTH and cortisone-induced regression of lymphoid tumors in man. Cancer 2, 943-945 (1949).
11. Pearson, O., Eliel, L.: Use of pituitary adrenocorticotropic hormone and cortisone in lymphomas and leukemias. J. Am. med. Ass. 144, 1349-1353 (1950).
12. Wolff, J., Brubaker, C., Murphy, M., Pierce, M., Severo, N.: Prednisone therapy of acute childhood leukemia: prognosis and duration of response in 330 treated patients. J. Pediat. 70, 626-631 (1967).

13. Bernard, J., Boiron, M., Weil, M., Levy, J.P., Seligman, M., Najean, Y.: Etude de la rémission complète des leucemies aigues. Nouvelle Revue Francaise Hématologie 2, 195-222 (1962).

14. Hyman, C., Borda, E., Brubaker, C., Hammond, D., Sturgeon, P.: Prednisone in childhood leukemia. Pediatrics 24, 1005-1008 (1959).

15. Mauer, A., Simone, J.: The current status of the treatment of childhood acute lymphoblastic leukemia. Cancer Treat. Rev. 3, 17-41 (1976).

16. George, S., Aur, R., Mauer, A., Simone, J.: A reappraisal of the results of stopping therapy in childhood leukemia. New Engl. J. Med. 300, 269-273 (1979).

17. Cline, M., Rosenbaum, E.: Prediction of *in vivo* toxicity of chemotherapeutic agents by their *in vitro* effect on leukocytes from patients with acute leukemia. Cancer Res. 28, 2516-2521 (1968).

18. Lippman, M., Halterman, R., Leventhal, B., Perry, S., Thompson, E.B.: Glucocorticoid-binding proteins in human acute lymphoblastic leukemic blast cells. J. clin. Invest. 52, 1715-1725 (1973).

19. Crabtree, G., Smith, K., Munck, A.: Glucocorticoid receptors and sensitivity of isolated human leukemia and lymphoma cells. Cancer Res. 38, 4268-4272 (1978).

20. Thompson, E.B., Lippman, M.: Mechanism of action of glucocorticoids. Metabolism 23, 159-202 (1974).

21. Harris, A.W.: Differentiated functions expressed by cultured mouse lymphoma cells. Exp. Cell Res. 60, 341-353 (1970).

22. Bourgeois, S., Newby, R.: Diploid and haploid states of the glucocorticoid receptor gene of mouse lymphoid cell lines. Cell 11, 423-430 (1977).

23. Salmon, S., Hamburger, A., Soehnlen, B., Durie, B., Alberts, D., Moon, T.: Quantitation of differential sensitivity of human tumor stem cells to anti-cancer drugs. New Engl. J. Med. 298, 1321-1327 (1978).

24. Adams, W., Valentine, W., Bassett, S., Lawrence, J.: The effect of cortisone and ACTH in leukaemia. J. Lab. clin. Med. 39, 570-581 (1952).

25. Fessas, P., Wintrobe, M., Thompson, R., Cartwright, G.: Treatment of acute leukemia with cortisone and corticotropin. Arch. intern. Med. 94, 384-401 (1954).

26. Sandberg, A., Cartwright, G., Wintrobe, M.: Studies on leukemia. I. Uric acid excretion. Blood 11, 154-166 (1956).

27. Fauci, A.S.: Effect of hydrocortisone on guinea-pig peripheral blood lymphocyte subpopulations. Fed. Proc. 33, 750 (1974).

28. Cohen. J.J.: Thymus-derived lymphocytes sequestered in the bone marrow of hydrocortisone-treated mice. J. Immunol. 108, 841-844 (1972).

29. Fauci, A.S., Dale, D.: The effect of hydrocortisone on the kinetics of normal human lymphocytes. Blood 46, 235-243 (1975).

30. Yu, D., Clements, P.J., Paulus, H.E., Peter, J.B., Levy, J., Barnett, E.V.: Human lymphocyte subpopulations. J. clin. Invest. 53, 565-571 (1974).

31. King, R.J., Mainwaring, W.I.P.: "Steroid-cell Interactions" Butterworth, London (1974).

32. Baxter, J.D., Rousseau, G.G.: "Glucocorticoid Hormone Action", Springer-Verlag, Berlin (1979).

33. Higgins, S., Gehring, U.: Molecular mechanisms of steroid hormone action. Adv. Cancer Res. 28, 313-397 (1978).

34. McGuire, W.: Steroid receptors in human breast cancer. Cancer Res. 38, 4289-4291 (1978).

35. Allegra, J.C., Lippman, M.E., Thompson, E.B., Simon, R., Barlock, A., Green, L., Huff, K.K., Do, H.M.T., Aitken, S., Warren, R.: The relationship between the progesterone, androgen and glucocorticoid receptor and response rate to endocrine therapy in metastatic breast cancer. Cancer Res. 39, 1973-1979 (1979).

36. Leclercq, G., Henson, J.C.: Quantitative aspects of estrogen receptors in relation to therapeutic response. In: "Steroid Receptors and the Management of Cancer", vol. 2, Eds. Thompson, E.B., Lippman, M., CRC Press, Boca Raton, FL (1979).

37. Jensen, E.V.: Estrogen receptors in hormone-dependent breast cancers. Cancer Res. 35, 3362-3364 (1975).

38. Lippman, M., Konior Yarbro, G., Leventhal, B.: Practical implications of glucocorticoid receptors in human leukemia. Cancer Res. 38, 4251-4256 (1978).

39. Lippman, M., Perry, S., Thompson, E.B.: Cytoplasmic glucocorticoid-binding proteins in glucocorticoid-unresponsive human and mouse leukemic cell lines. Cancer Res. 34, 1572-1576 (1974).

40. Homo, F., Duval, D., Meyer, P., Belas, F., Debre, P., Binet, J.-L.: Chronic lymphatic leukaemia: cellular effects in vitro. Br. J. Haematol. 38, 491-499 (1978).

41. Dausse, J., Duval, D., Meyer, P., Gaignault, J., Marchandeau, C., Raynaud, J.: The relationship between glucocorticoid structure and effects upon thymocytes. Mol. Pharmacol. 13, 948-955 (1977).

42. Sibley, C., Tomkins, G.: Isolation of lymphoma cell variants resistant to killing by glucocorticoids. Cell 2, 213-220 (1974).

43. Yamamoto, K., Gehring, U., Stampfer, M., Sibley, C.: Genetic approaches to steroid hormone action.Recent Prog. Horm. Res. 32, 3-32 (1976).

44. Pfahl, M., Kelleher, R., Bourgeois, S.: General features of steroid resistance in lymphoid cell-lines. Mol. and Cell Endocrinol. 10, 193-207 (1978).

45. Uribe, M., Shalm, S., Summerskill, W., Go, V.: Effect of liquid diet on serum protein binding and prednisolone concentrations after oral prednisolone. Gastroenterology 71, 362-364 (1976).

46. Plagemann, P., Renner, E.: Glucocorticoids: competitive inhibition of glucose transport. Biochem. biophys. Res. Commun. 46, 816-823 (1972).

47. Blackburn, E.: Effect of stilboestrol in acute leukaemia. Br. J. Cancer 8, 255-258 (1954).

48. Ernst, P., Killman, S-A.: Effect of anti-leukemic drugs on cell cycle of human leukemic blast cells *in vivo*. Acta med. scand. 186, 239-240 (1969).

49. Ernst, P., Killman, S-A.: Perturbation of generation cycle of human leukemic blast cells by cytostatic therapy *in vivo*: effect of corticosteroids. Blood 36, 689-696 (1970).

50. Lampkin, B., Nagao, T., Mauer, A.: Drug effect in acute leukemia. J. clin. Invest. 48, 1124-1130 (1969).

51. Goldstone, A., McVerry, B., Janossy, G., Walker, H.: Clonal identification in acute lymphoblastic leukaemia. Blood 53, 892-898 (1979).

52. Gunz, F., Baikie, A.:"Leukemia", 3rd ed., Grune and Stratton New York (1974).

53. Chessels, J., Hardisty, R., Rapson, N., Greaves, M.: Acute lymphoblastic leukaemia in children: classification and prognosis. Lancet II, 1307-1309 (1977).

54. Goldin, A., Sandberg, J., Henderson, E., Newman, J., Frei, E., Holland, J.: The chemotherapy of human and animal acute leukemia. Cancer Chemother. Rep. 55, 309-507 (1971).

55. Claman, H.: Corticosteroids and lymphoid cells. New Engl. J. Med. 287, 388-397 (1972).

56. Hirshaut, Y., Weiss, G., Perry, S.: The use of long-term human leukocyte cell cultures as models for the study of antileukemic agents. Cancer Res. 29, 1732-1740 (1969).

57. Bird, C.C., Waddell, A., Robertson, A., Currie, A., Steel, C., Evans, J.: Cytoplasmic receptor levels and glucocorticoid response in human lymphoblastoid cell lines. Br. J. Cancer 33, 700-707 (1976).

58. Gailan, S., Minowada, J., Silvernail, P., Nussbaum, A., Kaiser, N., Rosen, F., Shimaoka, K.: Specific glucocorticoid binding in human hemopoietic cell lines and neoplastic tissue. Cancer Res. 33, 2653-2657 (1973).

59. Rosner, F., Hirshaut, Y., Grunwald, H., Dietrich, M.: In vitro combination chemotherapy demonstrating potentiation of Vincristine cytotoxicity by Prednisolone. Cancer Res. 35, 700-705 (1975).

60. Drewinko, B., Loo, T.L., Freireich, E.: Combination chemotherapy in vitro. III BCNU Cancer Treatment Rep. 63, 373-375 (1979).

61. Lippman, M., Perry, S., Thompson, E.B.: Glucocorticoid binding proteins in myeloblasts of acute myelogenous leukemia. Am. J. Med. 59, 224-227 (1975).

62. Duval, D., Homo, F.: Prognostic value of steroid receptor determinations in leukemia. Cancer Res. 38, 4263-4267 (1978).

63. Foley, G., Lazarus, H., Farber, S., Uzman, B.G., Boone, B., McCarthy, R.: Continuous culture of human lymphoblasts from peripheral blood of a child with acute leukemia. Cancer 18, 522-529 (1965).

64. Kaplan, M.R., Peterson, W.: Childhood lymphoblastic lymphoma, a cancer of thymus-derived lymphocytes. Cancer Res. 34, 521-525 (1974).

65. Smith, R., Blaese, R., Hathcock, K., Buell, D., Edelson, R., Lutzner, M.: T and B lymphocyte markers in lymphoid cell research and in human diseases. In: "Lymphocyte Recognition and Effector Mechanisms", Eds. Lindahl-Kiessling, K., Osoba, D., Academic Press, New York, pp. 127-146 (1974).

66. Hayata, I., Oshimura, M., Minowada, J., Sandberg, A.: Chromosomal banding of cultured T and B lymphocytes. In Vitro 11, 361-368 (1975).

67. Norman, M., Thompson, E.B.: Characterization of a glucocorticoid-sensitive human lymphoid cell line. Cancer Res. 37, 3785-3791 (1977).

68. Roper, P., Drewinko, B.: Comparison of in vitro methods to determine drug-induced cell lethality. Cancer Res. 36, 2182-2188 (1976).

69. Thompson, E.B., Norman, M.R., Lippman, M.E.: Steroid hormone actions in tissue culture cells and cell hybrids - their relation to human malignancies. Recent Prog. Horm. Res. 33, 571-615 (1977).

70. Noll, H.: Polysomes: analysis of structure and function. In: "Techniques in Protein Biosynthesis", vol. 2, Eds. Campbell, P.N., Sargent, J.R., Academic Press, New York, pp. 101-179 (1969).

71. Wiernak, P., Macleod, R.: The effect of a single large dose of 9 α-fluoroprednisolone on nucleodepolymerase activity and nucleic acid content of the rat thymus. Acta endocr. 49, 138-144 (1965).

72. Harmon, J., Norman, M., Thompson, E.B.: Human leukemic cells in culture - a model system for the study of glucocorticoid-induced lymphcytolysis. In: "Steroid Receptors and the Management of Cancer", Eds. Thompson, E.B., Lippman, M., CRC Press, Boca Raton, FL (1979).

73. Clarkson, B.: Review of recent studies of cellular proliferation in acute leukemia. In: "Human Tumor Cell Kinetics, Monograph No. 30", National Cancer Institute, Bethesda (1969).

74. Harmon, J., Norman, M., Fowlkes, B.J., Thompson, E.B.: Dexamethasone induces irreversible G_1 arrest and death of a human lymphoid cell line. J. cell comp. Physiol. 98, 267-278 (1979).

75. Norman, M., Harmon, J., Thompson, E.B.: Use of a human lymphoid cell line to evaluate interactions between prednisolone and other chemotherapeutic agents. Cancer Res. 38, 4273-4278 (1978).

76. Hill, B., Baserga, A.R.: The cell cycle and its significance for cancer treatment. Cancer Treatment Rev. 2, 159-175 (1975).

77. Royston, I., Graze, P., Pitts, R.: Failure of cultured human T-cell lymphoid lines to stimulate in mixed leukocyte culture. J. natn. Cancer Inst. 53, 361-367 (1974).

78. Nakazawa, S., Minowada, J., Tsubota, T., Sinks, L.: Profound radio-sensitivity in "leukemic" T-cell lines and T-cell-type acute lymphoblastic leukemia demonstrated by [^{51}Cr] chromate labelling. Cancer Res. 38, 1661-1666 (1978).

79. Roberts, D., Warmouth, E.: Methotrexate inhibition of CCRF-CEM cultures of human lymphoblasts. Europ. J. Cancer 11, 771-782 (1975).

80. Carson, D., Kaye, J., Matsumoto, S., Seegmiller, J., Thompson, L.: Biochemical basis for the enhanced toxicity of doxyribonucleosides towards malignant human T cell lines. Proc. natn. Acad. Sci. U.S.A. 76, 2430-2433 (1979).

81. Maca, R., Fry, G., Hakes, A.: Effects of glucocorticoids on the interaction of lymphoblastoid cells with human endothelial cells in vitro. Cancer Res. 38, 2224-2228 (1978).

REGULATION OF SOMATOSTATIN SECRETION AND ITS BIOLOGIC ACTIONS

J. E. Gerich
Endocrine Research Unit, Departments of Medicine and Physiology, Mayo Medical School and Mayo Clinic, Rochester, Minnesota 55901, U.S.A.

Somatostatin is a tetradecapeptide with a molecular weight of 1639 (Fig. 1) (1). In vivo, a disulfide bond between Cys^{3} and Cys^{14} renders the peptide cyclic. Confirmational studies (2)

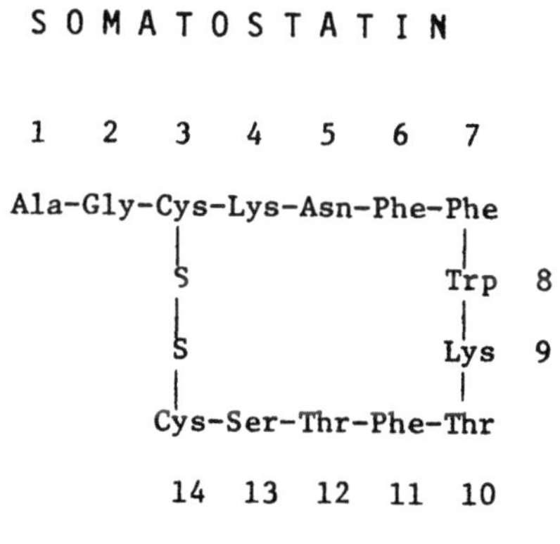

Fig. 1. Amino acid sequence of somatostatin

Hormones in Normal and Abnormal Human Tissues, Vol. II

suggest a type II^{1} turn from Phe^{6} to Thr^{10} and an antiparallel B-leated sheet structure involving Phe^{6}-Phe^{7} and Thr^{10}-Phe^{11}. It is currently thought (3) that the hydrophobic residues(Phe^{6}, Phe^{7}, Trp^{8}, Phe^{11}) and $lysine^{9}$ are involved in receptor binding and activation and that $threonine^{10}$ may be an essential spacer while cysteine and other amino acids determine the 3-dimensional structure of the active site of the molecule (4).

General Distribution and Actions

Somatostatin was discovered in 1971 by Guillemin and his colleagues during their search for the hypothalamic growth hormone (GH) releasing factor. A peptide was found in ovine hypothalamus which inhibited GH release from cultured anterior pituitary cells (5, 6). An identical peptide was later isolated from porcine hypothalamus by Schally and his coworkers (7). The peptide was named somatostatin in the belief that it was a hypothalamic releasing factor whose sole function was to inhibit the GH secretion. It soon became evident, however, that a peptide with identical immunologic characteristics and biologic activity was present in the D cells of pancreatic islets (8-12), in D-like cells of the gastro-intestinal tract (11-13), in parafollicular cells of the thyroid gland (14-16) and in extrahypothalamic neurons of both the central and peripheral nervous system (17-19). Moreover, studies employing synthetic somatostatin have demonstrated that the peptide possesses a wide spectrum of biologic activities in addition to GH inhibition.

Table 1 summarizes the tissue distribution of somatostatin in the rat. The peptide is found in highest concentration in the median eminence and pancreatic islets; the largest amounts are found in cerebral cortex, spinal cord, brain stem, and hypothalamus in the central nervous system and in the portions of the stomach, thyroid and pancreas. Lesser amounts of somatostatin have been reported in dorsal root ganglia and sympathetic ganglia (inferior and superior mesenteric, para-aortic, and

Table 1. Distribution of somatostatin in the rat

	Patel and Reichlin[20]			Arimura et al[21] Brownstein et al[22]		Kronheim et al[8]	
	ng/ region	ng/mg wet wt	ng/mg protein	ng/mg wet wt	ng/mg protein	ng/mg wet wt	ng/mg protein
CNS structures							
Hypothalamus	77	2.3	26.1	2.12		1.10	216.4
Median eminence			248.0		309.1		
Ventromedial nucleus		0.44	17.5		14.6		
Brain stem	128	0.67	5.1	0.05		0.13	53.4
Spinal cord	317	0.08	10.4			0.45	165.2
Olfactory lobe	7	0.52	1.1	0.02		0.15	21.1
Cerebral cortex	516	0.03	6.7	0.03	2.4	0.09	35.7
Cerebellum	7		0.4	0.02		0.04	28.4
Pineal			0.1		0.5		0
Pituitary							
Anterior		0					
Posterior			5.6				
Gut and visceral structures							
Stomach	306	0.37	2.4	0.17	11.7	Body of stomach	1.6
Pylorus	116	0.52	6.4	0.43	9.7	Antrum of stomach	20.2
Duodenum	42	0.15	1.9	0.03	1.6		2.1
Jejunum (10 cm)	50	0.07	1.9	0.03	1.6		2.3
Pancreas (whole)	137	0.17	1.8	0.14	33.8		26.4
Pancreatis			786.0				
Liver			0		0		0.1
Lung			0		0		0
Kidney			0		0		0.2
Submandibular glands			0				

superior cervical) in the guinea pig and rat (17) and also in Auerbach's plexus of the rat intestine (18). Somatostatin immunoreactivity which behaves chromatographically similar to synthetic somatostatin has been found in human cerebrospinal fluid (22, 23) and urine (24); increased amounts of cerebrospinal fluid somatostatin are present in various neurologic disorders e.g. nerve root compression, spinal cord, and cerebral disease, suggesting that increases in cerebrospinal fluid levels may be a non-specific index of brain damage (22).

Consistent with the view that somatostatin located at extrahypothalamic sites in the nervous system may function as a neurotransmitter, the peptide has been found to alter neuronal function in various parts of the central nervous system and to modify behavior in experimental animals (25-35). In man, somatostatin administered intravenously has a mild tranquilizing action but no other major behavioral or motor effects (36-38).

There is extensive evidence that hypothalamic somatostatin released from nerve terminals into the pituitary portal vessels acts as a physiological GH regulator and perhaps also of thyrotropic (TSH) secretion. Release of somatostatin and hypothalamic neural elements is stimulated by potassium, dopamine, and norepinephrine and is calcium dependent (39-43). Somatostatin does not affect posterior pituitary hormone secretion. The peptide inhibits GH release at concentrations as low as 10^{-9} M _in vitro_ and is also a potent inhibitor of GH secretion _in vivo_. Abnormally elevated circulating GH levels found in acromegaly (44-49), poorly-controlled diabetes (36, 50, 51), protein malnutrition (49) and Laron dwarfism (52) are decreased during intravenous infusion of somatostatin. Observations in experimental animals that administration of antiserum against somatostatin augments circulating GH levels (53-55) and prevents stress and starvation induced suppression of serum GH hormone levels (55, 56), that serum GH levels are increased in baboons actively immunized against somatostatin (57) and that the decrease in hypothalamic somatostatin content after hypophysectomy is restored by GH administration (58-61) provide convincing evidence that somatostatin released into the hypothalamic pituitary portal vessels acts as a physiologic regulator of GH secretion.

Somatostatin is also a potent inhibitor of TSH secretion both *in vivo* and *in vitro* (62-66). Systemic administration of antiserum against the peptide augments basal serum TSH levels and TSH responses to both cold exposure and thyrotropin releasing factor in the rat (54, 67-69) suggesting that it might act as a physiologic modulator of TSH secretion.

Somatostatin does not normally affect circulating prolactin (44, 63, 64, 70), adrenocorticotrophin (ACTH) (44, 71, 72), luteinizing hormone (44, 70) or follicle stimulating hormone (44, 70) levels. However, in certain patients with acromegaly (48), somatostatin has been reported to inhibit prolactin secretion. Moreover, in patients with hypersecretion of ACTH due to pituitary tumors (Nelson-Salassa syndrome) or to suboptimal corticosteroid replacement for Addison's disease (72-74), somatostatin decreases circulating ACTH levels. There are conflicting data concerning the effects of somatostatin on parathyroid hormone, calcitonin and thyroid hormone release (75-80), since somatostatin antiserum increases parathyroid hormone and calcitonin secretion *in vitro* (81) and since hypercalcaemia induced by vitamin D administration causes depletion of thyroidal somatostatin content (82). Possibly the peptide acts as a local regulator of parathyroid hormone and/or calcitonin secretion.

In the gastrointestinal tract, somatostatin is found in D-like cells in stomach, duodenum, jejunum and salivary glands (83-87), in saliva (83), gastric juice (88), duodenal aspirates (89), in neurons of Auerbach's plexus (18) and in fibres of the vagus nerve (90). Various gastro-intestinal tract functions are affected by somatostatin: secretion of gastrin (91-95), pancreozymin (92, 96, 97), vasoactive intestinal peptide (98), gut glucagon (99), motilin (100), gastric inhibitory polypeptide (101), secretin (92, 96, 102, 103) and pancreatic polypeptide (104, 105) as well as gastric acid, pepsin and intrinsic factor secretion, gastric motility (91, 93, 94, 104-111), gall bladder contraction (112, 113) and both small and large intestinal motility (114,

115), absorption (116, 117) and secretion (118) are inhibited by somatostatin in various species. Despite these numerous effects of somatostatin on gastrointestinal function, to date no malabsorption has been reported during long-term infusions of somatostatin in man (36).

Intra-aortic administration of somatostatin to rats was reported to cause a prompt increase in urine flow and in free water clearance without concomitant changes in renal blood flow, osmolar clearance, electrolyte excretion and cyclic AMP excretion (119). In dogs, somatostatin was shown to increase free water clearance during infusion of arginine vasopressin (120). Since the peptide does not affect antidiuretic hormone secretion in this species (121), the above results can be best explained on the basis of antagonism of the action of antidiuretic hormone. In the isolated toad bladder preparation, somatostatin antagonized the hydro-osmotic effect of vasopressin and enhanced water flow induced by cAMP (122). However, no effect was found on serum electrolytes, urine volume and electrolyte balance during prolonged infusion of somatostatin in man (36).

Increases in plasma renin activity after furosemide administration (123, 124) or infusion or a β-adrenergic agonist (125) in man are decreased by somatostatin but basal circulating plasma renin activity is not affected. These results suggest that somatostatin may inhibit secretion of renin by the kidney. Transient increases in blood pressure (5-10 mm Hg) and pulse (5-10 beats/min) have been occasionally observed after bolus injection of somatostatin but in normal men, somatostatin did not affect cardiac output, stroke volume, cardiac index, stroke index or total peripheral resistance (126).

Administration of somatostatin usually has no effect on circulating leukocyte, erythrocyte or platelet concentrations (26, 127-130); however, a 25% reduction in leukocyte count was found in patients with acute bacterial leukocytosis (127). In baboons with chronically implanted intravenous catheters profound thrombocytopenia was found after infusions of large quantities of somatostatin (131). In rats, somatostatin apparently prevents pyromen and endotoxin-induced leukocytosis (132). Diminished aggregation of platelets was reported in baboons (131), rabbits (133) and man (134) but in most studies no effect was found on platelet aggregation, bleeding time, prothrombin time, partial thromboplastin time, fibrinogen, fibrin split production, factor VII, and Von Willebrand factor (36, 128-130, 135, 136).

Somatostatin also inhibits insulin and glucagon secretion (Fig. 2). It is as potent an inhibitor of insulin and glucagon secretion _in vivo_ and _in vitro_ as it is of GH secretion (137, 138). The degree to which somatostatin inhibited insulin and glucagon secretion varied depending upon the dose of the peptide employed and the stimulus used for insulin and glucagon secretion. _In vitro_, using the perfused rat pancreas with arginine (19 nM) plus glucose (5.5 nM) as a stimuli, somatostatin

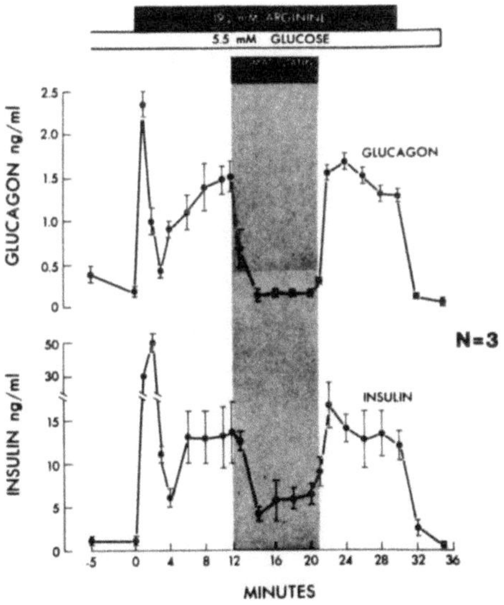

Fig. 2. Effect of somatostatin on insulin and glucagon release from rat pancreas perfused _in vitro_.

was a more effective inhibitor of glucagon than of insulin release (139). Under other conditions insulin release is more sensitive to somatostatin inhibition than is glucagon secretion (140-142).

The response of insulin and glucagon to all known secretagogues is inhibited by an appropriate concentration of somatostatin; among these are orciprenaline (143), glucose (139, 144-152), glucagon (153-156), arginine (140, 143, 151, 152, 157-159), secretin (153), theophylline (139, 144, 148), tolbutamide (145, 148, 154, 156), isoproterenol (139, 153), calcium (140, 148, 160), potassium (144), epinephrine (161-163), meals (36, 51, 164-166), 3-isobutyl-methyl-xynthine (160), the divalent ionophore A23187 (160, 167), cyclic AMP (155) and dibutyryl cyclic AMP (168). Onset of inhibition is virtually immediate and is reversible upon withdrawal of somatostatin. In general, increasing the concentration of a given secretagogue can overcome the inhibitory effect of a given dose of somatostatin as in the case of glucose (148, 156) and calcium (140). Of interest is the observation that *in vitro*, the first phase of glucose-stimulated insulin appears to be 25-50 times more sensitive to inhibition by somatostatin than is the second phase (146).

The ability of somatostatin to inhibit insulin and glucagon secretion and its presence in pancreatic islets suggests that this peptide may be important in regulating insulin and glucagon secretion. This concept is supported by studies showing that under appropriate conditions, antiserum against somatostatin can augment glucagon (169, 170) and insulin (170, 171) release from isolated pancreatic islets (Fig. 3). It seems that locally released somatostatin, rather than circulating somatostatin, is involved in this process since neither active (57) nor passive immunization (172) of animals against somatostatin alters circulating insulin and glucagon levels.

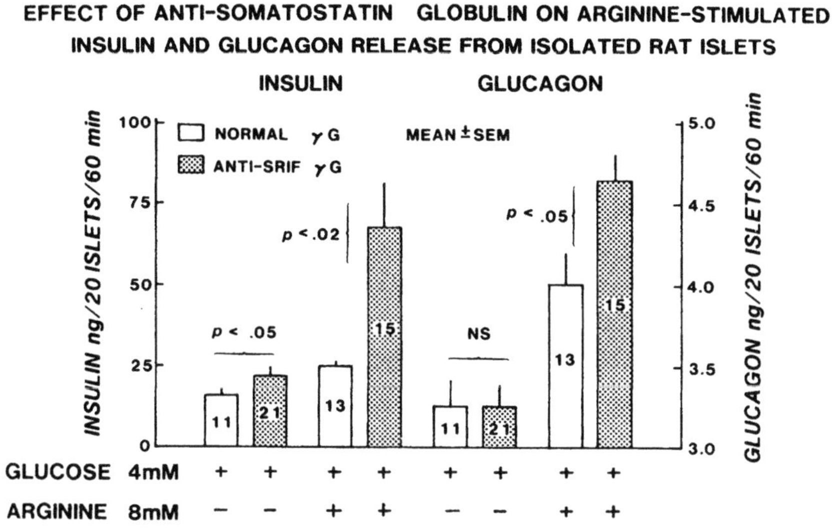

Fig. 3. Effect of somatostatin antiserum on insulin and glucagon release from rat islets incubated *in vitro* (from Itoh et al. 170).

Mechanism of Action

It is generally assumed that somatostatin acts by a similar mechanism in the various tissues in which it acts. The most extensively studied action of somatostatin has been its inhibition of pancreatic islet hormone secretion. The onset of somatostatin action is rapid and does not depend on protein synthesis (173, 174) suggesting that it may act like other peptide hormones via an interaction with plasma membrane receptors rather than like steroid or thyroid hormones which require intracellular translocation and are dependent on protein synthesis. High-affinity binding sites for somatostatin have been identified in cultured anterior pituitary cells (175) and in partially purified plasma membranes of pituicytes (176) and pancreatic β-cells (176, 177). Some of these tissues, however, were derived from tumors and thus characteristics of these receptors may not necessarily reflect those of normal tissue. The binding affinity for somatostatin receptors on cultured pituicytes was approximately 1×10^{10} M^{-1} and it has been estimated that these cells contained approximately 14,000 binding sites (175). These observations and the fact that somatostatin inhibits both neuronal (25, 26) and pancreatic β cell (178) electrical activity suggest a plasma membrane site for action of somatostatin. However, additional loci of action may be operative since cytosolic somatostatin binding proteins have been found in several tissues (179) and somatostatin has been reported to inhibit cyclic AMP stimulated protein kinase activity in secretory vesicles of isolated pancreatic islets and pituicytes (180). The observations that increases in extracellular calcium concentration (139, 148, 181, 182) and the addition of the divalent cation ionophore A23187 (182, 183) or theophylline (182, 183), which may mobilize intracellular calcium, can at least partly reverse somatostatin inhibition of insulin secretion suggest that somatostatin might act by intervening with cellular calcium fluxes or with an action of calcium. Initial reports of the diminution of pancreatic islet (139, 184) and pituitary cell (185) calcium uptake during inhibition of the release of their respective hormone by somatostatin supported this concept. However some of these results have not been subsequently confirmed (186, 187). Moreover, somatostatin has been shown to inhibit insulin (51), glucagon (160) and GH (188) secretion stimulated by the calcium ionophore A23187 in the presence of low extracellular calcium and also to inhibit insulin release stimulated by isobutylmethylxanthine in the absence of extracellular calcium (189).

Another potential mechanism by which somatostatin may inhibit hormone secretion is by interference with cellular cyclic nucleotide metabolism since cyclic nucleotides, particularly cyclic 3',5' adenosine monophosphate (cyclic AMP) are well known to be important in endocrine and exocrine secretion. Although somatostatin will decrease cyclic AMP levels in pituitary (190, 191) and pancreatic islets (192-194), several observations suggest that somatostatin may not inhibit secretion by lowering tissue cyclic AMP levels. Firstly, somatostatin inhibits GH response to prostaglandin E_2 and isobutylmethylxanthine without affecting pituitary cyclic AMP, cyclic GMP and protein kinase responses (195). Secondly, somatostatin can inhibit glucagon-stimulated insulin release without affecting activation of adenylate cyclase (155). Thirdly, somatostatin inhibits insulin and glucagon responses to arginine (139) which apparently stimulates islet hormone secretion by a mechanism independent of cyclic AMP. Fourthly, somatostatin uniformly blocks hormone responses to agents which increase tissue cyclic AMP levels by different means, e.g. adenylate cyclase activation (139) and phosphodiesterase inhibition (139). Fifthly, somatostatin inhibits pituitary and pancreatic hormone secretion in response to exogenous cyclic AMP and its analogues (155, 168, 184); the peptide does not alter islet phosphodiesterase (196) or ATPase activity (197).

Metabolism

The half-life of exogenously infused somatostatin is 1-2 minutes in man and dogs (198, 199). Its metabolic clearance rate (~30 ml/kg/min in normal man) is decreased in patients with chronic renal failure suggesting that the kidney may play a role in the metabolism of somatostatin (199). Arteriovenous differences in somatostatin levels during infusion of the peptide in baboons and rats indicate that tissues such as liver, muscle and kidney may be major sites of degradation (200-201). Crude brain and hypothalamic extracts (202-204), isolated guinea pig pancreatic islet cells (205), perfused rat pancreas (205) and both rat and human serum degrade synthetic somatostatin (206). Rat serum contains both an aminopeptidase and an endopeptidase which appear to be involved in degrading somatostatin (206). Peptidases present in brain extracts cleave the amino terminal alanine and glycine residues and also the internal residues (Phe^6-Phe^7,

Trp^{8-}-Lys^{9}, Thr^{9},-Phe^{10}) (202). Induction of hypothyroidism was reported to decrease degradation of somatostatin by rat hypothalamus (207). Decreased degradation of somatostatin might explain the increased concentrations of somatostatin found in the pancreas and other tissues of hypothyroid and hypophysectomized rats (208).

Regulation of Pancreatic Somatostatin Secretion *In Vitro*

Only a few studies have examined secretion or release of somatostatin from tissues other than the pancreas; in this section, primarily studies of secretion of pancreatic somatostatin will be reviewed (209-231).

A. Substrates

Glucose stimulates biphasic release of somatostatin from perfused dog (213), rat (216, 220) and cat pancreas and from perifused and incubated rat islets (Fig. 4) (210, 220, 214). Both phases of somatostatin release coincide with corresponding phases of insulin release. The magnitude of both phases of somatostatin responses of glucose appear to be less than those of insulin regardless of the species studied (213, 220, 222) but no dose-response studies have been performed comparing each phase of somatostatin and insulin responses to glucose.

To what extent stimulation of somatostatin secretion by glucose is dependent upon metabolism of glucose is unclear. Galactose, which is not metabolized by islets and which does not stimulate insulin release, has been reported not to cause release of somatostatin from neonatal rat islet monolayers (227). Mannoheptulose, a blocker of glucose phosphorylation in islets and which inhibits glucose-stimulated insulin release, was reported to inhibit glucose-stimulated somatostatin release from incubated rat islets (210). These results could be due to either the fact that a substrate used as stimulus must be metabolized

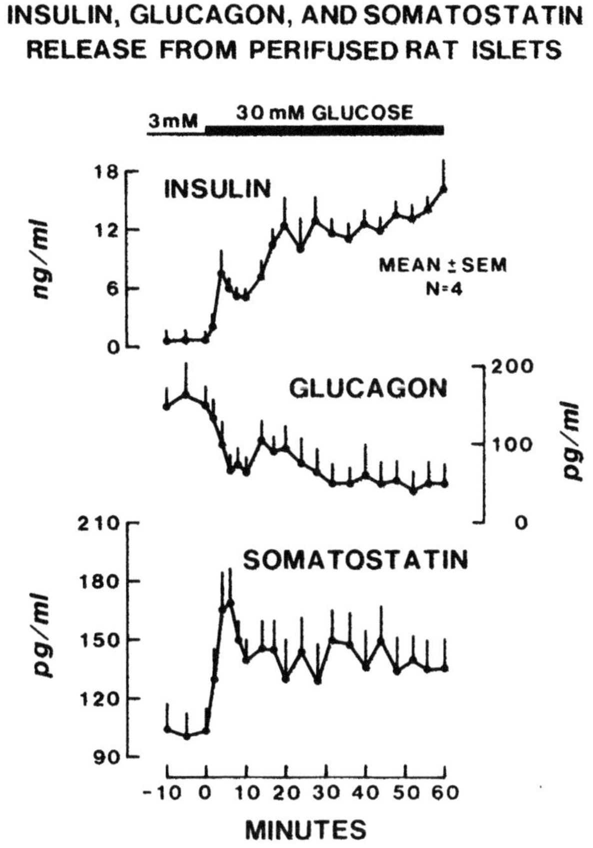

Fig. 4. Effect of glucose on somatostatin, insulin and glucagon release from rat islets perifused in vitro (from Gerich et al. unpublished observations).

in order to stimulate somatostatin release or that an energy source must be available for somatostatin secretion to occur. Of great interest is the observation that D-glyceraldehyde, a metabolite of glucose, inhibits somatostatin release and stimulates insulin release from incubated rat islets (213); this represents the first instance of a dissociation between somatostatin and insulin release and would suggest that stimulation of somatostatin release by glucose may not simply be the direct consequence of the metabolism of glucose. The effects of carbohydrates other than glucose, galactose, and D-glyceraldehyde on somatostatin release have not been examined.

Arginine (211, 212, 216, 221, 222), leucine (214, 215) and the metabolite of leucine, α-ketoisocaproic acid (215), have been demonstrated to stimulate somatostatin release in several systems. In perfusion systems such as the perfused cat pancreas (Fig. 5) both arginine and leucine cause biphasic somatostatin release in the presence of basal levels (2-5 mM) of glucose.

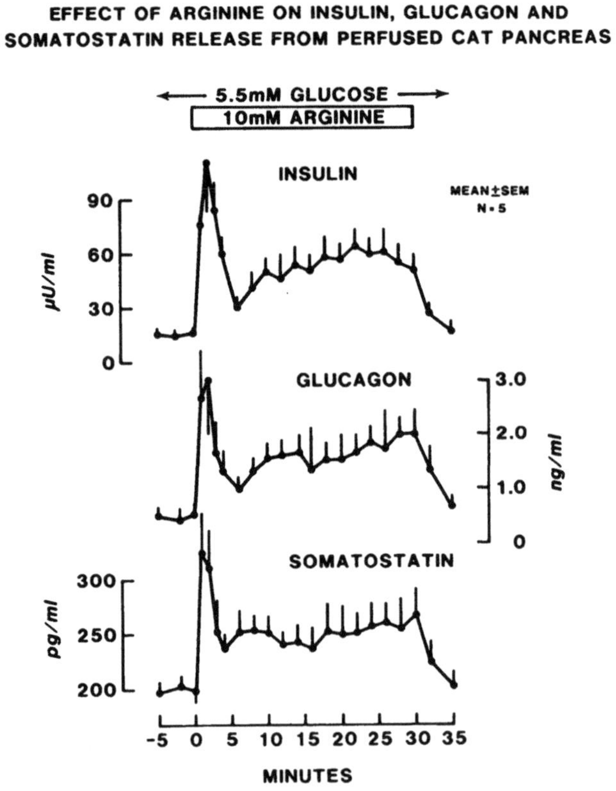

Fig. 5. Effect of arginine on somatostatin, insulin and glucagon release from cat pancreas perfused *in vitro* (from Gerich et al. unpublished observations).

B. Ionic change

It is well established that the ionic composition of extracellular fluid exerts an important influence on both insulin and glucagon release. The presence of extracellular calcium is essential for release of both insulin and glucagon and, over a given range, increases in the extracellular calcium or potassium concentrations increase insulin release while increases in the extracellular magnesium concentrations decrease insulin release. The effects of extracellular ionic concentrations on somatostatin secretion have not been studied in detail. It appears that, like insulin and glucagon release, secretion of somatostatin from the pancreas is increased by increasing the extracellular calcium concentrations (Fig. 6) (232, 233). Magnesium inhibits and potassium augments somatostatin release from the perfused cat pancreas (233).

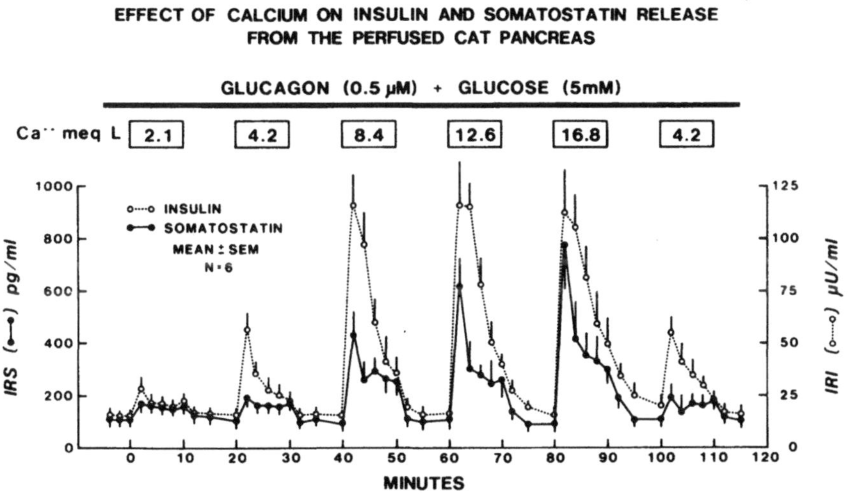

Fig. 6. Effect of calcium on somatostatin and insulin release from cat pancreas perfused *in vitro* (from Mandarino et al. 233)

C. Neurotransmitters and other Monoamines

The effects of catecholamines and monoamines on somatostatin release from the pancreas have been investigated by several groups (210, 219, 224, 230). Epinephrine inhibits release of somatostatin from the pancreas (Fig. 7). Samols et al. (224), using the perfused dog pancreas, concluded that β-adrenergic mechanisms increased somatostatin release while α-adrenergic mechanisms inhibited somatostatin release. This conclusion is consistent with the findings that isoproterenol (232) and agents such as theophylline and cAMP derivatives (209, 231) augment somatostatin release.

Acetylcholine stimulates pancreatic somatostatin release (Fig. 7) (224). Vagal stimulation causes release of somatostatin

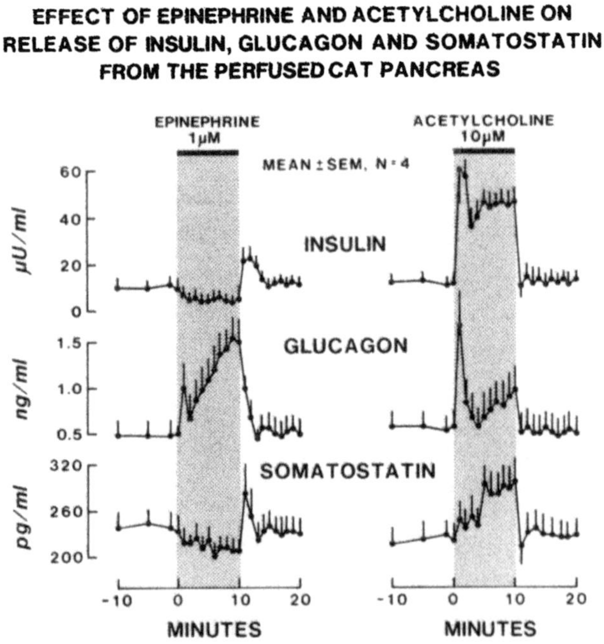

Fig. 7. Effect of epinephrine and acetyl choline on somatostatin, insulin and glucagon release from cat pancreas perfused _in vitro_ (from Gerich et al. unpublished observations).

into the gastric antrum of cats (88). Dopamine inhibits somatostatin release from incubated rat islets (219, 234). Of interest is the report (235) that apomorphine, a relatively specific dopaminergic agonist, increases somatostatin release into the gastric antrum of cats and dopamine, norepinephrine and acetylcholine increase somatostatin release from rat hypothalamus (40-42). The discrepancy between the effects of dopamine (stomach and pancreas) and norepinephrine (hypothalamus and pancreas) on somatostatin release in different tissues is not unique since opposite effects of these agents have been reported on somatostatin release from synoptosomes from different parts of the brain (cerebral cortex and hypothalamus) (219). Serotonin has been reported to increase release of somatostatin.

D. Hormones

Various peptide hormones alter pancreatic somatostatin secretion: glucagon (212, 213, 219, 222, 233), pancreozymin (213), gastrin (215), secretin (216) and gastric inhibitory polypeptide (215) stimulate somatostatin release. β-Endorphin, an opioid peptide, and morphine inhibit somatostatin release from the perfused dog pancreas (218) while neurotensin stimulates somatostatin release from isolated rat islets at low glucose concentrations (3 mM) but inhibits somatostatin responses at 23 mM glucose or 20 mM arginine (230). The physiological significance of these observations are unclear since in virtually all instances what would be considered pharmacologic doses of each hormone were employed. However, based on the observations that all the gastrointestinal hormones studied increased somatostatin secretion, that exogenous somatostatin inhibited release of each of these hormones and that somatostatin is found in the gastrointestinal tract, it has been proposed that gastrointestinal somatostatin may act in some feedback inhibition axis to regulate nutrient absorption.

Although the ability of physiologic concentrations of glucagon to augment pancreatic somatostatin has not been demonstrated, the recent report that somatostatin release from islet monolayers is augmented by antiglucagon serum (227) strongly suggests that glucagon may play a physiologic role in the regulation of islet D cell function. Conceivably, the prolonged hyperglucagonemia associated with alloxan diabetes may explain in part the D cell hyperplasia and increased somatostatin release from pancreas of alloxan diabetic rats perfused in vitro (221). No studies have demonstrated an acute effect of insulin on mammalian islet somatostatin release.

Somatostatin Secretion In Vivo

A number of potential problems make the interpretation of studies measuring somatostatin in plasma difficult: The tissue of origin of the somatostatin cannot be ascertained with certainty. Plasma somatostatin is heterogeneous, consisting of at least two moieties - one with a molecular weight greater than 100,000 daltons and one similar to synthetic somatostatin (237-242). Plasma degrades endogenous and I^{125}-labeled somatostatin (206, 243, 244) and contains proteins which interfere in its radioimmunoassay (244-246). Thus somatostatin-free plasma causes marked reduction in binding (247) and not all somatostatin-like immunoreactivity in unextracted plasma is removed by affinity chromatography (238). Because of these problems, most investigators have resorted to extraction of plasma prior to assay (239, 243, 247-249).

Studies employing extracted plasma generally have found circulating somatostatin levels in peripheral and portal venous plasma which are much lower than those using unextracted plasma (250-258). Normal values for somatostatin levels in extracted plasma of fasting subjects are from 20 to 140 pg/ml (247, 259) whereas in rats levels are between 10 and 50 pg/ml (244, 248, 260). Plasma somatostatin concentrations in hypophyseal portal blood (150-1500 pg/ml) (243, 260) and abdominal portal venous blood (70-150 pg/ml) (244, 211, 260) are several fold greater than those found in peripheral venous plasma.

Studies employing extracted plasma have found the release of somatostatin from the hypothalamus to be influenced by catecholamines and other putative neurotransmitters (43). Abdominal portal venous somatostatin levels, presumably reflecting primarily gastric and pancreatic secretion, are increased by infusion of glucose (243) arginine (243, 248) and glucagon (243) and are decreased by infusion of pancreatic polypeptide (260) in rats; increased levels have been found in rats made diabetic by streptozotocin (248) confirming prior evidence for D cell hyperfunction based on studies of pancreas of alloxan diabetic rats perfused *in vitro* (221).

Pancreatic D Cell Function in Diabetes

Abnormalities in islet D cell morphology in human diabetes and in alloxan diabetes in the rat were recognized more than 25 years ago using conventional histochemical methods (261-265). Recently, these have been studied using more sophisticated immunohistochemical and radioimmunoassay techniques. In rats with alloxan or streptozotocin-induced diabetes, there is an increase in the number of islet D cells and in the content of pancreatic or islet somatostatin (266-270). These types of diabetes are characterized by hypoinsulinemia and hyperglucagonemia *in vivo*. Two studies, one *in vitro* (226) and one *in vivo* (248) have documented that there is hypersecretion of somatostatin in this type of diabetes. In the *in vitro* study, two weeks after induction of alloxan diabetes in rats, a time at which pancreatic somatostatin content should still be normal, there was excessive release of somatostatin from pancreas perfused *in vitro* during arginine stimulation accompanied by markedly decreased insulin and slightly decreased glucagon responses. These results indicate that D cell function is abnormal in alloxan diabetes, that it could precede gross changes in D cell mass and that it may contribute to concomitant abnormalities of insulin and glucagon release.

In contrast to the above insulinopenic types of induced diabetes, that caused by the M variant of the encephalomyocarditis virus results in a decrease in islet D and B cells and an increase in islet A cells (271). A similar decreased pancreatic somatostatin content associated with decreased insulin and increased glucagon content was found in the spontaneously diabetic Chinese hamster (272). This animal in contrast to most other widely studied animals with spontaneous diabetes is not obese. The importance of the decrease in islet somatostatin content and islet D cell number to the abnormalities of insulin and glucagon release in the above two animal models of diabetes is unclear since there are no studies of somatostatin secretion in either of these models.

Variable changes in pancreatic or islet somatostatin content have been found in other closely related models of spontaneous diabetes - OBOB and DBDB mice (273-276). Decreased pancreatic somatostatin content or decreased numbers of islet D cells and increases in the number of D cells or in pancreatic somatostatin content have been found. Reasons for these discrepancies have not been completely resolved although factors related to differences in the ages of the animals studied and the severity of their diabetes have been suggested as possible explanations.

Somatostatin-Producing Tumors

To date, seven cases of somatostatin producing tumors, somatostatinomas, have been reported (277-283); all but one (279) were malignant and all but one (281) originated in the pancreas. Plasma somatostatin was markedly increased (277, 278, 280, 283) and could be resolved by chromatography into several immunoreactive fractions (277, 278, 280). The tumors occurred were associated with non-specific features usually including cholelithiasis, diabetes mellitus, steatorrhea, hypochloridria, weight loss and excessive secretion of another hormone (277, 278, 281-283). Usually insulin, glucagon and GH secretion were suppressed and the associated diabetes mellitus was mild. Diagnosis of the syndrome has been late since in all malignant cases, hepatic metastases were evident at the time of presentation. Conceivably with wider availability of assays for plasma somatostatin and the recognition of a characteristic constellation of symptoms, earlier diagnosis and therapeutic intervention may be possible.

Physiologic Role of Endogenous Somatostatin

Four functions for somatostatin have been proposed depending on its location: a neurotransmitter, a neurohormone, a parahormone and a hormone. The location of somatostatin in extrahypothalamic neurons in the central nervous system, the biological actions of somatostatin on behavior and neuronal function and the release of somatostatin from synaptosomes by agents such as dopamine and norepinephrine provide considerable evidence that somatostatin may function as a peptidergic neurotransmitter. There is also considerable evidence that somatostatin GH acts as a neurohormone regulating the secretion of GH and TSH; the peptide is present in hypothalamic neurons of the median eminence; it is released into the hypophyseal portal vessels; it is a potent inhibitor of all known stimuli for GH and TSH release; its hypothalamic concentration is altered by hypophysectomy, GH administration and hypothyroidism; and its neutralization by either passive or active immunization increases GH and TSH secretion.

The location of somatostatin in the mucosa of the gastrointestinal tract and in pancreatic islets and the ability of exogenous somatostatin to alter the function of adjacent cells in these locations suggest that endogenous somatostatin may play a role in the regulation of gastrointestinal and pancreatic islet function. The failure of active immunization and passive immunization to alter insulin and glucagon secretion _in vivo_ whereas direct application of antisomatostatin serum to pancreatic islets in vitro can increase insulin and/or glucagon release suggests that, at least with respect to pancreatic islets, endogenous somatostatin probably acts as a local regulator (parahormone) rather than a classical hormone.

In view of the above likely physiologic roles of somatostatin, it seems possible that abnormalities in the metabolism of endogenous somatostatin could be involved in the pathogenesis of a variety of psychiatric, neurological, gastro-intestinal and endocrine disorders in man.

References

1. Burgus, R., Ling, N., Butcher, M., Guillemin, R.: Primary structure of somatostatin, a hypothalamic peptide that inhibits the secretion of pituitary growth hormone. Proc. natn. Acad. Sci. U.S.A. 70, 684-688 (1973).
2. Arison, B.H., Hirschman, R., Veber, D.F.: Inferences about the conformation of somatostatin at a biologic receptor based on NMR studies. Bioorganic Chem. 7, 447-451 (1978).
3. Brown, M., Rivier, J., Vale, W.: Somatostatin analogs with selected biologic activities. Metabolism 25 (suppl. 1), 1491-1494 (1976).
4. Holladay, L.A., Puett, D.: Somatostatin conformation: Evidence for a stable intramolecular structure from circular dichroism, diffusion and sedimentation equilibrium. Proc. natn. Acad. Sci. U.S.A. 73, 1199-1202 (1976).
5. Burgus, R., Brazeau, P., Vale, W.: Isolation and determination of the primary structure of somatostatin of ovine hypothalamic origin. DHEW Publications, 74, (NIH) 144-158 (1973).
6. Vale, W., Brazeau, P., Rivier, C., Brown, M., Boss, B., Rivier, J., Bergus, R., Ling, N., Guillemin, R.: Somatostatin. Recent Prog. Horm. Res. 34, 365-397 (1975).
7. Schally, A.V., DuPont, A., Arimura, A., Redding, T., Nishi, N., Linthicum, G., Schlessinger, D.: Isolation and structure of somatostatin from porcine hypothalami. Biochemistry 15, 509-514 (1976).
8. Kronheim, S., Berelowitz, M., Pimstone, B.L.: A radioimmunoassay for growth hormone release-inhibiting hormone: Method and quantitative tissue distribution. Clin. Endocr. 5, 619-630 (1976).

9. Orci, L., Baetens, D., Dubois, M.P., Rufener, C.: Evidence for the D-Cell of the pancreas secreting somatostatin. Horm. Metab. Res. 7, 400-402 (1975).

10. Goldsmith, P.C., Rose, J.C., Arimura, A., Ganong, W.F.: Ultrastructural localization of somatostatin in pancreatic islets of the rat. Endocrinology 97, 1061-1064 (1975).

11. Polak, J.M., Grimelius, L., Pearse, A.G.E., Bloom, S.R., Arimura, A.: Growth-hormone release-inhibiting hormone in gastrointestinal and pancreatic D cells. Lancet 1, 1220-1222 (1975).

12. Hökfelt, T., Efendic, S., Hellerström, C., Johansson, O., Luft, R., Arimura, A.: Cellular localization of somatostatin in endocrine-like cells and neurons of the rat with special references to the A_1-cells of the pancreatic islets and to the hypothalamus. Acta Endocrinol. 80 (suppl. 200) 1-41 (1975).

13. Rufener, C., Dubois, M.P., Malaisse-Lagae, F., Orci, L.: Immunofluorescent reactivity to anti-somatostatin in the gastrointestinal mucosa of the dog. Diabetologia 11, 321-324 (1975).

14. Sundler, F., Alumets, J., Hakanson, R., Bjorklund, L., Lundberg, O.: Somatostatin-immunoreactive cells in medullary carcinoma of the thyroid. Am. J. Path. 88, 381-386 (1977).

15. Van Noorden, S., Polak, J.M., Pearse, A.G.E.: Single cellular origin of somatostatin and calcitonin in the rat thyroid gland. Histochem. 53, 243-247 (1977).

16. Yamada, Y., Ito, S., Matsubara, Y., Kobayashi, S.: Immunohistochemical demonstration of somatostatin-containing cell in the human, dog and rat thyroids. Tohoku J. Exp. Med. 122, 87-92 (1977).

17. Hökfeldt, T., Elfvin, L.G., Elde, R., Schultzberg, M., Goldstein, M., Luft, R.: Occurrence of somatostatin-like immunoreactivity in some peripheral sympathetic noradrenergic neurons. Proc. natn. Acad. Sci. U.S.A. 74, 3587-3591 (1977).

18. Hökfeldt, T., Johansson, O., Efendic, S., Luft, R., Arimura, A.: Are there somatostatin-containing nerves in the rat gut? Immunohistochemical evidence for a new type of peripheral nerve. Experientia 31, 852-854 (1975).

19. Parsons, J.A., Erlandsen, S.L., Hegre, O.D., McEvoy, R., Elde, R.P.: Central and peripheral localization of somatostatin: Immunoenzyme immunohistochemical studies. J. Histochem. Cytochem. 24, 872-882 (1976).

20. Patel, Y.C., Reichlin, S.: Somatostatin in hypothalamus, extrahypothalamic brain and peripheral tissues of the rat. Endocrinology 102, 523-530 (1978).

21. Arimura, A., Sato, H., DuPont, A., Nishi, N., Schally, A.V.: Somatostatin; Abundance of immunoreactive hormone in rat stomach and pancreas. Science 189, 1007-1008 (1975).

22. Brownstein, M., Arimura, A., Sato, H., Schally, A.V., Kizer, J.S.: The regional distribution of somatostatin in the rat brain. Endocrinology 96, 1456-1461 (1975).

22a. Patel Y.C., Rao, K., Reichlin, S.: Somatostatin in human cerebrospinal fluid. New Engl. J. Med. 296, 529-533 (1977).

23. Kronheim, S., Berelowitz, M., Pimstone, B.L.: The presence of immunoreactive growth hormone release-inhibiting hormone in normal cerebrospinal fluid. Clin. Endocr. 6, 411-415 (1977).

24. Kronheim, S., Berelowitz, M., Pimstone, B.L.: The characterization of growth hormone release inhibiting hormone-like immunoreactivity in normal urine. Clin. Endocr. 7, 343-347 (1977).

25. Renaud, L.P., Martin, J.B., Brazeau, P.: Depressant action of TRH, LH-RH and somatostatin on activity of central neurons. Nature 255, 233-235 (1975).

26. Randic, M., Miletic, V.: Depressant actions of methionine-enkaphalin and somatostatin in cat dorsal horn neurons activated by noxious stimuli. Brain Res. 152, 196-202 (1978).

27. Tan, A.T., Tsang, D., Renaud, L.P., Martin, J.B.: Effect of somatostatin on calcium transport in guinea pig cortex synaptosomes. Brain Res. 123, 193-196 (1977).

28. Havlicek, V., Rezek, M., Friesen, H.: Somatostatin and thyrotropin releasing hormone: Central effect on sleep and motor systems. Pharmacol. Biochem. Behav. 4, 455-459 (1976).

29. Cohn, M.L., Cohn, M.: Barrel rotation induced by somatostatin in the non-lesioned rat. Brain Res. 96, 138-141 (1975).

30. Brown, M., Vale, W.: Central nervous system effects of hypothalamic peptides. Endocrinology 96, 1333-1336 (1975).

31. Koranyi, L., Whitmoyer, D.I., Sawyer, C.H.: Effect of thyrotropin-releasing hormone, luteinizing hormone-releasing hormone and somatostatin on neuronal activity of brain stem reticular formation and hippocampus in the female rat. Expl.Neurol. 57, 807-816 (1977).

32. Plotnikoff, N.P., Kastin, A.J., Schally, A.V.: Growth hormone release inhibiting hormone: Neuropharmacological studies. Pharmacol. Biochem. Behav. 2, 693-696 (1974).

33. Guillemin, R.: Somatostatin inhibits the release of acetyl choline induced electrically in the myenteric plexus. Endocrinology 99, 1653-1654 (1976).

34. Resek, M., Havlicek, V., Hughes, K.R., Friesen, H.: Central site of action of somatostatin (SRIF): Role of hippocampus. Neuropharmacology 15, 499-504 (1976).

35. Cohen, M.L., Rosing, E., Wiley, K.S., Slater, I.H.: Somatostatin inhibits adrenergic and cholinergic neurotransmission in smooth muscle. Life Sci. 23, 1659-1664 (1978).

36. Gerich, J.E., Schultz, T.A., Lewis, S.B., Karam, J.H.: Clinical evaluation of somatostatin as a potential adjunct to insulin in the management of diabetes mellitus. Diabetologia 13, 537-544 (1977).

37. Ashton, H., Millman, J.E., Telford, R., Thompson, J.W.: An electro-encephalographic investigation of short-term effects of three hypothalamic hormones (TRH, LH/FSH-RH, GH-RIH) in normal subjects. Brit. J. Clin. Pharmacol. 3, 523-531 (1976).

38. DuPont, E., Hansen, A.P., Juul-Jensen, P., Lundbaek, K., Magnussen, I., de Fine Olivarius, B.: Somatostatin in the treatment of patients with extra pyramidal disorders and patients with EEG abnormalities. Acta Neurol. Scand. 57, 488-493 (1978).

39. Wakabayashi, I., Miyazaki, Y., Kanda, M., Miki, N., Demura, R., Demura, H., Shizume, K.: Stimulation of immunoreactive somatostatin release from hypothalamic synaptosomes by high K^+ and dopamine. Endocrinol. jap. 24, 601-604 (1977).

40. Negro-Villar, A., Ojeda, S., Arimura, A., McCann, S.: Dopamine and norepinephrine stimulate somatostatin release by median eminence fragments in vitro. Life Sci. 23, 1493-1498 (1978).

41. Patel, Y.C., Zingg, H.H., Dreifuss, J.J.: Calcium-dependent somatostatin secretion from rat neurohypophysis in vitro. Nature 267, 852-853 (1977).

42. Berelowitz, M., Kronheim, S., Pimstone, B., Sheppard, M.: Potassium stimulated calcium dependent release of immunoreactive somatostatin from incubated rat hypothalamus. J. Neurochem. 31, 1537-1539 (1978).

43. Chihara, K., Arimura, A., Schally, A.V.: Effect of intraventricular injection of dopamine, norepinephrine, acetylcholine, and 5-hydroxytryptamine on immunoreactive somatostatin release into rat hypophysical portal blood. Endocrinology 104, 1656-1662 (1979).

44. Hall, R., Besser, G.M., Schally, A.V., Coy, D.H., Evered, D., Goldie, D.J., Kastin, A.J., McNeilly, A.S., Mortimer, C.H., Phenekos, C., Tunbridge, W.M.G., Weightman, D.: Action of growth-hormone-release inhibitory hormone in healthy men and in acromegaly. Lancet 2, 581-584 (1973).

45. Besser, G.M., Mortimer, C.H., McNeilly, A.S., Thorner, M.O., Batistoni, G.A., Bloom, S.R., Kastrup, K.W., Hanssen, K.F., Hall, R., Coy, D.H., Kastin, A.J., Schally, A.V.: Long-term infusion of growth hormone release inhibiting hormone in acromegaly: Effects on pituitary and pancreatic hormones. Brit. med. J. 4, 622-627 (1974).

46. Besser. G.M., Mortimer, C.H., Carr, D., Schally, A.V., Coy, D.H., Evered, D., Kastin, A.J., Tunbridge, W.M.G., Thorner, M.O., Hall, R.: Growth hormone release inhibiting hormone in acromegaly. Brit. med. J. 1, 352-355 (1974).

47. Peracchi, M., Reschini, E., Cantalamessa, L., Guistina, G., Cavagnini, F., Pinto, M., Bulgheroni, P.: Effect of somatostatin on blood glucose, plasma growth hormone, insulin, and free fatty acids in normal subjects and acromegalic patients. Metabolism 23, 1009-1015 (1974).

48. Yen, S.S.C., Siler, T.M., De Vane, G.W.: Effect of somatostatin in patients with acromegaly. New Engl. J. Med. 290, 935-938 (1974).

49. Pimstone, B.L., Becker, D., Kronheim, S.: Disappearance of plasma growth hormone in acromegaly and protein-calorie malnutrition after somatostatin. J. clin. Endocrinol. Metab. 40, 168-171 (1975).

50. Gerich, J.E., Lorenzi, M., Bier, D.M., Schneider, V., Tsalikian, E., Karam, J.H., Forsham, P.H.: Prevention of human diabetic ketoacidosis by somatostatin: Evidence for an essential role of glucagon. New Engl. J. Med. 292, 985-989 (1975).

51. Christensen, S.E., Hansen, A.P., Weeke, J., Lundbaek, K.: 24-Hour studies of the effects of somatostatin on the levels of plasma growth hormone, glucagon, and glucose in normal subjects and juvenile diabetics. Diabetes 27, 300-306 (1978).

52. Laron, Z., Pertzelan, A., Doron, M., Assa, S., Keret, R.: The effect of dihydrosomatostatin in dwarfism with high plasma immunoreactive growth hormone. Horm. Metab. Res. 9, 338-339 (1977).

53. Arimura, A., Smith, W.D., Schally, A.V.: Blockade of the stress-induced decrease in blood GH by anti-somatostatin serum in rats. Endocrinology 98, 540-543 (1976).

54. Ferland, L., Labrie, F., Jobin, M., Arimura, A., Schally, A.V.: Physiological role of somatostatin in the control of growth hormone and thyrotropin secretion. Biochem. biophys. Res. Commun. 68, 149-156 (1976).

55. Terry, L.C., Willoughby, J.O., Brazeau, P., Martin, J.B., Patel, Y.C.: Antiserum to somatostatin prevents stress-induced inhibition of growth hormone secretion in the rat. Science 192, 565-567 (1976).

56. Tannenbaum, G.S., Epelbaum, J., Colle, E., Brazeau, P., Martin, J.B.: Antiserum to somatostatin reverses starvation-induced inhibition of growth hormone but not insulin secretion. Endocrinology 102, 1909-1914 (1978).

57. Steiner, R.A., Stewart, J.K., Barber, J., Koerker, D., Goodner, C.J., Brown, A., Illner, P., Gale, C.C.: Somatostatin: A physiological role in the regulation of growth hormone secretion in the adolescent male baboon. Endocrinology 102, 1587-1594 (1978).

58. Baker, B.L., Yen, Y.Y.: The influence of hypophysectomy on the stores of somatostatin in the hypothalamus and pituitary stem. Proc. Soc. exp. Biol. Med. 151, 599-602 (1976).

59. Wakabayashi, I., Demura, R., Kanda, M., Demura, H., Shizume, K.: Effect of hypophysectomy on hypothalamic somatostatin content in rats. Endocrinol. jap. 23, 439-442 (1976).

60. Fernandez-Durango, R., Arimura, A., Fishback, J., Schally, A.V.: Hypothalamic somatostatin and LH-RH after hypophysectomy in hyper- or hypothyroidism and during anesthesia in rats. Proc. Soc. exp. Biol. Med. 156, 265-271 (1977).

61. Fernandez-Durango, R., Arimura, A., Fishback, J., Schally, A.V.: Hypothalamic somatostatin and LH-RH after hypophysectomy, in hyper- or hypothyroidism and during anesthesia in rats. Proc. Soc. exp. Biol. Med. 157, 235-240 (1978).

62. Weeke, J., Hansen, A.P., Lundbaek, K.: The inhibition by somatostatin of the thyrotropin response to thyrotropin-releasing hormone in normal subjects. Scand. J. clin. Lab. Invest. 33, 101-103 (1974).

63. Siler, T.M., Yen, S.S.C., Vale, W., Guillemin, R.: Inhibition by somatostatin of the release of TSH induced in man by thyrotropin-releasing factor. J. clin. Endocrinol. Metab. 38, 742-745 (1974).

64. Carr, D., Gomez-Pan, A., Weightman, D.R., Roy, V.C.M., Hall, R., Besser, G.M., Thorner, M.O., McNeilly, A.S., Schally, A.V., Kastin, A.J., Coy, D.H.: Growth hormone release inhibiting hormone: Action on thyrotropin and prolactin secretion after thyrotrophin-releasing hormone. Brit. med. J. 3, 67-69 (1975).

65. Weeke, J., Hansen, A.P., Lundbaek, K.: Inhibition by somatostatin of basal levels of serum thyrotropin (TSH) in normal men. J. clin. Endocrinol. Metab. 41, 168-171 (1975).

66. Lucke, C., Höffken, B., von zur Mühlen, A.: The effect of somatostatin on TSH levels in patients with primary hypothyroidism. J. clin. Endocrinol. Metab. 41, 1082-1084 (1975).

67. Florsheim, W.H., Kozbur, X.: Physiological modulation of thyrotropin secretion by somatostatin and thyroliberin. Biochem. biophys. Res. Commun. 72, 603-609 (1976).

68. Tanjasiri, P., Kozbur, X., Florsheim, W.H.: Somatostatin in the physiologic feedback control of thyrotropin secretion. Life Sci. 19, 657-660 (1976).

69. Chihara, K., Arimura, A., Chihara, M., Schally, A.V.: Studies on the mechanism of growth hormone and thyrotropin responses to somatostatin antiserum in anesthetized rats. Endocrinology 103, 1916-1923 (1978).

70. Siler, T.M., Vandenberg, G., Yen, S.S.C.: Inhibition of growth hormone release in humans by somatostatin. J. clin. Endocrinol. Metab. 37, 632-634 (1973).

71. Gerich, J., Davis, J., Lorenzi, M., Rizza, R., Bohannon, N., Karam, J., Lewis, S., Kaplan, R., Schultz, T., Cryer, P.: Hormonal mechanisms of recovery from insulin-induced hypoglycemia in man. Am. J. Physiol. 236, 380-385 (1979).

72. Tyrrell, J.B., Lorenzi, M., Gerich, J.E., Forsham, P.H.: Inhibition by somatostatin of ACTH secretion in Nelson's syndrome. J. clin. Endocrinol. Metab. 40, 1125-1127 (1975).

73. Benker, G., Hackenberg, K., Hamburger, B., Reinwein, D.: Effects of growth hormone release inhibiting hormone and bromocryptine (CB-154) in states of abnormal pituitary-adrenal function. Clin. Endocr. 5, 187-190 (1976).

74. Fehm, H.L., Voigt, K.H., Lang, R., Beinert, K.E., Raptis, S., Pfeiffer, E.F.: Somatostatin: A potent inhibitor of ACTH-hypersecretion in adrenal insufficiency. Klin. Wschr. 54, 173-175 (1976).

75. Deftos, L.J., Lorenzi, M., Bohannon, N., Tsalakian, E., Schneider, V., Gerich, J.E.: Somatostatin does not suppress plasma parathyroid hormone. J. clin. Endocrinol. Metab. 43, 205-207 (1976).

76. Gordin, A., Lamberg, B.A., Pelkonen, R., Almquist, S.: Somatostatin inhibits the pentagastrin-induced release of serum calcitonin in medullary carcinoma of the thyroid. Clin. Endocr. 8, 289-293 (1978).

77. Metz, S.A., Deftos, L.J., Baylink, D.J., Robertson, R.P.: Neuroendocrine modulation of calcitonin and parathyroid hormone in man. J. clin. Endocrinol. Metab. 47, 151-159 (1978).

78. Ahrén, B., Hedner, P., Melander, A., Westgren, W.: Inhibition by somatostatin of mouse thyroid activity following stimulation by thyrotropin, isoprenaline and dibutyryl cyclic AMP. Acta Endocrinol. 86, 323-329 (1977).

79. Loos, U., Raptis, S., Birk, J., Escobar-Jimenez, F., Meyer, G., Voigt, K., Rothenbuchner, G., Pfeiffer, E.F.: Inhibition of TSH-mediated secretion of T_4 , T_3 , and reverse-T_3 in vivo and in isolated thyroid cells by somatostatin. Metabolism 27 (suppl. 1) 1269-1274 (1978).

80. Faber, J., Gormsen, J., Friis, Th., Kirkegaard, C., Lauridsen, U.B., Nerup, J., Rogowski, P., Siersbaek-Nielsen, K.: Lack of effect of somatostatin on TSH induced T_3 release and platelet function in normal man. Horm. Metab. Res. 9, 165-166 (1977).

81. Williams, G.A., Hargis, G.K., Ensinck,J.W., Kukreja, S.C., Bowser, E.N., Chertow, B.S., Henderson, W.J.: Role of endogenous somatostatin in the secretion of parathyroid hormone and calcitonin. Metabolism 28, 950-954 (1979).

82. Yamada, Y., Ito, S., Kayamori, R., Shibata, A.: The effects of vitamin D_2 on the somatostatin and calcitonin concentration in the rat thyroid. Horm. Metab. Res. 11, 184-185 (1979).

83. Molnar, J., Arimura, A., Kastin, A.J.: Presence of immunoreactive somatostatin in the salivary gland and saliva. Fed. Proc. 35, 782 (1976).

84. Forssman, W.G., Helmstaedter, V., Metz, J., Mühlmann, G., Feurle, G.E.: Immunohistochemistry and ultrastructure of somatostatin cells with special reference to the gastroenteropancreatic system. Metabolism 27 (suppl. 1) 1179-1192 (1978).

85. Falkmer, S., Elde, R.P., Hellerström, C., Petersson, B.: Phylogenetic aspects of somatostatin in the gastro-enteropancreatic endocrine system. Metabolism 27 (suppl. 1) 1193-1196 (1978).

86. Helmstaedter, V., Feurle, G.E., Forssman, W.G.: Relationship of glucagon-somatostatin and gastrin-somatostatin cells in the stomach of the monkey. Cell Tissue Res. 177, 29-46 (1977).

87. McIntosh, C., Arnold, R., Bothe, E., Becker, H., Kobberling, J., Creutzfeld, W.: Gastrointestinal somatostatin in man and dog. Metabolism 27 (suppl. 1) 1317-1320 (1978).

88. Uvnäs-Wallensten, K., Efendic, S., Luft, R.: Vagal release of somatostatin into the antral lumen of cats. Acta physiol. scand. 99, 126-128 (1977).

89. Uvnäs-Wallensten, K., Efendic, S., Luft, R.: Release of gastrointestinal hormones into the duodenal lumen of cats. Horm. Metab. Res. 10, 173 (1978).

90. Uvnäs-Wallenstein, K., Efendic, S., Luft, R.: The occurrence of somatostatin-like immunoreactivity in the vagal nerves. Acta physiol. scand. 102, 248-250 (1978).

91. Bloom, S.R., Mortimer, C.H., Thorner, M.O., Besser, G.M., Hall, R., Gomez-Pan, A., Roy, V.M., Russell,R.C.G., Coy, D.H., Kastin, A.J., Schally, A.V.: Inhibition of gastrin and gastric acid secretion by growth-hormone release-inhibiting hormone. Lancet 2, 1106-1109 (1974).

92. Schlegel, W., Raptis, S., Dollinger, H., Pfeiffer, E.F.: Inhibition of secretin, pancreozymin and gastrin release and their biological activities by somatostatin. In: "First International Symposium on Hormonal Receptors in Digestive Tract Physiology, INSERM Symposium No.3", Eds. Bonfils, S., Fromageat, P., Rosselin, G., Elsevier/North Holland Publishing Co.,New York, pp. 361-377 (1977).

93. Schrumpf, E., Vatn, M.H., Hanssen, K.F., Semb, L.S., Myren, J.: Somatostatin inhibits insulin-stimulated gastrin release and gastric secretion of acid, pepsin and intrinsic factor (IF) in duodenal ulcer patients. Scand. J. Gastroenterol. 11, 517-520 (1976).

94. Creutzfeldt, W., Arnold, R.: Somatostatin and the stomach: Exocrine and endocrine aspects. Metabolism 27 (suppl. 1) 1309-1316 (1978).

95. Konturek, S.J., Tasler, J., Cieszkowski, M., Coy, D.H., Schally, A.V.: Effect of growth hormone release-inhibiting hormone on gastric secretion, mucosal blood flow, and serum gastrin. Gastroenterology 70, 737-741 (1976).

96. Raptis, S., Schlegel, W., Lehmann, E., Dollinger, H.C., Zoupas, C.: Effects of somatostatin on the exocrine pancreas and the release of duodenal hormones. Metabolism 27 (suppl. 1) 1321-1328 (1978).

97. Schlegel, W., Harvey, R.F., Raptis, S., Oliver, J.M., Pfeiffer, E.F.: Inhibition of cholecystokinin-pancreozymin release by somatostatin. Lancet 2, 166-167 (1977).

98. Lennon, J.R., Sircus, W., Bloom, S.R., Mitchell, S.J., Polak, J.M., Besser, G.M., Hall, R., Coy, D.H., Kastin, A.J., Schally, A.V.: Investigation and treatment of a recurrent vipoma. Gut 16, 821-822 (1975).

99. Sakurai, H., Dobbs, R.E., Unger, R.H.: The effect of somatostatin on the response of GLI to intraduodenal administration of glucose, protein and fat. Diabetologia 11, 427-430 (1975).

100. Bloom, S.R., Ralphs, D.N., Besser, G.M., Hall, R., Coy, D.H., Kastin, A.J., Schally, A.V.: Effect of somatostatin on motilin levels and gastric emptying. Gut 16, 834 (1975).

101. Pederson, R.A., Dryburgh, J.R., Brown, J.C.: The effect of somatostatin on release and insulinotropic action of gastric inhibitory polypeptide. Can. J. Physiol. Pharmacol. 53, 1200-1205 (1975).

102. Boden, G., Sivitz, M.C., Owen, O.E., Essa-Koumar, N., Landor, J.: Somatostatin suppresses secretin and pancreatic exocrine secretion. Science 190, 163-165 (1975).

103. Hanssen, L.E., Hanssen, K.F., Myren, J.: Inhibition of secretin release and pancreatic bicarbonate secretion by somatostatin infusion in man. Scand. J. Gastroenterol. 12, 391-394 (1977).

104. Marco, J., Hedo, J.A., Villanueva, M.L.: Inhibitory effect of somatostatin on human pancreatic polypeptide secretion. Life Sci. 21, 789-792 (1977).

105. Kayasseh, L., Haecki, W.H., Gyr, K., Stalder, G.A., Rittman, W.W., Halter, F., Girard, J.: The endogenous release of pancreatic polypeptide by acid and meals in dogs: Effect of somatostatin. Scand. J. Gastroenterol. 13, 385-391 (1978).

106. Barros, D'Sa, A.A.J., Bloom, S.R., Baron, J.H.: Direct inhibition of gastric acid by growth-hormone release-inhibiting hormone in dogs. Lancet 1, 886-887 (1975).

107. Konturek, S.J., Radecki, T., Pucher, A., Coy, D.H., Schally, A.V.: Effect of somatostatin on gastrointestinal secretions and peptic ulcer production in cats. Scand. J. Gastroenterol. 12, 379-383 (1977).

108. Gomez-Pan, A., Reed, J.D., Albinus, M., Shaw, B., Hall, R., Besser, G.M., Coy, D.H., Kastin, A.J., Schally, A.V.: Direct inhibition of gastric acid and pepsin secretion by growth-hormone release-inhibiting hormone in cats. Lancet 1, 888-890 (1975).

109. Schrumpf, E., Vatn, M.H., Hanssen, K.F., Myren, J.: A small dose of somatostatin inhibits the pentagastrin stimulated gastric secretion of acid, pepsin and intrinsic factor in man. Clin. Endocr. 8, 391-395 (1978).

110. Dollinger, H., Raptis, S., Pfeiffer, E.F.: Effects of somatostatin on exocrine and endocrine pancreatic function stimulated by intestinal hormones in man. Horm. Metab. Res. 8, 74-78 (1976).

111. Wilson, R.M., Boden, G., Shore, L.S., Essa-Koumar, N.: Effect of somatostatin on meal-stimulated pancreatic exocrine secretions in dogs. Diabetes 26, 7-10 (1977).

112. Creutzfeldt, W., Lankisch, P.G., Fölsch, U.R.: Hemmung der sekretin und cholezystokinin-pancreozymin-induzierten saft- und enzymesekretion des pankreas und der gallenblasenkotraktion beim menschen durch somatostatin. Dt. med. Wschr. 100, 1135-1138 (1975).

113. Holm, I., Thulin, L., Samnegard, H., Efendic, S., Tydén, G.: Anticholeretic effect of somatostatin in anesthetized dogs. Acta physiol scand. 104, 241-243 (1978).

114. Tansy, M.F., Martin, J.S., Landin, W.E., Kendall, F.M.: The differential action of somatostatin on the motor effector system of the canine gastrointestinal tract. Metabolism 27 (suppl.1)1353-1358 (1978).

115. Thor, P., Krol, R., Konturek, S.J., Coy, D.H., Schally, A.V.: Effect of somatostatin on myoelectrical activity of small bowel. Am. J. Physiol. 235, 249-254 (1978).

116. Scholz, D., Schwille, P.O.: Somatostatin and intestinal calcium absorption in man. Metabolism 27 (suppl. 1) 1349-1352 (1978).

117. Krejs, G.J., Raskin, P., Fordtran, J.S.: Inhibition of jejunal sugar and amino acid absorption in man: A nonspecific effect of somatostatin. Clin. Res. 26, 420A (1978).

118. Carter, R.F., Bitar, K.N., Zfass, A.M., Makhlouf, G.M.: Inhibition of VIP-stimulated intestinal secretion and cyclic AMP production by somatostatin in the rat. Gastroenterology 74, 726-730 (1978).

119. Reid, I.A., Rose, J.C.: An intrarenal effect of somatostatin on water excretion. Endocrinology 100, 782-785 (1977).

120. Brautbar, N., Levine, B.S., Coburn, J.W., Kleeman, C.R.: Interaction of somatostatin with PTH and AVP: Renal effects. Am. J. Physiol. 237, 428-436 (1979).

121. Le Roith, D., Bark, H., Glick, S.M.: Somatostatin and antidiuretic hormone secretion in dogs. Horm. Metab. Res. 11, 177-178 (1979).

122. Strandhoy, J.W., Zook, T.E.: Antagonism of vasopressin-induced water flow by somatostatin. Res. Commun. Chem. Pathol. Pharmacol. 24, 599-602 (1979).

123. Gomez-Pan, A., Snow, M.H., Piercy, D.A., Robson, V., Wilkinson, R., Hall, R., Evered, D.C., Besser, G.M., Schally, A.V., Kastin, A.J., Coy, D.H.: Actions of growth hormone-release inhibiting hormone on the renin angiotensin system. J. clin. Endocrinol. Metab. 43, 240-243 (1976).

124. Rosenthal, J., Escobar-Jimenez, F., Raptis, S., Pfeiffer, E.F.: Inhibition of frusemide-induced hyperreninaemia by growth-hormone release-inhibiting hormone in man. Lancet 1, 772-774 (1976).

125. Rosenthal, J., Escobar-Jimenez, F., Raptis, S.: Prevention by somatostatin of rise in blood pressure and plasma renin mediated by beta-receptor stimulation. Clin. Endocr. 6, 455-462 (1977).

126. Rosenthal, J., Raptis, S., Zoupas, C., Escobar-Jimenez, F.: Hemodynamic and renin responses to somatostatin in essential hypertension. Metabolism 27, (suppl. 1) 1361-1364 (1978).

127. Zierden, E., Hengst, K., Wagner, H.: Leukocyte response to somatostatin in normals and patients with bacterial leukocytosis. Klin. Wschr. 55, 503-505 (1977).

128. Mielke, C.H., Gerich, J.E., Lorenzi, M., Tsalikian, E., Rodvien, R., Forsham, P.H.: The effect of somatostatin on coagulation and platelet function in man. New Engl. J. Med. 293, 480-483 (1975).

129. Rasche, H., Raptis, S., Scheck, R., Pfeiffer, E.F.: Coagulation studies and platelet function after somatostatin. Klin. Wschr. 54, 977-982 (1976).

130. Bensoussan, D., Levy-Toledano, S.L., Passa, Ph., Caen, J., Canivet, J.: Effect of somatostatin on platelet aggregation and plasma factor. VIII. Level in normal man. Diabète et Métabolisme 3, 223-227 (1977).

131. Koerker, D.J., Harker, L., Goodner, C.J.: Effects of somatostatin on hemostasis in baboons. New Engl. J. Med. 293, 476-479 (1975).

132. Zierden, E., Hengst, K., Wagner, H.: Influence of somatostatin on peripheral leukocyte count and granulation tissue in man and rats. Horm. Metab. Res. 9, 378-384 (1977).

133. Chiang, T.M., Duckworth,W.C., Beachey, E.H., Kang, A.H.: The effect of somatostatin on platelet aggregation. Endocrinology 97, 753-756 (1975).

134. Besser, G.M., Paxton, A.M., Johnson, S.A., Moody, E., Mortimer, C.H., Hall, R., Gomez-Pan, A., Schally, A.V., Kastin, A.J., Coy, D.H.: Impairment of platelet function by growth-hormone release-inhibiting hormone. Lancet 1, 1166-1169 (1975).

135. Mielke, C.H., Rodvien, R.: Somatostatin: Influence on hemostasis. A review. Metabolism 27 (suppl. 1) 1369-1375 (1978).

136. Scheck, R., Raptis, S., Rasche, H., Escobar-Jimenez, F.: The effect of somatostatin on platelets in vivo and in vitro studies. Diabète et Métabolisme 3, 219-222 (1977).

137. Guillemin, R., Gerich, J.E.: Somatostatin: Physiological and clinical significance. Ann. Rev. Med. 27, 379-388 (1976).

138. Giustina, G., Peracchi, M., Reschini, E., Panerai, A.E., Pinto, M.: Dose-response study of the inhibiting effect of somatostatin on growth hormone and insulin secretion in normal subjects and acromegalic patients. Metabolism 24, 807-815 (1975).

139. Gerich, J.E., Lovinger, R., Grodsky, G.M.: Inhibition by somatostatin of glucagon and insulin release from the perfused rat pancreas in response to arginine, isoproterenol and theophylline: Evidence for a preferential effect on glucagon secretion. Endocrinology 96, 749-754 (1975).

140. Bhathena, S.J., Perrino, P.V., Voyles, N.R., Smith, S.S., Wilkins, S.D., Coy, D.H., Schally, A.V., Recant, L.: Reversal of somatostatin inhibition of insulin and glucagon secretion. Diabetes 25, 1031-1040 (1976).

141. Johnson, D.G., Ensinck, J.W., Koerker, D., Palmer, J., Goodner, C.J.: Inhibition of glucagon and insulin secretion by somatostatin in the rat pancreas perfused in situ. Endocrinology 96, 370-374 (1975).

142. Lorenzi, M., Karam, J.H., Schmitt, J.K., Burns, A., Forsham, P.H.: Hormonal, metabolic and gastrointestinal effects of low- and high-dose somatostatin in man. Diabetes 27, (suppl. 2) 442 (1978).

143. Raptis, S., Escobar-Jimenez, F., Rosenthal, J., Ditschuneit, H., Pfeiffer, E.F.: Somatostatin modulation of pancreatic glucagon, insulin, glucose and free fatty acids following beta-adrenergic stimulation. J. clin. Endocrinol. Metab. 44, 1088-1093 (1977).

144. Efendic, S., Luft, R., Grill, V.: Effect of somatostatin on glucose induced insulin release in isolated perfused rat pancreas and isolated rat pancreatic islets. FEBS Lett. 42, 169-172 (1974).

145. Turcot-Lemay, L., Lemay, A., Lacy, P.E.: Somatostatin inhibition of insulin release from freshly isolated and organ cultured rat islets of Langerhans in vitro. Biochem. biophys. Res. Commun. 63, 1130-1138 (1975).

146. Curry, D.L., Bennett, L.L.: Does somatostatin inhibition of insulin secretion involve two mechanisms of action ? Proc. natn. Acad. Sci. U.S.A. 73, 248-251 (1976).

147. Curry, D.L., Bennett, L.L., Li, C.H.: Direct inhibition of insulin secretion by synthetic somatostatin. Biochem biophys. Res. Commun. 58, 885-889 (1974).

148. Fujimoto, W.Y.: Somatostatin inhibition of glucose-, tolbutamide-, theophylline, cytochalasin B-, and calcium-stimulated insulin release in monolayer cultures of rat endocrine pancreas. Endocrinology 97, 1494-1500 (1975).

149. Leblanc, H., Yen, S.S.C.: Comparison of cyclic and linear forms of somatostatin in the inhibition of growth hormone, insulin and glucagon secretion. J. clin. Endocrinol. Metab. 40, 906-908 (1975).

150. Leblanc, H., Anderson, J.R., Sigel, M.B., Yen, S.S.C.: Inhibitory action of somatostatin on pancreatic α and β cell function. J. clin. Endocrinol. Metab. 40, 568-572 (1975).

151. Alberti, K.G.M.M., Christensen, S.E., Iversen, J., Seyer-Hansen, K., Christensen, N.J., Hansen, A.P., Lundbaek, K., Orskov, H.: Inhibition of insulin secretion by somatostatin. Lancet 2, 1299-1301 (1973).

152. Koerker, D.J., Ruch, W., Chideckel, B., Palmer, J., Goodner, C.J., Ensinck, H., Gale, C.C.: Somatostatin: Hypothalamic inhibitor of the endocrine pancreas. Science 184, 482-484 (1974).

153. Chideckel, E.W., Palmer, J., Koerker, D.J., Ensinck, J., Davidson, M.B., Goodner, C.J.: Somatostatin blockade of acute and chronic stimuli of the endocrine pancreas and the consequences of this blockade on glucose homeostasis. J. clin. Invest. 55, 754-762 (1975).

154. Gerich, J.E., Lorenzi, M., Schneider, V., Forsham, P.H.: Effect of somatostatin on plasma glucose and insulin responses to glucagon and tolbutamide in man. J. clin. Endocrinol. Metab. 39, 1057-1060 (1974).

155. Shapiro, S., Sumiya, E., Fleischer, N., Baum, S.G.: Regulation of in vitro insulin release from a transplantable Syrian hamster insulinoma. Endocrinology 97, 442-447 (1975).

156. Efendic, S., Luft, R., Claro, A.: Studies on the mechanism of somatostatin action on insulin release in man. II. Comparison of the effects of somatostatin on insulin release induced by glucose, glucagon, and tolbutamide. Acta Endocrinol. 81, 743-752 (1976).

157. Mortimer, C.H., Carr, D., Lind, T., Bloom, S.R., Mallinson, C., Schally, A.V., Tunbridge, W., Yeomans, L., Coy, D.H., Kastin, A.J., Besser, G.M., Hall, R.: Effects of growth-hormone release-inhibiting hormone on circulating glucagon, insulin, and growth hormone in normal, diabetic, acromegalic and hypopituitary patients. Lancet 1, 697-701 (1974).

158. Efendic, S., Claro, A., Luft, R.: Studies on the mechanism of somatostatin action on insulin release. III. Effect of somatostatin on arginine induced release of insulin and glucagon in man and perfused rat pancreas. Acta Endocrinol. 81, 753-761 (1976).

159. Iversen, J.: Inhibition of pancreatic glucagon release by somatostatin: In vitro. Scand. J. clin. Lab. Invest. 33, 125-129 (1974).

160. Wollheim, C.B., Blondel, B., Renold, A.E., Sharp, G.W.G.: Somatostatin inhibition of pancreatic glucagon release from monolayer cultures and interactions with calcium. Endocrinology 101, 911-919 (1977).

161. Weir, G.C., Knowlton, S.D., Martin, D.B.: Somatostatin inhibition of epinephrine-induced glucagon secretion. Endocrinology 95, 1744-1746 (1974).

162. Chideckel, E.W., Goodner, C.J., Koerker, D.J., Johnson, D., Ensinck, J.: Role of glucagon in mediating metabolic effects of epinephrine. Am. J. Physiol. 232, 464-470 (1977).

163. Gerich, J.E., Lorenzi, M., Tsalikian, E., Karam, J.H.: Studies on the mechanism of epinephrine-induced hyperglycemia in man: Evidence for participation of pancreatic glucagon secretion. Diabetes 25, 65-71 (1976).

164. Gerich, J.E., Lorenzi, M., Karam, J.H., Schneider, V., Forsham, P.H.: Abnormal pancreatic glucagon secretion and postprandial hyperglycemia in diabetes mellitus. JAMA 234, 159-165 (1975).

165. Ward, F.R., Leblanc, H., Yen, S.S.C.: The inhibitory effect of somatostatin on growth hormone, insulin and glucagon secretion in diabetes mellitus. J. clin. Endocrinol. Metab. 41, 527-532 (1975).

166. Christensen, S.E., Hansen, A.P., Lundbaek, K.: Somatostatin in maturity-onset diabetes. Diabetes 27, 1013-1019 (1978).

167. Griffey, M.A., Conway, H.H., Harshfield, D.L., Whitney, J.: Effect of somatostatin on insulin secretion induced by Ionophore A23187. Proc. Soc. exp. Biol. Med. 154, 198-200 (1977).

168. Taminato, T., Seino, Y., Goto, Y., Imura, H.: Interaction of somatostatin and calcium in regulating insulin release from isolated pancreatic islets of rats. Biochem. biophys. Res. Commun. 66, 928-934 (1975).

169. Barden, N., Lavoie, M., Dupont, A., Cote, J., Cote, J-P.: Stimulation of glucagon release by addition of anti-somatostatin serum to islets of Langerhans in vitro. Endocrinology 101, 635-638 (1977).

170. Itoh, M., Mandarino, L., Gerich, J.E.: Antisomatostatin γ-globulin augments secretion of both insulin and glucagon in vitro: Evidence for a physiologic role for endogenous somatostatin in the regulation of pancreatic A and B cell function. Diabetes 29 (1980) (in press).

171. Taniguchi, H., Utsumi, M., Hasegawa, M., Kobayashi, T., Watanabe, Y., Murakami, K., Seki, M., Tsutou, A., Makimura, H., Sakoda, N., Baba, S.: Physiologic role of somatostatin: Insulin release from rat islets treated by somatostatin antiserum. Diabetes 26, 700-702 (1977).

172. Schusdziarra, V., Rouiller, D., Arimura, A., Unger, R.H.: Anti-somatostatin serum increases levels of hormones from the pituitary and gut but not from the pancreas. Endocrinology 103, 1956-1959 (1978).

173. Olsson, S.E., Andersson, A., Petersson, B., Hellerström, C.: Effects of somatostatin on the biosynthesis and release of insulin from isolated pancreatic islets. Diabète et Métabolisme 2, 199-202 (1976).

174. Lin, B.J.: Effects of somatostatin on insulin biosynthesis, glucose oxidation and cyclic guanosine monophosphate level. Metabolism 27, (suppl. 1) 1295-1298 (1978).

175. Schonbrunn, A., Tashjian, H.: Characterization of functional receptors for somatostatin in rat pituitary cells in culture. J. biol. Chem. 253, 6473-6483 (1978).

176. Rifkin, R.M., Leitner, J.W., Maman, A., Sussman, K.E.: Localization of somatostatin binding in somatostatin-responsive tissues. Clin. Res. 27, 87A (1979).

177. Rizza, R., Gerich, J.: Somatostatin receptors in pancreatic islet plasma membrane. (Unpublished observations).

178. Pace. C.S., Murphy, M., Conant, S., Lacy, P.E.: Somatostatin inhibition of glucose-induced electrical activity in cultured rat islet cells. Am. J. Physiol. 233, C165-171 (1977).

179. Ogawa, N., Thompson, T., Friesen, H.G., Martin, J.B., Brazeau, P.: Properties of soluble somatostatin-binding protein. Biochem. J. 165, 269-277 (1977).

180. Sussman, K.E., Leitner, J.W., Rifkin, R.M.: Somatostatin: Selective inhibition of cyclic AMP stimulated protein kinase activity in isolated pancreatic islet and pituitary secretory vesicles. Clin. Res. 26, 563A (1978).

181. Curry, D.L., Bennett, L.L.: Reversal of somatostatin inhibition of insulin secretion by calcium. Biochem. biophys. Res. Commun. 60, 1015-1019 (1974).

182. Basabe, J.C., Cresto, J.C., Aparicio, N.: Studies on the mode of action of somatostatin on insulin secretion. Endocrinology 101, 1436-1443 (1977).

183. Fujimoto, W.Y., Ensinck, J.W.: Somatostatin inhibition of insulin and glucagon secretion in rat islet culture. Endocrinology 98, 259-262 (1976).

184. Oliver, J.R.: Inhibition of calcium uptake by somatostatin in isolated rat islets of Langerhans. Endocrinology 99, 910-913 (1976).

185. Schofield, J.G., Bicknell, R.J.: Effect of somatostatin and verapamil on growth hormone release and ^{45}Ca fluxes. Molec. Cell Endocrinol. 9, 255-268 (1978).

186. Shapiro, S., Kaneko, Y., Baum, S.G., Fleischer, N.: The role of calcium in insulin release from hamster insulinoma cells. Endocrinology 101, 485-493 (1977).

187. Wollheim, C.B., Kikuchi, M., Renold, A.E., Sharp, G.W.G.: Somatostatin- and epinephrine-induced modification of $^{45}Ca^{++}$ fluxes and insulin release in rat pancreatic islets maintained in tissue culture. J. clin. Invest. 60, 1165-1173 (1977).

188. Bicknell, R.J., Schofield, J.G.: Mechanism of action of somatostatin: Inhibition of ionophore A23187-induced release of growth hormone from dispersed bovine pituitary cells. FEBS Lett. 68, 23-26 (1976).

189. Mandarino, L., Itoh, M., Blanchard, W., Patton, G., Gerich, J.: Stimulation of insulin release in the absence of extracellular calcium by isobutylmethylxanthine and its inhibition by somatostatin. Endocrinology 106 (1980) (in press).

190. Borgeat, P., Labrie, F., Drouin, J., Belanger, A., Immer, H., Sestanj, K., Ivelson, V., Gotz, M., Schally, A., Coy, D., Coy, E.: Inhibition of adenosine 3',5' monophosphate accumulation in anterior pituitary gland in vitro by growth hormone release inhibiting hormone. Biochem. biophys. Res. Commun. 56, 1052-1059 (1974).

191. Kaneko, T., Oka, H., Munemura, M., Suzuki, S., Yasuda, H., Oda, T., Yanaihara, N.: Stimulation of Guanosine 3',5' cyclic monophosphate accumulation in rat anterior pituitary gland in vitro by synthetic somatostatin. Biochem. biophys. Res. Commun. 61, 53-57 (1974).

192. Efendic, S., Grill, V., Luft, R.: Inhibition by somatostatin of glucose induced 3',5'-monophosphate (cyclic AMP) accumulation and insulin release in isolated pancreatic islets of the rat. FEBS Lett. 55, 131-133 (1975).

193. Oliver, J.R., Wagle, S.R.: Studies on the inhibition of insulin release, glycogenolysis, and gluconeogenesis by somatostatin in the rat islets of Langerhans and isolated hepatocytes. Biochem. biophys. Res. Commun. 62, 772-777 (1975).

194. Oliver, J.R., Wright, P.H., Ashmore, J.: The effect of somatostatin on glucose stimulated adenosine 3',5'-monophosphate accumulation and glucose oxidation by isolated rat islets of Langerhans. Proc. Soc. exp. Biol. Med. 158, 458-461 (1978).

195. Bicknell, R.J., Young, P.W., Schofield, J.G.: Mechanism of action of somatostatin: Growth hormone release ^{45}Ca ion efflux and cyclic nucleotide metabolism of bovine anterior pituitary slices in the presence of prostaglandin E_2 and 1-methyl-3-isobutylxanthine. Biochem. Soc. Trans. 5, 219-222 (1977).

196. Claro, A., Grill, V., Efendic, S., Luft, R.: Studies on the mechanisms of somatostatin action on insulin release. IV. Effect of somatostatin on cyclic AMP levels and phosphodiesterase activity in isolated rat pancreatic islets. Acta Endocrinol. 85, 379-388 (1977).

197. Kemmler, W., Löffler, G.: NaK-ATPase in rat pancreatic islets. Diabetologia 13, 235-238 (1977).

198. Schusdziarra, V., Harris, V., Unger, R.H.: Half-life of somatostatin-like immunoreactivity in canine plasma. Endocrinology 104, 109-110 (1979).

199. Sheppard, M., Shapiro, B., Pimstone, B., Kronheim, S., Berelowitz, M., Gregory, M.: Metabolic clearance and plasma half disappearance time of exogenous somatostatin in man. J. clin. Endocrinol. Metab. 48, 50-53 (1979).

200. Ensinck, J., Laschansky, E., Chideckel, E., Palmer, J., Goodner, C.: Somatostatin kinetics during infusion in the baboon. Clin. Res. 24, 155A (1976).

201. Shapiro, B., Sheppard, M., Kronheim, S., Pimstone, B.: Transrenal gradient of serum somatostatin-like immunoreactivity in the rat. Horm. Metab. Res. 10, 356 (1978).

202. Marks, N., Stern, F.: Inactivation of somatostatin (GH-RIH) and its analogs by crude and partially purified rat brain extracts. FEBS Lett. 55, 220-224 (1975).

203. Griffiths, E.C., Jeffcoate, S.L., Holland, D.T.: Inactivation of somatostatin by peptidases in different areas of the rat brain. Acta Endocrinol. 85, 1-10 (1977).

204. Marks, N., Stern, F., Benuck, M.: Correlation between biological potency and biodegradation of a somatostatin analogue. Nature 261, 511-512 (1976).

205. Patton, G., Rizza, R., Gerich, J.: Degradation of synthetic somatostatin by isolated guinea pig pancreatic acinar cells and by the perfused rat pancreas. (Unpublished observations).

206. Benuck, M., Marks, N.: Differences in the degradation of hypothalamic releasing factors by rat and human serum. Life Sci. 19, 1271-1276 (1976).

207. Dupont, A., Mérand, Y., Barden, N.: Effect of propylthiouracil and thyroxine on the inactivation of somatostatin by rat hypothalamus. Life Sci. 23, 2007-2012 (1978).

208. Berelowitz, M., Pimstone, B., Shapiro, B., Kronheim, S., De Wit, D.: Tissue growth hormone release inhibiting hormone-like immunoreactivity in experimental hypothyroidism and hypopituitarism. Clin. Endocr. 9, 185-191 (1978).

209. Barden, N., Alvarado-Urbina, G., Cote, J.P., DuPont, A.: Cyclic AMP-dependent stimulation of somatostatin secretion by isolated rat islets of Langerhans. Biochem. biophys. Res. Commun. 71, 840-844 (1976).

210. Schauder, P., McIntosh, C., Arends, G., Arnold, R., Ferichs, H., Creutzfeldt, W.: Somatostatin and insulin release from isolated rat pancreatic islets stimulated by glucose. FEBS Lett. 68, 225-227 (1976).

211. Patton, G.S., Ipp, E., Dobbs, R.E., Orci, L., Vale, W., Unger, R.H.: Response of pancreatic immunoreactive somatostatin to arginine. Life Sci. 19, 1957-1960 (1976).

212. Patton, G.S., Ipp, E., Dobbs, R.E., Orci, L., Vale, W., Unger, R.H.: Pancreatic immunoreactive somatostatin release. Proc. natn. Acad. Sci. U.S.A. 74, 2140-2143 (1977).

213. Ipp, E., Dobbs, R.E., Arimura, A., Vale, W., Harris, V., Unger, R.H.: Release of immunoreactive somatostatin from the pancreas in response to glucose, amino acids, pancreozymin-cholecystokinin and tolbutamide. J. clin. Invest. 60, 760-765 (1977).

214. Schauder, P., McIntosh, C., Arends, J., Arnold, R., Frerichs, H., Creutzfeldt, W.: Somatostatin and insulin release from isolated rat pancreatic islets in response to D-glucose, L-leucine, and α-ketoisocaproic acid or D-glyceraldehyde: Evidence for a regulatory role of adenosine-3',5'-cyclic monophosphate. Biochem. biophys. Res. Commun. 75, 630-635 (1977).

215. Ipp, E., Dobbs, R.E., Harris, V., Arimura, A., Vale, W., Unger, R.H.: The effects of gastrin, gastric inhibitory polypeptide, secretin, and the octapeptide of cholecystokinin upon immunoreactive somatostatin release by the perfused canine pancreas. J. clin. Invest. 60, 1216-1219 (1977).

216. Efendic, S., Nylén, A., Roovete, A., Uvnäs-Wallensten, K.: Effects of glucose and arginine on the release of immunoreactive somatostatin from the isolated perfused rat pancreas. FEBS Lett. 92, 33-35 (1978).

217. Ipp, E., Dobbs, R.E., Unger, R.H.: Vasoreactive intestinal peptide stimulates pancreatic somatostatin release. FEBS Lett. 90, 76-78 (1978).

218. Ipp, E., Dobbs, R.E., Unger, R.H.: Morphine and β-endorphin influence on the secretion of the endocrine pancreas. Nature 276, 190-191 (1978).

219. Barden, N., Cote, J.P., Lavoie, M., DuPont, A.: Secretion of somatostatin by rat islets of Langerhans and gastric mucosa and a role for pancreatic somatostatin in the regulation of glucagon release. Metabolism 27, (suppl. 1) 1215-1218 (1978).

220. Gerich, J., Greene, K., Hara, M., Rizza, R., Patton, G.: Radioimmunoassay of somatostatin and its application in the study of pancreatic somatostatin secretion in vitro. J. Lab. clin. Med. 93, 1009-1018 (1979).

221. Hara, M., Patton, G., Gerich, J.: Increased somatostatin release from pancreases of alloxan diabetic rats perfused in vitro. Life. Sci. 24, 625-628 (1979).

222. Weir, G.C., Samols, E., Loo, S., Patel, Y.C., Gabbay, K.H.: Somatostatin and pancreatic polypeptide secretion: Effects of glucagon, insulin and arginine. Diabetes 28, 35-40 (1979).

223. Schauder, P., McIntosh, C., Arends, J., Frerichs, H.: Effect of fasting on the release of insulin and somatostatin from perfused islets of Langerhans. Diabetes 28, 204-207 (1979).

224. Samols, E., Weir, G.C.: Adrenergic modulation of pancreatic A, B and D cells: α-Adrenergic suppression of β-adrenergic stimulation of somatostatin secretion, α-adrenergic stimulation of glucagon secretion in the perfused dog pancreas. J. clin. Invest. 63, 230-238 (1979).

225. Ipp, E., Rivier, J., Dobbs, R.E., Brown, M., Vale, W., Unger, R.H.: Somatostatin analogs inhibit somatostatin release. Endocrinology 104, 1270-1273 (1979).

226. Petersson, B., Lundqvist, G., Anderson, A.: Somatostatin content and release of isolated pancreatic islets from obese-hyperglycemic mice. Experientia 35, 127-128 (1979).

227. Patel, Y.C., Amherdet, M., Orci, L.: Somatostatin secretion from monolayer cultures of neonatal rat pancreas. Endocrinology 104, 676-679 (1979).

228. Honey, R.N., Weir, G.C.: Insulin stimulates somatostatin and inhibits glucagon secretion from the perfused chicken pancreas-duodenum. Life Sci. 24, 1747-1750 (1979).

229. Barden, N., Dube, D., Cote, J.P., Leclerc, R., Pelletier, G.: Immunohistochemical characterization of monolayer cell cultures of embryonic chicken pancreas and measurement of somatostatin release. J. Histochem. Cytochem. 27, 939-941 (1979).

230. Dolais-Kitabgi, J., Kitabgi, P., Brazeau, P., Freychet, P.: Effect of neurotensin on insulin, glucagon and somatostatin release from isolated pancreatic islets. Endocrinology 105, 256-260 (1979).

231. Goto, Y., Seino, Y., Taminato, T., Kadowaki, S., Chiba, T., Note, S., Imura, H.: Theophylline: Potentiation of arginine-induced somatostatin release from the isolated rat pancreas. Diabetes 28, 457-459 (1979).

232. Hermansen, K., Christensen, S.E., Orskov, H.: Characterization of somatostatin release from the pancreas: The role of calcium and acetylcholine. Diabetologia 16, 261-266 (1979).

233. Mandarino, L., Itoh, M., Blanchard, W., Gerich, J.: Effect of calcium, magnesium and potassium on pancreatic D cell function in vitro. Diabetes (in press).

234. Itoh, M., Mandarino, L., Gerich, J.: Characterization of cholinergic, adrenergic, and dopaminergic regulation of pancreatic somatostatin secretion. Clin. Res. (in press).

235. Uvnäs-Wallensten, K., Lundberg, J., Efendic, S.: Dopaminergic control of antral gastrin and somatostatin release. Acta physiol. scand. 103, 343-345 (1978).

236. Kadowaki, S., Taminato, T., Chiba, T., Mori, K., Abe, H., Goto, Y., Seino, Y., Matsukura, S., Nozawa, M., Fujita, T.: Somatostatin release from isolated perfused rat pancreas: Possible role of endogenous somatostatin on insulin release. Diabetes 28, 600-603 (1979).

237. Berelowitz, M., Kronheim, S., Pimstone, B., Shapiro, B.: Somatostatin-like immunoreactivity in rat blood: Characterization, regional differences and responses to oral and intravenous glucose. J. clin. Invest. 61, 1410-1414 (1978).

238. Harris, V., Conlon, J.M., Srikant, C.B., McCorkle, K., Schusdziarra, V., Ippe, E., Unger, R.H.: Measurements of somatostatin-like immunoreactivity in plasma. Clinica chim. Acta. 87, 275-283 (1978).

239. Abe, H., Kato, Y., Chiba, T., Taminato, T., Fujita, T.: Plasma immunoreactive somatostatin levels in rat hypophysial portal blood: Effects of glucagon administration. Life Sci. 23, 1647-1654 (1978).

240. Kronheim, S., Berelowitz, M., Pimstone, B.L.: The characterization of somatostatin-like immunoreactivity in human serum. Diabetes 27, 523-529 (1978).

241. Conlon, J.M., Srikant, C.B., Ipp, E., Schusdziarra, V., Vale, W., Unger, R.H.: Properties of endogenous somatostatin-like immunoreactivity and synthetic somatostatin in dog plasma. J. clin. Invest. 62, 1187-1193 (1978).

242. Patel, Y.: Measurement and characterization of somatostatin-like immunoreactivity in extracted portal and peripheral plasma of normal and diabetic rats. Program 61st Annual Meeting of the Endocrine Society, Anaheim, California, p. 143 (1979).

243. Utsumi, M., Makimura, H., Ishihara, K., Morita, S., Baba, S.: Determination of immunoreactive somatostatin in rat plasma and responses to arginine, glucose and glucagon infusion. Diabetologia 17, 319-323 (1979).

244. Arimura, A., Sato, H., Coy, D.H., Schally, A.V.: Radioimmunoassay for GH-release inhibiting hormone. Proc. Soc. exp. Biol. Med. 148, 784-789 (1975).

245. Kronheim, S., Sheppard, M.C., Shapiro, B., Pimstone, B.L.: Ultracentrifugation evidence for a somatostatin-binding protein in serum. Biochim. biophys. Acta 586, 568-573 (1979).

246. Penman, E., Wass, J.A.H., Lund, A., Lowry, P.J., Stewart, J., Dawson, A.M., Besser, G.M., Rees, L.H.: Development and validation of a specific radioimmunoassay for somatostatin in human plasma. Ann. Clin. Biochem. 16, 15-25 (1979).

247. Arimura, A., Lundqvist, G., Rothman, J., Chang, R., Fernandez-Durango, R., Elde, R., Coy, D.H., Meyers, C., Schally, A.V.: Radioimmunoassay of somatostatin. Metabolism 27 (suppl. 1) 1139-1144 (1978).

248. Kazumi, T., Utsumi, M., Yoshino, G., Ishihara, K., Hirose, Y., Makimura, H., Baba, S.: Somatostatin concentration responds to arginine in portal plasma: Effects of fasting, streptozotocin diabetes and insulin administration in diabetic rats. Diabetes 29, 71-73 (1978).

249. Schusdziarra, V., Harris, V., Conlon, J.M., Arimura, A., Unger, R.: Pancreatic and gastric somatostatin release in response to intragastric and intraduodenal nutrients and HCl in the dog. J. clin. Invest. 62, 509-518 (1978).

250. Schusdziarra, V., Rouiller, D., Harris, V., Unger, R.H.: Release of gastric somatostatin-like immunoreactivity during acidification of the duodenal bulb. Gastroenterology 76, 950-953 (1979).

251. Schusdziarra, V., Rouiller, D., Harris, V., Unger, R.H.: Plasma somatostatin-like immunoreactivity in depancreatized dogs. Endocrinology 105, 595-599 (1979).

252. Schusdziarra, V., Harris, V., Unger, R.: Response of plasma somatostatin-like immunoreactivity to the administration of alloxan in dogs. Horm. Metab. Res. 11, 457-459 (1979).

253. Schusdziarra, V., Rouiller, D., Harris, V., Conlon, J.M., Unger, R.H.: The response of plasma somatostatin-like immunoreactivity to nutrients in normal and alloxan diabetic dogs. Endocrinology 103, 2264-2273 (1978).

254. Schusdziarra, V., Rouiller, D., Pietri, A., Harris, V., Zyznar, E., Conlon, J.M., Unger, R.H.: Pancreatic and gastric release of somatostatin-like immunoreactivity during the intestinal phase of a meal. Am. J. Physiol. 237, 555-560 (1979).

255. Schusdziarra, V., Dobbs, R.E., Harris, B., Unger, R.H.: Immunoreactive somatostatin levels in plasma of normal and alloxan diabetic dogs. FEBS Lett. 81, 69-72 (1977).

256. Schusdziarra, V., Harris, V., Unger, R.H.: Half-life of somatostatin-like immunoreactivity in canine plasma. Endocrinology 104, 109-110 (1979).

257. Schusdziarra, V., Rouiller, D., Harris, V., Unger, R.H.: Gastric and pancreatic release of somatostatin-like immunoreactivity during the gastric phase of a meal: Effect of truncal vagotomy and atropine in anesthetized dog. Diabetes 28, 658-663 (1979).

258. Lundqvist, G., Gustavsson, S., Hällgren, R.: Plasma levels of somatostatin-like immunoreactivity-independence of kidney function. Clin. Endocr. 10, 489-492 (1979).

259. Chihara, K., Arimura, A., Schally, A.V.: Immunoreactive somatostatin in rat hypophyseal portal blood: Effects of anesthetics. Endocrinology 104, 1434-1441 (1979).

260. Arimura, A., Meyers, C.A., Case, W.L., Murphy, W.A., Schally, A.V.: Suppression of somatostatin levels in the hepatic portal and systemic plasma of the rat by synthetic human pancreatic polypeptide. Biochem. biophys. Res. Commun. 89, 913-918 (1979).

261. Creutzfeldt, W.: Zur deutung des silberzellbildes und anderer pankreasbefund beim diabetes mellitus und inseladonom. Beitr. Pathol. Anat. 113, 133-168 (1953).

262. Gepts, W.: Die histopathologischen veranderungen des Langerhansschen inseln und ihrer bedeutung in der frage der pathogenese des menschlichen diabetes. Endokrinologie 36, 185-211 (1958).

263. Ferner, H.: Beitrage zur histologic der Langerhansschen inseln des menschen mit besonderer berucksichtung der silberzellen und ihrer beziehung zum pankreasdiabetes. Virchows Arch. Pathol. Anat. 309, 87-136 (1942).

264. Fujita, T.: D-zellern der pankreasinseln beim diabetes mellitus mit besonderer berucksichtung ihrer argyrophibe. Z. Zellforsch. mikrosk. Anat. 69, 363-370 (1976).

265. Koyayaski, K., Takahashi, Y., Yoshita, T.: Influences of alloxan administration and hypophysectomy on the pancreatic islets of the rat. Arch. Histol. Japon 25, 199-216 (1964).

266. Matsushima, Y., Makino, H., Kanatsuka, A., Yamamoto, M., Kumagai, A.: Immunohistochemical changes of somatostatin cells in the pancreatic islets of rats after streptozotocin administration. Endocrinol. jap. 25, 111-115 (1978).

267. Orci, L., Baetens, D., Rufener, C., Amherdt, M., Ravazzola, M., Studer, P., Malaisse-Lagae, F., Unger, R.H.: Hypertrophy and hyperplasia of somatostatin-containing D cells in diabetes. Proc. natn. Acad. Sci. U.S.A. 73, 1338-1342 (1976).

268. Patel, Y.C., Cameron, D.P., Bankier, A., Malaisse-Lagae, F., Ravazzola, M., Studer, P., Orci, L.: Changes in somatostatin concentration in pancreas and other tissues of streptozotocin diabetic rats. Endocrinology 103, 917-924 (1978).

269. Makino, H., Matsushima, Y., Kanatsuka, A., Yamamoto, M., Kumagai, A., Nishimura, M.: Changes in pancreatic somatostatin content in spontaneously diabetic mice, as determined by radioimmunoassay and immunohistochemical methods. Endocrinology 104, 243-247 (1979).

270. Berelowitz, M., Shapiro, B., Pimstone, B., Kronheim, S.: Growth hormone release inhibitory hormone-like immunoreactivity in pancreas and gut in streptozotocin diabetes in the rat and response to insulin administration. Clin. Endocr. 10, 195-198 (1979).

271. Stefan, Y., Malaisse-Lagae, F., Yoon, J.W., Notkins, A.L., Orci, L.: Virus-induced diabetes in mice: A quantitative evaluation of islet cell population by immunofluorescence technique. Diabetologia 15, 394-401 (1978).

272. Petersson, B., Elde, R., Efendic, S., Hökfelt, T., Johansson, O., Luft, R., Cerasi, E., Hellerström, C.: Somatostatin in the pancreas, stomach and hypothalamus of the diabetic Chinese hamster. Diabetologia 13, 463-466 (1977).

273. Baetens, D., Stefan, Y., Ravazzola, M., Malaisse-Lagae, F., Coleman, D.L., Orci, L.: Alteration of islet cell population in spontaneously diabetic mice. Diabetes 27, 1-7 (1978).

274. Patel, Y.C., Orci, L., Bankier, A., Cameron, D.P.: Decreased pancreatic somatostatin (SRIF) concentration in spontaneously diabetic mice. Endocrinology 99, 1415-1418 (1976).

275. Patel, Y.C., Cameron, D.P., Stefan, Y., Malaisse-Lagae, F., Orci, L.: Somatostatin: Widespread abnormality in tissues of spontaneously diabetic mice. Science 198, 930-931 (1977).

276. Orci, L.: The microanatomy of the islets of Langerhans. Metabolism 25 (suppl. 1) 1303-1314 (1976).

277. Pipeleers, D., Somers, G., Gepts, W., De Nutte, N., De Vroede, M.: Plasma pancreatic hormone levels in a case of somatostatinoma: Diagnostic and therapeutic implications. J. clin. Endocrinol. Metab. 49, 572-579 (1979).

278. Krejs, G.J., Orci, L., Conlon, J.M., Ravazzola, M., Davis, G.R., Raskin, P., Collins, S.M., McCarthy, D.M., Baetens, D., Rubenstein, A., Aldor, T.A.M., Unger, R.H.: Somatostatinoma syndrome: Biochemical, morphologic and clinical features. New Engl. J. Med. 301, 285-292 (1979).

279. Ganda, O.P., Weir, G.C., Soeldner, J.S., Legg, M.A., Chick, W.L., Patel, Y.C., Ebeid, A.M., Gabbay, K.H., Reichlin, S.: "Somatostatinoma": A somatostatin-containing tumor of the endocrine pancreas. New Engl. J. Med. 296, 963-967 (1977).

280. Larsson, L.I., Holst, J.J., Kühl, C., Lundqvist, G., Hirsch, M.A., Ingemansson, S., Jensen, S.L., Rehfeld, J.F., Schwartz, T.W.: Pancreatic somatostatinoma: Clinical features and physiologic implications. Lancet 1, 666-668 (1977).

281. Alumets, J., Ekelund, G., Hakanson, R., Ljungberg, O., Ljungqvist, U., Sundler, F., Tibblin, S.: Jejunal endocrine tumor composed of somatostatin and gastrin cells and associated with duodenal ulcer disease. Virchows Arch. A. Path. Anat. Histol. 378, 17-22 (1978).

282. Kovacs, K., Horvath, E., Ezrin, C., Sepp, H., Elkan, I.: Immunoreactive somatostatin in pancreatic islet-cell carcinoma accompanied by ectopic ACTH syndrome. Lancet 1, 1365-1366 (1977).

283. Galmiche, J.P., Colin, R., DuBois, P.M., Chayvialle, J.A., Descos, F., Paulin, C., Geffroy, Y.: Calcitonin secretion by a pancreatic somatostatinoma. New Engl. J. Med. 299, 1252 (1978).

THE THYROTROPHIN RECEPTOR IN GRAVES' DISEASE

B. Rees Smith, *Sandra M. McLachlan, Jody Ginsberg, Carole Rickards, R. Hall
Department of Medicine, Welsh National School of Medicine, Cardiff, CF4 4XN, U.K.

*Department of Medicine, University of Newcastle upon Tyne, Newcastle upon Tyne, NE1 4LP, U.K.

Introduction

The presence of thyroid stimulating immunoglobulins in the serum of patients with Graves' disease was established by Adams and Purves in the mid 1950's (1, 2). Subsequently, these antibody molecules were shown to be of the IgG class[2] with the thyroid-stimulating site formed by combination of heavy and light chains in the Fab part of the molecule (3). The effects of the thyroid-stimulating autoantibodies on the thyroid appeared to be virtually identical to those of TSH[2] with the principal activities of both stimulators being mediated by the adenylate cyclase-cyclic AMP system (4, 5). More recently, analysis of the effects of Graves' IgG on labelled TSH binding to the TSH receptor has provided compelling evidence that thyroid-stimulating antibodies are antibodies to the TSH receptor (6-9) and that Graves' hyperthyroidism is due to these TSH receptor antibodies (10-13).

This review considers the TSH receptor in Graves' disease and in particular the nature of the receptor and receptor antibodies and the role of TSH receptor antibodies in Graves' disease.

Hormones in Normal and Abnormal Human Tissues, Vol. II

The TSH Receptor

When highly purified preparations of biologically active TSH became available in the early 1970's it was possible, for the first time, to study the interaction between TSH and its receptor directly. These investigations were carried out using isolated cells (14) or crude or partially purified membranes from porcine (14), guinea pig (15) or human thyroid tissue (7, 16) and ^{125}I-labelled bovine or porcine TSH. Labelled TSH binding to these preparations was found to be a saturable partially reversible process. Analysis of binding data in terms of Scatchard transformation gave linear plots in the case of guinea pig (15) and porcine thyroid (14) tissue and conventional interpretation of this data suggested association constants in the region of 10^9-10^{10} molar^{-1}. Human thyroid membranes gave curved Scatchard plots (7, 16). The reason for this is not clear at present but detailed studies have indicated that negative co-operativity is not involved (16).

Thyrotrophin has been shown to stimulate lipolysis in isolated fat cells (17, 18) and TSH receptors are readily demonstrable in adipose tissue (19, 20). These receptors have similar TSH binding characteristics to those in thyroid tissue. Thyroid stimulation by TSH appears to be mediated by the adenylate cyclase - cyclic AMP system and studies with thyroid membrane preparations have demonstrated a good correlation between receptor binding and stimulation of cyclic AMP synthesis (14, 15). In the case of the extremely rapid effects of TSH, such as stimulation of iodine release from isolated cells, changes in cyclic AMP levels are undetectable at the time of the effect (21). This could reflect limitations in the ability to detect adenylate cyclase activation rather than a non-cyclic AMP mediated phenomenon. However, iodine release could also be stimulated by cyclase independent events such as ion movement across the plasma membrane.

Thyrotrophin receptors can readily be extracted from thyroid tissue preparations by the use of non-ionic detergents such as Triton X-100 or Lubrol (6, 9, 22). The detergent solubilized receptors have similar TSH binding characteristics to membrane bound receptors but appear to be much less stable (9, 22). Analysis of detergent solubilized porcine and human TSH receptors by isoelectric focusing indicates that the molecule has an isoelectric point of about 4.5 (22). Gel filtration of complexes of labelled TSH, TSH receptor and Lubrol micelles on Sephacryl S-300 indicate that the complex has a Kav of 0.25. Making very approximate corrections for the size of the hormone and detergent micelle, this type of analysis suggests that the receptor itself has a molecular weight in the region of 1.5 x 10 (5).

The nature of the TSH receptor has been investigated indirectly by using a variety of chemical, enzymatic and affinity probes. Thyrotrophin binding activity of thyroid membranes is readily inactivated by proteolytic enzymes such as trypsin and reducing agents such as dithioethreitol and mercaptoethanol. These effects are also observed on detergent solubilised receptors (Table 1) suggesting that the probes are acting directly on the receptor. Consequently the TSH receptor appears to be a protein with at least one functionally important disulphide bridge. Disulphide blocking agents such as iodoacetamide do not influence the TSH binding properties of membrane bound or detergent solubilised receptors indicating that free sulphydryl groups are not important in forming the active site.

Detergent solubilised TSH receptors can be reversibly bound by columns of Sepharose coupled to Lentil Lectin or Concanavalin A (Fig. 1). As well as providing a useful means of purifying the receptor these observations suggest that sugar groups (particularly glucosyl and mannosyl residues) are an integral part of the receptor. However, neuraminidase in amounts ranging from 10 µU to 1 unit and phospholipases A_2, C and D in amounts up to 10 mU had no effect on detergent solubilised TSH receptors which suggests that sialic acid residues and phospholipids are not important components of the TSH binding site. Solubilised TSH receptors can also be absorbed by columns of Sepharose

Table 1.

Effect of trypsin and dithiothreitol on ^{125}I - labelled TSH binding to Lubrol solubilised porcine thyroid membranes

	Trypsin concentration (% w/v)				Dithiothreitol concentration (mM)		
	10^{-5}	10^{-4}	10^{-3}	10^{-2}	.05	0.5	5
% inhibition of TSH binding	0	40	75	100	10	80	100

The receptor preparations were incubated with enzyme or reducing agent for 15 min at 20° and then treated with a 1.5 fold excess of trypsin inhibitor or iodacetamide prior to addition of labelled TSH.

coupled to TSH (Fig. 2) and this procedure together with lectin chromatography are clearly promising approaches to the purification and further characterisation of the receptor.

An interesting and probably important feature of the TSH-TSH receptor interaction is that hormone and receptor show a reduced tendency to dis-sociate with increasing time of contact (15, 23). Similar characteristics have been observed with other systems including the growth hormone (24) and luteinising hormone receptors (25). In the case of TSH-TSH receptor complexes, the process of reduced dis-sociation rate with time has been studied in isolated cells, particulate membrane preparations and detergent solubilised membranes (23). These observations suggest that the hormone receptor complex (HR) undergoes a configurational change to a more stable form (HR)´. The rate of formation of the more stable form is slowest in isolated intact cells, more rapid in membranes and fastest in solubilised receptor preparations. This suggests that the rate of conversion of

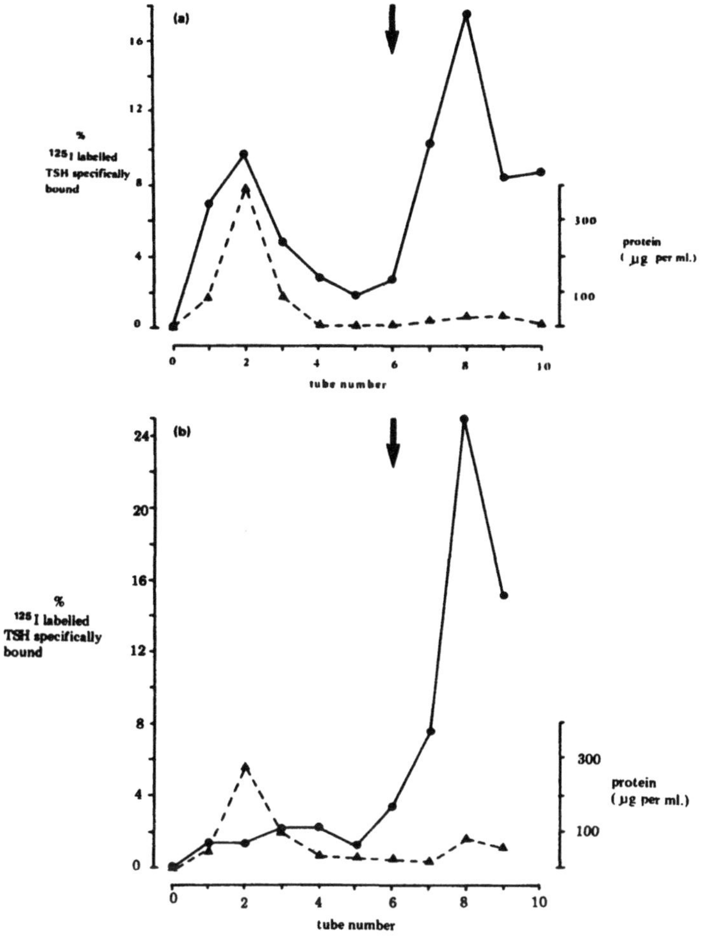

Fig. 1. Fractionation of Lubrol (1.0% ^{w}/v) solubilised TSH receptors (1.7 ml) on 2 ml lectin affinity columns. a=Sepharose-lentil lectin; b=Sepharose-concanavalin A. Sepharose-lectin preparations were obtained from Pharmacia. Flow rate=4 ml per h. Samples were run into the columns at 20° and eluted with 0.1% Lubrol in 50 mM NaCl; 10 mM Tris pH 7.5 followed by 1Mα-methyl-D-Glucoside in 0.1% Lubrol buffer at the point indicated by a vertical arrow; 2 ml fractions were collected and dialysed overnight at 0° against 0.1% Lubrol buffer and analysed for TSH binding activity. Recovery of receptor from the columns by elution with 1M sugar was nearly 100% and in the case of con A-Sepharose, this gave a preparation of receptors with about 7 times the specific activity of unfractionated material in terms of binding activity per mg of protein.

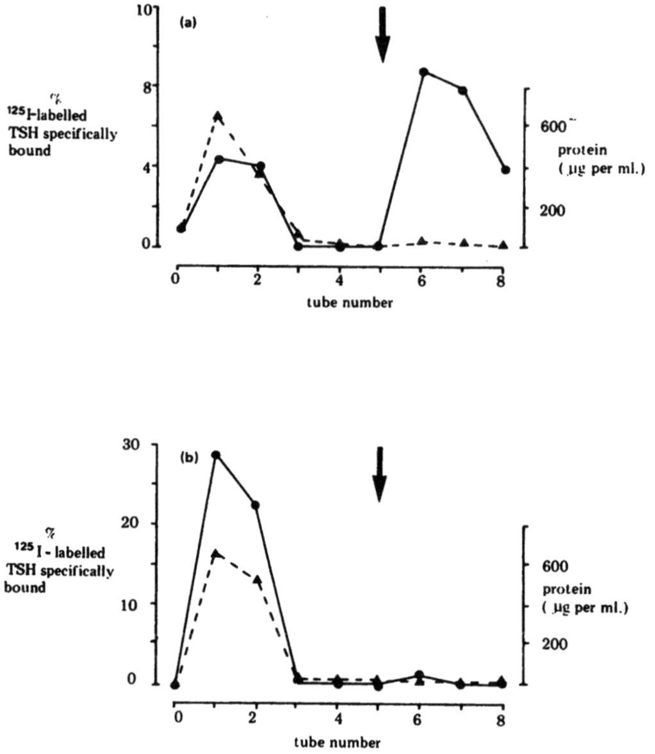

Fig. 2. Fractionation of Lubrol solubilised TSH receptors (1.7 ml) on columns of Sepharose-TSH (a) and Sepharose-BSA (b). Experimental details were as described in the legend to figure 1 except that both TSH and BSA were coupled to CNBr activated Sepharose (Pharmacia) by the method recommended by the manufacturer; 1 ml of gel contained approximately 1 mg of protein. After sample application and elution with 0.1% Lubrol buffer, 1M NaCl in 0.1% Lubrol was run through the columns (vertical arrows) and the fractions dialysed overnight prior to assay for TSH binding activity. Virtually all the receptor binding activity was eluted from the Sepharose-BSA columns with 0.1% Lubrol. However, Sepharose-TSH absorbed about 90% of the activity and about 30% of the bound material was recovered after elution with 1M NaCl. The specific activity of the 1M NaCl eluted receptors was about 4 times that of the unfractionated material in terms of binding activity per mg of protein.

(HR) to (HR)´ is influenced by the degree of disruption of membrane structure. Similar observations have been made on the rate of dis-sociation of labelled human chorionic gonadotrophin from rat testis membranes, detergent solubilised testis membranes and isolated Leydig cells (26, 27).

The role of a stable hormone-receptor complex in the actions of hormones such as TSH and hCG is not clear at present. They are clearly not important in the acute actions of TSH and hCG but may be involved in events which require prolonged contact of hormone and receptor such as internalisation or shedding from the cell surface.

The Interaction of Graves' IgG with the TSH Receptor

The ability of Graves' IgG to inhibit TSH binding to thyroid membranes (6-8) could result from interaction between the IgG and TSH or an effect of the Graves' IgG on thyroid membranes. Studies using gel filtration and polyethylene glycol precipitation have failed to show any interaction between TSH and Graves' IgG. Furthermore, when thyroid membranes are incubated with Graves' IgG and then washed prior to addition of labelled TSH, inhibition of hormone binding is still observed. Consequently, the Graves' IgG must act by binding to the membrane and not by interacting with TSH. The Graves' IgG could possibly interact directly with the TSH receptor; alternatively binding to a different membrane component could occur and this process could somehow result in transmission of a signal through the membrane which inactivated the TSH binding site. One way of deciding between these two possibilities is to disperse the membrane components in an excess of non-ionic detergent micelles and reexamine the effects of Graves' IgG on TSH binding. When this is carried out, the Graves' IgG are found to inhibit TSH binding to the detergent solubilised receptors in a very similar manner to TSH binding to membrane-bound receptors (6, 9). Consequently the Graves' IgG appear to interact directly with a component of the TSH receptor and it would seem therefore that they contain antibodies to the TSH receptor. Furthermore, preliminary studies have shown that Graves' IgG inhibit labelled TSH binding to TSH receptors purified by affinity chromatography on Sepharose - TSH or Sepharose - lectin columns (Table 2).

The regions of the TSH receptor which are involved in receptor antibody binding are unknown at present. A molecule as large as the receptor would be expected to have multiple antigenic sites and Graves' IgG probably contain antibodies to several different antigenic determinants on the receptor. In this respect, however, it is of interest that the Fab fragments of receptor antibodies are equally effective in inhibiting TSH binding as the intact IgG (28, 29). Furthermore, the binding of TSH and TSH receptor antibodies to the TSH receptor appear to be mutually exclusive in so far as there is no evidence for the formation of a complex consisting of all three components (6, 4, 30). It would appear therefore that although the receptor antibodies may not bind directly to the TSH binding site on the receptor, the antibody binding sites are closely linked to the hormone binding site.

Freezing and thawing of human thyroid particulate preparations has been shown to release a water soluble substance which will reversibly bind and inactivate the thyroid-stimulating activity of Graves' IgG (31, 32). This material has a molecular weight in the region of 30,000 and isoelectric point of about 4.5 (33). The relationship between this binding protein and the TSH receptor is not clear at present. It would seem likely however that it is a hydrophilic fragment of the amphilic TSH receptor cleaved off by enzymes released during freezing and thawing of thyroid tissue (22, 34).

Thyroid Stimulation and TSH Receptor Antibodies

As Graves' IgG contain antibodies to the TSH receptor, a likely mechanism for the thyroid stimulating action of Graves' IgG is

Table 2.

The interaction of Graves' IgG with TSH receptors purified by Sepharose-TSH affinity chromatography

Test Material		^{125}I-labelled TSH bound (%)	
		Non-purified detergent solubilized TSH receptors	Affinity-purified TSH receptors
Unlabelled TSH (uU)			
	0	48.0	19.0
	10^2	23.4	6.6
	10^4	6.4	4.6
Graves' IgG (µg)			
	0	48.0	19.0
	6	35.1	9.8
	60	12.6	6.3

Affinity-purified (3 x 150 µl aliquots) or non-purified receptors (3 x 100 µl aliquots) were incubated with unlabelled TSH (100 µl aliquots) or Graves' IgG (100 µl aliquots diluted in normal IgG so that the total IgG content of each tube was constant) for 10 min. at 20°. Labelled TSH (100 µl; 5000 cpm) was then added, incubation continued for 1 h at 37° and then bound and free hormone separated by polyethylene glycol precipitation. The methods used were principally those described by Petersen et al. (9). Receptors were purified by affinity chromatography using Sepharose-TSH as outlined in Fig. 2.

that these antibodies act as TSH agonists. This hypothesis is very difficult to prove absolutely at the present time as it is always possible to propose that the IgG preparations also contain another antibody which stimulates the thyroid cell by interacting with another receptor. If a non-TSH receptor is involved, however, this has to be a rather specialized molecule able to undergo a complex coupling reaction with adenylate cyclase (35). The simplest explanation for the thyroid-stimulating properties of Graves' IgG is to attribute them to TSH receptor antibodies acting as TSH agonists. Strong circumstantial support for this hypothesis is provided by the observation that both Graves' IgG and TSH interact with TSH receptors in fat and stimulate lipolysis (17-20). If thyroid stimulation by Graves' IgG is due to the effects of an antibody interaction with a membrane component other than the TSH receptor this hypothesis would have to propose that this membrane component is also present on fat cells.

Biochemical Characteristics of TSH Receptor Antibodies

Biochemical analysis of TSH receptor antibodies has been carried out using both receptor binding and thyroid-stimulating systems to assess antibody activity. Studies using the mouse bioassay demonstrated that the thyroid stimulating activity of Graves' serum was exclusively associated with the IgG fraction (36, 37). Furthermore, the activity was formed by combination of heavy and light chains in the Fab part of the IgG molecule (2, 3). Isolated heavy chains also showed a small amount of thyroid-stimulating activity (3). Ion exchange (38) and isoelectric focusing (33, 39, 40) studies demonstrated that the thyroid stimulating activity of Graves' IgG showed a wide range of isoelectric points indicating that the antibodies were of polyclonal origin. Studies with immunoglobulin light chain antisera have also demonstrated that the stimulating activity is distributed approximately equally between antibody molecules with

Kappa and Lamda light chains (37, 41, 42) In addition, stimulating activity in one Graves' serum has been shown to be associated with IgG subclasses 1, 2 and 4 but not IgG 3 (43).

Analysis of the properties of Graves' IgG using assay systems other than the mouse bioassay have been less extensive. Stimulation of human thyroid adenylate cyclase has been demonstrated with the Fab fragment of Graves' IgG (29) and the activity has been shown to be polyclonal (44). Similarly, the ability of Graves' IgG to inhibit TSH binding to thyroid membranes has been localized in the Fab fragment (28, 29). The property of antibodies to the receptor to stimulate the thyroid rather than induce cell lysis by way of the complement system is of interest. However, as the number of receptors on the surface of the thyroid cell is small (in the region of 10^3 sites per cell) and the receptor antibodies are of the IgG class, complement activation might not be expected to occur.

The binding of Graves' IgG to thyroid preparations is not readily reversible (45) in contrast to the easily dissociable characteristics of the TSH-TSH receptor complex (14-16). However, dissociation of antibody-receptor complexes can be effected by treatment with the chaotropic agent sodium thiocyanate (33, 45) and this suggests that hydrophobic bonding is a major factor in the antibody-receptor interaction.

Levels of Receptor Antibody in Different Groups of Patients

Initial studies suggested that nearly 100% of patients with Graves' disease contained detectable levels of TSH receptor antibodies (10). However, these observations were made on patients selected on the basis of age (over 45 yr) because of their inclusion in ^{131}I uptake studies and subsequent studies on 150 unselected Graves' patients in the Newcastle upon Tyne area indicate that about 75% have detectable serum TSH receptor antibodies. A recent report from Hong Kong indicates that 84% of Chinese patients with Graves' disease (46) have detectable receptor antibodies. Lower incidences have been reported in other areas (12, 47-49). These variations must reflect several factors including geographical location, clinical and biochemical criteria used to define Graves' disease, patient selection and assay methodology.

About 10% of patients with Hashimoto's thyroiditis have detectable TSH receptor antibodies (10) and in some cases these can act as TSH agonists and stimulate thyroid function (11) (hyperthyroidism does not occur because of extensive autoimmune destruction). The absence of detectable receptor antibody levels in 90% of Hashimoto patients provides good evidence for the specificity of the receptor assay system. High titres of antibodies to thyroglobulin and thyroid microsomes do not influence TSH binding to its receptor (7). There has been one report of TSH receptor antibody activity in patients with toxic multinodular goitre (50). In our own experience (51) and those of other laboratories (52) this does not appear to be the case and the reasons for the discrepancy are not clear.

Assays for TSH receptor antibody activity are usually carried out with concentrates of serum immunoglobulins. Unfortunately normal serum immunoglobulins non-specifically inhibit labelled TSH binding to a certain extent (28) and the effects of test immunoglobulins must always be considered relative to those of immunoglobulins from an appropriate normal control population. It is possible that serum TSH could interfere in the measurements of receptor antibody activity. However, serum levels of 100 μU per ml or less do not influence the effect of immunoglobulins on TSH binding to thyroid membranes but it is advisable to consider serum TSH activity when assessing the results of receptor assays. Thyroglobulin has also been reported to inhibit TSH binding to thyroid membranes (53) but in our own experience, the concentrations found in serum even after destructive therapy to the thyroid or in thyroid cancer do not influence the effects of serum immunoglobulins on TSH binding.

Thyroid Function in Graves' Disease and TSH Receptor Antibodies

In normal subjects, thyroid function is under the control of a feedback system involving pituitary TSH and thyroid hormones (28). Perturbation of the system by administration of thyroid hormones or thyrotropin releasing hormone can be used to assess the state of the pituitary-thyroid axis and the effects of serum TSH receptor antibodies (28). When this is carried out in patients who have been treated, the presence of receptor antibodies correlates well with the loss of TSH control of thyroid function (11, 12) suggesting that when the antibodies are present, they are involved in thyroid stimulation.

The relationship between levels of receptor antibodies and the extent of thyroid stimulation is difficult to assess as Graves' thyroid tissue is usually subject to some autoimmune destruction as well as autoimmune stimulation. However, the iodine trapping mechanism is not markedly influenced by autoimmune destruction and, consequently, early ^{131}I uptake measurements are probably one of the most useful assessments of the ability of receptor antibodies to stimulate the thyroid. Indeed in untreated Graves' patients (carefully selected for absence of iodine contamination in their diets) levels of receptor antibodies are found to show a significant correlation with the ^{131}I uptake (10). In addition, Endo and associates (13) have shown that levels of TSH receptor antibodies correlate significantly with 30 min ^{99m}Tc uptake by the thyroid in untreated Graves' patients. These investigators also demonstrated a good relationship between the levels of receptor antibodies and the extent of thyroid follicle hyperplasia in needle biopsy samples.

These initial observations on the relationship between receptor antibody levels and control of thyroid function suggested that when the antibodies were present, they stimulated the thyroid. Consideration of the complexity of the immune response and the heterogeneity of antibody affinity and specificity however might suggest that some receptor antibodies could act as TSH antagonists as well as TSH agonists. Subsequently good evidence for the existence of receptor antibodies which were unable to stimulate thyroid function was obtained in a few patients with Hashimoto's thyroiditis (11) and Ophthalmic Graves' disease (54) (eye signs of Graves' disease in the absence of hyperthyroidism or a past history of hyperthyroidism). More recently further support for these observations has been provided by a report of a euthyroid mother with high levels of receptor antibody (which crossed the placenta) giving birth to a euthyroid child (55). It is also possible that under some circumstances, receptor antibodies acting as TSH antagonists could induce hypothyroidism and again there has recently been some evidence that this can occur in the neonate (56).

As mentioned earlier in this section, Graves' disease usually has the features of both autoimmune stimulation and autoimmune destruction. In hyperthyroid Graves' disease the stimulatory process is clearly predominant. In some patients with ophthalmic Graves' disease, however, there appears to be a stable balance between autoimmune stimulation and destruction (54). A further factor in the process of thyroid stimulation by TSH receptor antibodies is the ability of thyroid tissue to become refractory to stimulation (5, 57, 8, 31).

Receptor antibodies can be of both TSH agonist and TSH antagonist types and most Graves' sera probably contain a mixture of antibodies with agonist, partial agonist and antagonist properties. In our own experience the agonist or stimulating properties virtually always predominate and induce a stimulating signal in the receptor. This stimulating signal usually leads to thyroid stimulation and hyperthyroidism. Sometimes however the stimulating signal is rendered ineffective or at least attenuated by autoimmune destruction and tissue refractoriness.

Clinical values of TSH-receptor antibody measurements

Diagnosis of hyperthyroid Graves' disease is usually carried out on the basis of clinical signs and various biochemical assessments including serum thyroid hormone levels (28). Measurement of TSH receptor antibody activity would appear to be unnecessary in order to make the initial diagnosis. However, receptor antibody determinations can be of value in the diagnosis of ophthalmic Graves' disease (58). Furthermore, measurements of these antibodies would be expected to be of considerable value in predicting the occurrence of neonatal Graves' disease.

Prediction of disease course following an initial treatment schedule with antithyroid drugs also appears to be possible in some patients from measurements of receptor antibody levels by TSH receptor assay immediately prior to drug withdrawal as patients with high levels of receptor antibodies tend to relapse (46, 59). McGregor et al. (60) have recently improved their success in predicting disease course following carbimazole treatment to over 90% by using a combination of receptor antibody determinations and HLA assessment. Patients who were HLA DRw3 positive relapsed whereas patients who were DRw3 negative but showed detectable levels of receptor antibodies also relapsed.

Synthesis of TSH Receptor Antibodies by Lymphocytes Localised in the Thyroid

In this section, Hashimoto's thyroiditis as well as Graves' disease will be considered. Hashimoto's disease is characterized by the presence of serum autoantibodies to thyroglobulin and thyroid microsomes and extensive autoimmune destruction (58). Lymphocytic infiltration of the thyroid is a feature of both autoimmune disorders and the immune cells in Hashimoto thyroid tissue show many of the organizational features of lymph nodes (61). In Graves' disease, lymphocytic infiltration is less extensive but aggregates of lymphoid cells are a frequent finding (62).

It is quite possible that the lymphocytes localized in the thyroid are involved in the synthesis of thyroid autoantibodies in Graves' disease and Hashimoto's thyroiditis. In the case of Hashimoto's disease there is some direct evidence for this possibility (63) including studies which have demonstrated that lymphocytes extracted from Hashimoto thyroid tissue synthesise relatively large amounts of thyroglobulin and microsomal antibodies (64). With regard to Graves' disease, there is considerable indirect evidence that thyroid lymphocytes are also a major site of TSH receptor antibody production. This evidence comes principally from studies of the effects of treatment for Graves' disease on serum levels of TSH receptor antibodies and other thyroid antibodies (about 80% of patients with Graves' disease have serum microsomal antibodies detectable by the tanned red cell haemagglutination inhibition technique).

If lymphocytes localized in the thyroid are a major site of autoantibody synthesis, antithyroid treatment for Graves' hyperthyroidism might be expected to influence autoantibody production by thyroid lymphocytes as well as thyroid hormone synthesis by thyroid tissue.

Three types of antithyroid treatment are generally used in Graves' hyperthyroidism:

1) Antithyroid drugs such as Carbimazole or Propylthiouracil which are concentrated by the thyroid and block iodine organification.
2) Destructive therapy with ^{131}I.
3) Removal of a large part of the thyroid by surgery (subtotal thyroidectomy).

In addition, treatment directed against the effects of thyroid hormones at the tissue level is also used in the form of the β blocking drug propranolol.

These different forms of therapy are followed in most, but not all patients, by characteristic changes in serum levels of microsomal and TSH receptor antibodies.

1) Antithyroid drug therapy is accompanied by a marked fall in both autoantibodies (10, 46, 65-70) and this appears to be independent of changes in thyroid status such as serum thyroid hormone levels (70).

2) ^{131}I treatment is followed by a marked increase in thyroid autoantibody synthesis (66-69). Serum levels are maximal about 3 months after therapy and then fall away over the succeeding months.
3) The effects of surgery are more difficult to analyse because some patients are treated with antithyroid drugs until immediately before thyroidectomy. However, in patients who have detectable microsomal or TSH receptor antibodies, serum levels tend to fall after surgery and remain low or undetectable (10, 68, 69).
4) Treatment of patients for short periods (2 months) with propranolol or placebo is not accompanied by any significant change in serum autoantibody levels (69, 70).

These observations indicate that:

a) Spontaneous changes in autoantibody levels do not tend to occur frequently over short periods of time.
b) Antithyroid drugs inhibit autoantibody synthesis directly or indirectly.
c) Irradiation of the thyroid transiently stimulates autoantibody production.
d) Removal of a large proportion of the thyroid results in reduced production of thyroid autoantibody synthesis.

Studies in vitro have demonstrated that concentrations of antithyroid drugs similar to those found in the thyroid during treatment readily inhibit autoantibody synthesis by lymphocyte cultures (69, 70). Furthermore, lymphocytic infiltration of the thyroid is markedly reduced during antithyroid drug treatment (62). Consequently, antithyroid drugs concentrated in the thyroid and acting directly on thyroid lymphocytes to inhibit autoantibody production appears to be a likely explanation for the fall in serum autoantibody levels during treatment.

Similarly, irradiation of lymphocytes in vitro can be shown to generate a population of cells capable of stimulating autoantibody synthesis (71) and such a mechanism could be important in the increase in autoantibody synthesis observed after irradiation of the thyroid. With regard to surgery, the removal of a large proportion of the lymphocytes synthesising thyroid autoantibodies would be expected to result in a marked reduction in serum levels.

The role of antigen release which probably occurs during ^{131}I treatment and surgery on autoantibody synthesis is not clear. Both procedures probably result in similar marked elevations in concentrations of autoantigen as evidenced by estimations of serum thyroglobulin levels (72). However, the changes in serum autoantibody levels are opposite following the two procedures (increase after ^{131}I treatment, decrease after surgery) and this suggests that antigen release does not have a major role in the acute changes in autoantibody levels observed following surgery or ^{131}I treatment. In addition, stimulation of autoantibody production in vitro by irradiated lymphocytes can be demonstrated to occur in the absence of autoantigen (71).

In summary therefore, the evidence for lymphocytes localized in the thyroid being a major site of autoantibody production is as follows:

1) Relatively large amounts of microsomal antibodies are produced by lymphocytes isolated from Hashimoto thyroid tissue.
2) Microsomal and TSH receptor antibody syntheses in Graves' disease are influenced by antithyroid treatment in a parallel fashion.
3) The effects of antithyroid drugs, ^{131}I and surgery on microsomal and TSH receptor antibody production are consistent with the autoantibodies being synthesized by thyroid lymphocytes.

Future Developments

TSH receptor antibodies are a heterogeneous population of immunoglobulins present in serum in small amounts. Purification and detailed characterisation of these and other organ specific autoantibodies would provide us with useful analytical probes and considerable information about the whole process of autoimmunity. Until recently, the possibility of obtaining relatively large amounts of TSH receptor antibodies and other autoantibodies, particularly in the form of non-heterogeneous immunoglobulins, seemed remote. However, the recent demonstration by Kohler and Milstein (73) that fusion of specifically immune B cells from mice to murine myeloma cells can produce hybrid cells that will grow in continuous culture (and thereby immortalise the secretion of homogeneous antibodies with the specificity for a single antigen) has indicated a possible technique to obtain relatively large amounts of monoclonal autoantibodies.

An alternative approach has also been suggested by the observation that B lymphocytes infected in culture with Epstein Base Virus (EBV) develop into immunoglobulin secreting cells and can become immortalised (74). Recently, we have used this technique to stimulate immunoglobulin and thyroid antibody production by cultures of peripheral blood lymphocytes. As our preliminary results are encouraging and suggest that this may be a useful method of obtaining monoclonal thyroid autoantibodies, they will be discussed briefly in this section. Furthermore, Steinitz et al. (75) have very recently observed continuous production of monoclonal rheumatoid factor by EBV transformed lymphocytes from a patient with rheumatoid arthritis.

Initially it was important to establish a technique for analysing immunoglobulin and specific autoantibody production by cultured human peripheral blood lymphocytes. As TSH receptor antibodies are difficult to measure in small amounts and purified antigen is not yet available, we chose to study thyroglobulin antibody synthesis by lymphocytes from patients with Hashimoto's disease. Specific antibody and total immunoglobulin production by individual cells are most conveniently investigated using the Jerne plaque method (76). This depends on coating sheep red blood cells (SRBC) with antigen (in our case immunoglobulin or thyroglobulin) and incubating the coated cells with antibody synthesising lymphocytes in an agar plate. After appropriate development with complement, using where necessary a developing antisera, plaques of lysed red cells are observed around specific antibody secreting or immunoglobulin secreting lymphocytes and the numbers of these plaques can readily be counted to give a quantitative estimate of the number of secreting lymphocytes.

Earlier, we had demonstrated that peripheral blood lymphocytes from Hashimoto patients would only secrete detectable levels of microsomal or thyroglobulin autoantibody when cultured under special conditions (77). In particular it was necessary to use relatively long periods of culture (1-2 weeks), Marbrook culture flasks and stimulation with pokeweed mitogen. Similarly, we were unable to detect specific thyroglobulin antibody plaque forming cells in lymphocytes immediately after isolation. However, after 10-14 days in Marbrook culture flasks with pokeweed mitogen, specific antibody plaques were readily detectable (Fig. 3). When the cells were infected with EBV and cyclosporin included in the medium to inhibit cytotoxic T cell development, a marked increase in the numbers of both immunoglobulin and specific thyroglobulin antibody synthesising cells occurred. An example, typical of experiments with 4 Hashimoto patients, is shown in Figure 4.

These observations together with those of Steinitz et al. (75) on rheumatoid factor synthesis, suggest that infecting lymphocytes with EBV may provide a general technique for immortalising the cells and producing monoclonal autoantibodies. It should be possible therefore to extend the studies with thyroglobulin antibodies synthesis to TSH receptor antibody production. Different monoclonal TSH receptor antibodies would be particularly interesting to study in terms of their ability to act as TSH agonists or antagonists. In addition, the availability of relatively large amounts of monoclonal organ specific autoantibodies should allow analysis and comparison of their primary structures. This type of investigation could well lead to a much greater understanding of the fundamental relationship between different autoimmune disorders and the mechanisms involved in the control of autoantibody synthesis.

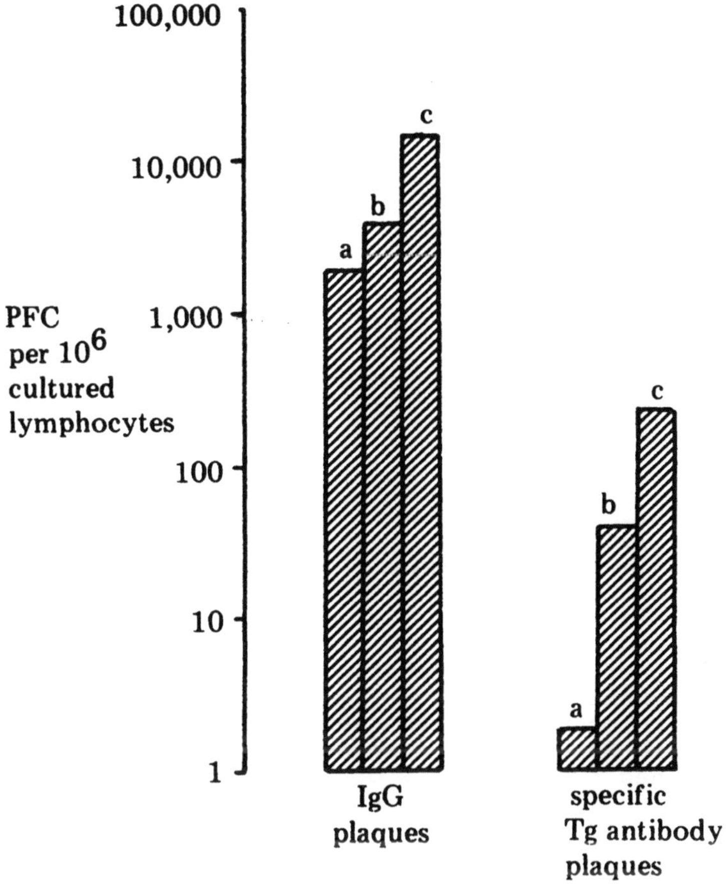

Fig. 3. Synthesis of total IgG and specific thyroglobulin antibody assessed by plaque forming cell (PFC) assays. IgG plaques were determined with a reverse plaque system involving protein-A coated sheep red blood cells (SRBC). Specific thyroglobulin antibody plaques were enumerated using SRBC, to which thyroglobulin had been coupled by the chromic chloride method. In both systems a developing anti human γ chain antisera was employed. Normal and Hashimoto lymphocytes were cultured for 10-14 days in Marbrook flasks with pokeweed mitogen (ref) prior to assessing plaque formation. Geometric means and 95% confidence limits are shown

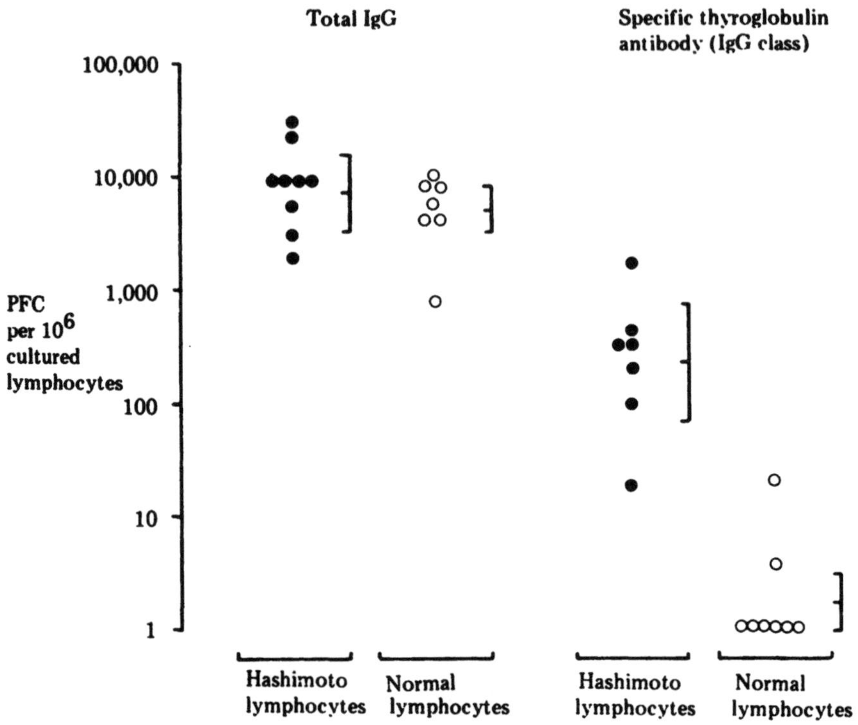

Fig. 4. Stimulation of IgG and specific thyroglobulin (Tg) antibody synthesis by EBV.
Peripheral blood lymphocytes were isolated from a patient with Hashimoto's disease and incubated with EBV, obtained from cultures of the B 95-8 cell line. After 1 h, the lymphocytes were transferred to Marbrook flasks and cultured for 10-14 days in the presence or absence of cyclosporin A (0.02 µg per ml). After this period, the cells were assessed for their ability to synthesise total IgG or specific IgG thyroglobulin antibody, using the PFC methods as described in the legend to Fig. 3.
a=cells cultured in medium only; b=cells infected with EBV and cultured; c=cells infected with EBV and cultured with cyclosporin A.

Acknowledgements

We should like to acknowledge the generosity of Dr. J.G. Pierce who provided highly purified preparations of biologically active TSH. Our thanks are also due to Sandoz for the generous gift of Cyclosporin A.

References

1. Adams, D.D., Purves, H.D.: Abnormal responses in the assay of thyrotropin. Proc. Univ. Otago. Med. Sch. 34, 11-12 (1956).
2. Dorrington, K.J., Munro, D.S.: The long-acting thyroid stimulation. Clin. Pharm. Ther. 7, 788-806 (1966).
3. Smith, B.R., Dorrington, K.J., Munro, D.S.: The thyroid-stimulating properties of long-acting thyroid stimulator γG-globulin subunits. Biochim. biophys. Acta 192, 277-285 (1969).
4. Kendall-Taylor, P.: Effects of long-acting thyroid-stimulator (LATS) and LATS protector on human thyroid adenyl cyclase activity. Brit. med. J. 3, 72-75 (1973).
5. Kendall-Taylor, P.: Adenyl cyclase activity in the mouse thyroid. J. Endocrinol. 52, 533-540 (1972).
6. Manley, S.W., Bourke, J.R., Hawker, R.W.: The thyrotrophin receptor in guinea pig thyroid homogenate: Interaction with the long-acting thyroid stimulator. J. Endocrinol. 61, 437-445 (1974).
7. Smith, B.R., Hall, R.: Thyroid-stimulating immunoglobulins in Graves' disease. Lancet ii, 427-431 (1974).
8. Mehdi, S.Q., Nussey, S.S.: A radio-ligand receptor assay for the long-acting thyroid stimulator. Biochem. J. 145, 105-111 (1975).
9. Petersen, V.B., Dawes, P.J.D., Rees Smith, B., Hall, R.: The interaction of thyroid-stimulating antibodies with solubilised human thyrotrophin receptors. FEBS Lett. 83, 63-67 (1977).
10. Mukhtar, E.D., Rees Smith, B., Pyle, G.A., Hall, R., Vice, P.: Relation of thyroid-stimulating immunoglobulin to thyroid function and effects of surgery, radioiodine and antithyroid drugs. Lancet i, 713-715 (1975).
11. Clague, R., Mukhtar, E.D., Pyle, G.A., Nutt, J., Clark, F., Scott, M., Evered, D., Rees Smith, B., Hall, R.: Thyroid stimulating immunoglobulins and the control of thyroid function. J. clin. Endocrinol. Metab. 43, 550-556 (1976).

12. Kuzuya, N., Chiu, S.C., Ikeda, H., Uchimura, H., Ito, K., Nagataki, S.: Correlation between thyroid stimulators and 3,5,3'-triiodothyronine suppressibility in patients during treatment for hyperthyroidism with thionamide drugs: Comparison of assays by thyroid-stimulating and thyrotropin-displacing activities. J. clin. Endocrinol. Metab. 48, 706-711 (1979).

13. Endo, K., Kasagi, K., Konishi, J., Ikekubo, K., Okuno, T., Takeda, Y., Mori, T., Torizuka, K.: Detection and properties of TSH-binding inhibitor immunoglobulins in patients with Graves' disease and Hashimoto's thyroiditis. J. clin. Endocrinol. Metab. 46, 734-739 (1978).

14. Verrier, B., Fayet, G., Lissitzky, S.: Thyrotropin binding properties of isolated thyroid cells and their purified plasma membranes. Europ. J. Biochem. 42, 355-365 (1974).

15. Manley, S.W., Bourke, J.R., Hawker, R.W.: The thyrotrophin receptor in guinea pig thyroid homogenate: General properties. J. Endocrinol. 61, 419-436 (1974).

16. Rees Smith, B., Pyle, G.A., Petersen, V.B., Hall, R.: Interaction of thyrotrophin with the human thyrotrophin receptor. J. Endocrinol. 75, 391-400 (1977).

17. Kendall-Taylor, P., Munro, D.S.: Lipolytic activity of long-acting thyroid stimulator. Biochim. biophys. Acta 231, 314-319 (1971).

18. Hart, I., McKenzie, J.M.: Comparison of the effects of thyrotropin and long-acting thyroid stimulator on guinea pig adipose tissue. Endocrinology 88, 26-30 (1971).

19. Teng, C.S., Rees Smith, B., Anderson, J., Hall, R.: Comparison of thyrotrophin receptors in membranes prepared from fat and thyroid tissue. Biochem. biophys. Res. Commun. 66, 836-841 (1975).

20. Gill, D.L., Marshall, N.J., Ekins, R.P.: Binding of thyrotropin to membranes from adipose tissue. Biochem. Soc. Trans. 5, 1064-1067 (1977).

21. Povey, P.M., Rees Smith, B., Davies, T.F., Hall, R.: Thyrotrophin receptor binding, intracellular cyclic AMP levels and iodine release in isolated thyroid cells. FEBS Lett. 72, 251-255 (1976).

22. Dawes, P.J.D., Petersen, V.B., Rees Smith, B., Hall, R.: Solubilization and partial characterization of human and porcine thyrotrophin receptors. J. Endocrinol. 78, 89-102 (1978).

23. Brennan, A., Petersen, V.B., Petersen, M.M., Rees Smith, B., Hall, R.: Time-dependent stabilisation of the TSH-TSH receptor complex. FEBS Lett. 111, 35-38 (1980).

24. Donner, D.B., Casadei, J., Hartstein, L., Martin, D., Sonenberg, M.: Characterization of the slowly dissociable human growth hormone binding component of isolated rat hepatocytes. Biochemistry 19, 3293-3300 (1980).

25. Ketelslegers, J.M., Knott, G.D., Catt, K.J.: Kinetics of gonadotrophin binding by receptors of the rat testis. Analysis by a multilinear curve-fitting method. Biochemistry 14, 3075-3083 (1975).

26. Karem, S.: The binding of human chorionic gonadotrophin to the rat testis. MSc Thesis, University of Newcastle Upon Tyne (1979).

27. Karem, S., Rees Smith, B., Hall, R.: Time dependent stabilisation of the hcg-hcG receptor complex. J. Endocrinol. (1980) (in press).

28. Hall, R., Rees Smith, B., Mukhtar, E.D.: Thyroid stimulators in health and disease. Clin. Endocr. 4, 213-230 (1975).

29. Rees Smith, B., Pyle, G.A., Petersen, V.B., Hall, R.: Interaction of thyroid-stimulating antibodies with the human thyrotrophin receptors. J. Endocrinol. 75, 401-407 (1977).

30. Rees Smith, B., Hall, R.: Proceedings of the VIII International Thyroid Congress, Sydney, Australia, Eds. Stockight, J.R., Nagataki, S., Australian Academy of Science, Canberra, Australia, pp. 715-716 (1980).

31. Smith, B.R.: The interaction of the long-acting thyroid stimulator with thyroid tissue in vitro. J. Endocrinol. 46, 45-54 (1970).

32. Dirmikis, S., Munro, D.S.: Studies on the binding activity for long acting thyroid stimulator. J. Endocrinol. 59, 579-592 (1973).

33. Smith, B.R.: Characterization of long acting thyroid stimulator γ G binding protein. Biochim. biophys. Acta. 229, 649-662 (1971).

34. Adlkofer, F., Kotulla, P., Schleusener, H.: Binding of thyrotrophin to low molecular weight fragments of human thyroid membranes. Acta Endocrinol. 94, 58-63 (1980).

35. Baxter, J.D., Funder, J.W.: Hormone receptors. New Engl. J. Med. 301, 1149-1161 (1979).

36. Benhamou-Glynn, N., El Kabir, D.J., Roitt, I.M., Doniach, D.: Studies on the antigen reacting with the thyroid stimulating immunoglobulin (LATS) in thyrotoxicosis. Immunology 16, 187-204 (1969).

37. Maisey, M.N.: The Ig class and light chain type of the long acting thyroid stimulator. Clin. Endocr. 1, 189-198 (1972).

38. Smith, B.R., Munro, D.S., Dorrington, K.J.: The distribution of the long-acting thyroid stimulator among γG-immunoglobulins. Biochim. biophys. Acta. 188, 89-100 (1969).

39. Adlkofer, F., Schleusener, H., Uher, L., Ananos, A.: Heterogeneity of long-acting thyroid stimulating (LATS)-activity, thyroglobulin antibodies and thyroid microsomal antibodies. Acta Endocrinol. 73, 483-488 (1973).

40. Lonergan, D., Babiarz, D., Burke, G.: Isoelectric focusing of long-acting thyroid stimulator immunoglobulin G. J. clin. Endocrinol. Metab. 36, 439-444 (1973).

41. Ochi, Y., De Groot, E.J.: Studies on the immunological properties of LATS. Endocrinology 83, 845-854 (1968).

42. Kriss, J.P.: Inactivation of long-acting thyroid stimulator (LATS) by anti-kappa and anti-lamda antisera. J. clin. Endocrinol. Metab. 28, 1440-1457 (1968).

43. Ochi, Y., Yoshimura, M., Hachiya, T., Miyazaki, T.: Distribution of LATS activity in immunoglobulin G subclass. Acta Endocrinol. 85, 791-798 (1977).

44. Zakarija, M., McKenzie, J.M.: Isoelectric focusing of thyroid-stimulating antibody of Graves' disease. Endocrinology 103, 1469-1475 (1978).

45. Smith, B.R., Munro, D.S.: The nature of the interaction between thyroid stimulating γG-globulin and thyroid tissue. Biochim. biophys. Acta. 208, 285-293 (1970).

46. Teng, C.S., Yeung, R.T.T.: Changes in thyroid-stimulating antibody activity in Graves' disease treated with antithyroid drug and its relationship to relapse: A prospective study. J. clin. Endocrinol. Metab. 50, 144-147 (1980).

47. Docter, R., Bos, G., Visser, T., Hennemann, G.: Thyrotrophin binding inhibiting immunoglobulins in Graves' disease before, during and after antithyroid therapy, and its relation to long-acting thyroid stimulation. Clin. Endocr. 12, 143-153 (1980).

48. O'Donnell, J., Trokoudes, K., Silverberg, J., Row, V., Volpé, R.: Thyrotropin displacement activity of serum immunoglobulins from patients with Graves' disease. J. clin. Endocrinol. Metab. 46, 770-777 (1978).

49. Schleusener, H., Kotulla, P., Finke, R., Sörjee, H., Meinhold, H., Adlkofer, F., Wenzel, K.W.: Relationship between thyroid status and Graves' disease-specific immunoglobulins. J. clin. Endocrinol. Metab. 47, 379-384 (1978).

50. Brown, R.S., Jackson, I.M.D., Pohl, S.L., Reichlin, S.: Do thyroid-stimulating immunoglobulins cause non-toxic and toxic multinodular goitre ? Lancet i, 904-906 (1978).

51. McGregor, A.M., Petersen, M.M., Capiferri, R., Evered, D.C., Rees Smith, B., Hall, R.: Effects of radioiodine on thyrotrophin binding inhibiting immunoglobulins in Graves' disease. Clin. Endocr. 11, 437-444 (1979).

52. Bolk, J.H., Elte, J.W.F., Bussemaker, J.K., Haak, A., van der Heide, D.: Thyroid-stimulating immunoglobulins do not cause non-autonomous, autonomous, or toxic multinodular goitres. Lancet ii, 61-63 (1979).

53. Hashizume, K., Fenzi, G., De Groot, L.J.: Thyroglobulin inhibition of thyrotropin binding to thyroid plasma membrane. J. clin. Endocrinol. Metab. 46, 679-685 (1978).

54. Teng, C.S., Rees Smith, B., Clayton, B., Evered, D.C., Clark, F., Hall, R.: Thyroid-stimulating immunoglobulins in opthalmic Graves' disease. Clin. Endocr. 6, 207-211 (1977).

55. Hales, I.B., Luttrell, B.M., Saunders, D.M.: Proceedings of the VIII International Thyroid Congress, Sydney, Australia, Eds. Stockight, J.R., Nagataki, S., Australian Academy of Sciences, Canberra, Australia, pp. 591-593 (1980).

56. Konishi, J., Kasagi, K., Endo, K., Mori, T., Torizuka, K., Yamada, Y., Nohara, Y., Matsuura, N., Kojima, H.: Proceedings of the VIII International Thyroid Congress, Sydney, Australia, Eds. Stockight, J.R., Nagataki, S., Australian Academy of Sciences, Canberra, Australia, pp. 555-558 (1980).

57. Shuman, S.J., Zor, U., Chayoth, R., Field, J.B.: Exposure of thyroid slices to thyroid-stimulating hormone induces refractoriness of the cyclic AMP system to subsequent hormone stimulation. J. clin. Invest. 57, 1132-1141 (1976).

58. Hall, R., Rees Smith, B.: The role of thyroid autoantibodies in thyrotoxicosis. In: Clinical Immunology Update, Ed. Franklin, E.C., Elsevier, New York, pp. 291-304 (1980).

59. Davies, T.F., Yeo, P.P.B., Evered, D.C., Clark, F., Rees Smith, B., Hall, R.: Value of thyroid-stimulating-antibody determinations in predicting short-term thyrotoxic relapse in Graves' disease. Lancet ii, 1181-1182 (1977).

60. McGregor, A.M., Rees Smith, B., Hall, R., Petersen, M.M., Miller, M., Dewar, P.J.: Prediction of relapse to hyperthyroid Graves' disease. Lancet i, 1101-1103 (1980).

61. Söderström, N., Biörklund, A.: Organization of the invading lymphoid tissue in human lymphoid thyroiditis. Scand. J. Immunol. 3, 295-302 (1974).

62. Swanson Beck, J., Young, R.J., Simpson, J.G., Gray, E.S., Nicol, A.G., Pegg, C.A.S., Michie, W.: Lymphoid tissue in the thyroid gland and thymus of patients with primary thyrotoxicosis. Brit. J. Surg. 60, 769-771 (1973).

63. Davoli, C., Salabe, G.B.: Tissue-specific gamma-globulins in human thyroid. Clin. Exp. Immunol. 23, 242-247 (1976).

64. McLachlan, S.M., McGregor, A.M., Rees Smith, B., Hall, R.: Thyroid-autoantibody synthesis by Hashimoto thyroid lymphocytes. Lancet i, 162-163 (1979).

65. Pincherra, A., Liberti, P., Martino, E., Fenzi, G., Grasso, L., Rovis, L., Baschieri, L., Doria, C.: Effects of antithyroid therapy on the long-acting thyroid stimulator and the antithyroglobulin antibodies. J. clin. Endocrinol. Metab. 29, 231-238 (1969).

66. Einhorn, J., Einhorn, N., Fagraeus, A., Jonsson, J.: Observations on the chemical structure of the long-acting thyroid stimulator and its function in thyrotoxicosis. In: "Thyrotoxicosis", Ed. Irvine, W.J., Livingstone, Edinburgh, pp. 123-134 (1967).

67. Fenzi, G.F., Hashizume, K., Roudebush, C.P., De Groot, L.J.: Changes in thyroid-stimulating immunoglobulins during anti-thyroid therapy. J. clin. Endocrinol. Metab. 48, 572-578 (1979).

68. McGregor, A.M., Petersen, M.M., Capifferi, R., Evered, D.C., Rees Smith, B., Hall, R.: A prospective study of the effects of radio-iodine therapy on thyroid-stimulating antibody synthesis in Graves' disease. J. Endocr. 81, 114P-115P (1978).

69. McGregor, A.M., Petersen, M.M., McLachlan, S.M., Rees Smith, B., Hall, R.: Treatment and the autoimmune response in Graves' disease. J. Mol. Med. 4, 119-127 (1980)

70. McGregor, A.M., Petersen, M.M., McLachlan, S.M., Rooke, P., Rees Smith, B., Hall, R.: Carbimazole and the autoimmune response in Graves' disease. New Engl. J. Med. 303, 302-307 (1980).

71. McGregor, A.M., McLachlan, S.M., Rees Smith, B., Hall, R.: Effect of irradiation on thyroid-autoantibody production. Lancet ii, 442-444 (1979).

72. Van Herle, A.J., Vassart, G., Dumont, J.E.: Control of thyroglobulin synthesis and secretion. New Engl. J. Med. 301, 307-315 (1979).

73. Köhler, G., Milstein, G.: Continuous cultures of fused cells secreting antibody of predefined specificity. Nature 256, 495-497 (1975).

74. Steinitz, M., Klein, G., Koskimies, S., Makela, O.: EB virus induced B lymphocyte cell lines producing specific antibody. Nature 269, 420-422 (1977).

75. Steinitz, M., Izak, G., Cohen, S., Ehrenfeld, M., Flechner, J.: Continuous production of monoclonal rheumatoid factor by EBV-transformed lymphocytes. Nature 287, 443-445 (1980).

76. Bird, A.G., Britton, S.: A live human B-cell activator operating in isolation of other cellular influences. Scand. J. Immunol. 9, 507-510 (1979).

77. McGregor, A.M., McLachlan, S.M., Clark, F., Rees Smith, B., Hall, R.: Thyroglobulin and Hashimoto peripheral blood lymphocytes. Immunology 36, 81-85 (1979).

Subject Index

Hormones in Normal and Abnormal Human Tissues Vol. 1

Editor K. Fotherby S. B. Pal

Errata

page 22

23. Brooksbank. B.W.L., Gower, D.B.: The use of thin-layer and gas-liquid chromatography in the identification of 5β-androst-16-en-3α-ol and androsta-5,16-dien-3β-ol in human urine. Steroids 4, 787-800 (1964).

24. Brooksbank, B.W.L., Gower, D.B.: The estimation of 3α-hydroxy-5α-androst-16-ene and other C_{19} -Δ^{16}-steroids in urine by gas-liquid chromatography. Acta Endocr.(Kbh.) 63, 79-90 (1970).

Walter de Gruyter · Berlin · New York 1981

Bei Fragen zur Produktsicherheit wenden Sie sich bitte an:
If you have any questions regarding product safety,
please contact:

Walter de Gruyter GmbH
Genthiner Straße 13
10785 Berlin
productsafety@degruyterbrill.com